nts

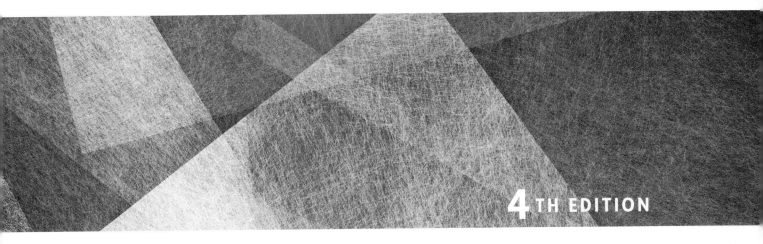

4TH EDITION

FAMILY NURSE PRACTITIONER
CERTIFICATION REVIEW

JoAnn Zerwekh, EdD, RN
President/CEO
Nursing Education Consultants, Inc.
Chandler, Arizona

Adjunct Faculty
Upper Iowa University
Mesa, Arizona

Faculty
University of Phoenix Online
Phoenix, Arizona

ELSEVIER

Elsevier
3251 Riverport Lane
St. Louis, MO 63043

FAMILY NURSE PRACTIONER CERTIFICATION REVIEW, FOURTH EDITION ISBN: 978-0-323-67399-0

Notices

Knowledge and best practice in this field are constantly changing. As new research and experience broaden our understanding, changes in research methods, professional practices, or medical treatment may become necessary.

Practitioners and researchers must always rely on their own experience and knowledge in evaluating and using any information, methods, compounds, or experiments described herein. In using such information or methods they should be mindful of their own safety and the safety of others, including parties for whom they have a professional responsibility.

With respect to any drug or pharmaceutical products identified, readers are advised to check the most current information provided (i) on procedures featured or (ii) by the manufacturer of each product to be administered, to verify the recommended dose or formula, the method and duration of administration, and contraindications. It is the responsibility of practitioners, relying on their own experience and knowledge of their patients, to make diagnoses, to determine dosages and the best treatment for each individual patient, and to take all appropriate safety precautions.

To the fullest extent of the law, neither the Publisher nor the authors, contributors, or editors, assume any liability for any injury and/or damage to persons or property as a matter of products liability, negligence or otherwise, or from any use or operation of any methods, products, instructions, or ideas contained in the material herein.

Library of Congress Control Number: 2020942471

Senior Content Strategist: Sandra Clark
Senior Content Development Manager: Lisa Newton
Senior Content Development Specialist: Sara Hardin
Publishing Services Manager: Julie Eddy
Project Manager: Andrew Schubert
Designer: Brian Salisbury

Printed in United States of America

Last digit is the print number: 9 8 7 6 5 4 3 2 1

Working together
to grow libraries in
developing countries

www.elsevier.com • www.bookaid.org

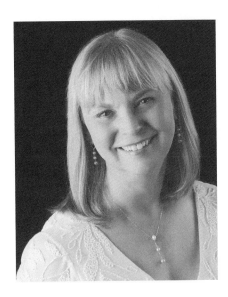

JoAnn Zerwekh has worked as a family nurse practitioner at Carondelet Health Care primary health care clinics in southern Arizona. She taught FNP students at the University of Phoenix and worked briefly as the advance practice consultant for the Arizona Board of Nursing. She is the author of numerous publications, including *Nursing Today: Transition & Trends*, NCLEX® RN and PN review books, and the popular *Memory NoteCards of Nursing and Memory Notebooks of Nursing*. She is the President/CEO of Nursing Education Consultants, Inc.

Contributors

WENDY BIDDLE, PhD, RN, MSN-FNP
Former Program Director
FNP Program
South University
Virginia Beach Campus
Virginia Beach, Virginia

JANEEN DAHN, PhD, FNP-C
Arizona State Board of Nursing
NP House Calls
Chandler, Arizona

JOHN DISTLER, DPA, MBA, MS, FNP, FAANP
Professor, FNP Track, Master Instructor
Chamberlain University
Downers Grove, Illinois

ASHLEY GARNEAU, PhD, RN
Nursing Faculty
GateWay Community College
Phoenix, Arizona

ANNIE M. GERHARDT, DNP, APRN, FNP-C
FNP Clinical Coordinator, Assistant Professor
University of Mary
Bismarck, North Dakota

MELLISA A. HALL, DNP, AGPCNP-BC, FNP-BC
Graduate Nursing Chair
University of Southern Indiana
Evansville, Indiana

JACQUIE HANKS, DNP, APRN-NP PC/AC
Assistant Professor
Creighton University College of Nursing
Omaha, Nebraska

ELAINE KAUSCHINGER, PhD, ARNP, FNP-BC
Assistant Professor of Clinical Nursing
Duke University School of Nursing
Durham, North Carolina

NATALIE L. MURPHY, PhD, APRN, FNP-BC
Interim Associate Dean for Academic Programs & Associate
Teaching Professor
Coordinator–Family Nurse Practitioner Program
College of Nursing
University of Missouri–St. Louis
St. Louis, Missouri

RICHARD M. PRIOR, DNP, FNP-BC, FAANP
Associate Professor
University of Cincinnati
Cincinnati, Ohio

MARYLOU ROBINSON, PhD, FNP-C
Associate Professor
School of Nursing
Pacific Lutheran University
Tacoma, Washington

DARYLE WANE, PhD, ARNP, FNP-BC
BSN Program Director
Professor of Nursing, BSN Faculty
Department of Nursing and Health Programs
Pasco-Hernando State College
New Port Richey, Florida

ERICH WIDEMARK, PhD, RN, FNP-BC
Curriculum and Instruction Developer
Chamberlain University
Downer's Grove, Illinois

MARIE ELENA BOTTE, FNP, APRN-BC, CDE
Family Nurse Practitioner, Diabetes Educator
Boston Children's Hospital
Boston, Massachusetts

JOHN DISTLER, DPA, MBA, MS, FNP, FAANP
Professor, FNP Track, Master Instructor
Chamberlain University
Downers Grove, Illinois

CAITLIN GREENBURG, DO
Internal Medicine Hospitalist
University of Vermont Medical Center
Burlington, Vermont

MELLISA A. HALL, DNP, AGPCNP-BC, FNP-BC
Professor of Nursing
University of Southern Indiana
Evansville, Indiana

WENDY HALM, DNP, APNP, FNP-BC, CNE
Clinical Associate Professor
University of Wisconsin–Madison School of Nursing
Madison, Wisconsin

KIMBRA KENNEY, MD
Associate Professor
Department of Neurology
Uniformed Services University of the Health Sciences
Bethesda, Maryland

ATNENA LUSTER, DNP, FNP
Family Nurse Practitioner
The Tall Trees Health Initiative
Selmer, Tennessee

SHEILA MEDINA, DNP, MBA
Family Nurse Practitioner
Fairfax, Virginia

SUSAN SANNER, PhD, APRN, FNP-BC
Associate Professor of Nursing
Chamberlain University
Morrow, Georgia

VANESSA VOTYPKA, MSN, RN, CPNP, FNP-C
Certified Nurse Practitioner
Cleveland Clinic
Cleveland, Ohio

KAREN J. WHITT, PhD, FNP-C, AGN-BC, FAANP
Associate Professor
George Washington University
Washington, DC

Preface

With the proliferation of new DNP programs, there is an increasing need for additional reference information and study materials for certification examinations. Nurse practitioners are playing a vital role in the health care delivery system in the United States. With the assistance of certified nurse practitioners and my editorial expertise in test item writing, *Family Nurse Practitioner Certification Review*, Fourth Edition, has been developed to assist the advanced practice nurse to prepare for the FNP certification exam. Extensive efforts have been made to include current information that is representative of the content based on the blueprints for the certification exams. This book of questions is not intended to be an exhaustive review of the content, but rather an adjunct to the review process.

Test-taking strategies are included in Chapter 1. As a candidate prepares for the exam, it is vitally important to be familiar with and to practice good testing strategies. Testing strategies can prevent the candidate from making mistakes and selecting the wrong answer. As the review process begins, a review of the test-taking strategies chapter and the practice of good testing strategies is critical. With many years' experience in the field of testing, I consistently have identified the importance that practice testing plays in the review process. Practice questions give the candidate an opportunity to review questions written from different perspectives. To enhance the review process, answers with complete rationales are provided at the end of each chapter. Not only does the candidate increase his/her knowledge of the subject area, but also, with more practice, testing skills become fine-tuned. Good testing skills make the candidate more comfortable and help decrease the stress associated with certification exams.

This book also includes chapters reviewing important concepts related to Growth & Development and Health Promotion & Maintenance. These chapters provide questions that test information related to growth and development, general health supervision, and health maintenance. The clinical chapters are developed using a systems approach (e.g., cardiovascular, respiratory, and endocrine). In each of these chapters, the test questions are divided into three areas: Physical Examination & Diagnostic Tests, Disorders, and Pharmacology. This format assists the candidate to easily locate specific questions. Separate content chapters on mental health, pediatrics, and maternity are included. The last two chapters in the text are on Research & Theory and Professional Issues. The test questions in these chapters focus on professional competencies inherent in the role and function of the FNP.

My thanks to the many nurse practitioners across the country who provided questions and insight into the role of the nurse practitioner. I wish to thank Sara Hardin, my Content Development Specialist, and Sandy Clark, Senior Content Strategist at Elsevier, for their support and suggestions in the preparation of the manuscript. Thank you also goes to the nurse practitioners who took time from their busy schedules to review the questions for content correctness and clarity.

Acknowledgments

I want to express my appreciation to Sandy Clark at Elsevier and her "can-do" attitude that made the realization of this fourth edition possible.

I am especially grateful to the many people at Elsevier who assisted with this major revision effort, including the folks who assisted with the online practice exams and the alternate item formats. In particular, I want to thank Sara Hardin in Content, Andrew Schubert in Production, Erica Kelley in Marketing, and Brian Salisbury in Design.

I want to thank the contributors and reviewers for their assistance in the revision process. Your current practice and clinical expertise are surely noted in your contribution to updating this edition.

I am particularly appreciative of the many nurse practitioners who used the previous editions to pass their certification exams and the faculty who requested a new edition of this test question review book.

I want to thank my adult children, Ashley Garneau and Tyler Zerwekh, and their spouse and significant other (Brian Garneau and Julie Goehring) for their love and support. You make your mother proud by all that you do as successful health care professionals. I would also like to thank my stepchildren, Carrie Parks and Matt Masog, for their great friendship and to express my sorrow at the loss of their father, John Masog, my late husband, who was loved and is missed by all of us.

A special note to my amazing grandchildren (Maddie and Harper Zerwekh; Ben Garneau; Brooklyn and Alexis Parks; and Owen, Emmett, and Cole Masog) who have such bright futures; you always put a smile on Grandma's face and make her proud.

JoAnn Zerwekh

Contents

Test-Taking Strategies

Certification Examination Information

For the family nurse practitioner certification examination, there are two credentialing bodies, the American Nurses Credentialing Center (ANCC) and the American Academy of Nurse Practitioners Certification Board (AANPCB). Both groups provide detailed information in handbooks available for download at their respective websites. This information includes the application process, testing procedure, test content outline, bibliography of references, and other relevant information for the examination candidate. Certification from both agencies is recognized by the U.S. Department of Veterans Affairs, Centers for Medicare & Medicaid (CMS), health insurance companies, the National Council State Boards of Nursing (NCSBN), and state boards of nursing. Both examinations are computer based, and the candidate will schedule the examination at a designated testing center.

ANCC

The ANCC certification examination consists of multiple-choice test questions, drag and drop (ordered response or a proper sequence), hot spot (click on a particular feature or area of a graphic image), and multiple responses (asked to select a specific number of correct responses). There is a total of 175 questions on the family nurse practitioner examination with 150 items scored and 25 pilot test items that do not count toward the final score. The passing score is a scale score of 350 or higher. The raw score (number of test items answered correctly, e.g., 122 out of 175) is converted to a scale score using a conversion formula before the results are given to the examination candidate at the testing site. Candidates who successfully complete the ANCC certification examination may use the credential, Family Nurse Practitioner-Board Certified (FNP-BC).

AANPCB

Each AANPCB examination consists of 150 multiple-choice questions (135 test items are scored and 15 pretest items are not counted in the final score). A "preliminary" examination score is provided to the candidate at the completion of the examination. The scaled score ranges from 200–800 points with a minimum passing score of 500. Candidates who successfully complete the AANPCB certification examination may use the credential, Nurse Practitioner-Certified (NP-C).

Testing Strategies

Knowing how to take an examination is a skill that is developed through practice and experience. Being able to take an examination effectively is almost as important as the basic knowledge required to answer the question. Everyone has taken an examination only to find in the review of the examination that questions were missed because of inadequate testing skills.

Nurse practitioner programs provide the graduate student with a comprehensive base of knowledge; how you use this knowledge will determine your success on a certification examination. The certification examination is an objective test that covers knowledge, understanding, and application of professional nursing theory and practice.

Read the information in this chapter carefully and make sure you understand the strategies discussed. This chapter is designed to help you identify problem areas in testing skills and learn how to use strategy and judgment in selecting correct answers. It is important for you to practice testing skills if you are going to be able to use these skills on the certification examination.

1. Do not read extra meaning into the question. The question is asking for specific information; if it appears to be simple "common sense," then assume it is simple. Do not look for a hidden meaning in what appears to be an easy question.

The family nurse practitioner understands that the most common form of facial paralysis in the adult patient is:

1. Facial nerve fasciitis.
2. Trigeminal neuralgia.

3. Bell's palsy.
4. Herpes zoster.

The correct answer is Option #3. Be careful not to "read into" the question and add pain to the facial paralysis symptom. Instead, concentrate on the question's key words, "the most common form of facial paralysis," which is Bell's palsy, a disorder that affects the facial nerve and is characterized by muscle flaccidity of the affected side of the face. Trigeminal neuralgia is a disorder of cranial nerve V that is characterized by an abrupt onset of pain in the lower and upper jaw, cheek, and lips. Herpes zoster affects the dermatomes and does not cause a paralysis, but it causes pain, herpetic grouped skin vesicles, and possibly postherpetic neuralgia.

2. Read the stem correctly. Make sure you understand exactly what information the question is asking. It is important to understand the question before reviewing the options for the correct answer.

EXAMPLE

The family nurse practitioner would refer a child with the following findings to a pediatric cardiologist for workup and evaluation in 1–2 weeks:

1. Signs of exercise intolerance, dyspnea, and elevated pulse.
2. Poor feeding, increased cyanosis with crying, and dizziness.
3. Nonfunctional heart murmur, respiratory crackles, and retarded growth and development.
4. Systolic ejection murmur, grade II, which disappears on sitting.

The question asks you to determine which child's symptoms would require a referral to a pediatric cardiologist in the next 1–2 weeks. Options #1, #2, and #3 are considered unstable and acute, and should be immediately referred to a pediatric cardiologist. Option #4 is not considered an emergency, as long as the child who has the murmur is asymptomatic, has normal activity and exercise, and is growing normally.

3. Before considering the options, think about the characteristics of this condition and the critical concepts to consider. Begin by assessing each option with regard to the concepts of the condition.

EXAMPLE

A mother who is 3 days' postpartum has been complaining of soreness and fullness in her breasts, and that she wants to stop breast-feeding her infant until her breasts feel better. The family nurse practitioner:

1. Shows the patient how to apply a breast binder to decrease the discomfort and the production of milk.
2. Tells the patient that breast fullness may be a sign of infection and to stop breast-feeding.
3. Suggests to the patient that she decrease her fluid intake for the next 24 hours to suppress lactation temporarily.
4. Explains to the patient that the breast discomfort is normal and that the infant's sucking will promote the flow of milk.

Formulate in your mind critical information for the care of this patient. Think to yourself, "Is it normal to have fullness and soreness in the breasts during the first 3 days of lactation?" If you are unsure,

go back and reassess the question. In this instance Option #4 is correct. Initially, breast soreness may occur for about 2–3 minutes during each feeding until the let-down reflex is established.

4. Identify what type of response the question is asking. A positive stem requires identification of three false items and one correct answer.

EXAMPLE

How soon after exposure should patients who believe they have been exposed to human immunodeficiency virus (HIV) have an HIV antibody test?

1. The next day and 2 months later.
2. 6 months after exposure and again at 12 months.
3. 6–12 weeks after exposure and again at 6 months.
4. 4 weeks and 12 weeks later.

The correct answer is Option #3. This question requires you to identify three incorrect responses and one correct response. The HIV antibody develops between 6 and 12 weeks after exposure. Because of the variability of antibody development, it is recommended that the test be repeated in 6 months to confirm the findings.

5. Identify questions that require identification of something the family nurse practitioner should not or would not do (i.e., an unsafe action, contraindication, or inappropriate action).

EXAMPLE

An older adult patient is diagnosed with chronic open-angle glaucoma. The patient has a past history of bradycardia and first-degree atrioventricular block. In consideration of her treatment, what medication is to be avoided?

1. Pilocarpine (Isopto Carpine).
2. Timolol (Timoptic).
3. Hydrochlorothiazide (HydroDiuril).
4. Acetazolamide (Diamox).

The correct answer is Option #2. Topical beta blockers, such as timolol, lower intraocular pressure but can be absorbed systemically. The major side effects are similar to those associated with systemic beta-blocker therapy, which can include a worsening of heart failure, bradycardia, and heart block. Topical beta blockers are contraindicated in some patients who have cardiac or pulmonary disease.

6. Questions may also be analytical. These questions may ask the nurse practitioner to identify findings and statements that are consistent or inconsistent with the patient's presenting problem, and/or differentiate between them.

EXAMPLE

A child is being evaluated for attention deficit hyperactivity disorder (ADHD). Which test is helpful in evaluating the difference between ADHD and a learning disability?

1. Standardized IQ achievement test.
2. Denver Developmental Screening Test.
3. Audiologic and visual testing.
4. Complete neurologic examination.

Before you examine the options in this question, it is important to think about the differences between ADHD and learning disabilities. The correct answer is Option #1. Children who have learning disabilities and ADHD are often impulsive, inattentive, and overactive. Usually, children with ADHD do not have lower IQ achievement scores; however, children with a learning disability usually demonstrate a level of educational achievement substantially below that of the IQ.

7. Identify key words that affect your understanding of the question. Make sure you understand exactly what information the question is asking. Be aware of words in the stem such as *except, contraindicated, avoid, least, not applicable,* and *does not occur.* These words change the direction of the question. It may help to rephrase the question in your own words to better understand what information is being requested.

> **EXAMPLE**

A patient complains of intolerable itching in the pubic hair. On examination, the family nurse practitioner notes erythematous papules and tiny white specks in the pubic hair. The differential diagnosis includes all except:

1. Pediculosis pubis.
2. Scabies.
3. Impetigo.
4. Atopic dermatitis.

Rephrase the question and look for the three conditions associated with itching, "What are the three differential diagnoses for pruritus or itching in the pubic hair?" Intense itching is characteristic of pediculosis pubis, scabies, and atopic dermatitis. Impetigo starts out as a tender erythematous papule and progresses through a vesicular to a honey-crusted stage with no itching. The correct answer is Option #3, because impetigo is not in the differential diagnosis with conditions that are characterized by itching.

8. As you read the options, eliminate the options you know are not correct. This will help narrow the field of choice. When you select an answer or eliminate a distracter, you should have a specific reason for doing so. Do not try to predict a correct answer; it is distressing if the answer you want is not a selection.

> **EXAMPLE**

A 45-year-old female patient complains of knee pain while kneeling and a "clicking" noise when walking up steps. On examination, there is a slight knee effusion and tenderness when palpating the patella against the condyles. The diagnosis for this patient is:

1. Anterior cruciate tear. (No, the patient generally cannot bear weight on the extremity without it buckling or giving way.)
2. Dislocated patella. (No, there would be considerable effusion and locking of the knee in flexion.)
3. Chondromalacia patella. (Yes, there is clicking and anterior knee pain around or under the kneecap, aggravated by knee extensor stress.)
4. Patellar tendonitis. (No, there would be no clicking sound with movement.)

After systematically evaluating the options, Option #3 is the correct answer.

9. Identify similarities in the distracters. Frequently, three distracters will contain similar information, and one will be different. The different one may be the correct answer.

> **EXAMPLE**

An older adult patient is encouraged to increase protein intake. The addition of which of these foods to 100 mL of milk will provide the greatest amount of protein?

1. 50 mL of light cream and 2 tbsp of corn syrup.
2. 30 g of powdered skim milk and 1 egg.
3. 1 small scoop (90 g) of ice cream and 1 tbsp of chocolate syrup.
4. 2 egg yolks and 1 tbsp of sugar.

Options #1, #3, and #4 all contain a simple sugar. The correct answer, Option #2 has the greatest amount of protein. Notice that three of the options are similar and the one that is different is the correct answer. This strategy is not a substitute for basic knowledge but may help you figure out the answer.

10. Select the most comprehensive answer. All options may be correct, but one will include the other three options or will need to be considered first.

> **EXAMPLE**

The family nurse practitioner is planning to teach a client with newly diagnosed gestational diabetes about the condition. Before the family nurse practitioner provides instruction, what is most important to evaluate? The patient's:

1. Required dietary modifications.
2. Understanding of carbohydrate counting.
3. Ability to administer insulin.
4. Present understanding of diabetes.

Options #1, #2, and #3 are certainly important considerations in diabetic education for the newly diagnosed pregnant patient. However, they cannot be initiated until the family nurse practitioner evaluates the patient's knowledge of gestational diabetes, which is the reason that Option #4 is the correct answer. When two options appear to say the same thing, only in different words, look for another answer; that is, eliminate the options that you know are incorrect. Options #1 and #2 both refer to the client's understanding of nutrition.

11. Select the best answer that is most specific to what the question asks. All options may be correct, but one is more specific or essential to the question being asked.

> **EXAMPLE**

When a child visits a health maintenance clinic, what is essential for the family nurse practitioner to do?

1. Order routine laboratory tests.
2. Perform vision and auditory screening.
3. Plot height and weight on charts.
4. Review immunization record.

The correct answer is Option #4. It is absolutely essential that the immunization record be reviewed, because of the importance of having a child protected from infection and childhood communicable diseases. The other options are important but are not essential or a priority for a health maintenance visit. Recognize key words that identify the question that is asking for a priority of care—first, initial, essential, best, and most.

12. Watch questions in which the options contain several items to consider. After you are sure you understand what information the question is requesting, evaluate each part of the option. Is it appropriate to what the question is asking? If an option contains one incorrect item, the entire option is incorrect. All items listed in the selection must be correct if the option is to be the answer to the question.

EXAMPLE

Which diagnostic tests are typically abnormal when ruling in systemic lupus erythematosus (SLE) as a differential diagnosis?

1. Complete blood count (CBC), electrolyte panel, and erythrocyte sedimentation rate (ESR).
2. Chest x-ray and coagulation profile.
3. Antinuclear antibodies (ANA), ESR, and C-reactive protein.
4. CBC, urinalysis (UA), and chest x-ray.

The correct answer is Option #3. In a methodical evaluation of the diagnostic tests in the options, you can eliminate Options #1, #2, and #4. Although all tests included in the answer may be included in a complete physical examination, the laboratory test specific to the diagnosis of SLE includes the ANA, ESR, and C-reactive protein. During flares, ESR and C-reactive protein are elevated. The ANA titer in a patient with SLE is positive at a 1:80 ratio.

13. Be alert to relevant information contained in previous questions. Sometimes as you are answering questions, you will find information similar to the question being tested. Previous questions may assist you in identifying relevant information in the current question. This strategy is particularly helpful when the student is answering paper-and-pencil tests.

EXAMPLE

The Advisory Committee of Immunization Practices (ACIP) recommends that healthy older adults receive the Tdap vaccination:

1. Every 5 years.
2. At age 75.
3. At age 65.
4. Every 10 years.

The correct answer to this question is Option #3. On February 22, 2012, ACIP approved the use of Tdap (tetanus toxoid, reduced diphtheria toxoid, and acellular pertussis) for all adults aged 65 years and older. Boostrix should be used for adults aged 65 years and older; however, ACIP concluded that either vaccine (Boostrix or Adacel) administered to a person 65 years or older is immunogenic and would provide protection. In another question involving immunizations, you read the following question (see next example).

EXAMPLE

In taking the history of an alert older adult, the family nurse practitioner determines the patient is an avid gardener and spends much time outside. The patient had a pneumococcal vaccination last year but cannot remember whether a tetanus vaccination was ever administered. A health maintenance recommendation for this patient would be to obtain:

1. Pneumococcal vaccine.
2. Tdap/Td vaccine.
3. Hepatitis B vaccine.
4. No recommendation.

The correct answer is Option #2. A clue to the correct answer may be found in the previous question. Older adults who enjoy gardening and outdoor activities should have a Tdap/Td booster once, as recommended by the ACIP. As part of standard wound management care to prevent tetanus, a tetanus toxoid–containing vaccine might be recommended for wound management in adults aged 19 years and older if 5 years or more have elapsed since last receiving the vaccine. If a tetanus booster is indicated, Tdap is preferred over Td for wound management in adults aged 19 years and older who have not received Tdap previously. Td should be administered every 10 years.

When you are taking the test on a computer, it is more difficult to remember previous questions because you may not be able to go back and change answers or review previous questions; therefore this strategy is often most helpful for those students taking paper-and-pencil tests.

14. Multiple-choice mathematical computations may be included in the examination. Mathematical computations may include calculations of IM, PO, and IV dosages; calculations of pediatric dosage; determining creatinine clearance; and conversion of units of measurement.

EXAMPLE

The nurse practitioner is ordering amoxicillin (Amoxil) for a 15-month-old child who has otitis media. The child weighs 22 lb. How would the order be written?

1. Amoxicillin 250 mg/5 mL Sig: 5 mL PO tid × 10 days.
2. Amoxicillin 500 mg/5 mL Sig: 1 tab PO tid × 3 days.
3. Amoxicillin 350 mg/5 mL Sig: 5 mL PO bid × 14 days.
4. Amoxicillin 125 mg/5 mL Sig: 5 mL PO tid × 10 days.

The correct answer is Option #4. First, you must convert pounds (lb) to kilograms (kg). By using the formula 2.2 lb = 1 kg, the child who weighs 22 lb is 10 kg (22 lb/2.2 = 10 kg). The dose for amoxicillin is 20–40 mg/kg/day given every 8 hours for a child older than 3 months and less than 40 kg (10 kg × 40 mg/kg/day = 400 mg/day). Dosing 3 times a day would be approximately 133 mL for each dose. Amoxicillin is supplied in 125 mg/5 mL. The easiest to administer for the parent and closest correct dose for this child would be the 5 mL PO every 8 hours.

15. Evaluate priority questions carefully. Frequently, all answers are appropriate to the situation. You need to decide which actions you should do first.

While attending a rural public school, a 7-year-old child was bitten on the hand by a raccoon. At the rural clinic, the family nurse practitioner cleansed the wound. The next action is:

1. Administer tetanus antitoxin.
2. Contact local animal control authorities.
3. Administer rabies immune globulin (RIG) and human diploid cell vaccine (HDCV).
4. Teach the family how to do hourly soaks to the hand using normal saline and peroxide.

The correct answer is Option #3. Any type of animal bite that might be associated with an animal that may harbor rabies (skunks, bats, raccoons, foxes, coyotes, rats) should be treated with both active and passive rabies immunization. The priority action is to prevent rabies. Tetanus antitoxin would be indicated if the child was not current on the immunization. Animal authorities would be called after the initial treatment to locate the animal and sacrifice it so that the brain can be examined for rabies.

Techniques to Increase Critical Thinking Skills

Memory aids and Mindmapping™ are tools that assist in drawing associations from other ideas with the use of visual images. **Mnemonics** are words, phrases, or other techniques that help you remember information. **Imagery** is a tool that helps you identify a problem and visualize a mental picture. Learning content that uses these techniques will assist you to recall information more effectively.

Mindmapping™ is a method of organizing important information that is in sharp contrast to the traditional outline format. A thought or concept is written in the center of the page, and images and color are added to information as ideas begin to flow from the center focus (Figure 1-1).

Acronyms help you recall specific information through word associations or letter arrangements. Examples of these are the "6-Ps" of dyspnea (Figure 1-2), the "6-Ps" of circulatory assessment (Figure 1-3), and the "ABCDE" of malignant melanoma (Figure 1-4).

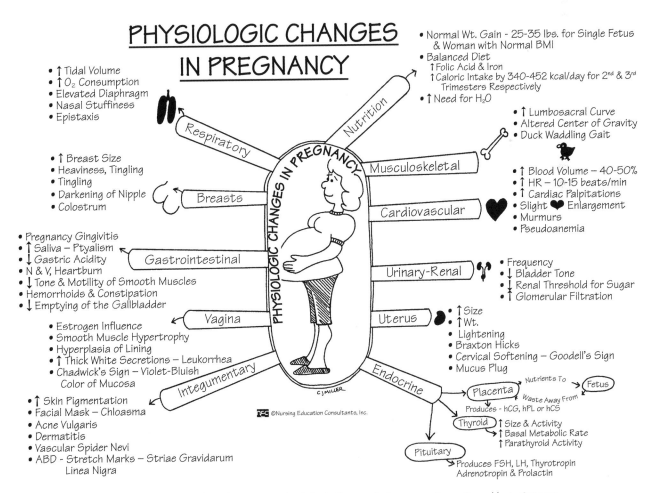

Figure 1-1 Example of Mindmapping™: Physiologic Changes in Pregnancy. From: Zerwekh, J., Garneau, A., & Miller, C. J. (2017). *Digital Collection of the Memory Notebook of Nursing* (4th ed.). Chandler, AZ: Nursing Education Consultants Publishing, Inc.

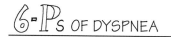

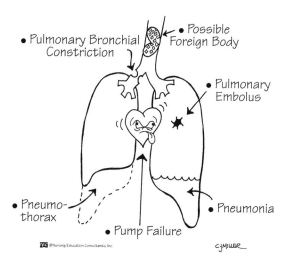

Figure 1-2 Acronym Memory Aid: The "6-Ps" of Dyspnea. From: Zerwekh, J., Garneau, A., & Miller, C. J. (2017). *Digital Collection of the Memory Notebook of Nursing* (4th ed.). Chandler, AZ: Nursing Education Consultants Publishing, Inc.

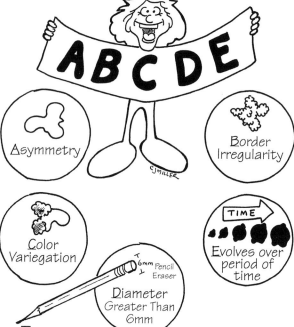

Figure 1-4 Indications of Possible Malignant Melanoma: "ABCDE." From: Zerwekh, J., Garneau, A., & Miller, C. J. (2017). *Digital Collection of the Memory Notebook of Nursing* (4th ed.). Chandler, AZ: Nursing Education Consultants Publishing, Inc.

NEUROVASCULAR ASSESSMENT

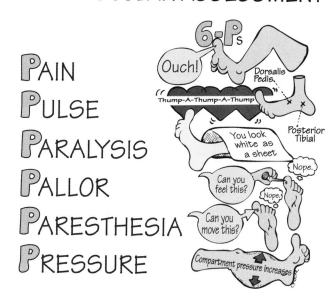

Figure 1-3 Circulation Assessment: The "6-Ps." From: Zerwekh, J., Garneau, A., & Miller, C. J. (2017). *Digital Collection of the Memory Notebook of Nursing* (4th ed.). Chandler, AZ: Nursing Education Consultants Publishing, Inc.

Acrostics are catchy phrases in which the first letter of each word stands for something to recall. For example, in remembering the use of canes and walkers, think of "Wandering Wilma's Always Late" (**W**alker **W**ith **A**ffected **L**eg) (Figure 1-5). Everyone remembers the cranial nerve mnemonic (Figure 1-6).

Memory aids/images are pictures or caricatures that help you recall information more effectively (Figure 1-7).

Rhymes are phrases or words spoken in a rhythmic or musical manner that increase recall, such as the rhyme for hypoglycemia versus hyperglycemia (Figure 1-8). Another rhyme, "fingers, nose, penis, toes," identifies the areas where lidocaine with epinephrine is contraindicated as a local anesthetic. "Two is too much" may help you remember toxic levels of lithium, digoxin, and theophylline, which have a narrow margin of safety (Figure 1-9). Books and electronic resources are available on these helpful aids (see References in the back of the book).

Testing Skills for Paper-and-Pencil Tests

Because your certification examinations are available on computer, the following skills are applicable for **paper-and-pencil tests**, which you may encounter as a student in your program.

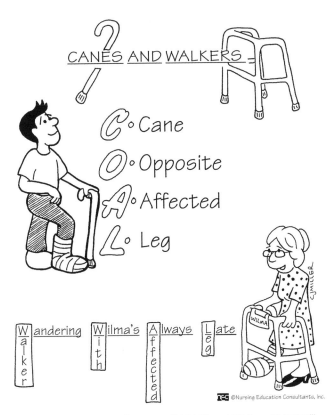

Figure 1-5 Mnemonics for Canes ("COAL") and Walkers ("WWAL"). From: Zerwekh, J., Garneau, A., & Miller, C. J. (2017). *Digital Collection of the Memory Notebook of Nursing* (4th ed.). Chandler, AZ: Nursing Education Consultants Publishing, Inc.

1. Go through the examination and mark all answers that you know are correct. This ensures you have adequate time to answer the questions you know. Then, go back and evaluate those questions for which you did not readily recognize the answer.
2. Do not indiscriminately change answers. If you go back and change an answer, you should have a specific reason for doing so. You may remember information and realize you answered the question incorrectly. Frequently, test takers "talk themselves out of" the correct answer and change it to an incorrect one.
3. After you have completed the examination, go back and check your booklet and make sure all questions are answered. Be sure to answer all questions, even if you must guess at some.

Successful Test Taking

1. Listen carefully to the instructions given at the beginning of the examination. Make sure you understand all information given and exactly how to mark your answers and/or how to use the keyboard and mouse. Adjust the computer screen for optimum viewing.
2. Watch your timing. Do not spend too much time on one question. It is very important that you practice your timing on the sample examinations. You may not be able to review your questions and answers on completion of the computerized test; therefore watch your timing on the computerized tests and make use of a computer clock if it is available.
3. Be aware of your "first hunch" because it is frequently the correct answer. Sometimes information is processed by the brain without your awareness. If something about an answer "feels right" or if you have a "gut feeling" about an answer, pay attention to it.
4. Eliminate options that assume the patient "would not understand" or "is ignorant of" the situation or those that "protect them from worry." For example, "The patient should not be told she has cancer because it would upset her too much."
5. Be aware of options that contain the words *always* and *never*.
6. There is no pattern of correct answers. Both computerized and paper-and-pencil examinations are compiled by a computer, and the position of the correct answers is selected at random.
7. Watch the length of the options to consider. The number of words required to adequately state the correct answer is sometimes longer than the other options.

Decrease Anxiety

Your activities on the day of the examination strongly influence your level of anxiety. By carefully planning ahead, you will be able to eliminate some anxiety-provoking situations. If you are a diabetic or have special needs, contact

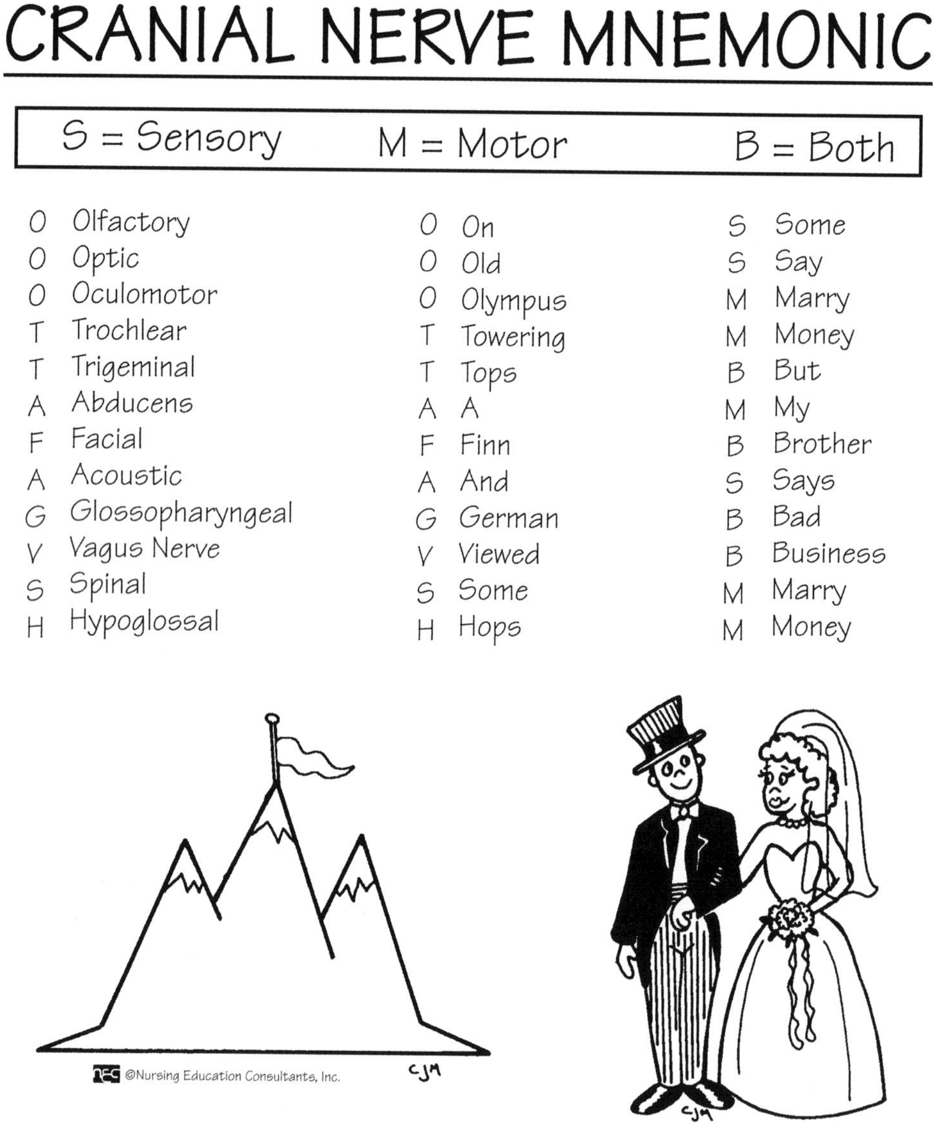

CRANIAL NERVE MNEMONIC

S = Sensory	M = Motor	B = Both

O	Olfactory	O	On	S	Some
O	Optic	O	Old	S	Say
O	Oculomotor	O	Olympus	M	Marry
T	Trochlear	T	Towering	M	Money
T	Trigeminal	T	Tops	B	But
A	Abducens	A	A	M	My
F	Facial	F	Finn	B	Brother
A	Acoustic	A	And	S	Says
G	Glossopharyngeal	G	German	B	Bad
V	Vagus Nerve	V	Viewed	B	Business
S	Spinal	S	Some	M	Marry
H	Hypoglossal	H	Hops	M	Money

©Nursing Education Consultants, Inc.

Figure 1-6 Cranial Nerve Mnemonic. From: Zerwekh, J., Garneau, A., & Miller, C. J. (2017). *Digital Collection of the Memory Notebook of Nursing* (4th ed.). Chandler, AZ: Nursing Education Consultants Publishing, Inc.

the certification agency ahead of time to make arrangements to have accommodations that you may require.

1. Visit the examination site before the day of the examination. Evaluate travel time, parking, and time to reach the designated area. Be sure to get an early start to allow for extra time.
2. If you have to travel some distance to the examination site, try to spend the night in the immediate vicinity.
3. Do something pleasant the evening before the examination. This is not the time to "crash study."
4. Anxiety is contagious. If those around you are extremely anxious, avoid contact with them before the examination.
5. Make your meal before the test a light, healthy one.
6. Avoid eating highly spiced or different foods. This is not the time for a gastrointestinal upset.
7. Wear comfortable clothes. This is not a good time to wear tight clothing or new shoes.

8. Wear clothing of moderate weight. It is difficult to control the temperature to keep everyone comfortable. Take a sweater or wear layered clothes. You may not be allowed to remove any garments once you are seated for the examination.
9. Wear soft-soled shoes; this decreases the noise in the testing area.
10. Make sure you have the papers and proper identification that are required to gain admission to the examination site. If you wear reading glasses, do not forget to bring them with you.
11. Do not take study materials to the examination site. You will not be able to take such materials with you into the examination area.
12. Do not panic when you encounter content with which you are unfamiliar in a question. Use good test-taking strategies, select an answer, and continue. Remember, you are not going to know all of the correct answers.

HYPERTHYROIDISM

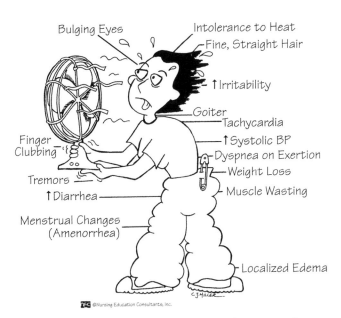

Figure 1-7 Image as Memory Aid for the Signs/Symptoms of Hyperthyroidism. From: Zerwekh, J., Garneau, A., & Miller, C. J. (2017). *Digital Collection of the Memory Notebook of Nursing* (4th ed.). Chandler, AZ: Nursing Education Consultants Publishing, Inc.

BLOOD SUGAR MNEMONIC

HOT & DRY = SUGAR HIGH

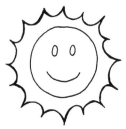

COLD & CLAMMY = NEED SOME CANDY

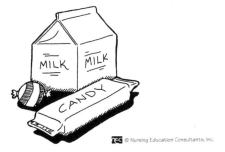

Figure 1-8 Blood Sugar Rhyme. From: Zerwekh, J., Garneau, A., & Miller, C. J. (2017). *Digital Collection of the Memory Notebook of Nursing* (4th ed.). Chandler, AZ: Nursing Education Consultants Publishing, Inc.

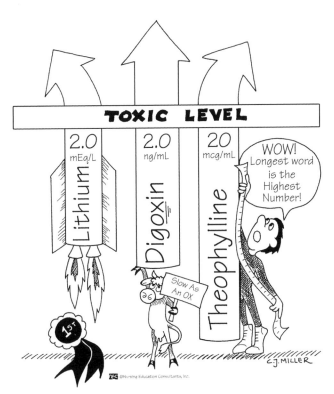

Figure 1-9 Two is Too Much: Toxic Levels of Lithium, Digoxin, and Theophylline. From: Zerwekh, J., Garneau, A., & Miller, C. J. (2017). *Digital Collection of the Memory Notebook of Nursing* (4th ed.). Chandler, AZ: Nursing Education Consultants Publishing, Inc.

13. Reaffirm to yourself that you know the material. It is not time for any self-defeating behavior or negative self-talk. You will pass! Build your confidence by visualizing yourself in 6 months working in the area you desire. Create that mental picture of where you want to be and who you want to be—a certified family nurse practitioner. Use your past successes to bring positive energy and "vibes" to your certification. You can do it!

Study Habits

ENHANCING STUDY SKILLS

- Decide on a realistic study schedule; write it down and stick with it.
- Divide the review material into segments—pediatrics, well woman, cardiac, and so forth.
- Prioritize the segments; review first the areas in which you seem deficient or weak.
- Identify areas that will require additional review.
- Establish a realistic schedule; study in short segments or "bursts." Avoid marathon sessions.
- Plan on achieving your study goal several days before the examination.
- Do not study when you are tired or when there are frequent distractions or interruptions.
- Review general concepts of practice from a variety of resources.

GROUP STUDY

- Keep the group limited to three to five people.
- Group members should be mature and serious about studying.
- The group should agree on the planned study schedule.
- If the group makes you anxious, or if you do not think the group meets your study needs, do not continue to participate.

TESTING PRACTICE

- Include testing practice in your schedule.
- Select about 50 questions for a practice testing session of 1 hour. This will allow you to evaluate the pace of the examination (i.e., approximately 1 question per minute).
- Try to answer the questions as if you were taking the real examination. Do not look up the correct answer immediately after answering the question. Complete all questions you have selected, then go back and grade the questions.
- Use the testing strategies described in this chapter.
- Evaluate the practice examination for problem areas: testing skills and knowledge base.
- Evaluate the questions you answered incorrectly. Review the rationale for the right answer and understand why you missed it.
- Use the questions at a later point to review the information again.

Growth & Development

Physical Assessment

1. The following sequence is recommended for well-child examinations up to the age of 5 years:
   1. 2 weeks, 2 months, 4 months, 6 months, 1 year, 15 months, 18 months, and every year from ages 2–5.
   2. 2 months, 4 months, 6 months, 9 months, and annually from years 1–5.
   3. 2 weeks, 2 months, 4 months, 6 months, 9 months, 12 months, 15 months, 18 months, and annually years 2–5.
   4. The same intervals recommended for immunizations.

2. An appropriate treatment for overweight children under 8 years of age would be to:
   1. Administer an appetite suppressant.
   2. Eliminate all carbohydrates in the diet.
   3. Plan a program of activity, balanced diet, and exercise.
   4. Use vitamin therapy and herbal teas.

3. The family nurse practitioner examines a 2-week-old newborn during a first clinic visit. The family nurse practitioner notes dysmorphic facial features. The family nurse practitioner's evaluation includes:
   1. Ordering a chromosome analysis.
   2. Completing a postnatal history.
   3. Writing a detailed physical exam and perinatal history.
   4. Avoiding discussion with parents until diagnostic studies are completed.

4. An 18-month-old's feet turn inward. The mother is concerned, although the child is unaware of the problem. The differential diagnosis includes all **except**:
   1. Femoral anteversion.
   2. Metatarsus adductus.
   3. Legg-Calvé-Perthes disease.
   4. Adducted great toe.

5. The characteristics of an innocent heart murmur in children include:
   1. Asymptomatic, loud diastolic rumble, grades I to V.
   2. Midsystolic, no thrill, and asymptomatic.
   3. Asymptomatic with an S4 heard at lower left sternal border.
   4. May disappear on sitting and after any type of physical activity.

6. The family nurse practitioner is examining a 6-month-old infant. What would be the anticipated findings on examining the infant's fontanels?
   1. Both anterior and posterior should be open.
   2. The anterior should be open, the posterior closed.
   3. Both anterior and posterior should be closed.
   4. The anterior should be closed, the posterior open.

7. Genu varum up to 20 degrees is normal until age:
   1. 18 years.
   2. 5 years.
   3. 18 months.
   4. 6 months.

8. When approaching a toddler to complete a cardiac assessment, the family nurse practitioner would:
   1. Allow the toddler to handle the stethoscope while the history is being taken.
   2. Explain in detail what procedures will take place and get the toddler involved.
   3. Keep the child warm and covered to minimize discomfort.
   4. Approach the child by cheerfully calling out his name.

9. In performing a physical exam, the family nurse practitioner allows the child to touch the medical equipment first, and then begins by examining the extremities. This sequence would be most appropriate for a patient in what age group?
   1. Infant.
   2. Toddler.
   3. School-age child.
   4. Adolescent.

10. An appropriate test to check for color perception in a preschooler would be:
    1. Ishihara's test.
    2. Brückner's test.
    3. Hirschberg's test.
    4. Jaeger's test.

11. When assessing the cranial nerves in a young child, the family nurse practitioner should:
    1. Obtain help from the parents to enlist the child's cooperation.
    2. Defer assessing the cranial nerve until the child is older.
    3. Modify the physical exam technique based on the child's developmental level.
    4. Expect minimal variations among age groups.

12. Genu valgum is considered normal from:
    1. 1–2 years old.
    2. 2–6 years old.
    3. 8–10 years old.
    4. 12–16 years old.

13. An African American mother and her newborn are seen by the family nurse practitioner for a well-baby visit. The mother is responsive to the baby's cries, and the baby comforts easily and makes frequent eye contact with the mother. On examination, the family nurse practitioner notes the following: height and weight are at the 75th percentile on growth charts, there is a strong sucking reflex, and there is a large blue-black macular area over the lumbosacral area. The family nurse practitioner should:
    1. Contact a social worker and report the mother to Child Protective Services immediately.
    2. Refer the mother and infant to a dermatologist.
    3. Recognize that the blue-black spot is a congenital skin spot, and counsel the mother that no treatment is necessary.
    4. Prescribe clotrimazole cream 1% (Mycelex) bid for 4 weeks.

14. The plantar fat pad, which makes a young child appear to have pes planus, is normal until:
    1. 6 months–1 year old.
    2. 1–2 years old.
    3. 2–5 years old.
    4. 6–8 years old.

15. Growth hormone secretion tests, along with a history and physical exam, have indicated a positive diagnosis for delayed puberty. The next step for the family nurse practitioner is to:
    1. Treat with hormone replacement.
    2. Refer to a pediatric endocrinologist.
    3. Treat with hormone stimulation therapy.
    4. Refer for possible pituitary tumor.

16. The family nurse practitioner is performing a physical exam on a 13-year-old female. It is important for the family nurse practitioner to incorporate developmental principles such as:
    1. Maintain a comfortable silence.
    2. Verbally affirm normalcy of physical findings.
    3. Discuss only the major areas of abnormality.
    4. Verbally address problems of sexually transmitted diseases.

17. At a school clinic, a 14-year-old girl comes in complaining of dizziness midmorning, and then later that morning. The family nurse practitioner should question the adolescent regarding diet, drug use, and:
    1. Asthma.
    2. Pregnancy.
    3. Heart disease.
    4. Stress.

18. **QSEN** The family nurse practitioner understands that sulfonamide medications are not recommended for children under which age?
    1. 18 months.
    2. 12 months.
    3. 6 months.
    4. 2 months.

19. What are common findings noted when assessing the skin of an older adult patient? (Select 3 responses.)
    1. Petechiae.
    2. Thick, brittle nails.
    3. Senile lentigines.
    4. Sebaceous gland hyperplasia.
    5. Chloasma.

20. Which statement is accurate about conducting a physical exam on an older adolescent?
    1. Provide a previsit screening tool or questionnaire to allow the adolescent to identify and write down concerns before the start of the visit.
    2. Have the adolescent's parent remain in the room during the health history and review of systems.
    3. Explain to the adolescent that everything that is discussed will remain confidential.
    4. Use a gentle confrontational approach when the adolescent is silent or unable to express specific words about physical changes occurring.

21. The family nurse practitioner is assessing immediate recall or new learning. A healthy adult patient should be able to repeat a series of how many numbers?
    1. More than 15 numbers.
    2. 10–14 numbers.
    3. 5–8 numbers.
    4. 3–5 numbers.

22. **QSEN** As part of a Medicare annual wellness visit, screening for cognitive deficits or impairment is an important component of the visit. Which three tests can be used to assess the progression of cognitive impairment?
    1. Short Portable Mental Status Questionnaire.
    2. Folstein Mini-Mental State Examination.
    3. Index of Independence of Activities of Daily Living.
    4. Katz Index.
    5. AD8 Dementia Screening Interview.
    6. 15 Minute Screen (15MS).

23. The family nurse practitioner is constructing a pedigree chart during a clinical visit. What is the purpose of obtaining a pedigree diagram?
    1. Record of growth and development milestones.
    2. Sexual orientation (LGBTQ) and sexual development.
    3. Genetic and familial health problems.
    4. Cultural variation and ethnic background.

24. In assessing the nutritional status of an older adult patient, the family nurse practitioner identifies the common physiologic changes in the gastrointestinal system to be: (Select 2 responses.)
    1. Increased peristalsis.
    2. Decreased absorption of iron.
    3. Maintenance of normal fat metabolism.
    4. Overgrowth of certain bacteria.
    5. Increased elasticity of the stomach.

25. When an 88-year-old patient who has short-term memory loss is interviewed, the patient states that she cannot remember what she ate for breakfast a few hours earlier. What would be an appropriate action for the family nurse practitioner?
    1. Order laboratory work and stop all medications.
    2. Consult with the patient's family member and/or caregivers to validate the patient's concerns.
    3. Refer the patient to a neurologist.
    4. Consider the short-term memory loss finding as a normal age-related change associated with aging.

26. Which statement is accurate about pain assessment in the very old adult?
    1. Pain perception varies from what is usually expected in the adult patient.
    2. Pain symptoms are more dramatic and specific as the patient ages.
    3. Older adults often exaggerate pain symptoms.
    4. Dull pain is often felt as sharp, stabbing pain.

27. Which statement is accurate about common changes occurring because of aging that are considerations during a physical exam?
    1. Tenting of the skin is a good indicator of hydration status.
    2. The whispered voice test is a helpful aid in screening for loss of hearing.
    3. Third and fourth heart sounds are uncommon.
    4. Increased sensitivity to touch and exaggerated vibratory sense in the lower extremities is noted.

28. **QSEN** During the physical exam of an older patient, the family nurse practitioner indicates an understanding of deviations in the neurologic system from the normal aging process with which clinical finding?
    1. Decrease in short-term memory.
    2. Decrease in deep tendon and superficial reflexes.
    3. Decreased sense of touch.
    4. Positive Romberg's sign.

29. A family nurse practitioner is interviewing an older adult with a physical disability requiring the use of a wheelchair. What are important considerations? (Select 3 responses.)
    1. Have an uncluttered surrounding, so that the patient has room to maneuver the wheelchair.
    2. Start the interview with a written questionnaire and have the patient take notes on the form.
    3. Speak clearly and with higher volume because of the patient' significant hearing impairment.
    4. Face the patient at eye level while communicating.
    5. Use a conversational tone of voice to promote a sense of ease with the patient.

30. **QSEN** A family nurse practitioner is assessing a 47-year-old patient who has come to the office for an annual physical examination. One of the first physical signs of aging is:
    1. Having more frequent aches and pains.
    2. Diminished eyesight, especially close vision.
    3. Increasing loss of muscle tone.
    4. Diminished hearing or taste.

31. The family nurse practitioner is asking questions during a review of systems and understands that constitutional symptoms include:
    1. Increased heart rate, bounding pulse, dizziness.
    2. Pruritic rash, malaise, diminished visual acuity.
    3. Weight, height, body mass index.
    4. Pain, fever, malaise.

32. Which of the following tools are available to assist with evaluating polypharmacy in the older adult patient? (Select 3 responses.)
    1. Medication Appropriateness Index (MAI).
    2. Screening Tool to Alert Medical Practitioners (STAMP).
    3. Katz Index.
    4. Screening Tool of Older Persons' Potentially Inappropriate Prescriptions (STOPP).
    5. Beers List.

33. When assessing the dehydration status of an older adult, which finding resulting from aging may provide unreliable physical assessment evidence?
    1. Poor skin turgor.
    2. Slight elevated temperature.
    3. Very dry mucous membranes.
    4. Swollen, furrowed tongue.

34. An adult patient with cerebral palsy and minimal cognitive dysfunction is seen at the clinic. The family nurse practitioner understands that health history information should:
    1. Be obtained only from the past medical record.
    2. Be obtained from the patient's family member and/or caregiver.
    3. Involve the patient to the limit of their ability.
    4. Involve the community group home where the patient resides.

35. **QSEN** Which functional assessment tool should the family nurse practitioner use to evaluate the safety of a patient who had a stroke and is planning to return to a home environment?
    1. Older American Resources and Services Activities of Daily Living (OARS ADL) Scale.
    2. Bennet Social Isolation Scale.
    3. Mini-Mental State Examination.
    4. Norton Scale.

36. When communicating with adolescents, the family nurse practitioner needs to be sensitive to the adolescent's:
    1. Reluctance to talk.
    2. Desire to be in control.
    3. Need for detailed instructions.
    4. Urge to communicate.

37. Which assessment would make the family nurse practitioner consider a developmental delay in a 6-month-old infant?
    1. Persistent tonic neck reflex.
    2. Absence of the Moro reflex.
    3. Inability to sit unsupported.
    4. Poor pincer grasp.

Growth and Development

38. The major influence on the timing of puberty is:
    1. Exposure to light.
    2. Genetics.
    3. General health.
    4. Nutrition.

39. A 14-year-old girl is seen in the clinic by the family nurse practitioner because she has not achieved menarche. Physical exam reveals axillary and pubic hair and breast buds with increased size of areola. Based on these findings, the most appropriate intervention would be:
    1. Bone age studies.
    2. Labs for luteinizing hormone (LH) and follicle-stimulating hormone (FSH) levels.
    3. Chromosome analysis to rule out Turner's syndrome.
    4. Reassurance that she is developing normally.

40. A 13-year-old male is seen by the family nurse practitioner for a sports physical. The genital exam reveals straight dark pubic hair at the base of the penis and testicular enlargement. Using the Tanner scale, the family nurse practitioner would record these findings as:
    1. Tanner stage I.
    2. Tanner stage II.
    3. Tanner stage III.
    4. Tanner stage IV.

41. An 11-year-old girl who has just begun to show signs of breast development asks the family nurse practitioner when she will start having periods like her friends. The family nurse practitioner's response is based on the knowledge that:
    1. The average age of menarche is 12.8 years.
    2. Most girls will have a growth spurt after the onset of menarche.
    3. Menarche usually occurs about 3–6 months after the onset of breast development.
    4. Menarche usually occurs about 18–24 months after the onset of breast development.

42. A teenage girl with curly pubic hair on the mons pubis and breast enlargement without secondary contour would be classified on the Tanner scale as:
    1. Tanner stage I.
    2. Tanner stage II.
    3. Tanner stage III.
    4. Tanner stage IV.

43. A routine well-child visit for a healthy full-term infant should include a hemoglobin and hematocrit test at:
    1. 1 month of age.
    2. 4 months of age.
    3. 6–9 months of age.
    4. 1 year of age.

44. During a routine well-child exam, a mother reports that her 5-month-old, who weighs 15 lb and was sleeping all night at 3 months of age, is now waking up hungry in the middle of the night. A diet history reveals that the infant is taking six 6-oz bottles of formula in a 24-hour period and has 2 tbsp of rice cereal in the morning. What teaching should the family nurse practitioner give the mother?
    1. Increase the amount of formula at each feeding to 8 oz.
    2. Take the child off formula and switch to homogenized milk.
    3. Decrease the amount of formula to 32 oz in 24 hours and add fruits, cereals, and juices.
    4. Continue the same amount of formula and introduce a variety of baby foods.

45. The father of a 12-year-old male tells the family nurse practitioner that he is afraid that his son is "getting fat." The child is at the 50th percentile for height and the 75th percentile for weight on the growth chart. The most appropriate response would be:
    1. Reassure the father that the son is not "fat."
    2. Assess family for the presence of obesity and genetic factors.
    3. Suggest a low-calorie, low-fat diet.
    4. Explain that this is typical of the growth pattern of boys at this age and encourage exercise and a healthy diet.

46. **QSEN** The mother of a 6-month-old infant tells the family nurse practitioner that the baby was spitting up his formula so she put him on goat milk. The family nurse practitioner is concerned because goat milk places the infant at risk of developing:
    1. Rickets.
    2. Scurvy.
    3. Megaloblastic anemia secondary to folic acid deficiency.
    4. Botulism.

47. A 1-year-old reaches for the family nurse practitioner's stethoscope with his left hand and the father says, "It looks like he's going to be a lefty, just like his old man!" The nurse's response is based on the knowledge that:
    1. Male infants usually have the same hand preference as their fathers.
    2. Hand preference is well established by 9 months of age.
    3. Children will not demonstrate a hand preference until about age 6.
    4. Children usually develop handedness by 18–24 months of age.

48. A mother is concerned that her 7-month-old breastfed infant is not getting enough to eat. The infant weighed 7 lb, 8 oz at birth and was 19 inches long. At 6 months of age, he weighed 15 lb and was 25 inches long. He now weighs 15 lb and is 25½ inches long. The family nurse practitioner's response is based on the knowledge that:
    1. Infants should gain 2–4 oz per week and ½ inch in height per month during the first 6 months of life.
    2. Infants should triple their birth weight by 6 months of age.
    3. Infants should gain 3–4 oz per week and ½ inch in height per month from 6–12 months of age.
    4. Infants should gain 1–2 oz per week and 1 inch in height per month from 6–12 months of age.

49. A child will be able to do which of the following fine motor skills first?
    1. Imitate a circle.
    2. Imitate a square.
    3. Copy a triangle.
    4. Copy a diamond.

50. The family nurse practitioner would expect a child to follow a one-step command that is given without a gesture and with only four to six individual words at what age?
    1. 7 months.
    2. 9 months.
    3. 14 months.
    4. 20 months.

51. The family nurse practitioner knows that language is the best single measure of normal cognitive development in early childhood. At what age do children begin to combine two words together?
    1. 8–10 months.
    2. 10–12 months.
    3. 12–15 months.
    4. 14–23 months.

52. A mother of 2-year-old twins is concerned that the twins do not talk very much and seem to have their own "private" language. The family nurse practitioner should:
    1. Tell the mother to spend some individual time with the twins so that they learn language skills.
    2. Perform a pure-tone audiometry.
    3. Tell the mother that this is normal for twins or siblings that are close in age.
    4. Refer to a speech pathologist for further testing.

53. The family nurse practitioner notices that a 9-month-old infant who was born 2 months prematurely reaches for an object only with his left hand. The nurse would:
    1. Record these findings as normal for a premature infant.
    2. Refer the infant for further evaluation.
    3. Order a muscle biopsy to rule out muscular dystrophy.
    4. Make a note on the chart that the child will probably be left-handed.

54. The mother of a 6-month-old infant tells the family nurse practitioner that her infant is now taking homogenized milk instead of an iron-fortified infant formula. The family nurse practitioner's response would be based on the knowledge that:
    1. Homogenized milk has the same solute load as formula and is a safe alternative to iron-fortified formula if vitamin supplements are given.
    2. There is an increased incidence of occult gastrointestinal bleeding and the development of iron-deficiency anemia in infants fed homogenized milk before 1 year of age.
    3. Once the infant is taking solid foods regularly, there is no need to continue offering iron-fortified formula.
    4. Homogenized milk has too high of a fat content and needs to be diluted 2:1 with water.

55. **QSEN** A 16-year-old adolescent with diabetes is noncompliant with consuming a healthy diet. In addition, the family nurse practitioner notes that he seems unconcerned about any consequences of his activities, such as riding a motorcycle without a helmet. Which factor is typical of adolescence and pertinent to this adolescent's overall health?
    1. Less involvement with parents.
    2. Less dominant role with peer group.
    3. Secure sense of self and high self-esteem.
    4. Experimenting with risky behaviors.

56. What is true about the developmental process of sperm or spermatozoa?
    1. Each mature sperm contains 23 chromosomes.
    2. Sperm become motile immediately at maturation.
    3. Spermatogenesis takes place in the prostate.
    4. Higher than normal body temperature contributes to sperm production.

57. Which statement is correct concerning healthy sexual developmental tasks?
    1. At 9 years of age, children are less self-conscious and readily expose themselves to younger children or parents of the opposite sex.
    2. At 16 years of age, adolescents are significantly influenced by the media in terms of sexual content and conduct.
    3. At 4 years of age, children distinguish organs associated with each sex and demonstrate increased sexual curiosity.
    4. At 5 years of age, children begin to have concerns about body image and begin to investigate their own sexual organs.

58. An adolescent female with breast budding and sparse, straight, lightly pigmented pubic hair along the medial border of labia is at which Tanner stage of sexual maturity?
    1. Stage I.
    2. Stage II.
    3. Stage III.
    4. Stage IV.

59. Precocious puberty is defined as:
    1. Onset of puberty before age 8 in females and 9 in males.
    2. Onset of puberty before age 5 in females and 7 in males.
    3. Onset of puberty before age 10 in females and 12 in males.
    4. Onset of puberty for either gender before older siblings enter into puberty.

60. The mother of a 5-month-old infant brings her child to the clinic because the infant awakens frequently at night and cries. The family nurse practitioner understands that the most common cause of night awakening in healthy infants is:
    1. Night terrors and nightmares.
    2. Separation anxiety.
    3. Trained night crying.
    4. Hunger pain and wet diaper.

61. A 10-day-old breastfed infant is brought to the clinic because the mother is concerned about the infant's "yellow-orange" color. History and findings are as follows: mother's blood type is AB-positive; infant's blood type is B-negative and total bilirubin 15 mg/dL. The family nurse practitioner understands that this is most likely caused by:
    1. Hemolytic jaundice.
    2. Breastfed jaundice.
    3. Obstructive jaundice.
    4. Physiologic jaundice.

62. A new mother presents to the clinic inquiring about when she should start feeding her 2-month-old infant solid foods. The family nurse practitioner should recommend that the mother:
    1. Start the infant on meat and eggs now.
    2. Wait until the infant is 1 years old before introducing solid foods.
    3. Start the infant on cereals now.
    4. Introduce one new food at a time when the infant is 4–6 months old.

Aging

63. As an individual ages, dehydration becomes a more prevalent problem. The family nurse practitioner understands this issue is related to which normal aging changes? (Select 2 responses.)
    1. Increased glomerular filtration.
    2. Ineffective water conservation.
    3. Decreased solute/water ratio.
    4. Decreased thirst drive.
    5. Increased vasopressin release.

64. As an individual ages, which physiologic change would affect responses to pharmacologic agents?
    1. Increased gastric emptying.
    2. Increased glomerular filtration rate.
    3. Decreased percentage of body fat.
    4. Decreased albumin concentration.

65. **QSEN** Although driving is an important task that allows the older adult to be mobile and independent, it is important when counseling an older adult driver to include the following:
    1. Drive only during the day when it is bright and sunny.
    2. Drive with headlights on at dusk and at night.
    3. Avoid driving in inclement weather.
    4. Use the bright headlights when driving at night.

66. **QSEN** The number one cause of accidental death in patients older than 65 years of age is:
    1. Motor vehicle accidents.
    2. Poisoning.
    3. Falls.
    4. Drowning.

67. What are the normal physiologic changes in the thyroid gland that occur with aging?
    1. Hypertrophy with a decrease in triiodothyronine (T_3) and thyroxine (T_4).
    2. Normal size with increase in thyroid-stimulating hormone (TSH) and decrease in T_4.
    3. Atrophy of the gland with a decrease in TSH, T_3, and T_4.
    4. Increase in nodularity with normal TSH and T_4.

68. The aging process causes what normal physiologic changes in the heart?
    1. Heart size stays the same, and the valves thicken and become rigid secondary to fibrosis and sclerosis.
    2. Cardiomegaly occurs along with the prolapse of the mitral valve and regurgitation.
    3. Dilation of the right ventricle with sclerosis of pulmonic and tricuspid valves.
    4. Hypertrophy of the right ventricle with decreasing capacity and compromised efficiency of the coronary arteries.

69. Which pulmonary physiologic change is commonly associated with the aging process?
    1. Increased cough response.
    2. Decrease in vital capacity.
    3. Decreased anteroposterior (AP) diameter of the thorax.
    4. Increase in residual Po_2.

70. During a teaching session, the family nurse practitioner instructs the patient regarding normal skin lesions in the older population. These would include:
    1. Seborrheic dermatitis.
    2. Senile keratosis.
    3. Senile lentigo.
    4. Squamous cell.

71. As an individual ages, which three findings are associated with normal age-related visual changes?
    1. Increased sensitivity to glare and sunlight.
    2. Loss of peripheral vision.
    3. Diminished color discrimination with colors appearing faded.
    4. Difficulty in focusing on objects far away.
    5. Decreased tear production.

72. Based on changes in hepatic function in older adult patients, which adjustment should the family nurse practitioner expect for oral medications that undergo extensive first-pass metabolism?
    1. The interval between doses should be increased.
    2. The metabolism of the oral medication will not be affected.
    3. A higher dose should be used with the same time schedule.
    4. The interval between doses should be reduced.

73. What is a general principle regarding drug absorption in the older adult?
    1. Rate of absorption is slowed.
    2. Amount or percentage of absorption is greatly reduced.
    3. Absorption responses are enhanced.
    4. Absorption and bioavailability are increased.

74. Which two statements are accurate regarding pharmacokinetics in the older adult patient?
    1. Older adults are less sensitive to drugs than younger adults.
    2. Reduced renal function, with resultant drug accumulation, is the most important cause of adverse drug reactions in older adults.
    3. The rate of absorption is increased.
    4. Reduced liver function may prolong drug effects.
    5. Serum creatinine tests should be performed on all medications primarily eliminated by the kidneys.

75. Which physiologic factor of aging contributes to incontinence in older adults?
    1. Decreased vascularity of the bladder mucosa.
    2. Increased urethral closing pressure.
    3. Increased ability to concentrate urine.
    4. Decreased bladder capacity.

76. What is the pathophysiologic age-related change that predisposes an older adult to dehydration?
    1. A decrease in body fat along with a significant decrease in lean muscle mass makes the older adult more susceptible to minute changes in blood volume.
    2. Thirst is normally experienced when there is a loss of 2% of the client's body weight or when osmolality is increased; this mechanism is significantly diminished in the older adult.
    3. With aging, the glomeruli reduce in number, which leads to a corresponding increase in glomerular filtering surface, which causes the kidney to increase its ability to concentrate urine in the older adult.
    4. Antidiuretic hormone (ADH) increases as the kidney loses function, leading to diminished ability to maintain osmolality.

77. The aging process causes what normal physiologic changes in the nervous system? (Select 2 responses.)
    1. Increase vibratory sense.
    2. Increase in tendon reflexes.
    3. Progressive deficits in smell and taste.
    4. Skeletal muscle hypertrophy.
    5. Changes in gait and posture.

78. What normal physiologic changes occur in the hematologic system with aging?
    1. Blood composition changes dramatically with aging.
    2. Levels of total serum iron are low, and intestinal absorption of iron is decreased.
    3. Lymphocyte function improves with age.
    4. Thrombus formation and platelet aggregation diminish.

2 Growth & Development Answers & Rationales

Physical Assessment

1. Answer: 3

Rationale: These are the recommended health evaluation intervals for children to obtain regular assessment information regarding growth and development and to administer recommended immunizations.

2. Answer: 3

Rationale: An approach with a well-balanced diet, activity, and exercise is necessary for weight reduction. This allows for a slow approach to weight loss that incorporates healthy behavior habits.

3. Answer: 3

Rationale: The first and most important part of all data gathering starts with a detailed history and physical exam. A detailed, objective description of the dysmorphic features is essential for comparison to textbook descriptions and other data. Although chromosome analysis will probably be ordered, it is not done initially. Parents should be included in the discussion of the findings and kept informed of the progress throughout the evaluation process.

4. Answer: 3

Rationale: In-toeing is a common problem in children and can result from femoral anteversion, adduction of the great toe, medial tibial torsion, and metatarsus adductus. Legg-Calvé-Perthes disease is commonly seen in older children (ages 4–8 years) who have loss of hip medial rotation.

5. Answer: 2

Rationale: Characteristics of innocent murmurs include midsystolic; asymptomatic; less than a grade III; loudest in pulmonic area (2–3 left intercostal space at the left sternal border); no radiation to other areas; may disappear on sitting; and may intensify with fever, activity, anemia, and stress. Any loud S4 sound is considered pathologic in children and in adults and deserves further evaluation.

6. Answer: 2

Rationale: The posterior fontanel is usually closed by 2 months of age; the anterior fontanel closes at about 24 months of age.

7. Answer: 3

Rationale: Genu varum (bowleg) of up to 20 degrees is a normal finding in children until the age of 18 months.

8. Answer: 1

Rationale: Toddlers like to make the first move (i.e., let them move closer and initiate eye contact first; do not call out their name because this might frighten them). Allowing them to handle the stethoscope will decrease their fear. Detailed explanations and involvement are more appropriate when assessing a school-age child.

9. Answer: 2

Rationale: Allow a toddler to explore the instruments and start with the extremities. Save the most invasive exam (of the head) for last. In infants, auscultate the heart and lungs while the infant is quiet, then proceed to do a head-to-toe assessment. In school-age and adolescent children, a head-to-toe sequence is preferred.

10. Answer: 1

Rationale: Ishihara's test checks for color perception. Brückner's test checks for the red reflex. Hirschberg's test checks for corneal light reflex, and Jaeger's test checks for near vision.

11. Answer: 3

Rationale: Because assessing cranial nerves can be a challenging task, the family nurse practitioner should use techniques that consider the child's developmental level.

12. Answer: 2

Rationale: Genu valgum (knock knee) is considered normal from age 2–6 years.

13. Answer: 3

Rationale: Congenital dermal melanocytosis, also known as Mongolian spots, are often found in infants of African American, Hispanic, Native American, and Asian descent. These spots are benign and tend to fade and disappear by age 3, requiring no intervention or treatment. Abuse is not suspected because signs of a healthy mother–infant relationship are noted (e.g., mother and infant respond positively to each other, and the baby is thriving).

14. Answer: 3

Rationale: Most children are flat-footed (pes planus) up to 2–5 years of age because of the plantar fat pad under the medial longitudinal arch, which protects it while the arch develops.

15. Answer: 2

Rationale: Once the tentative diagnosis is made, the family nurse practitioner should refer to a pediatric endocrinologist for further workup. It is beyond the scope of the family nurse practitioner's practice to treat the patient at this point.

16. Answer: 2

Rationale: Early adolescence is a time when the child undergoing great physical changes continually wonders if these changes are normal. Verbal affirmation of areas of normalcy during the physical exam can decrease anxiety.

17. Answer: 2

Rationale: Although all areas would be assessed, pregnancy is a common reason for midmorning syncope in adolescents associated with altered nutrition.

18. Answer: 4

Rationale: Newborns and infants up to 2 months of age may develop kernicterus because sulfonamides displace bilirubin from the plasma proteins.

19. Answer: 2, 3, 4

Rationale: Both structural and functional changes occur in the skin. Older adults often have senile lentigines (liver spots), which are brown macules found on the backs of the hands, forearms, and face caused by localized mild epidermal hyperplasia in association with increased numbers of melanocytes and increased melanin production. Sebaceous gland hyperplasia is found especially on the forehead and nose, with a raised area from 1–3 mm in size with a central pore. Petechiae are reddish, purple spots (usually 1–2 mm) of bleeding under the skin that may occur from numerous causes but is not affected by age. The nails, particularly the toenails, become thick, brittle, hard, and yellowish with marked longitudinal ridges and are prone to splitting into layers. Chloasma is hyperpigmentation occurring on the face of a pregnant woman and usually disappears in the postpartum period, although it does persist in a small percentage of women.

20. Answer: 1

Rationale: Providing a previsit screening tool or questionnaire to allow the older adolescent to identify and write down concerns before the start of the visit is a helpful open-ended approach to assist the family nurse practitioner to phrase questions in an appropriate way to promote a sense of partnership that encourages communication. Adolescents may be reluctant to talk and have a clear need for confidentiality. All adolescent patients should be given the opportunity to discuss their concerns privately. Every effort should be made to maintain confidentiality; however, it is important to explain

that there are limits on what can be kept confidential during the clinical visit. It should be explained that information that suggests that the adolescent's safety or the safety of another is at risk may be a reason for the family nurse practitioner to "break" confidentiality. Adolescents do not respond well to confrontation or any type of "forced" conversation to express how they are feeling.

21. Answer: 3

Rationale: When assessing immediate recall or new learning, a healthy adult patient without cognitive decline should be able to repeat a series of 5–8 numbers.

22. Answer: 1, 2, 5

Rationale: The following tests can be used to assess cognitive impairment and dementia: the Folstein Mini-Mental State Examination, the Mini-Cog screen for dementia, the Short Portable Mental Status Questionnaire, the AD8 Dementia Screening Interview, and the Montreal Cognitive Assessment (MoCa). The Index of Independence of Activities of Daily Living helps identify daily activities with which the patient needs assistance, as does the Katz Index. The Seven Minute Screen (7MS) (not 15MS) is a quick and common test used to assess temporal orientation, enhanced cued recall, clock drawing, and verbal fluency. The 7MS has been shown to be useful for detecting Alzheimer's disease in a patient with memory problems.

23. Answer: 3

Rationale: A pedigree chart is a diagram of family information using a standardized set of symbols (squares representing males and circles females). A dark symbol is used to indicate someone affected with a genetic condition, and unfilled symbols for those who are unaffected; carriers of a condition are often indicated by a gray symbol. The pedigree chart should have at least three generations noted. The pedigree chart is an important component of a family history and can provide information regarding diseases that are transmitted or occur in family generations. It can be used as a diagnostic tool to help guide decisions about genetic testing for the patient and at-risk family members.

24. Answer: 2, 4

Rationale: Decreased hydrochloric acid, which occurs with aging, leads to decreased absorption of iron and vitamin B_{12}. Excessive growth of certain bacteria (bacterial overgrowth syndrome) becomes more common with age and can lead to pain, bloating, and weight loss. Bacterial overgrowth may also lead to decreased absorption of certain nutrients, such as vitamin B_{12}, iron, and calcium. The stomach cannot accommodate as much food (because of decreased elasticity), and the rate at which the stomach empties food into the small intestine decreases with aging. Fat absorption will decrease, as would peristalsis.

25. Answer: 2

Rationale: Older adults may be confused or experience recent memory loss. Recent memory for important events and conversations is usually not impaired. Consultation with the patient's family member and/or caregivers to validate the patient's concerns is important to determine whether this is an isolated incident or a pattern of decline of memory loss. Although a careful review of medications is important, as changes in memory can be associated, for instance, with use of opiates, benzodiazepines, antidepressants, corticosteroids, and muscle relaxants, the patient's medications should not be stopped until further assessment is obtained. Loss of immediate and recent memory with retention of remote memory suggests dementia. Referral to a neurologist would be appropriate after concerns of the patient's memory loss are validated with the family member and/or caregiver.

26. Answer: 1

Rationale: Pain is both highly prevalent and undertreated in the older adult population. There is an increase in pain threshold that occurs in some older adults and a decrease in pain tolerance. Pain may be unreliably reported because, with age, its perception varies from the expected. Pain symptoms may be less dramatic, vague, or nonspecific. The severe pain usually associated with pancreatitis, for example, may be perceived as a dull ache, and the perception of pain during a cardiac event (myocardial infarction) may be minimal. Some patients may not report chronic pain symptoms because they attribute them to getting older or feel that nothing can be done to relieve the pain, especially because they have lived with the chronic pain for such a long time that it becomes part of their daily living.

27. Answer: 2

Rationale: High-frequency hearing loss (presbycusis) is a common age-related change with hearing. The whispered voice test is a simple test that can be useful in hearing assessment during a clinic visit, if older patients do not identify that they have difficulty hearing. It is the only test that does not require any equipment. Older adult patients with sensorineural hearing loss will have difficulty with the whispered voice test because their hearing loss is usually in the high frequency range. A whisper is a high-frequency sound and is used to detect high-tone loss. Because of thinning of the skin, tenting is not a good indicator of hydration status. The third heart sound is normal in adults but may indicate heart failure in older adults. The fourth heart sound is rarely a normal finding. If there is a decreased or absent vibratory sense of the lower extremities, testing is unnecessary.

28. Answer: 4

Rationale: Positive Romberg's sign indicates the inability to maintain balance, which indicates a need for further evaluation.

A decrease in short-term memory, deep tendon and superficial reflexes, and sense of touch are normal age-related changes. If it affects the patient's functional ability, a decrease in short-term memory would be considered a deviation. Also, the testing strategy of looking for similarities in the options applies here, as the three incorrect responses all relate to a decrease in a body function with age.

29. Answer: 1, 4, 5

Rationale: When interviewing an older adult who uses a wheelchair because of a physical disability, it is important to have the environment setting for the interview conducive to making the patient comfortable. This means having an uncluttered room that the patient can easily move around in a wheelchair, facing the patient at eye level to assist with eye contact while communicating, and using a conversational tone of voice to promote a sense of ease with the patient. It is not necessary to speak loudly, but better to face the patient while talking. Written questionnaires may be useful but should be given in advance of the interview visit.

30. Answer: 2

Rationale: Refractive errors are the most frequent eye problems in the United States. Blurred vision results from an inappropriate length of the eye and/or shape of the eye or cornea, and almost all errors—myopia (nearsightedness), hyperopia (farsightedness), astigmatism (distorted vision at all distances), and presbyopia (a form of farsightedness that usually occurs between 40 and 45 years of age)—can be corrected by eyeglasses, contact lenses, or, in some cases, surgery.

31. Answer: 4

Rationale: A constitutional symptom is defined as a symptom that affects the general well-being or general status of a patient. Examples include weight loss, shaking, chills, fever, pain, and vomiting. Constitutional symptoms tend to be nonspecific to a particular disease, and because of this, they are not useful in diagnosis of conditions as nonconstitutional symptoms.

32. Answer: 1, 4, 5

Rationale: The following screening tools are available for the family nurse practitioner to use to assess for polypharmacy in the older adult patient: MAI, STOPP, and the most familiar and recommended—Beers List, which is updated by experts in geriatric care (American Geriatrics Society) and pharmacology using Institute of Medicine standards. The Katz Index helps identify daily activities where the patient needs assistance.

33. Answer: 1

Rationale: Because of changes in skin collagen and loss of skin elasticity with aging, poor skin turgor, which is often used as a sign of dehydration in younger individuals, is unreliable in older adults. The patient's body temperature may be elevated because of dehydration or the elevation may be a result of an inflammatory or infectious process. Mucous membranes are often not noticeably dry until severe dehydration is present. The tongue may be swollen and furrowed in the older adult who is dehydrated.

34. Answer: 3

Rationale: The patient with a history of cerebral palsy with minimal cognitive dysfunction should be fully involved in the health history interview to the best of their ability. Support from the patient's family and/or caregiver may be encouraged; however, the focus should be on the patient by speaking directly to them. Additional information from past medical records and the community group home can be obtained either before (preferable) or after the health history interview.

35. Answer: 1

Rationale: The OARS ADL Scale is the more appropriate screening tool for identifying at-risk populations. The Bennet Social Isolation Scale would be appropriate to evaluate social interactions and resources. The Mini-Mental State Examination is used to evaluate memory, orientation, and attention. The Norton Scale is used to evaluate pressure ulcer risk.

36. Answer: 1

Rationale: Adolescents may be reluctant to talk with a health care provider and if they are willing to communicate, they often have a need for confidentiality. All adolescent patients should be given the opportunity to discuss their concerns privately. Explain to the adolescent and parent that during the clinical visit, you will be asking the parent to leave the room to provide an opportunity for the adolescent to communicate confidentially. It is important with motivational interviewing to show concern for the adolescent's perspective, as often it has not been acknowledged, which leads to a desire to be in control. Avoid assumptions, judgments, and lectures. When possible, ask open-ended questions beginning with less sensitive issues and then proceeding to more sensitive ones.

37. Answer: 1

Rationale: The tonic neck reflex should diminish around 4 months and disappear by 6 months of age. If any newborn reflex persists, developmental delay should be anticipated. The Moro reflex disappears by 6 months of age as well.

Infants at 6 months of age should still need support to maintain an upright sitting position until 8–9 months. A well-developed pincer grasp is not expected until age 10–12 months.

Growth and Development

38. Answer: 2

Rationale: Genetics is the primary determinant of the timing of puberty. Factors such as geographic location, exposure to light, nutritional status, and health status play a role, but genetics is the major influence.

39. Answer: 4

Rationale: Menarche usually occurs about 18–24 months after the onset of breast development. Bone age and laboratory studies are not necessary because development is within normal limits. Findings do not indicate a chromosomal abnormality, so chromosome analysis is unnecessary.

40. Answer: 2

Rationale: The following is a table reviewing the Tanner stages for males.

Tanner Stage	Pubic Hair
I	None
II	Countable; straight; increased pigmentation and length
III	Darker; begins to curl; increased quantity
IV	Increased quantity; coarser texture; covers most of pubic area
V	Adult distribution; spread to medial thighs and lower abdomen
Genital Development	
I	Prepubertal
II	Testicular enlargement; slight rugation of scrotum
III	Further testicular enlargement; penile lengthening begins
IV	Testicular enlargement continues; increased rugation of scrotum; increased penile length
V	Adult genitalia

41. Answer: 4

Rationale: Menarche usually occurs about 18–24 months after the onset of breast development. Although the average age of menarche is 12.8 years, this should not be the basis for the family nurse practitioner's response. Most girls have a growth spurt at Tanner stage IV.

42. Answer: 3

Rationale: The following is a table reviewing the Tanner Stages for females.

Tanner Stage	Pubic Hair
I	None
II	Countable; straight; increased pigmentation and length
III	Darker; begins to curl; increased quantity on mons pubis
IV	Increased quantity; coarser texture; labia and mons well covered
V	Adult distribution; with feminine triangle and spread to medial thighs
Breast Development	
I	None
II	Breast bud present; increased areolar size
III	Further enlargement of breast; no secondary contour
IV	Areolar area forms secondary mound on breast contour
V	Mature; areolar area is part of breast contour; nipples project

43. Answer: 4

Rationale: It is important in a healthy infant to check the hemoglobin and hematocrit levels at 1 year, as per current American Academy of Pediatrics recommendations (2018). A risk assessment for anemia should be performed at 4 months of age with appropriate action to follow, if positive (indicating anemia). For the first 4–6 months, the healthy infant can rely on their body's own storage supply of iron.

44. Answer: 3

Rationale: Consumption of 32 oz of formula per day is usually an indicator of the need for solids. Formula is recommended for the first year of life. Nutritional requirements are 110–120 cal/kg/day. Introduction of solids usually occurs between 4 and 6 months of age.

45. Answer: 4

Rationale: It is normal for boys at this age to appear heavier before they have their "growth spurt." Reassuring the father, although appropriate, is not the best response. Although the findings are within normal limits, it would not be necessary to assess the family for the presence of obesity. Low-calorie, low-fat diets are contraindicated for the growing child. Encouraging exercise and a healthy diet would be important to prevent obesity.

46. Answer: 3

Rationale: Goat milk can cause folic acid deficiency, which can lead to megaloblastic anemia. Rickets is caused by the lack of vitamin D. Scurvy is caused by a lack of ascorbic acid (vitamin C)

in the diet. Botulism is food poisoning caused by an endotoxin produced by the bacillus *Clostridium botulinum*. Most botulism cases occur after eating improperly canned or cooked foods. Infants have been known to develop botulism from raw honey that is placed on their pacifiers.

47. Answer: 4

Rationale: Children usually develop handedness by 18–24 months of age. The hand preference is usually fixed after 5 years of age.

48. Answer: 3

Rationale: Infants should gain 3–4 oz per week and ½ inch in height per month from 6–12 months of age. This child also doubled his birth weight by 6 months of age, as expected.

Age	Weight	Length/Height
0–6 months	6–8 oz/week (doubles birth weight by 5–7 months)	1 in./month
6–12 months	3–4 oz/week (triples birth weight by 1 year)	½ in./month

49. Answer: 1

Rationale: A child should be able to imitate a circle at 2½ years, copy a square at 4 years, copy a triangle at 5 years, and copy a diamond at 6 years. The ability to draw a shape after watching someone else draw it first is called imitation. Children are always able to imitate a shape or form before being able to copy it.

50. Answer: 3

Rationale: A child should be expected to follow a one-step command (using no gestures and only four to six individual words) between 10½ and 16½ months of age.

51. Answer: 4

Rationale: Two-word combinations are expected at 14–23 months of age.

52. Answer: 3

Rationale: It is normal for twins or siblings close in age to develop a "private" language understood only by them. Although it is important for the mother to spend individual time with each child, this is not what the question is asking. Pure-tone audiometry is done after age 3. There is no need for a referral to a speech pathologist at this time.

53. Answer: 2

Rationale: The infant should be referred for further evaluation. Handedness before 1 year of age may be an early sign of cerebral palsy. The history of prematurity could be an indication of anoxia at birth and would warrant further investigation. The earlier a child is diagnosed, the earlier intervention can be started.

54. Answer: 2

Rationale: There is an increased incidence of occult gastrointestinal bleeding and iron-deficiency anemia in infants fed homogenized milk before 1 year of age. Homogenized milk does not have the same solute load as formula and is not a safe alternative to iron-fortified formula, even if vitamin supplements are given. The solute load of whole milk is too much for the infant's immature kidneys. The infant needs to continue taking iron-fortified formula for the first year of life, if possible.

55. Answer: 4

Rationale: The peer group is important and influences the adolescent, which often manifests as experimentation with risky behaviors (riding a motorcycle without a helmet, not eating healthily to manage diabetes). Later on, as the adolescent approaches young adulthood, more thought is given to risky behaviors and the consequences, and a more secure sense of self develops.

56. Answer: 1

Rationale: Each mature sperm develops from mitotic division of diploid (46-chromosome) germ cells (spermatogonium) found on the basement membrane of each seminiferous tubule and becomes primary spermatocytes with 23 chromosomes each. Each of these two cells further divides into two more cells (spermatids), each of which has 23 chromosomes. Motility depends on the biochemicals in semen and in the female reproductive tract. Sperm production needs a temperature that is less than normal body temperature by at least 1°–2°F.

57. Answer: 2

Rationale: Adolescents are greatly influenced by the media and tend to identify with their parents as sexually functioning people. At age 9, children are more interested in their own body and are quite self-conscious. Children distinguish organs associated with each sex and demonstrate increased sexual curiosity at age 6, not age 4. The 10-year-old begins to have concerns about body image and begins to investigate his or her own sexual organs, not a 5-year-old.

58. Answer: 2

Rationale: Tanner has five stages of sexual maturity for both males and females. Stage I for both is preadolescent, and stage V for both is mature or adult development. Stages II, III, and IV chronicle development of breasts, pubic hair distribution, penis, and testes. This young female is demonstrating characteristics of Tanner stage II.

Tanner Stage	Pubic Hair
I	None
II	Countable; straight; increased pigmentation and length
III	Darker; begins to curl; increased quantity on mons pubis
IV	Increased quantity; coarser texture; labia and mons well covered
V	Adult distribution; with feminine triangle and spread to medial thighs
Breast Development	
I	None
II	Breast bud present; increased areolar size
III	Further enlargement of breast; no secondary contour
IV	Areolar area forms secondary mound on breast contour
V	Mature; areolar area is part of breast contour; nipples project

59. Answer: 1

Rationale: Precocious puberty is defined as beginning at age 8 for females and at age 9 for males.

60. Answer: 3

Rationale: Trained night crying can become a problem in infants who are not allowed to learn to "self-quiet." Activities such as rocking to sleep, exciting play activities before bedtime, and picking up the infant as soon as he cries can lead to trained night crying. Separation anxiety occurs in infants after 6 months of age. The majority of infants after 4 months of age are able to sleep throughout the night. Nightmares and night terrors occur at a later age.

61. Answer: 2

Rationale: This is a type of exaggerated physiologic jaundice that occurs frequently in breastfed babies because of the infant's inadequate caloric intake before the mother's milk comes in. It typically occurs between 7 and 15 days of life, whereas physiologic jaundice occurs most often between the second and fourth day of life. Hemolytic jaundice occurs in an Rh-negative mother who has an Rh-positive infant who becomes isoimmunized.

62. Answer: 4

Rationale: Solid foods are not recommended until the infant is 4–6 months old. Cereals should be introduced first, followed by fruits, vegetables, meats, and eggs. All foods should be introduced based on the readiness of the child.

Aging

63. Answer: 2, 4

Rationale: The thirst response is diminished, which results in an increased solute/water ration. Decreased renal plasma flow (glomerular filtration) leads to reduced ability to concentrate urine. The inability to concentrate urine prevents the body from retaining fluid leading to dehydration. Vasopressin release is decreased because of low fluid volume. These changes lead to ineffective water conservation.

64. Answer: 4

Rationale: Medications are often protein bound (not fat bound); albumin decreases with age. A low albumin level decreases the number of protein-binding sites, causing an increase in the amount of free drug in the plasma. Drug overdose may occur in older adult patients. Gastric emptying and glomerular filtration rate *decrease* with the aging process.

65. Answer: 3

Rationale: It is important to have the older driver recognize unsafe driving conditions, which include inclement weather, driving in bright sunlight or at dusk, and driving at night. Older adults should avoid interstate driving and driving long distances.

66. Answer: 3

Rationale: Falls are the major cause of morbidity and mortality in the older adult. A fall is often the precipitating event for a cascade of problems leading to death. Complications from falls include fractures, pneumonia, pressure ulcers, pain, and immobility.

67. Answer: 4

Rationale: There is usually adequate secretion of TSH and a normal serum concentration of T_4. Aging may produce fibrosis and increased nodularity, but overall the thyroid function remains within normal limits.

68. Answer: 1

Rationale: The heart does not increase in size with normal aging. An enlarged heart is a result of cardiac dysfunction. Dilation of the left ventricle occurs with myocardial infarction and altered cardiac functioning secondary to cardiac

disease, not from normal aging. The aging process does cause fibrosis and sclerosis of the cardiac valves; all valves are equally affected.

69. Answer: 2

Rationale: A decrease in the vital capacity, along with a 50% increase in residual volume, occurs during the aging process. Other aging changes include a less effective cough, impaired ciliary action, and weaker respiratory muscles. Increased AP diameter is associated with aging and in chronic obstructive pulmonary disease. P_{O_2} usually decreases, but P_{CO_2} usually remains unchanged or slightly increased.

70. Answer: 3

Rationale: The senile lentigo is a gray-brown, irregular, macular lesion on sun-exposed areas of the face, arms, and hands that are normal skin lesions. The other lesions are common abnormal skin lesions in the older adult.

71. Answer: 1, 3, 5

Rationale: Normal vision changes that occur with aging include increased sensitivity to glare and sunlight, diminished color vision with colors appearing faded, difficulty in focusing on objects close-up, need for more light for reading, and decreased tear production. Any sudden decrease or loss of peripheral vision can be indicative of a detached retina, which requires immediate treatment by an ophthalmologist.

72. Answer: 1

Rationale: In the older adult patient liver function is diminished, which may increase the half-lives of certain drugs, leading to prolonged responses. Responses to oral drugs that ordinarily undergo extensive first-pass metabolism may be enhanced because fewer drugs are inactivated before entering the systemic circulation. Consequently, the interval between doses should be increased.

73. Answer: 1

Rationale: With aging, the rate of absorption is slowed because of delayed gastric emptying and reduced splanchnic blood flow. Amount or percentage of absorption does not usually change with age. Drug responses are delayed, not enhanced because of aging. Bioavailability is the degree to which a drug or other substance becomes available to the target tissue after administration.

74. Answer: 2, 4

Rationale: Older adult patients are generally more sensitive to drugs than are younger adults, and they show wider individual variation. Drug accumulation secondary to reduced renal excretion is the most important cause of adverse drug reactions in older adults. In older adults, the proper index of renal function is creatinine clearance, not serum creatinine levels. Serum creatinine levels do not adequately reflect kidney function in older adults because the source of serum creatinine, lean muscle mass, declines in parallel with the decline in kidney function. Consequently, serum creatinine levels may be normal even though renal function is greatly reduced. The rate of absorption is slowed because of delayed gastric emptying and reduced splanchnic blood flow. Rates of hepatic drug metabolism tend to decline with age because of reduced hepatic blood flow, reduced liver mass, and decreased activity of some hepatic enzymes, which may prolong the drug effects.

75. Answer: 4

Rationale: Decreased bladder capacity, decreased ability to concentrate urine, and decreased urethral closing pressure after menopause lead to incontinence. Other factors are depression, decreased mobility, decreased vision, and lack of attention to bladder cues of feelings of fullness.

76. Answer: 2

Rationale: The older adult experiences significant hypodipsia and diminished thirst sensations, which leads to problems associated with adequate fluid intake. The older adult has increased body fat and less lean muscle mass. In addition, the quantity of total body water as a proportion of body weight decreases. The functional decline of the aging kidney leads to a gradual loss of glomeruli that results in a diminished filtering surface. The kidney does not concentrate urine effectively, and there is a decreased effect of ADH.

77. Answer: 3, 5

Rationale: The functional changes in the nervous system that occur with aging include progressive deficits in smell and taste, as well as changes in gait and posture. Vibratory sense is decreased along with tendon reflexes. Skeletal muscle atrophy occurs.

78. Answer: 2

Rationale: Values of total serum iron, total iron-binding capacity, and intestinal iron absorption are all decreased in older adults. Iron deficiency is often responsible for the low hemoglobin levels noted in older adults. Blood composition changes little with age. Lymphocyte function appears to decrease, with age affecting a decrease in cellular immunity. Platelet adhesiveness may increase with age, as do clotting factors, which leads to an increased risk for thromboembolism.

Health Promotion & Maintenance

3

1. The family nurse practitioner is preparing to provide an education class on medication compliance to a group of older adult individuals. Which strategies could lead to potential barriers that would affect the group's ability to receive the information?
   1. Assume that mental deficits exist in the group; therefore repetition of information should be strongly encouraged.
   2. Use handouts that contain easily understood language.
   3. Provide pill boxes as a demonstration technique to help engage the audience.
   4. Ensure that the room in which the teaching session is taking place has good lighting.

2. **QSEN** The family nurse practitioner is assessing an older adult patient using the Stopping Elderly Accidents, Deaths, & Injuries (STEADI) initiative algorithm called the Algorithm for Fall Risk Assessments & Interventions. Which documentation is representative of moderate risk?
   1. The patient has not fallen within the past year and has no gait, balance, or strength deficits.
   2. The patient has sustained more than two falls within the past year with injuries.
   3. The patient has fallen once in the past year without injury, gait and balance deficits present.
   4. The patient indicates that she is concerned about falling but does not exhibit balance problems on ambulation.

3. What is an example of a secondary level of prevention measure for an older adult patient?
   1. Dietary counseling.
   2. Focus on preventing complications related to disease processes.
   3. Assessment of vitamin D level.
   4. Identification of smoking based on self-report of patient.

4. What are the current American Cancer Society (ACS) dietary recommendations for cancer prevention?
   1. Maintaining a desirable body weight and eating a variety of foods, including fruits and vegetables and foods that are high in fiber.
   2. Increasing the amount of protein in the diet.
   3. Alcohol use in small to moderate amounts.
   4. Increase in consumption of fresh fruits, fish, and dairy products.

5. The family nurse practitioner is developing a plan of care for a group of adolescents who have a history of being unsupervised after school. Which three factors of adolescence should the family nurse practitioner consider when planning care?
   1. Have no symptoms of depression.
   2. Use alcohol and smoke marijuana.
   3. Adjust and perform well in school.
   4. Be involved in risky behavior.
   5. Are more likely to smoke tobacco.

6. In the presence of dyslipidemia and diabetes, the National Cholesterol Education Program guidelines set the goals for lipid levels as follows:
   1. LDL <100 mg/dL and triglyceride levels <150 mg/dL.
   2. LDL <160 mg/dL and triglyceride levels <240 mg/dL.
   3. LDL <100 mg/dL and triglyceride levels <180 mg/dL.
   4. LDL <150 mg/dL and triglyceride levels <220 mg/dL.

7. Which of the following is recommended as an annual screening test for colorectal cancer in a patient who is 51 years old?
   1. Guaiac-based fecal occult blood test (gFOBT) at-home test.
   2. Digital rectal exam.
   3. Sigmoidoscopy.
   4. Stool sample (gFOBT) collected at the office.

8. The American Diabetes Association recommends screening adults starting at age 45 with a fasting plasma glucose (FPG) test every:
   1. 1 year.
   2. 3 years.
   3. 5 years.
   4. 10 years.

9. What are tertiary prevention activities for an older adult woman who has had a stroke?
   1. Annual influenza vaccination.
   2. Physical therapy program.
   3. Annual mammogram.
   4. Annual ophthalmologic examination to evaluate for glaucoma.

10. The family nurse practitioner is conducting an admission assessment interview with an adult Native American client. Which therapeutic approach would be most effective?
    1. Use a soft voice with open-ended statements and reflective technique; avoid direct constant eye contact.
    2. Convey an open, friendly attitude; ask direct questions; touch the client occasionally for reassurance.
    3. Touch the client frequently for reassurance as a nonverbal supportive behavior, along with smiling or making a sardonic face to express a negative comment.
    4. Talk in a loud voice; maintain unbroken eye contact when asking direct questions and use minimal gestures.

11. For an older adult patient who has an alteration in the sensory-perceptual function of hearing, which plan would be most appropriate for the family nurse practitioner to implement during a health promotion session?
    1. Increase the pitch of the voice.
    2. Stand behind the patient when speaking.
    3. Speak in a tone that does not include shouting.
    4. Use typical complex sentences to prevent insulting the patient.

12. **QSEN** Which of the following management plans demonstrates an understanding of primary prevention of falls among older adults?
    1. Evaluate the need for assistive devices for ambulation after the patient has been injured in a fall.
    2. Provide resources to correct hazards that contributed to falling in the home environment.
    3. Reinforce the need to use prescribed eyeglasses to prevent further injury resulting from falls.
    4. Provide information about medications, side effects, and interactions.

13. Which of these health promotion screenings should be completed annually for the patient who is over age 50?
    1. Chest x-ray.
    2. Pneumococcal vaccination.
    3. Colonoscopy.
    4. Guaiac-based fecal occult blood test (gFOBT).

14. The family nurse practitioner is preparing to conduct an interview with a non-English-speaking client. An interpreter is scheduled. Which of the following actions are appropriate?
    1. Watch the client's verbal and nonverbal communication.

2. Speak to and look directly at the interpreter.
3. Use accurate medical terminology so the client understands the situation.
4. Have the interpreter paraphrase the client's communication to facilitate the pace of the interview.

15. Which of the following describes how cultural diversity may affect a client's health?
    1. Diabetes and cancer have higher occurrence rates among Caucasians than among African Americans.
    2. Asian Americans have a low incidence of stomach and liver cancers.
    3. African Americans have an increased incidence of hypertension, which is easily controlled by the beta-adrenergic blocker propranolol.
    4. Caucasians and other ethnic groups may self-treat their depression with over-the-counter alternative remedies, such as St. John's wort.

16. While teaching a class to a group of senior citizens, which would be most important for the family nurse practitioner to consider during the presentation?
    1. Provide increased overhead lighting to enhance visualization.
    2. Provide handouts on blue paper with black print.
    3. Review a video narrated by a woman.
    4. Recognize that past life experiences are beneficial in learning new information.

17. **QSEN** What is the most common occupationally related health problem?
    1. Repetitive motion injury.
    2. Hearing loss.
    3. Lung disease.
    4. Cancer.

18. The family nurse practitioner answers a phone call from an Asian American client who is experiencing a fever. The client wants to self-treat first before taking an antipyretic medication. What would the family nurse practitioner suggest to the client?
    1. Ingest yin foods.
    2. Meditate and pray.
    3. Have a massage.
    4. Ingest yang foods.

19. The family nurse practitioner is scheduled to provide health promotion teaching on oral health for a group of older patients who reside in an assisted-living community. Which four content areas should be included in the discussion?
    1. Excessive salivation.
    2. Periodontal irritation.
    3. Tooth loss.
    4. Decreased taste perception.
    5. Maintaining hydration.

20. Which of the following best describes the benefit of sports screening physicals?
    1. Screening for undiagnosed musculoskeletal deformities.
    2. Assessment of drug and alcohol use.
    3. Estimation of aerobic capacity.
    4. Identification of risk for an adverse cardiovascular event.

21. According to U.S. Department of Health and Human Services guidelines, which test is considered an important screening test to be done every 2 years for women between the ages of 50 and 64?
    1. HIV test.
    2. Colonoscopy.
    3. Mammogram.
    4. Chlamydia test.

22. A 48-year-old man presents to the clinic after having his cholesterol checked at a health fair. He states that his results were over 300 mg/dL and that he needs to see his primary care provider for further testing. An appropriate intervention for the family nurse practitioner to include is:
    1. Prescribing a cholesterol-lowering agent.
    2. Ordering an electrocardiogram (ECG) and an exercise stress test.
    3. Starting the patient on an exercise program.
    4. Performing a thorough history and physical and drawing a lipid profile.

23. In preparing a patient for a colorectal screening, the family nurse practitioner should instruct the patient to:
    1. Eat at least two servings of meat daily before collecting samples.
    2. Avoid aspirin, iron, and antiinflammatory medications.
    3. Avoid taking extra vitamin and mineral supplements before the test.
    4. Eat extra servings of high-fiber foods and water to ensure good samples.

24. **QSEN** The family nurse practitioner is performing an annual Medicare exam on a 77-year-old patient. Which of the following recommendations would be of greatest benefit in maintaining optimal health?
    1. "Exercise your arms and legs as much as you can each day."
    2. "Sleeping at least 9 hours will improve your energy level."
    3. "Urinate every 2 hours while awake to prevent accidents."
    4. "You should avoid soda and other types of junk food."

25. According to ChooseMyPlate, which two foods are included in the vegetable group?
    1. Chickpeas.
    2. Quinoa.
    3. Beans.
    4. Popcorn.
    5. Wild rice.

26. At what age should a routine screening mammography begin for women who have average risk of breast cancer, according to the U.S. Preventive Services Task Force (USPSTF) 2016 recommendations?
    1. 30 years old.
    2. 35 years old.
    3. Begin at age 40.
    4. After age 50.

27. Which of the following components should be included when taking a history from a patient who is new to the clinic?
    1. Past medical and surgical history, family medical and surgical histories, psychosocial history, diet and exercise habits, chemical use, sexual practices, and review of systems.
    2. Interval history, past medical history, family medical history, dietary habits, substance use, and sexual practices.
    3. Past medical and surgical histories, family medical history, psychosocial history, physical activity, tobacco and other substance use, and sexual practices.
    4. The history listed on the form provided to patients for completion before the physical exam is sufficient, and no interview needs to be done.

28. **QSEN** A family nurse is prescribing a narcotic analgesic for pain relief to an 82-year-old patient who lives alone. Which three actions should the family nurse practitioner take to promote safety?
    1. Determine whether the patient has constipation.
    2. Conduct an assessment of the patient's cognitive and motor abilities.
    3. Start with a low dose of analgesic and increase slowly, if needed.
    4. Assess the patient's usual waking and sleeping patterns.
    5. Evaluate for polypharmacy before ordering the analgesic.

29. Which group is at greatest risk for alterations in immune functions related to nutritional status?
    1. Young adults.
    2. Adults.
    3. Premature infants.
    4. Older adults.

30. A family nurse practitioner is examining a 78-year-old man in an assisted-living facility who has exhibited decreased food intake for 1 day but is still taking fluids. Which priority assessment should the family nurse practitioner perform?
    1. Review medication profile, looking for potential adverse effects of medications that would lead to decreased food intake.
    2. Prescribe enteral nutritional support to maintain caloric intake.
    3. Inspect the patient's oral cavity to determine whether there are any structural or infectious processes.
    4. Switch the patient to a pureed diet.

31. The family nurse practitioner is discussing making lifestyle changes that will decrease the older adult's risks for cardiovascular disease. Which of the following is most important to include in this discussion?
    1. Decrease smoking, increase vitamin supplements, and increase protein intake.
    2. Control hypertension, stop smoking, maintain normal weight, and exercise regularly.
    3. Maintain normal levels of serum blood sugar and decrease cholesterol intake.
    4. Have a yearly physical exam, increase fiber in the diet, and exercise regularly.

32. The family nurse practitioner is seeing an 86-year-old patient diagnosed with postural hypotension. Which intervention would be recommended to reduce the patient's fall risk?
    1. Avoid excessive foot movement before standing.
    2. Encourage exercise in the early morning.
    3. Recommend wearing support stockings.
    4. Recommend walking away from the table within 10 minutes of eating.

33. A healthy 4-month-old infant weighing 13 lb, 3 oz has started waking up at night after previously sleeping for periods of 9–11 hours. The infant takes 32 oz of formula in a 24-hour period. The family nurse practitioner recommends:
    1. Increase the formula to 38 oz in a 24-hour period.
    2. Start introducing one food item at a time, beginning with vegetables.
    3. Maintain current formula intake and introduce small amounts of rice cereal.
    4. Switch to whole milk instead of formula.

34. The family nurse practitioner understands that the infant mortality rate is:
    1. The number of infant deaths per 1000 live births.
    2. The total number of infant deaths per 1000 persons in the population.
    3. The number of infant deaths attributed to specific illnesses.
    4. The monthly infant death rate per 100 live births.

35. Which of the following is most important for the family nurse practitioner to do each time a child comes in for a health maintenance clinic visit?
    1. Order routine laboratory tests.
    2. Perform vision and auditory screening.
    3. Plot height and weight on charts.
    4. Review immunization record.

36. An older adult patient reports being forgetful. The family nurse practitioner is planning a possible drug regimen. Which of the following would promote adherence to the drug regimen? (Select 3 responses.)
    1. Time doses of medications to mealtime.

2. Choose medications that are similar in size and color.
3. Prescribe the smallest number of medications.
4. Order medications that are dosed once daily whenever possible.
5. Provide detailed written instructions for each medication.
6. Teach the patient to reduce the dose if side effects occur.

37. Anticipatory guidance for the family with a 6-year-old child includes:
    1. Avoid fluoride supplements to prevent staining of teeth and dental caries.
    2. Continue to use a belt-positioning booster seat until the child has reached 4 feet, 9 inches tall and is between 8 and 12 years of age.
    3. Instruct parents to use bottled drinking water when traveling to different parts of the country.
    4. Serve only three regular meals with no snacks to prevent development of poor nutrition habits.

38. In teaching a new mother about fevers, the family nurse practitioner knows that:
    1. Fevers over 104°F (40°C) can cause brain damage.
    2. Most fevers over 104°F (40°C) are usually of bacterial origin.
    3. Children under 6 months of age are especially susceptible to brain damage from a fever.
    4. Fevers may precipitate convulsions in children between 6 months and 5 years of age.

39. A new mother asks about the differences between human milk and cow's milk. The family nurse practitioner explains that:
    1. Human milk has more lipase and linoleic acid.
    2. Human milk has more calcium, phosphorus, sodium, and potassium.
    3. Cow's milk has low protein and casein content.
    4. Cow's milk has high linoleic acid and low saturated fatty acids.

40. According to the American Academy of Pediatrics, infants may be fed whole cow's milk once they reach:
    1. 6 months of age.
    2. 8 months of age.
    3. 12 months of age.
    4. 18 months of age.

41. A mother states that the iron-fortified formula her 3-month-old is on has been causing the infant constipation. The family nurse practitioner recommends:
    1. Discontinuing the iron-fortified formula.
    2. Starting the infant on rice cereal.
    3. Adding 1–2 teaspoons of dark corn syrup to the formula.
    4. Adding ½ teaspoon of mineral oil to daily intake.

42. A 1-year-old child who had a normal physical exam has a lead level of 15 μg/dL. Which of the following actions should the family nurse practitioner take?
    1. Repeat the test because it may be a false result.
    2. Hospitalize for immediate chelation therapy.
    3. Investigate possible sources of lead and repeat in 3–4 months.
    4. Repeat the test in 1 year.

43. The recommended time for the introduction of solid foods into an infant's diet is:
    1. Age 2 months.
    2. Age 3 months.
    3. Age 4–6 months.
    4. Age 6–8 months.

44. In explaining the purpose of primary prevention programs to a group of nursing students, the family nurse practitioner states that primary prevention programs:
    1. Work to lower the incidence of birth defects.
    2. Emphasize early diagnosis and treatment of pediatric anomalies.
    3. Minimize the handicapping effect of mental retardation.
    4. Focus on the prevention of complications and rehabilitation.

45. Teaching testicular self-examination should be targeted to which age group?
    1. 10–14 years.
    2. 15–25 years.
    3. 30–40 years.
    4. 45–65 years.

46. A father (height 74 inches, onset of puberty at age 16) is concerned that his 15-year-old son is going to be short. In a physical examination, the family nurse practitioner finds the son is Tanner stage II, height 62 inches, and the results of the rest of the exam are essentially normal for a well-nourished adolescent. After reviewing his growth records, which indicate a growth pattern of height at the fifth percentile, the most likely diagnosis is:
    1. Constitutional growth delay.
    2. Familial short stature.
    3. Hypopituitarism.
    4. Idiopathic gonadotropin deficiency.

47. In the preparation of educational materials for patients and parents, the family nurse practitioner is aware that the reading level of most adults is at the:
    1. Twelfth-grade level.
    2. Tenth-grade level.
    3. Sixth-grade level.
    4. Fourth-grade level.

48. A child presenting with vague symptoms and a serum lead level of 28 μg/dL would be managed by:
    1. Removal of the child from the lead source.
    2. Removal of the environmental lead hazard.
    3. Chelation therapy treatment.
    4. Rescreening and referral to a physician.

49. Which of the following should be included when discussing primary injury prevention with the parents of a 2-month-old child?
    1. Set water heater thermostat at <120°F.
    2. Make sure crib rails are no more than 3¼ inches apart.
    3. Use a rear-facing car seat until the child is >40 lb.
    4. Apply sunscreen when child is outside and the temperature is 75°F.

50. An Hispanic child presents with symptoms of weakness, irritability, weight loss, constipation, and mild ataxia, and a history of elevated lead levels. Which of the following homeopathic substances would the family nurse practitioner suspect had been used?
    1. White willow bark.
    2. Arnica root.
    3. Mexican yam root.
    4. Azarcon and greta.

51. Which of the following is found in the LGBTQ young adult, compared with a heterosexual young adult? (Select 2 responses.)
    1. Increased rate of substance abuse.
    2. Increased rate of smoking tobacco.
    3. Increased anxiety and manic-type behavior.
    4. Decreased rates of suicide and depression.
    5. Decreased rate of drinking alcohol.

52. Which lifestyle modifications are most effective in controlling hypertension in the older adult patient?
    1. Maintain normal weight, decrease sodium in diet, and exercise regularly.
    2. Increase dietary protein, decrease weight, and use stress-reduction techniques.
    3. Consume a high complex carbohydrate, low-sodium diet and decrease stress.
    4. Reduce weight, increase vitamin supplements, and exercise regularly.

53. A family nurse practitioner is reviewing a 72-year-old patient's history in the clinical setting. Which finding, if noted, requires a priority action in terms of health promotion and maintenance?
    1. Patient is not current for flu vaccination.
    2. Smoking history of one pack per day (PPD) for 10 years but has not smoked for 30 years.
    3. Patient wears eyeglasses for reading.
    4. History of osteoarthritis bilaterally in the knees.

54. When screening for intimate partner violence (IPV), it is important for the family nurse practitioner to understand that the following statement is true:
    1. Only men with psychological problems abuse women.
    2. IPV occurs in a small percentage of the population.
    3. Only people who come from abusive families end up in abusive relationships.
    4. One-fourth of all women experience IPV.

55. The family nurse practitioner has been asked by a local high school to provide an education program on teaching adolescents about social networking and texting on phones. The family nurse practitioner identifies what four findings as being important?
    1. Mobile access to the Internet has become widespread among adolescents.
    2. Multitasking and using multiple media types at the same time have been associated with late nights and sleep deprivation in adolescents.
    3. Adolescents do not use the online social environment to interact with the same peers they spend their day with at school.
    4. Adolescent "sexting" has been linked to risky sexual behaviors in a few research studies.
    5. Adolescents texting on the phone while driving is outlawed in many states.
    6. Texting and emailing do not create opportunities for cyberbullying.

56. The family nurse practitioner who volunteers at a senior citizens center is planning activities for the members who attend the center. Which activity would best promote and maintain health for these senior citizens?
    1. Gardening every day for 1 hour.
    2. Cycling three times per week for 20 minutes.
    3. Sculpting once per week for 40 minutes.
    4. Walking three to five times per week for 30 minutes.

57. The family nurse practitioner is developing a plan of care for an Asian American client. Which two measures should be included in the client's plan of care?
    1. Maintain direct eye contact while explaining plan of care.
    2. Explain responses carefully to questions asked by client.
    3. Promote trust by holding the client's hand to provide comfort.
    4. Avoid the use of hand gestures to communicate.
    5. Consider that periods of silence indicate the client does not agree with the plan of care.

58. A client of Latino heritage is refusing treatment at the clinic and wants a curandero called. What should the family nurse practitioner understand about the practices of a curandero?
    1. Curanderos are folk healers who use holistic healing practices.
    2. Clients who believe in magic and witchcraft want the assistance of a curandero.
    3. Curanderos are religious leaders in Hispanic and Latino communities.
    4. Clients cannot receive medical treatment unless it is approved by the curandero.

Immunizations

59. A child is 6 years old. How many doses of inactivated poliovirus vaccine (IPV) will he have received?
    1. 2 doses.
    2. 3 doses.
    3. 4 doses.
    4. 5 doses.

60. Before giving a child the measles, mumps, and rubella (MMR) trivalent vaccine, it is recommended to wait how long after cancer chemotherapy has stopped?
    1. 30 days.
    2. 2 months.
    3. 3 months.
    4. 6 months.

61. The National Childhood Vaccine Injury Act requires standardized consent forms for the administration of vaccines to children. The content on the form for the medical record includes the vaccine lot number, nurse signature, injection/inoculation site, and:
    1. Signature of parent or legal guardian.
    2. Education provided.
    3. Absence of contraindications.
    4. Vaccine expiration date.

62. What would be an appropriate postexposure immunization for hepatitis A virus (HAV) for an adult over age 40 who has not been previously immunized?
    1. Immunoglobulin M (IgM).
    2. Twinrix.
    3. Shingrix.
    4. GamaSTAN S/D.

63. A person is concerned about travel to a hepatitis A virus (HAV) endemic area. What are the preexposure recommendations before travel?
    1. IM injection of immune globulin (IG).
    2. HAV vaccine and IG within 2 weeks of travel.
    3. HAV vaccine on return from the trip.
    4. Twinrix vaccine on return from the trip.

64. The mother of a 15-year-old child who has not had chickenpox is concerned and wants her daughter to be vaccinated. The recommendations are:
    1. Not recommended for children over age 12.
    2. One-time dose.
    3. Two doses at least 28 days apart.
    4. Three doses at 2 months apart.

65. Consultation with the mother of an 18-month-old who has received no immunizations reveals that the child was exposed to measles 48 hours before the visit. At this time, the family nurse practitioner would:
    1. Discharge the patient with care instructions.
    2. Administer the live attenuated measles vaccine.
    3. Administer 0.5 mL/kg immunoglobulin G (IgG).
    4. Administer half the regular measles vaccine dose.

66. Which statement about the polyvalent pneumococcal vaccine is true?
    1. It is recommended for children older than 2 years of age with chronic diseases, including diabetes.
    2. It is recommended to prevent otitis media (OM) and other pneumococcal infections in children younger than 2 years of age.
    3. It may not be given concurrently with other vaccines.
    4. Severe systemic reactions are common after immunization.

67. According to the Centers for Disease Control and Prevention (CDC), which two immunizations are recommended as primary prevention for adults ages 60 and over?
    1. Flu and shingles.
    2. Flu and HPV.
    3. Yearly tetanus prophylaxis.
    4. Adult who has had previous allergic reaction to an immunization.

68. Which of the following immunizations decreases the possibility of epiglottitis?
    1. Epstein-Barr virus.
    2. *Haemophilus influenzae* type B (Hib).
    3. *Streptococcus pyogenes.*
    4. Coxsackievirus.

69. The influenza vaccination is recommended annually for high-risk groups. The family nurse practitioner knows that the greatest need for this vaccination is for:
    1. Adults with chronic disease.
    2. Residents of long-term care facilities.
    3. Dialysis patients.
    4. Health care employees.

70. The family nurse practitioner understands that the only contraindication to hepatitis B vaccination is:
    1. Pregnancy and lactation.
    2. History of poliomyelitis.
    3. Prior anaphylaxis or severe hypersensitivity.
    4. Mild viral illness.

71. A female college student develops symptoms of hepatitis A virus (HAV) about 5 weeks after receiving a vaccination for HAV. The family nurse practitioner explains to the patient: (Select 3 responses.)
    1. HAV infections in the United States are most often acquired during travel to HAV-endemic countries.

2. HAV vaccine is effective only after the second dose.
3. Unprotected intercourse is the primary mode of transmission.
4. Symptoms occur primarily after consuming food or water contaminated with HAV or via direct contact with a person with HAV infection with poor hygiene.
5. A prevaccine exposure to HAV could be the reason for the patient's symptoms.

72. Immunizations and chemoprophylaxis offered routinely to patients 65 years of age or older are:
    1. Tdap/Td, influenza, shingles, and pneumococcal vaccine.
    2. Td, varicella, or shingles vaccine.
    3. Td and influenza; for those with a weakened immune system, offer the shingles vaccine.
    4. Offer influenza and Td vaccines to those who have not had these vaccines in the past 10 years.

73. The family nurse practitioner understands that the following is considered an attenuated live-virus vaccination:
    1. Rubella and measles.
    2. Mumps and hepatitis B.
    3. Poliomyelitis and hepatitis B.
    4. Rubella and rabies.

74. The family nurse practitioner understands that children who should not receive the measles vaccine are children who have severe allergic reactions to:
    1. Fungi.
    2. Pollen.
    3. Pets.
    4. Neomycin.

75. The family nurse practitioner is assessing an 8-month-old infant in an immunization clinic. By this time, the infant should have received which immunizations?
    1. All three hepatitis B injections, all rotavirus (RV) series, three doses of the pneumococcal conjugate series, and at least two doses of inactivated poliovirus (IPV).
    2. Hepatitis B first and second dose, all the DTaP, the polio series, and measles, mumps, and rubella (MMR).
    3. DTaP first and second dose, MMR first dose, all hepatitis B series.
    4. Varicella, acellular pertussis (Tdap) first dose, and hepatitis B first dose.

76. Based on 2020 recommendations for immunizations for individuals who are over the age of 65, which schedule may be recommended on the basis of individual risk assessment?
    1. Measles, mumps, and rubella (MMR).
    2. Chickenpox (varicella-zoster virus).
    3. Hepatitis B virus.
    4. Pneumococcal.

77. Which of the following patient situations requires the use of inactivated (not live) vaccines?
    1. History of nonspecific allergies.
    2. Immunocompromised adult.
    3. Concurrent antimicrobial therapy.
    4. Mild acute illness.

78. The family nurse practitioner performs a physical exam on a 75-year-old patient who is healthy. The patient remembers having chickenpox as a child and reports remembering a mild case of shingles on her back that occurred when she was in her 40s, with no postherpetic neuralgia. She has had no further episodes of shingles. What should the family nurse practitioner do?
    1. Administer the Zostavax vaccine.
    2. Order a varicella titer.
    3. Administer Twinrix vaccine.
    4. Do nothing, because the patient reports having had chickenpox.

79. In taking the history of a healthy 50-year-old man, the family nurse practitioner determines the patient is an avid gardener and spends much of his time enjoying outdoor activities. A health maintenance recommendation for this patient is to obtain a:
    1. Pneumococcal vaccine.
    2. Tdap/Td vaccine.
    3. Hepatitis B vaccine.
    4. Varicella vaccine.

80. At which patient age should the family nurse practitioner recommend routine use of the single-dose Pneumovax 23 (PPSV23) vaccination?
    1. 65 years of age or older.
    2. 60 years of age or older.
    3. 55 years of age or older.
    4. 50 years of age or older.

81. The Advisory Committee on Immunization Practices (ACIP) recommends that healthy older adults receive the Td or tetanus booster vaccination:
    1. Every 5 years.
    2. Every 10 years.
    3. At age 65.
    4. At age 50.

82. A 65-year-old woman inquires about her vaccination requirements regarding the pneumococcal vaccine. She received a single Pneumovax 23 (PPSV23) vaccination at age 57 because of the presence of risk factors. She has never received any other pneumococcal vaccinations. Which of the following should the family nurse practitioner recommend?
    1. Administer Pneumovax 23 (PPSV23) vaccine now.
    2. No further vaccination is necessary.
    3. Administer Prevnar (PPSV13) vaccine now.
    4. Administer PPSV23 vaccine at age 67.

83. Which statement most correctly describes tetanus toxoid?
    1. Tetanus toxoid is a bacterial toxin that has been changed to a nontoxic form.
    2. DTaP and DT are safe to give to adults.
    3. The recommended dose of tetanus toxoid for adults is 1 mL IM.
    4. Tetanus toxoid provides immunity from *Corynebacterium diphtheriae*.

84. Immunizations recommended for healthy young adults include:
    1. Measles, rubella, varicella, and hepatitis B.
    2. Pneumovax 23 (PPSV23), influenza, and rubella.
    3. Tetanus, influenza, varicella, PPSV23, and hepatitis B.
    4. Influenza, hepatitis B, rubella, measles, and tetanus.

85. A 2-month-old infant received his immunizations, and 12 hours later, the mother calls and says the infant has a fever of 101°F (38°C). What is the most likely cause of the fever?
    1. Vaccination for measles, mumps, and rubella (MMR).
    2. Combination of the diphtheria and the polio vaccinations.
    3. Presence of an infection when immunizations were given.
    4. Pertussis immunization.

86. Primary prevention of Neonatal Abstinence Syndrome (NAS) includes:
    1. Prescribing a reliable form of birth control for a patient being treated for chronic pain with opioids.
    2. Universally screen pregnant women for substance abuse and make referrals to treatment when appropriate.
    3. Never prescribe opioids to a woman of child-bearing age.
    4. Obtain a patient's records from the state prescription drug-monitoring program if you suspect she is getting opioids from another provider.

87. An elderly patient comes to your office 2 days after receiving the pneumococcal conjugate vaccine (PCV13). He complains of pain at the injection site, difficulty raising his arm without pain, and has a fever of 100.4°F (38°C). What should the family nurse practitioner suspect?
    1. This is a serious reaction to the immunization and that he may need hospitalization.
    2. The fever and the vaccination are likely unrelated.
    3. It is somewhat common to get a fever and localized reaction to this vaccine.
    4. The patient may be allergic to eggs.

88. Smallpox vaccine is offered to certain members of the military in anticipation of possible exposure caused by bioterrorism. What are two common side effects of smallpox vaccination?
    1. Myocarditis and pericarditis.
    2. Dime-sized blister lesion at the injection site that forms a scab and leaves a scar.
    3. Severe allergic reaction.
    4. Fatigue.
    5. Severe skin conditions.

89. In caring for school-age children, the family nurse practitioner should be aware that the number one reason for school absenteeism is:
    1. Sports injuries.
    2. Influenza.
    3. Asthma.
    4. Lack of sleep.

90. The human papilloma virus (HPV) vaccine should be recommended to:
    1. A 40-year-old man who did not finish the vaccine series as a teen.
    2. Girls age 11 or 12.
    3. At birth.
    4. Women with compromised immune systems (including HIV infection) through age 50, if they did not get the HPV vaccine when they were young.

91. Which person should not receive the Shingrix vaccine:
    1. A 62-year-old patient who previously had chickenpox.
    2. A 45-year-old patient who was exposed to chickenpox.
    3. A 50-year-old patient who has a history of having shingles.
    4. A 39-year-old patient who is pregnant.

92. An adult who works as a veterinarian has been administered a rabies vaccination. What are four possible side effects and risks of receiving the vaccination?
    1. Hives, fever, and joint pain.
    2. Soreness and redness at the injection site.
    3. Headache and dizziness.
    4. Abdominal pain and gastric distress.
    5. Diplopia and confusion.
    6. Severe allergic reaction.

93. Recommendations of the Advisory Committee on Immunization Practices (ACIP) and the Centers for Disease Control and Prevention for the hepatitis A vaccine (HAV) include: (Select 2 responses.)
    1. Vaccinate infants at 2 months of age.
    2. Only vaccinate those who live in HAV endemic countries.
    3. Testing for HAV immunity is not necessary before HAV vaccinations.
    4. Do not administer the HAV vaccine to a pregnant patient.
    5. If the interval between the first and second doses of HAV vaccine extends beyond 18 months, it is not necessary to repeat a dose.

94. Immunizations recommended for a healthy 40-year-old adult who has had his childhood series include:
    1. Measles, rubella, varicella, and hepatitis B.
    2. Pneumovax 23 (PPSV23), influenza, and rubella.
    3. Tetanus, influenza, varicella, PPSV23, oral polio vaccine (OPV), and hepatitis B.
    4. Influenza, hepatitis A, hepatitis B, varicella, measles mumps rubella (MMR), and tetanus.

1. Answer: 1

Rationale: With the older adult population, normal changes associated with aging may lead to potential sensory deficits (sensory losses) that can prove to be a barrier in providing and receiving information. Although information may have to be repeated, the assumption that this is caused by mental deficits associated with aging is a form of implicit bias. Handouts that contain easily understood language, providing examples to use in demonstration of content, and ensuring that the room in which teaching/learning occurs has good lighting will help promote educational learning.

2. Answer: 3

Rationale: Any patient with gait, balance, or sensory deficits is considered moderate or high risk, regardless of fall history. A patient with gait, balance, or sensory deficits who has not fallen, or a patient who has fallen one time without injury is classified as moderate risk. A patient who has fallen once with injury or fallen two or more times is considered at high risk. Only patients without gait and balance issues without a history of falls are classified as low risk and may need further evaluation with other assessment tools. A patient who had concerns about falling but did not exhibit any balance or ambulation problems would be considered at low risk.

3. Answer: 3

Rationale: Secondary prevention measures focus on detection and management of potential disease states through diagnostic testing and scheduled examinations; thus detection of vitamin D levels helps to establish a baseline. Dietary counseling and identifying smoking are examples of primary level of prevention measures because they focus on preventing the occurrence of disease and identifying relevant risk behaviors. Focusing on preventing complications related to disease is an example of a tertiary level of prevention because the disease process is already established.

4. Answer: 1

Rationale: The ACS recommends maintenance of a desirable body weight; research has shown an association between increased mortality resulting from various cancers and varying degrees of being overweight. Another recommendation is to eat a wide variety of foods, consistent with the ChooseMyPlate guide of the U.S. Department of Agriculture and U.S. Department of Health and Human Services. A variety of fruits and vegetables should be included in the daily diet (make half your plate fruits and vegetables) because research has shown an association between lower cancer rates and high fruit and vegetable consumption. High-fiber foods are also recommended; a lower risk of colon cancer is seen in those who consume a high-fiber diet. Currently, there are no recommendations to increase the amount of protein in the diet. Because of the high consumption of red meat in the American diet, many people are already receiving large quantities in their current diets. It is recommended that red meat and processed foods should be limited. The ACS recommends limiting the daily consumption of alcohol to two drinks for males, one drink for females, and no drinks for pregnant females. They also state that, ideally, no alcohol should be consumed; regular alcohol consumption has been shown to increase the risk of various cancers.

5. Answer: 2, 4, 5

Rationale: Adolescents most likely to smoke, abuse substances, perform poorly in school, be depressed, and engage in risky behavior are those who have a history of being unsupervised after school.

6. Answer: 1

Rationale: The recommendation is LDL <100 mg/dL and triglyceride levels <200 mg/dL for individuals with risk factors for coronary heart disease. Although 150 mg/dL is the ideal goal for triglyceride levels, treatment is started at >200 mg/dL in the diabetic and almost all other patients with risk factors. In a diabetic patient, the LDL goal is independently <100 mg/dL. If the patient has triglycerides >200 mg/dL, then the goal is <130 mg/dL non-LDL cholesterol. All other choices have inaccurate goals.

7. Answer: 1

Rationale: The U.S. Preventive Services Task Force recommends screening for colorectal cancer using high-sensitivity gFOBT, sigmoidoscopy, or colonoscopy beginning at age 50 years and continuing until age 75 years. Of course, a colonoscopy is the best test and it is okay to have a stand-alone screening of gFOBT, as long as colonoscopy is recommended first. The multiple gFOBT stool take-home test should be used. One gFOBT test obtained by the family nurse practitioner in the office is not adequate for testing. A colonoscopy should be scheduled if the gFOBT test result is positive.

8. Answer: 2

Rationale: The American Diabetes Association recommends screening adults starting at least by age 45 and repeating the FPG every 3 years. This is for all patients, and screening is indicated at 3-year intervals for patients with >25 body mass index or other risk factors at any age for an adult. The U.S. Preventive Services Task Force recommends screening for abnormal blood glucose as part of cardiovascular risk assessment in adults aged 40–70 years who are overweight or obese.

9. Answer: 2

Rationale: Tertiary prevention refers to reducing the impact of an ongoing illness or injury. The physical therapy program will assist the older adult woman in restoring her optimum level of functioning after a stroke. An annual influenza vaccination is a primary prevention activity nonspecific to the care of a patient with a stroke. An annual mammogram and ophthalmologic examination to evaluate for glaucoma are examples of secondary prevention activities nonspecific to the care of a patient with a stroke.

10. Answer: 1

Rationale: Indigenous cultures, such as the Native American culture, place special significance on the place of humans in the natural world. That culture emphasizes the importance of a holistic body-mind-spirit and living in harmony with nature. Using a soft voice with open-ended statements that reflect a cooperative, sharing style rather than competitive or intrusive approaches would be the preferred therapeutic approach (i.e., a passive style would be best received). Also, some Native American cultures use silence to a far greater degree, which should not be mistaken for belligerence or sullenness, but likened more to a common response in dealing with strangers or noted as a sign of wisdom. The other options would be more effective to use with clients of a Western culture orientation.

11. Answer: 3

Rationale: Shouting increases the pitch of the voice. In presbycusis, or hearing loss in older adults, high-pitched consonant sounds are the first to be affected, and the change may occur gradually. The family nurse practitioner should face the patient when speaking. If the nurse needs to stand behind the patient, touch is used to get the patient's attention. Simple sentences should be used to facilitate understanding.

12. Answer: 4

Rationale: The information about side effects and interactions of medication will prevent complications that may result in a fall. Evaluating for assistive devices following a fall

and providing resources to correct hazards in the home are appropriate for tertiary prevention. Reinforcing the need to wear prescribed eyeglasses is appropriate for secondary prevention, which is intended to prevent the patient from experiencing another fall.

13. Answer: 4

Rationale: The gFOBT will assist in identifying any problems with intestinal bleeding, polyps, and cancer and is recommended to be started at age 50. Pneumococcal vaccination is not a screening test. A colonoscopy is recommended at age 50 and then every 10 years thereafter, not annually. Annual chest x-rays are recommended for adults ages 55–80 years who have a 30 pack-year smoking history and currently smoke or have quit within the last 15 years.

14. Answer: 1

Rationale: Watch and listen to the client's nonverbal communication, when the client is talking. During the interview, look and speak with the client, not the interpreter. Pace a conversation so there is time for the client's response to be interpreted. Do not ask the interpreter to paraphrase or insert their meaning into the client's words. Ask the client for feedback and clarification at regular intervals. Use brief, concise sentences and simple language—avoid technical terms and slang language.

15. Answer: 4

Rationale: Many cultural factors affect a client's approach to health and health care. Alternative remedies, such as St. John's wort, are used for self-treatment of depression. For most cancers, certain racial and ethnic groups have lower survival rates than Caucasians. Hypertension has a higher rate of occurrence in African Americans, who are at greater risk of developing heart disease, end-stage renal disease, and stroke than the general population. Asian Americans have a higher incidence of stomach and liver cancers. Ethnic groups respond differently to medications. Caucasians are more sensitive to the effects of beta-adrenergic blockers, such as propranolol, whereas African Americans are less responsive to this drug group.

16. Answer: 4

Rationale: Using past life experiences applies the concept of adult educational principles. Overhead lighting may produce an increase in the glare, which can decrease visualization. There is an alteration of color perception (e.g., blue appears green-blue) as an individual ages. As individuals age, the ability to hear women's and children's voices decreases because these are generally at a higher pitch. The video would not enhance the program because the patients frequently have presbycusis as a result of the normal aging process.

17. Answer: 3

Rationale: All these disorders can be associated with workplace exposure, but lung disease is currently still the most common occupationally related disease. Representing approximately 10% of the chronic occupational diseases, lung disease has been named as 1 of 10 leading work-related disease and injury categories by the National Institute for Occupational Safety and Health. Musculoskeletal injuries are on the rise.

18. Answer: 1

Rationale: Yin foods are cold foods and yang foods are hot foods. With the client experiencing a fever, they will want to eat yin foods or cold foods. Having a massage and meditating and praying are not part of the yin and yang approach to address symptoms of illness.

19. Answer: 2, 3, 4, 5

Rationale: The older patient is at risk for oral health problems, and health promotion teaching should be focused on periodontal irritation, tooth loss, decreased taste perception, and maintaining hydration. Excessive salivation is typically not seen in the older patient; rather, dry mouth occurs because of decreased salivation.

20. Answer: 4

Rationale: The primary goal and benefit of a sports screening physical exam is to identify athletes at risk for an adverse cardiovascular event. The physical exam also screens for athletes at risk for orthopedic injuries secondary to previously unresolved injuries; however, this is not the primary benefit. Even with a thorough history obtained from the screening exam, performing the exam is unlikely to completely eliminate injuries or be able to identify all underlying health problems. The other options (assessing drug and alcohol use, estimating aerobic capacity, and assessing for undiagnosed musculoskeletal deformities) are not the benefit of the sports screening physical.

21. Answer: 3

Rationale: Starting at age 50, a screening mammogram should be performed every 2 years through age 74. At ages 75 and older, the patient needs to check with her doctor or family nurse practitioner to see if screening is required because of previous findings and current risk factors. Patients should be tested for chlamydia or HIV if they are sexually active and at increased risk. Starting at age 50, a patient should be screened for colorectal cancer every 10 years unless there are increased risk factors or polyps are present.

22. Answer: 4

Rationale: The patient's history and physical exam will reveal the presence of any coronary heart disease (CHD) risk factors (age, family, history of CHD, diabetes, current cigarette smoking, blood pressure, height/weight, cardiovascular exam). A lipid profile is also recommended to assess the level of risk and consists of total cholesterol, high-density lipoprotein, low-density lipoprotein, and triglyceride levels. It would be prudent to have a precise cholesterol measurement done because the previous measurement was done at a screening health fair, and no written record was taken. These parameters should be assessed first, before a cholesterol-lowering agent, ECG, or stress test is ordered. An exercise program is also important but should be done only after a history is taken and a physical exam is done and after lipid profile results are known. If the lipid profile or the history and physical exam results are abnormal, stress testing may be appropriate before undertaking a new exercise program.

23. Answer: 2

Rationale: Screening for colorectal cancer includes annual fecal occult blood screening for individuals over age 50. Avoiding medications that can cause gastrointestinal irritation and bleeding can help avoid false-positive results. Rare meats and vegetables that are high in peroxidase will cause false-positive results, whereas vitamin C can cause false-negative results.

24. Answer: 1

Rationale: Maintaining muscle strength reduces the risk of immobility. Immobility is a predictor of loss of independence, depression, reduced quality of life, falling, institutionalization, and death. Sleeping long hours is not associated with improved energy. Less-than-optimal nutrition and urinary incontinence are not as great a threat to loss of independence as is immobility. Preventing falls is a Healthy People 2020 goal.

25. Answer: 1, 3

Rationale: Beans and peas are legumes, which are included in the vegetable group and are excellent sources of plant proteins. Quinoa, popcorn, and wild rice belong to the grains group.

26. Answer: 4

Rationale: According to the 2016 USPSTF recommendations, screening mammography in women before age 50 years should be an individual decision. Women may choose to begin biennial screening between the ages of 40 and 49 years. Biennial screening mammography is recommended for women aged 50–74 with average risk. The American Cancer Society's current recommendations are that women aged 40–44 years should have the choice to start annual breast cancer screening with mammograms if they wish to do so, and women aged 45–54 years should get mammograms every year and switch to every 2 years at the age of 55.

27. Answer: 1

Rationale: All areas are important to probe in the initial interview of a new patient. The history will help determine the necessary components of the physical exam and laboratory or radiologic studies that are ordered and the counseling that is done during the appointment.

28. Answer: 2, 3, 5

Rationale: The family nurse practitioner should identify specific methods to improve safe use of medications in the older adult by conducting a thorough assessment of the patient's cognitive and motor abilities and presence of polypharmacy. Although many analgesics can contribute to constipation, it is assessment of kidney function that is most important because the older adult is less able to eliminate drugs, owing to the glomerular filtration rate gradually declining by about 40% from ages 20–80 years. The golden rule in prescribing to the older adult is to start with the lowest dose possible and titrate the medication dose slowly on the basis of the renal and hepatic function of the patient. Determining sleeping patterns does not focus on promoting drug safety in the older adult.

29. Answer: 4

Rationale: The older adult is at greatest risk for altered immune function related to nutrition. The older adult often does not receive enough nutrition for a variety of reasons, including altered taste, eating alone, ability to prepare meals, and malabsorption. Adequate nutrition in the older adult has been shown to improve immune status and antibody response to influenza vaccine.

30. Answer: 3

Rationale: Because the patient is experiencing a decrease in food intake but still taking fluids, there is no immediate need to prescribe enteral nutritional support or switching of diet. Best practice would be to inspect the oral cavity to see if there is any structural or infectious process that is preventing ingestion of food. Reviewing the medication profile of the patient may be needed but would not be the priority assessment at this time.

31. Answer: 2

Rationale: Hypertension, smoking, and hyperlipidemia are the major risk factors in the development of cardiovascular disease. Controlling hyperglycemia, increasing high dietary fiber intake, and taking vitamin supplements assist in maintaining a healthy lifestyle, but they are not as important in preventing cardiovascular disease.

32. Answer: 3

Rationale: Support stockings improve blood return to the central circulation, improving cardiac output and cerebral perfusion. Dorsiflexion of the feet and leg movement help

improve cardiac output. Exercise should be postponed until later in the afternoon or evening, when blood pressure is higher. Waiting for 20 minutes or longer to stand from the table helps reduce orthostatic hypotension following meals.

33. Answer: 3

Rationale: If the infant has been satisfied up to this point (by sleeping for long intervals), the infant probably needs additional calories in the form of rice cereal. Adding increased amounts of formula can lead to iron-deficiency anemia.

34. Answer: 1

Rationale: This frequently used ratio is calculated as follows:

$$\frac{\text{No. of deaths} <1 \text{ year of age in a year}}{\text{No. of live births in the same year} \times 1000} = \text{Infant mortality rate}$$

35. Answer: 4

Rationale: It is essential that the immunization record be reviewed. The other options are important but not essential for a health maintenance visit.

36. Answer: 1, 3, 4

Rationale: To promote patient adherence in prescribing medications, the following are effective measures: prescribe the lowest dose and the smallest number of medications with the simplest dose regimens, providing simple verbal and written instructions for each medication and what it is for. The scheduling of medications that is best for the patient who is forgetful is a once-a-day dose and timing the doses to mealtimes to support the older adult in remembering to take the medication. If side effects occur, the patient should be told to call the family nurse practitioner. The patient should not be taught to reduce or alter the dose of the medication without guidance from the family nurse practitioner. Medications that are similar in size and color can be difficult for the older adult to discriminate because of reduced vision or being forgetful.

37. Answer: 2

Rationale: Car safety and use of a forward-facing car seat continue to be a priority for the 6-year-old child. Belt-positioning booster seats are used until the child is 4 feet, 9 inches tall and is between 8 and 12 years of age. Bottled drinking water is not necessary when traveling, unless it is outside of the United States. A fluoridated dentifrice should be used in a small amount (pea size), and children under age 6 should be supervised so that they do not swallow too much toothpaste, which would put them at risk for fluorosis. Three regular meals and two snacks are recommended for the busy 6-year-old child. Snacks should be rich in complex carbohydrates and low in fat, such as in yogurt; children should avoid candy, chips, and soft drinks.

38. Answer: 4

Rationale: Febrile seizures are benign and do not lead to brain damage. Most febrile illnesses in children result from a virus rather than bacteria and are associated with a high fever.

39. Answer: 1

Rationale: Human milk has more lipase and linoleic acid. Cow's milk is not as good of a nutritional source as human milk because cow's milk has more mineral content (calcium, phosphorus, sodium, potassium), which causes a larger renal solute load. In addition, cow's milk is high in protein, casein, and saturated fat, and is lower in carbohydrates than human milk.

40. Answer: 3

Rationale: At 1 year of age, infants may be fed whole cow's milk. The purpose for waiting is that it has been shown that cow's milk is low in iron, linoleic acid, and vitamin E and high in protein, sodium, and potassium.

41. Answer: 3

Rationale: The American Academy of Pediatrics does not recommend low-iron formulas but does recommend, if stools are hard, to treat for constipation. Typical treatment includes giving 1–2 tsp of dark corn syrup, including fruit juices (prune, pineapple, apricot), nonstarchy vegetables, and water, and avoiding rice cereal. Mineral oil is not recommended at this age.

42. Answer: 3

Rationale: Although 15 µg/dL is an elevated lead level (normal is <10 µg/dL), chelation therapy in children with a normal exam is not usually conducted until the lead level is >25 µg/dL. It is important at this level to identify the source of the elevation and to monitor the child frequently.

43. Answer: 3

Rationale: Solid food does not need to be introduced before 4–6 months of age. The first foods introduced are cereals. New foods are introduced one at a time at weekly intervals. In this way, the infant's digestive system can adapt to the food, and any reaction can be easily detected.

44. Answer: 1

Rationale: Primary prevention programs exist to prevent disease, malfunctioning, or maladaptation from occurring (for example, work to lower the incidence of birth defects). Examples of these types of programs include the promotion of a healthy diet, practice of safe sex, and avoidance of alcohol and tobacco. Secondary prevention is early diagnosis and treatment

(for example, screening for tuberculosis or sickle cell disease, breast and testicular self-examination). Tertiary prevention is the prevention of complications and rehabilitation after the disease or condition has occurred (for example, cardiac rehabilitation, complete blood count done before chemotherapy).

45. Answer: 2

Rationale: The 15- to 25-year-old group is most often affected by testicular cancer.

46. Answer: 1

Rationale: Familial short stature is not indicated in this case, because the father is of normal height. Hypopituitarism would be associated with other findings (micropenis, small testes, immature facies, and olfactory defects). Gonadotropin deficiency might be a possibility but considering all findings in the situation and based on the father having a pubertal onset at age 16 and achieving an average height, the more likely diagnosis is constitutional growth delay.

47. Answer: 3

Rationale: The reading level of most American adults is from grades 6–8; therefore the sixth-grade level would be the most appropriate answer among the choices given.

48. Answer: 4

Rationale: Recommendations of the Centers for Disease Control and Prevention for a serum lead level greater than 10 µg/dL are for rescreening and referral to a physician. Rescreening is done before the removal of the child/family from the hazard, although a thorough environmental assessment is essential at rescreening.

49. Answer: 1

Rationale: The water heater should not be set over 120°F to prevent scald burns. Crib rails should be no more than 2⅜ inches apart. The rear-facing infant seat is applicable to 20 lb of weight or 1 year of age. Sunscreen should be applied whenever there is sun exposure.

50. Answer: 4

Rationale: Azarcon and greta are traditional Hispanic remedies that contain lead, which can result in increased lead levels and eventual poisoning. The other substances will not cause the symptoms described. Arnica root is used as a topical preparation to reduce inflammation, muscle pain, and bruising. The Mexican yam root is used for menopausal symptoms and is a source of natural progesterone. White willow bark action is similar to aspirin and is used for the relief of pain.

51. Answer: 1, 2

Rationale: LGBTQ is a common acronym that typically refers to lesbian, gay, bisexual, transgender, and queer or questioning individuals. LGBTQ young adults have increased rates of smoking, drinking alcohol, and substance abuse compared with their heterosexual peers. In addition, they also have increased rates of eating disorders, anxiety, depression, and suicidal thoughts.

52. Answer: 1

Rationale: Maintaining normal weight, decreasing sodium in the diet, and exercising regularly are three modifications that are most effective in maintaining normal blood pressure in the older adult.

53. Answer: 1

Rationale: When reviewing an older patient's history in the clinical setting, it is important to assess whether the patient is current (up-to-date) with immunizations. Older patients are especially susceptible to seasonal flu, which may end up compromising their health. Past smoking history, even with a recorded PPD, is not a priority assessment if it has been 30 years since active smoking. The fact that a patient wears reading glasses does not require a priority action. Similarly, a history of osteoarthritis does not require a priority action, unless there are known deficits related to ambulation and/or increases in pain.

54. Answer: 4

Rationale: One-fourth of all women experience IPV. IPV can occur in any adult-gerontology primary care setting. Most abused women report that their partner was the first person to abuse them. Many batterers are successful professionals, including politicians, ministers, physicians, and lawyers.

55. Answer: 1, 2, 4, 5

Rationale: The use of social media and access to the Internet are very prominent and widespread among adolescents. This promotes opportunities for developing interpersonal skills and in some environments (rural areas, adolescents with rare health conditions or shyness) provides an avenue for the adolescent to interact with others like themselves. Many states have outlawed the use of handheld mobile devices while an adolescent is actively driving a car. Sexting is the sending of sexually explicit or suggestive pictures or messages online and has been linked to risky sexual behaviors. Adolescents actually do use the online social environment to interact with the same peers they spend their day with at school and in extracurricular activities. The online environment can create

opportunities for cyberbullying. Cyberbullying is the communication of insults, harassment, and publicly humiliating statements via social media, that is, emails, online chat rooms, or texting on cell phones.

56. Answer: 4

Rationale: Exercise and activity are essential for health promotion and maintenance in the older adult and to achieve an optimal level of functioning. About half of the physical deterioration of the older patient is caused by disuse rather than by the aging process or disease. One of the best exercises for an older adult is walking, progressing to 30-minute sessions, three to five times each week. Swimming and dancing are also beneficial.

57. Answer: 2, 4

Rationale: It is important to check for understanding of what is being said about the plan of care for all clients, not just Asian Americans. Consider that periods of silence by the client are indicative of reflection on what has been said. Avoiding physical closeness, limiting eye contact, avoiding hand gestures, and clarifying responses to questions are all components of the plan of care for an Asian American client.

58. Answer: 1

Rationale: Latino clients may use home remedies and consult folk healers known as curanderos or curanderas rather than traditional Western health care providers. Curanderos provide a holistic form of healing, which combines prayer, herbal remedies, rituals, psychic healing, spiritualism, and massage. Curanderos believe in the hot and cold theory of disease.

Immunizations

59. Answer: 3

Rationale: It is recommended that the child receive the IPV at 2 months, 4 months, the third dose between 6 and 18 months, and the fourth dose between 4 and 6 years of age.

60. Answer: 3

Rationale: The MMR is a live-virus vaccine. Children severely immunosuppressed because of cancer therapy should not receive live-virus vaccines for 3 months after chemotherapy has been stopped.

61. Answer: 1

Rationale: The law calls for the parental signature to be maintained in the clinical record.

62. Answer: 4

Rationale: GamaSTAN S/D is the only IM preparation for immune globulin (IG). IG is administered to persons aged >40 years; however, vaccine may be used if IG cannot be obtained. Postexposure prophylaxis with IG or hepatitis A (HepA) vaccine prevents infection with HAV when administered within 2 weeks of exposure. Twinrix provides immunization for both HAV and hepatitis B virus. Shingrix is an immunization for herpes zoster. IgM, which is found mainly in the blood and lymph fluid, is the first antibody to be made by the body to fight a new infection.

63. Answer: 2

Rationale: Persons planning to depart to an area with high or intermediate endemic HAV in less than 2 weeks should receive the initial dose of HAV vaccine, and also simultaneously be administered IG at a separate anatomic injection site (e.g., separate limbs). The IG will provide immediate protection and the HAV vaccine will provide lifelong immunity. Twinrix provides immunization for both HAV and hepatitis B virus and should be administered before travel.

64. Answer: 3

Rationale: Children over the age of 13 years who have not had chickenpox and have not been previously immunized are recommended to have two doses at least 28 days apart for effective immunity.

65. Answer: 2

Rationale: If given within 72 hours of exposure, the live attenuated measles vaccine will provide protection in most cases. The dose of IgG would be 0.25 mL/kg, given within 6 days of exposure.

66. Answer: 1

Rationale: Polyvalent pneumococcal vaccine is recommended for children with chronic diseases. It is not recommended for use to prevent OM and other pneumococcal diseases. It can be given concurrently with other vaccines, and it does not cause severe systemic reactions. It will occasionally cause mild local reactions.

67. Answer: 1

Rationale: The CDC recommends that adults ages 60 and over should receive immunizations for seasonal flu and herpes zoster. Yearly tetanus prophylaxis is not indicated, because the required time interval for a booster is every 10 years and/or in response to an injury. An adult who has had a previous allergic reaction to an immunization should be further evaluated to determine potential adverse reactions to specific components before any immunization schedule is started.

68. Answer: 2

Rationale: Hib makes infection less likely. Hib vaccine successfully decreases the possibility of epiglottitis. A wide variety of viruses, bacteria, and even fungi can cause epiglottitis. There are no vaccines for Epstein-Barr virus, coxsackievirus, or *S. pyogenes*.

69. Answer: 2

Rationale: Influenza outbreaks may affect 60% of those in long-term care, and mortality rates are high. All the other groups listed are appropriate for the influenza vaccine but are not as high a priority. Poliomyelitis is not a contraindication.

70. Answer: 3

Rationale: Prior anaphylaxis and severe hypersensitivity would be considered a contraindication; a mild viral illness would not. The patient who is pregnant or lactating may be immunized.

71. Answer: 1, 4, 5

Rationale The primary transmission is fecal-oral; blood-borne transmission is rare. Men having sex with men is a risk factor. The incubation period is 2–6 weeks (mean 4 weeks). Infection occurs primarily after consuming food or water contaminated with HAV or via direct contact with a person with HAV infection with poor hygiene. The Advisory Committee on Immunization Practices recommends that one dose of single-antigen HAV vaccine administered within 2 weeks before travel departure may provide adequate protection for most healthy persons, along with passive immunization with immune globulin. The first dose should be followed by the second immunization within 6–12 months, if using Havrix. In this patient situation, prevaccine exposure to HAV was present.

72. Answer: 1

Rationale: ACIP continues to recommend that all adults aged ≥65 years receive 1 dose of PPSV23. A single dose of PPSV23 is recommended for routine use among all adults aged ≥65 years. Annual influenza immunizations are recommended for those who are age 65 years and older. Shingles vaccination is recommended as a 2-dose series (2-6 months apart). Tdap for all adults aged 65 years and older is recommended for those who never received a Tdap as an adult, because then they would just get a Td booster every 10 years as this is recommended at all ages >19 years. Boostrix should be used for adults aged 65 years and older; however, the ACIP concluded that either vaccine (Adacel or Boostrix) administered to a person 65 years or older is immunogenic and provides protection. Shingles vaccine is contraindicated in women who are pregnant and in individuals who have a weakened immune system.

73. Answer: 1

Rationale: Attenuated live-virus vaccines are available for the following communicable diseases: measles, mumps, rubella, poliomyelitis, yellow fever, and smallpox. Rabies vaccine is a killed virus, and hepatitis B is a purified viral antigen obtained from the blood of an infected patient, and then inactivated when manufactured into a vaccination.

74. Answer: 4

Rationale: Children who have a severe allergy to neomycin are at increased risk for the development of an allergic reaction to the measles vaccine.

75. Answer: 1

Rationale: Hepatitis B first dose should be given at birth. By 8 months of age, all three doses of the hepatitis B series should have been given. RV should be given at 2, 4, and 6 months. IPV should be given at 2 and 4 months, and the third dose anytime from 6–18 months. MMR first dose is given at 12 months and again at 4–6 years of age. Tetanus toxoid, diphtheria toxoid, and Tdap are given to children who are age 11 years and older; however, if children who are age 7 years and older are not fully immunized with the DTaP vaccine, they should receive the Tdap vaccine as one dose (preferably the first) in the catch-up series.

76. Answer: 3

Rationale: A hepatitis B series may be recommended for adults who are 65 years of age and older on the basis of clinical risk assessment, i.e., having chronic liver disease, HIV infection, incarcerated persons, travel in high risk countries, IV drug use, sexual exposure risk. MMR vaccination would not be required or recommended for this age group. Chickenpox (varicella-zoster virus) and pneumococcal immunization would be recommended for this age group.

77. Answer: 2

Rationale: The live vaccine can produce serious disseminated disease in patients with immunocompromised status (for example, leukemia, lymphoma, HIV/AIDS) and in those undergoing cancer chemotherapy. Mild acute illness, concurrent antimicrobial therapy, and a history of nonspecific allergies are not contraindications for use of a live vaccine.

78. Answer: 1

Rationale: People 60 years of age or older should get a shingles vaccine (Zostavax). They should get the vaccine regardless of whether they recall having had chickenpox. There is no maximum age for getting a shingles vaccine. Twinrix is a combined hepatitis A and hepatitis B virus vaccine that can be given to adults. There is no reason to order a varicella titer.

79. Answer: 2

Rationale: All adults (not just the ones who enjoy gardening and outdoor activities) should have a Tdap/Td booster once, as recommended by the Advisory Committee of Immunization Practice. As part of standard wound management care to prevent tetanus, a tetanus toxoid–containing vaccine might be recommended for wound management in adults aged 19 years and older if 5 years or more have elapsed since last receiving a Td vaccine. If a tetanus booster is indicated, Tdap is preferred over Td for wound management in adults aged 19 years and older who have not received Tdap previously. A pneumococcal vaccine is recommended for adults aged 65 or older and for those with a chronic illness or in an immunosuppressed state. Most older adults had chickenpox as a child and do not require the vaccine.

80. Answer: 1

Rationale: The pneumococcal polysaccharide vaccine Pneumovax 23 (PPSV23) is recommended in patients without risk factors starting at age 65. PPSV23 vaccination is indicated only for those ages 2–64 if additional risk factors or comorbidities are present, including smoking, immunosuppression, or serious disease.

81. Answer: 2

Rationale: Td is usually given as a booster dose every 10 years but it can also be given earlier after a severe and dirty wound or burn. For adults aged 19 through 64 years who previously have not received a dose of Tdap, a single dose of Tdap should replace a single decennial (occurring every 10 years) Td booster dose. Persons aged 65 years and older (e.g., grandparents, child-care providers, and health care practitioners) who have or who anticipate having close contact with an infant aged less than 12 months and who previously have not received Tdap should receive a single dose of Tdap to protect against pertussis and reduce the likelihood of transmission. For other adults aged 65 years and older, a single dose of Tdap vaccine may be administered instead of Td vaccine in persons who previously have not received Tdap. Boostrix should be used for adults aged 65 years and older; however, the ACIP concluded that either vaccine (Boostrix or Adacel) administered to a person aged 65 years or older is immunogenic and would provide protection.

82. Answer: 1

Rationale: PCV13 vaccination is no longer routinely recommended for all adults aged ≥65 years. ACIP continues to recommend that all adults aged ≥65 years receive 1 dose of PPSV23. A single dose of PPSV23 is recommended for routine use among all adults aged ≥65 years.

83. Answer: 1

Rationale: Tetanus toxoid is a bacterial toxin that has been changed to nontoxic form and produces persistent antitoxin antibody titers because the patient's immune system is stimulated to manufacture antitoxins (that is, antibodies directed against the bacterial toxin). *C. diphtheriae* is the organism that causes diphtheria, not tetanus. DTaP and DT are for use in children under age 7 years and should *not* be used in adults. DT does not contain pertussis and is given as a substitute for children who cannot tolerate the DTaP vaccine, which contains pertussis. The recommended dose of tetanus toxoid alone for an adult is 0.5 mL IM. To help you remember, look closely at the letters and keep the following in mind:

- Upper case "T" means there is about the same amount of tetanus in DTaP, Tdap, and Td. (DTaP is given to children, usually infants, under age 7.)
- Upper case "D" and "P" mean there is more diphtheria and pertussis in DTaP than in Tdap and Td; lower case letters ("d" and "p") mean there is less. (Tdap is a booster given at age 11 years and throughout life, usually every 10 years, and is recommended as a booster after age 65.)

84. Answer: 4

Rationale: A percentage of young adults (5%–20%) are susceptible to measles and/or rubella. Influenza and hepatitis B vaccinations are recommended for young adults who have exposure to a large number of people. Tetanus is recommended every 10 years, especially in high-risk situations (young adults who participate in outdoor sports). Pneumovax 23 (PPSV23) is indicated in a young adult who has a chronic disease (for example, diabetes, chronic pulmonary disease, chronic cardiovascular disease) and is also indicated for young adults who are immunocompromised.

85. Answer: 4

Rationale: The most common cause of fever at the 2-month immunization series is the pertussis. This vaccine causes reactions in about 75% of infants. The MMR vaccine is not given until 12–15 months of age.

86. Answer: 1

Rationale: Pregnancy prevention is the primary prevention for NAS. Universal screening and referrals to treatment are recommended, but they do not prevent NAS. There will be times when women of child-bearing age must be prescribed opioids. Although consulting the drug-monitoring program does help decrease doctor shopping, it does not prevent NAS.

87. Answer: 3

Rationale: According to the Centers for Disease Control and Prevention, one of three patients develops a mild fever and localized pain at the injection site. There is no indication that this patient requires hospitalization at this time. The fever is likely related to the vaccination. There is no contraindication about receiving this vaccine with an allergy to egg.

88. Answer: 2, 4

Rationale: The smallpox vaccination has the following common side effects: itching, swollen lymph nodes, sore arm resulting from the injection, fever, headache, body ache, mild rash, and fatigue. The injection site lesion starts as a red and itchy bump forming at the vaccination site within 2–5 days, then in the next few days, the bump becomes a blister and fills with pus. During the second week, the blister dries up, and a scab forms. The fluid from the lesion and the crust are contagious until a scab forms. The scab falls off after 2–4 weeks, leaving a scar. Serious side effects include heart problems (myocarditis and pericarditis), severe allergic reaction, swelling of the brain or spinal cord, and severe skin diseases.

89. Answer: 3

Rationale: The Centers for Disease Control and Prevention has identified that asthma is one of the leading causes of school absenteeism.

90. Answer: 2

Rationale: All boys and girls ages 11 or 12 years should get vaccinated. Catch-up vaccines are recommended for males through age 21 and for females through age 26. It is recommended for men and women with compromised immune systems (including those living with HIV infection) through age 26 years if they were not fully vaccinated when they were younger. The vaccine is also recommended for gay and bisexual men (or for any man who has sex with a man) through age 26 years. ACIP does not recommend the vaccine for patients >26 years of age but rather promotes shared decision making.

91. Answer: 4

Rationale: A person should not receive Shingrix if they have ever had a severe allergic reaction to any component of the vaccine or after a dose of Shingrix, tested negative for immunity to varicella zoster virus, currently have shingles, or currently are pregnant or breast-feeding. Women who are pregnant or breast-feeding should wait to get Shingrix. Healthy adults 50 years and older should get two doses of Shingrix, separated by 2–6 months. Patients should get Shingrix even if they already have had shingles, received Zostavax, or are not sure if they had chickenpox. There is no maximum age for getting Shingrix. If a patient had Zostavax (the other shingles vaccine) recently, then the patient should wait at least 8 weeks before getting Shingrix.

92. Answer: 1, 2, 3, 4

Rationale: The risk of the rabies vaccine causing serious harm or death is extremely small. Serious problems arising from the rabies vaccine are very rare, according to the Centers for Disease Control and Prevention. The family nurse practitioner recognizes the following as a mild problem after immunization: soreness, redness, swelling, or itching where the shot was given; headache; nausea; abdominal pain; muscle aches; and dizziness. Moderate problems after vaccination include hives, pain in the joints, and fever. Diplopia, confusion, and severe allergic reactions are not typical side effects or reactions.

93. Answer: 3, 5

Rationale: It is not necessary to test for HAV immunity before vaccinating. HAV vaccine is recommended for pregnant women with additional medical conditions or other indications for receiving the HAV vaccine. The vaccination schedule is two doses given 6 months apart, which is the minimum interval between the first and second doses. The antibody test for total anti-HAV measures both immunoglobin G (IgG) anti-HAV and immunoglobulin M (IgM) anti-HAV. The presence of IgM anti-HAV is found in the blood during an acute hepatitis A infection. Persons who are total anti-HAV positive and IgM anti-HAV negative have serologic markers indicating immunity consistent with either past infection or vaccination. IgG anti-HAV appears in the convalescent phase of HAV infection, remains present in serum for the lifetime of the person, and confers lifelong protection against disease. ACIP recommends that all children in the United States receive the hepatitis A vaccine at 1 year of age (i.e., 12–23 months) to avoid interference by passive maternal anti-HAV that may be present during the first year of life.

94. Answer: 4

Rationale: It would be important to start the hepatitis B series, considering his age, because this was not included as part of his childhood vaccination series. Hepatitis A is also recommended, especially if the person travels to foreign countries, along with varicella because these immunizations were not available during his childhood. An MMR immunization is required for adults born in 1957 or later who have no laboratory proof of immunity or documentation of either previous vaccination or a physician-documented case of measles. Tetanus vaccination is recommended every 10 years, especially in high-risk situations (adults who participate in outdoor sports). Pneumovax 23 (PPSV23) is indicated for an adult who has a chronic disease, such as diabetes, chronic pulmonary disease, or chronic cardiovascular disease, and it is also indicated for adults who are immunocompromised. If the adult did not receive the OPV series as a child, it is recommended to vaccinate the adult with injectable enhanced-potency inactivated poliovirus vaccine because the risk of vaccine-associated poliomyelitis is lower.

4

Cardiovascular

Physical Exam & Diagnostic Tests

1. The family nurse practitioner is taking a history and performing a physical examination on a female patient who is complaining of chest pain. Which of the following findings would increase suspicion for determination of an acute cardiac event?
   1. Patient denies drug use.
   2. Presence of adventitious lung sounds.
   3. Absent T waves on electrocardiogram.
   4. Absence of jaw pain.

2. The family nurse practitioner is providing instructions to a patient who is scheduled for a transthoracic echocardiogram (TTE). Which instructions should be included in the teaching session?
   1. Do not eat or drink for at least 12 hours before testing.
   2. Do not take any medication before the test, unless it is considered to be a cardiac medication.
   3. Take all regularly scheduled medications before testing.
   4. Increase fluids before testing.

3. The family nurse practitioner is performing a physical examination on a healthy adult male. On auscultation, the stethoscope would be placed in which areas to best hear the characteristic heart sounds S_1 and S_2?
   1. S_1 is best heard at the apex and S_2 at the base of the heart.
   2. Both are heard equally well at the right midclavicular line.
   3. On the left side, S_1 is at the area of the pulmonic valve and S_2 at the aortic valve.
   4. Both sounds are best heard at Erb point.

4. On the basis of a general assessment of an adult patient, the family nurse practitioner determines the presence of the apical impulse at the point of maximal impulse (PMI) on the patient's chest wall. Where on the chest wall is the PMI normally found?
   1. Second intercostal space at the midclavicular line on the left side.
   2. Right lower sternal border, fifth intercostal space.
   3. Left side at the fifth intercostal space on the midclavicular line.
   4. Left fifth intercostal space, lateral to the midclavicular line.

5. The family nurse practitioner is auscultating the carotid arteries for bruits. What is the correct procedure?
   1. Use the diaphragm of the stethoscope.
   2. Use the bell of the stethoscope.
   3. Place the stethoscope 1 inch off the area above the sternocleidomastoid muscle.
   4. Position the patient at a 30-degree angle and press firmly, using the bell of the stethoscope.

6. When inspecting the precordium, the family nurse practitioner's primary purpose in doing this inspection is to examine for:
   1. Scars and anatomic landmarks.
   2. Pulsations and retractions.
   3. Heaves and cardiac dullness.
   4. Pericardial friction rub and lifts.

7. While examining a patient in a left lateral position, the family nurse practitioner auscultates a third heart sound (S_3). From this examination, what does the family nurse practitioner know?
   1. This sound is considered normal in children and young adults.
   2. This rarely is associated with myocardial failure in the older adult.
   3. This patient should be immediately referred to a cardiologist for evaluation.
   4. This is considered a normal splitting of the S_2 during inspiration.

8. The family nurse practitioner knows that the correct auscultatory site for the aortic area is the:
   1. Midclavicular line, fifth interspace, left side.
   2. Left fourth interspace close to the sternum.
   3. Right second interspace close to the sternum.
   4. Midclavicular line, second interspace, left side.

9. The family nurse practitioner should include which statement in patient teaching when ordering a lipid profile on a patient? Eat a typical diet over the next week and:
   1. Eat a normal breakfast the morning of the lipid profile blood draw.
   2. Fast for 8–12 hours as directed before the lipid profile is drawn.
   3. There are no restrictions on alcohol consumption for this blood test.
   4. Take any current medications with a few sips of water before the blood test.

10. When auscultating the heart sounds of a 72-year-old patient with a history of hypertension (HTN), the family nurse practitioner notes an S_4 on auscultation. What does this finding indicate?
    1. Normal variant in people ages 65 years and older.
    2. Beginning of ventricular failure.
    3. Decreased resistance to ventricular filling.
    4. Severely failing heart.

11. Which of the following is an appropriate blood pressure (BP) goal for a 65-year-old male with no comorbidities?
    1. Systolic blood pressure (SBP) <150 mm Hg/diastolic blood pressure (DBP) <90 mm Hg.
    2. SBP <140 mm Hg/DBP <90 mm Hg.
    3. SBP <140 mm Hg/DBP <80 mm Hg.
    4. SBP <150 mm Hg/DBP <90 mm Hg.

12. The family nurse practitioner is examining a patient with a history of rheumatic fever who is being followed for the development of carditis. During cardiac auscultation, where on the chest wall is the stethoscope placed to determine the most common murmur associated with this condition?
    1. At the left sternal border, fourth left intercostal space.
    2. Fifth intercostal space, left side, at the midclavicular line.
    3. Second or third intercostal space at the left of the sternal border.
    4. Second intercostal space on the right of the sternal border.

13. A patient presents with unusual coolness in the left hand compared with the right hand. What is the next step in the exam?
    1. Palpate the radial pulse on both hands for a full minute.
    2. Perform the Allen test on both hands.
    3. Feel the forearms with the backs of the fingers.
    4. Hold the hand in a dependent position and then reexamine.

14. The first (S_1) and second heart sounds (S_2) are identified when the family nurse practitioner auscultates for cardiac sounds. What is the physiology responsible for the production of these heart sounds?
    1. Closure of atrioventricular (AV) valves produces S_1; closure of semilunar valves forms S_2.
    2. Closure of the aortic valve produces S_2; opening of the mitral valve produces S_1.
    3. Opening of AV valves produces S_1; closure of semilunar valves produces S_2.
    4. Opening of the tricuspid valve produces S_1; closure of the pulmonic valve forms S_2.

15. The family nurse practitioner is assessing a cardiac patient who is experiencing an atrial dysrhythmia. The patient's pulse rate is irregular at 110 beats/min, and there is concern regarding a pulse deficit. How is a pulse deficit determined in this patient?
    1. A 12-lead electrocardiogram is necessary to determine the presence and length of the PR intervals.
    2. The apical pulse is counted, and then the radial pulse is counted; the pulse deficit is determined by the difference between the two rates.
    3. The apical pulse is counted, and an increase or decrease is correlated with the phases of the respiratory cycle.
    4. The apical pulse and radial pulse are determined simultaneously; a pulse deficit is established if the apical rate is higher than the radial rate.

16. The family nurse practitioner notes a grade V systolic murmur while examining a patient's precordium. Which characteristics describe this type of murmur?
    1. Barely audible; faintly heard with the bell of the stethoscope.
    2. Heard only with the diaphragm of the stethoscope.
    3. Heard with the stethoscope partly off the chest.
    4. Heard without the aid of the stethoscope.

17. What are the normal physiologic changes in the geriatric population that affect conductivity and contractility of the myocardium?
    1. Increased automaticity and excitability.
    2. Increased contractility and conductivity.
    3. Decreased excitability and conductivity.
    4. Decreased automaticity and contractility.

18. When assessing the temperature of an extremity as part of a patient's peripheral vascular assessment, which part of the hand is the most sensitive for assessing temperature?
    1. Palm.
    2. Fingertips.
    3. Back of the wrist.
    4. Back of the fingers.

19. A 45-year-old male patient's lipid profile results are sent to the family nurse practitioner with the following levels: total cholesterol, 287 mmol/L; high-density lipoprotein, 30 mg/dL; and low-density lipoprotein, 165 mg/dL. On the basis of interpretation of these findings, the family nurse practitioner should do which of the following?
    1. Initiate treatment with low-dose statins.
    2. Discuss adherence to a heart-healthy diet and regular aerobic physical activity.
    3. Assess the 10-year arteriosclerotic cardiovascular disease (ASCVD) risk.
    4. Refer to cardiologist.

20. A patient returns to the clinic 3 weeks after myocardial infarction (post-MI) complaining of pericardial pain and elevated temperature. A physical exam reveals a pericardial friction rub. What diagnostic studies are indicated?
    1. 24-hour Holter monitoring.
    2. Echocardiogram.
    3. Complete blood count with differential.
    4. Cardiac enzymes with myoglobin.

21. On assessment of an older adult patient, the family nurse practitioner notes bilateral pulsations and distention of the jugular veins when the patient's head is elevated 45 degrees. What further assessment needs to be done at this time?
    1. Estimate the level of venous pressure by measuring from the sternal angle to the highest level of venous pulsations.
    2. Place the patient in a supine position and determine the effect of position change on distention and pulsations of the jugular vein.
    3. Measure carotid pulses because of the increased left ventricular pressure.
    4. Have the patient hold his or her breath to facilitate evaluation for the presence of carotid bruits.

22. The family nurse practitioner is examining a woman with a known history of mitral valve disease. What type of murmur heard on auscultation supports a history of mitral valve stenosis?
    1. Diastolic murmur, heard loudest at the apex with the patient on her left side.
    2. Midsystolic ejection murmur, heard loudest over the left lower sternal border.
    3. Holosystolic murmur, heard loudest over the apex and left axillary area.
    4. Diastolic murmur, heard loudest with the patient in a sitting position, leaning forward.

23. The family nurse practitioner is doing an assessment of a patient who is 2 weeks post-myocardial infarction (MI) affecting the left ventricle. The family nurse practitioner would pay particular attention to what area of the physical assessment?
    1. Lower extremities and the jugular vein.
    2. Area on the chest where the point of maximal impulse is heard.
    3. Presence of dyspnea and auscultation of crackles in the lungs.
    4. Level of dependent edema and fluid intake over the last 24 hours.

24. Which symptoms would indicate to the family nurse practitioner that the patient is experiencing intermittent claudication?
    1. Petechiae and itching of the lower part of the leg.
    2. Extensive discoloration and edema of the upper leg.
    3. Profuse rash and discoloration from the trunk down to the feet.
    4. Complaints of pain on walking, relieved by sitting down.

25. Stress testing, or the exercise tolerance test, without imaging is the most widely used diagnostic test for evaluation of ischemic heart disease. It is most accurate in what patient population?
    1. Males under age 40 with atypical angina pectoris.
    2. Asymptomatic premenopausal females without risk factors.
    3. Males over age 50 with typical angina pectoris.
    4. Males receiving digitalis with typical angina pectoris.

26. When palpating for the apical impulse of a 46-year-old female, the family nurse practitioner feels a hyperkinetic impulse. The nurse would auscultate for which additional finding?
    1. Pericardial friction rub.
    2. Pansystolic murmur.
    3. Pulsus paradoxus.
    4. Decreased intensity of heart sounds.

27. Which three predictor variables are included in the Thrombolysis in Myocardial Infarction (TIMI) risk score?
    1. Lipid profile.
    2. Aspirin use.
    3. Creatine kinase MB (CK-MB) level.
    4. ST segment elevation ≥ 0.5.
    5. Warfarin use.

28. While assessing a patient with a history of recent myocardial infarction, the family nurse practitioner notes pulsus alternans. The nurse would assess for other assessment changes most likely caused by:
    1. Unstable angina.
    2. Cardiogenic shock.
    3. Recurrent myocardial infarction.
    4. Left-sided heart failure (HF).

Disorders

29. A 70-year-old woman comes to the clinic with a complaint of severe aching of her legs after standing for 10 minutes. What other assessment finding of the lower extremities would support the family nurse practitioner's tentative diagnosis of chronic venous insufficiency?
    1. Pitting edema of 3+ and cyanosis on dependency.
    2. Shiny skin and dusky red appearance on dependency.
    3. Minimal hair and pallor on elevation.
    4. Pulses 1+ and ulceration involving the toes.

30. On what basis should the diagnosis of hypertension (HTN) be established?
    1. An average of two or more readings taken during at least two separate clinic visits.
    2. At least five readings 1 month apart.
    3. One reading of 140 mm Hg systolic blood pressure (SBP) and 90 mm Hg diastolic blood pressure (DBP) or higher.
    4. One reading taken in three different positions.

31. A patient has a 2-year history of hypertensive heart disease. What major pathophysiologic changes should the family nurse practitioner expect?
    1. Right ventricular hypertrophy.
    2. Left atrial dilation.
    3. Left ventricular hypertrophy.
    4. Right atrial dilation.

32. A 60-year-old female presents to the clinic for ongoing management of hypertension (HTN). Which physical finding, if noted by the family nurse practitioner, would warrant further inquiry?
    1. 20/20 vision screening.
    2. Presence of nosebleeds.
    3. Brisk capillary refill bilaterally.
    4. Occasional nonproductive cough in response to self-identified seasonal allergies.

33. Which clinical manifestation of a myocardial infarction (MI) is frequently not present in the older adult cardiac patient?
    1. Prolonged, severe chest pain.
    2. Diaphoresis, pallor, and syncope.
    3. Dyspnea and increasing anxiety.
    4. Gastrointestinal distress and orthopnea.

34. The family nurse practitioner is performing an assessment on a patient who is having difficulty controlling his left-sided heart failure (HF). The family nurse practitioner understands that the primary symptoms associated with this type of HF are:
    1. Systemic venous congestion.
    2. Dyspnea and pulmonary congestion.
    3. Increased peripheral edema and anorexia.
    4. Atrial fibrillation with a heart rate around 110 beats/min.

35. The family nurse practitioner is concerned that a post-myocardial infarction patient is developing a problem of constrictive pericarditis. What is a characteristic finding with constrictive pericarditis, and how is it evaluated?
    1. Cardiac tamponade, identified by muffled heart sounds and a paradoxical pulse.
    2. Pericardial triphasic friction rub, best heard at the apical area of the heart.

    3. Mitral valve prolapse, characterized by late systolic murmur at apex and left sternal borders.
    4. Altered waves on jugular venous pulse, as determined with a light directed tangentially to illuminate the shadows of the pulsations.

36. An older adult patient has a diagnosis of left-sided heart failure (HF). The family nurse practitioner would identify what common condition associated with HF?
    1. Peripheral vascular disease.
    2. Untreated hypertension (HTN).
    3. Ventricular dysrhythmias.
    4. Chronic obstructive pulmonary disease.

37. In evaluating the effectiveness of cardiopulmonary resuscitation (CPR) on the adult patient, what would the family nurse practitioner note?
    1. Dilated pupils.
    2. Palpable carotid pulse.
    3. Capillary refill.
    4. Pink and warm skin.

38. The family nurse practitioner is conducting a follow-up examination on a patient with coronary artery disease and a history of pericarditis. What is a characteristic physical finding in pericarditis, and how is it evaluated?
    1. Paradoxical pulse, identified by evaluating the changes in the amplitude of arterial pulse pressure associated with the respiratory cycle.
    2. Pulse deficit, as determined by counting the radial pulse and apical pulse at the same time and evaluating the difference.
    3. Pericardial friction rub, best heard using the diaphragm of the stethoscope and loudest to the left of the sternum at the fourth or fifth intercostal space.
    4. An S_4 is present, usually heard at the apex with the bell of the stethoscope and the patient in a left lateral position.

39. What are the symptoms of myocardial infarction (MI) usually experienced by the older adult patient?
    1. Dyspnea and diaphoresis.
    2. Back pain and muscle cramping.
    3. Numbness and tingling of the left arm.
    4. Epigastric pain and nausea.

40. What are the cardiovascular risk factors predisposing females to cardiovascular disease (CVD)?
    1. Absence of estrogen adversely affects lipoprotein metabolism.
    2. Fat deposited on the hips mobilizes, raising serum cholesterol.
    3. Coronary arteries are longer and wider in diameter.
    4. Resting ejection fraction is lower.

41. The family nurse practitioner is planning the treatment of an older adult patient newly diagnosed with hypertension (HTN). What parameters are most important in determining the appropriate pharmacologic therapy?
    1. Determine medications and dosage on the basis of the patient's weight, age, and drug availability.
    2. Begin treatment using diuretics.
    3. Initiate lifestyle changes before beginning medications.
    4. Determine other medical conditions for which the patient is being treated.

42. Which statement accurately describes coronary artery disease (CAD) in geriatric patients?
    1. Cardiovascular disease (CVD) is increased in the female patient receiving estrogen replacement therapy.
    2. A major risk factor for CVD in females and males is chronic hypertension.
    3. The majority of geriatric patients with CAD also have type 2 diabetes.
    4. Males over 60 years old continue to experience the highest level of CAD.

43. A patient with a history of chronic obstructive pulmonary disease comes to the clinic for his annual checkup with complaints of increasing difficulty breathing. Assessment findings include S_3 gallop; early systolic ejection click; and increased P-wave amplitude in leads II, III, and aVF of the electrocardiogram. The family nurse practitioner would expect to observe which change on the chest x-ray film?
    1. Hypertrophy of the left ventricle (LV).
    2. Hypertrophy of the right ventricle (RV).
    3. Hypertrophy of the left atrium and LV.
    4. Hypertrophy of the right atrium and RV.

44. When cardiac output falls in heart failure, the body attempts to compensate. What electrolyte imbalances result from this response?
    1. Hypernatremia and hyperkalemia.
    2. Hyponatremia and hypokalemia.
    3. Hypophosphatemia and hypercalcemia.
    4. Hyperphosphatemia and hypocalcemia.

45. When assessing the carotid pulse of a 72-year-old patient at a community-based clinic, the family nurse practitioner notes a bounding pulse with rapid rise and sudden collapse. The family nurse practitioner would include which additional assessment to support this finding?
    1. Auscultation for a diastolic murmur.
    2. Auscultation for paradoxical pulse.
    3. Blood pressure (BP) in both arms while lying, sitting, and standing.
    4. BP for an auscultatory gap.

46. The family nurse practitioner understands that the pain experienced with angina pectoris or myocardial infarction is caused by irritation of the myocardial nerve fibers by the increase in:
    1. Blood glucose.
    2. Lactic acid.
    3. Serum potassium.
    4. Serum magnesium.

47. New York Heart Association Functional Class III for patients with cardiac disease is characterized by:
    1. Symptoms present at rest, with any activity leading to increased discomfort.
    2. Slight limitation in ordinary activity, resulting in fatigue, palpitations, dyspnea, or angina.
    3. No physical limitation in activity.
    4. Marked limitation in activity, comfortable at rest, but ordinary activity leads to symptoms.

48. During the history and physical examination of a patient with suspected early heart failure (HF), which is the most prominent finding?
    1. Moist crackles in the lung bases bilaterally.
    2. Anorexia with weight loss of 3 lb in 1 week.
    3. Increased urine output and peripheral edema.
    4. Facial edema and distended neck veins.

49. What diagnosis is indicated with chest pain that is sudden and severe, described as "tearing," and accompanied by a decrease in peripheral pulses?
    1. Angina.
    2. Acute myocardial infarction (AMI).
    3. Aortic dissection.
    4. Pericarditis.

50. Which of the following would be appropriate dietary therapy recommendations for a patient with hyperlipidemia?
    1. Limiting intake of salt, sweets, and sugar-sweetened beverages.
    2. Increasing the average daily protein intake to 70 g/day.
    3. Decreasing total fat to <37% of the daily total calories per day.
    4. Limiting carbohydrate intake.

51. What is the most frequent life-threatening dysrhythmia experienced by a patient with acute myocardial infarction (AMI)?
    1. Atrial fibrillation.
    2. Ventricular tachycardia.
    3. Third-degree heart block.
    4. Ventricular fibrillation.

52. What is the first step in treatment for an overweight, older adult female patient with an elevated cholesterol level and abnormal lipoprotein profile?
    1. Prescribing a bile acid sequestrant agent.
    2. Initiation of a diet and exercise program.
    3. Prescribe statin therapy.
    4. Referral to a cardiologist.

53. Patients with chronic atrial fibrillation (AF) are at risk for which condition?
    1. Sudden cardiac death.
    2. Stroke.
    3. Ventricular tachycardia.
    4. Acute myocardial infarction.

54. The family nurse practitioner understands that the most common symptom of heart failure (HF) in adults is:
    1. Anorexia.
    2. Dependent edema.
    3. Dyspnea.
    4. Weight gain.

55. Which foods high in saturated fat does the family nurse practitioner teach the cardiac patient to avoid?
    1. Nuts, legumes, and seeds.
    2. Fish, shellfish, and mussels.
    3. Palm oil, coconut oil, and butter.
    4. Peanut oil, soybean oil, and olive oil.

56. An older adult male patient is complaining of chest pain. Which of the following is a parameter to assist the family nurse practitioner to differentiate the chest pain of angina from that of a myocardial infarction (MI)?
    1. Myocardial pain with an infarction is more severe.
    2. Anginal pain is more substernal and does not radiate to other areas.
    3. Anginal pain is frequently relieved by nitroglycerin.
    4. Pain from an infarction is always associated with other symptoms.

57. Which would **not** be considered as contributing to the development of thrombophlebitis?
    1. Excessive use of oral anticoagulants.
    2. Trauma to the leg or arm.
    3. Recent intravenous therapy.
    4. Secondary to pregnancy.

58. An older adult patient is being evaluated for a complaint of dizziness. What symptom/observation will make the family nurse practitioner consider that this is a life-threatening event?
    1. The dizziness occurs in certain positions.
    2. It is accompanied by tinnitus.
    3. The symptoms worsen when standing.
    4. It is preceded by rapid breathing.

59. A 28-year-old male presents to the family nurse practitioner with a history of chest pain that has been increasing over the past several days. The patient states that the pain worsens on lying down and denies any shortness of breath, cough, or radiation of the pain. The patient gives a history of a recent infection with coxsackievirus. An examination shows that the patient has a cardiac friction rub. What is one probable diagnosis the family nurse practitioner would consider?
    1. Acute myocardial infarction (AMI).
    2. Pleural effusion.
    3. Pericarditis.
    4. Esophageal reflux.

60. The family nurse practitioner would most likely suspect which differential diagnosis for an older adult patient presenting with atrial fibrillation (AF) and functional decline along with memory loss?
    1. Hyperthyroidism.
    2. Hypothyroidism.
    3. Sick sinus syndrome.
    4. Heart failure.

61. Which assessment made by the family nurse practitioner for an older patient would be a deviation from the normal changes of aging?
    1. Decreased exercise tolerance.
    2. Grade II/VI systolic ejection murmur.
    3. Prolongation of PR intervals on an electrocardiogram (ECG).
    4. Jugular venous pressure (JVP) of 14 cm H_2O.

62. Cardiac auscultation of an older patient reveals a grade II/VI murmur that is heard best at the right second intercostal space. The murmur is louder with squatting. There is a small carotid pulse with a delayed upstroke. The patient's history is benign, and his activity tolerance is within normal limits for his age. The family nurse practitioner would interpret this murmur to be indicative of:
    1. Aortic regurgitation.
    2. Aortic stenosis.
    3. Mitral valve prolapse.
    4. Mitral valve regurgitation.

63. What is the most frequently diagnosed valvular heart problem in older adult patients?
    1. Aortic stenosis.
    2. Mitral valve stenosis.
    3. Mitral valve regurgitation.
    4. Aortic regurgitation.

64. A patient has a history of heart failure (HF) and is currently taking an angiotensin-converting enzyme inhibitor combined with a beta blocker. Lifestyle modifications have been encouraged with some success. The patient has lost weight and stopped smoking. Which of the following are accurate statements about exercise therapy in patients with heart failure?
    1. Aerobic exercise should be avoided.
    2. Current recommendations are for 20 minutes of exercise three times a week.
    3. Use the talk test to gauge exercise intensity.
    4. Exercise is contraindicated, because it will worsen the heart failure.

65. A middle-aged man with no known risk factors for coronary artery disease presents with a total cholesterol level of 255 mg/dL. The family nurse practitioner would:
    1. Start him on a 3-hydroxy-3-methylglutaryl-coenzyme A reductase inhibitor.
    2. Start him on lifestyle changes and reevaluate the total cholesterol in 8–12 weeks.
    3. Repeat the total cholesterol and obtain high-density lipoprotein (HDL) and calculated low-density lipoprotein (LDL) levels.
    4. Do nothing because this patient demonstrates no coronary risk factors other than male sex.

Pharmacology

66. The family nurse practitioner is evaluating a patient in the office who is complaining of chest pain. The patient's blood pressure is 86/52 mm Hg, and electrocardiogram results reveal ischemia. The patient is to be transferred to the emergency department. What drug might the family nurse practitioner give the patient while awaiting transfer?
    1. Furosemide (Lasix) 40 mg intravenously.
    2. Morphine sulfate 5–10 mg intravenously.
    3. Nitroglycerin 0.3 mg sublingually.
    4. Aspirin 162–324 mg chewed and swallowed.

67. An adult patient who is being treated for hyperlipidemia prefers to take a "natural" medication approach. On the basis of this patient's request, the family nurse practitioner would order which medication?
    1. Ezetimibe (Zetia).
    2. Gemfibrozil (Lopid).
    3. Colesevelam (Welchol).
    4. Niacin (Niaspan).

68. A family nurse practitioner is reviewing a female patient's medication profile during her annual wellness examination. The patient's past medical history includes recent treatment for hypertension, which began 8 months ago, with a prescribed lisinopril (Prinivil) dosage of 10 mg daily. The patient now states that she may be considering having a child. Which action should be taken by the family nurse practitioner at this time?
    1. Immediate direct referral of the patient to a women's health care nurse practitioner.
    2. Maintain dosage of prescribed beta blocker.
    3. Discontinue lisinopril (Prinivil).
    4. Decrease the dosage of prescribed angiotensin-converting enzyme (ACE) inhibitor.

69. **QSEN** When prescribing a nonsteroidal antiinflammatory drug to control pain, which product would be the best choice for a patient with a comorbidity of cardiovascular disease?
    1. Celecoxib (Celebrex).
    2. Diclofenac (Voltaren).
    3. Ibuprofen (Advil).
    4. Naproxen (Aleve).

70. A 75-year-old male patient presents to the office complaining of "not feeling well." He has a history of chronic lung disease and heart failure. His vital signs are pulse 78 beats/min and irregular, respiration 26 breaths/min, and blood pressure of 158/100 mm Hg. An electrocardiogram indicates sinus rhythm and confirms the rate. The PR interval is 0.28 second, P-waves are present, and each is followed by a QRS complex. There are frequent premature atrial beats. The patient is taking digitalis, potassium, theophylline, hydrochlorothiazide, and a calcium channel blocker. What is the next best action to take?
    1. Obtain serum theophylline, digitalis, and potassium levels.
    2. Increase dosage of calcium blocker and diuretic.
    3. Order pulmonary function studies.
    4. Refer the patient to a cardiologist.

71. The family nurse practitioner is evaluating a patient who is "not feeling good." He has a history of coronary artery disease and heart failure. His vital signs are pulse 72 beats/min, respiration 20 breaths/min, blood pressure 130/88 mm Hg, and temperature normal. The patient has no complaints of chest pain or difficulty breathing. The patient has had some nausea but no vomiting over the last 2 days. His lower extremities are negative for edema. The patient states that he has been able to take his medications. His current medications are digoxin (Lanoxin) 0.5 daily, hydrochlorothiazide (HydroDIURIL) 100 mg twice daily, potassium (Micro-K) 10 mEq daily, and nitroglycerin transdermal patches. What is the priority of care for this patient?
    1. Immediate electrocardiogram and white blood cell count.
    2. Arterial blood gases and oxygen at 4 L/min.
    3. Serum digoxin and potassium levels.
    4. Serial cardiac enzymes now and every 6 hours ×2.

72. The family nurse practitioner has prescribed losartan (Cozaar) 50 mg by mouth daily. This medication promotes vasodilation by:
    1. Blocking the action of angiotensin II.
    2. Promoting release of aldosterone.
    3. Promoting synthesis of prostaglandin.
    4. Inhibiting calcium influx into smooth muscle cells.

73. Which medication would be prescribed by the family nurse practitioner for a 50-year-old female adult patient with no history of cardiac disease (but a calculated 10-year risk of a cardiovascular event >10%) who was placed on lisinopril (Zestril) 3 months ago for trended blood pressure readings of 150/92 mm Hg on two separate occasions that have responded to treatment?
    1. HMG-CoA reductase inhibitor.
    2. Loop diuretic.
    3. Low-molecular-weight heparin.
    4. Antihistamine.

74. A patient with a history of hypertension is started on spironolactone (Aldactone) 50 mg by mouth daily. The family nurse practitioner instructs the patient to call the clinic if which symptoms are experienced?
    1. Increased irritability, abdominal cramping, and lower extremity weakness.
    2. Decreased reflex response, nausea, and vomiting.
    3. Muscle twitching, numbness, tingling, burning sensations of the limbs, and diarrhea.
    4. Weight gain, excessive thirst, and fever.

75. A patient with a history of unstable angina is seen in the cardiac clinic for a checkup. The assessment reveals increased weight of 10 lb, distended jugular neck veins, and S₃. What changes in the pharmacologic treatment should be initiated?
    1. Discontinue beta blockers and calcium channel blockers.
    2. Initiate thrombolytic therapy.
    3. Discontinue nitrate and aspirin therapy.
    4. Initiate diuretic and vasoconstrictor therapy.

76. An 80-year-old patient with a history of glaucoma develops unstable angina. He is started on diltiazem (Cardizem) 30 mg by mouth four times daily and aspirin 325 mg by mouth daily in addition to timolol ophthalmic solution (Timoptic) one drop in the right eye twice daily. This patient would have an increased risk for:
    1. Bleeding episodes.
    2. Fainting episodes and falls.
    3. Rebound supraventricular tachycardia.
    4. Blurred vision.

77. What would the family nurse practitioner assess for when monitoring for the therapeutic effects of verapamil (Calan SR)?
    1. Increase in heart rate.
    2. Decrease in systemic vascular resistance.
    3. Increase in blood pressure (BP).
    4. Decrease in ventricular premature beats.

78. A 45-year-old African American male patient with essential hypertension (HTN) is treated by the family nurse practitioner with sodium restriction and chlorothiazide (Diuril) 25 mg by mouth daily. After 3 months of therapy, the patient's blood pressure is measured at 160/110 mm Hg. Which of the following is the next best step in the plan of care?
    1. Begin enalapril (Vasotec) 5 mg daily.
    2. Begin 50 mg of metoprolol (Toprol XL) daily.
    3. Add 5 mg of amlodipine (Norvasc) daily.
    4. Discontinue Diuril and change to captopril (Capoten) 50 mg three times daily.

79. The family nurse practitioner is prescribing antihypertensive drug therapy for older adult patients. Which class of antihypertensive agents should be used with great caution in the older adult?
    1. Calcium channel blockers.
    2. Diuretics.
    3. Beta blockers.
    4. Angiotensin-converting enzyme (ACE) inhibitors.

80. Medications used in managing ischemic heart disease include:
    1. Beta blockers, sedatives, and aspirin.
    2. Nitrates, beta blockers, calcium channel blockers, and aspirin.
    3. Vasoconstrictors, aspirin, and anxiolytics.
    4. Nitrates, angiotensin-converting enzyme (ACE) inhibitors, aspirin, and lipid-lowering drugs.

81. The family nurse practitioner initiates antihypertensive therapy for a middle-aged nonsmoking male. One week later, the patient returns for a follow-up visit and complains of a recurrent dry cough since initiating the medications. This is most likely a side effect of:
    1. Beta blocker.
    2. Thiazide diuretic.
    3. Angiotensin-converting enzyme (ACE) inhibitor.
    4. Calcium channel blocker.

82. The role of digoxin in the management of heart failure (HF) is indicated for patients with:
    1. Atrial fibrillation (AF).
    2. Mitral valve stenosis.
    3. Normal ejection fraction.
    4. Pericarditis.

83. The family nurse practitioner should monitor the older adult patient for which of the most common adverse reactions of digoxin?
    1. Blurred vision.
    2. Confusion.
    3. Diarrhea.
    4. Eating disorder.

84. The family nurse practitioner has been treating an older patient's hypertension successfully with diet, exercise, and hydrochlorothiazide (HydroDIURIL) 25 mg by mouth daily for 5 months. During today's clinic visit, the patient's blood pressure was 154/90 mm Hg and temperature was 99.9°F (37.7°C). The patient's physical exam revealed clear breath sounds; S_1 and S_2 with no murmurs, gallops, or rubs; and no JVD. The patient denied syncope, headaches, or visual changes but exhibited a tender and edematous right ankle. Which laboratory values would be most appropriate for evaluation?
    1. Blood urea nitrogen and sodium.
    2. Serum cholesterol and serum calcium.
    3. Serum potassium and complete blood count (CBC).
    4. Serum uric acid and CBC.

85. An older adult white male with a long history of chronic obstructive pulmonary disease has recently developed hypertension. Which class of antihypertensive agents should the family nurse practitioner avoid for this patient?
    1. ACE inhibitors.
    2. Beta blockers.
    3. Calcium channel blockers.
    4. Diuretics.

86. Which class of pharmacologic agents would the family nurse practitioner select for an older adult patient who has hypertension and is newly diagnosed with heart failure (HF)?
    1. Angiotensin-converting enzyme (ACE) inhibitors.
    2. Beta blockers.
    3. Calcium channel blockers.
    4. Diuretics.

87. A male patient who is mildly hypertensive and takes hydrochlorothiazide presents with red, painful swelling of the great toe. In addition to treating the gout, the family nurse practitioner also knows to:
    1. Order laboratory studies for diabetes.
    2. Explore for possible alcohol abuse.
    3. Advise him to lose weight.
    4. Change his thiazide antihypertensive medication.

88. An older adult male was diagnosed 3 months ago with systolic hypertension(HTN) and presents for follow-up care. He is on a no-added-salt diet and has lost 8 lb in 3 months. Weekly blood pressure (BP) checks at a senior center average in the 180s/70s. The patient's health history includes benign prostatic hyperplasia, diet-controlled type 2 diabetes, and coronary artery disease with a myocardial infarction 8 years ago. His chief complaint includes periodic angina, occasional heartburn, slowed urine stream with some dribbling, and decreasing energy level. His BP today is 188/78 mm Hg. His current medications are ranitidine 150 mg as needed, aspirin 325 mg daily, nitroglycerin, and aluminum hydroxide/magnesium hydroxide (Maalox) as needed. The patient is married and sexually active. Which medication would the family nurse practitioner initiate after a complete physical, including an electrocardiogram and all indicated blood work?
    1. Angiotensin-converting enzyme (ACE) inhibitor.
    2. Diuretic.
    3. α_1-adrenergic blocker.
    4. β-adrenergic blocker.

89. Secondary prophylaxis for acute rheumatic fever in a 25-year-old schoolteacher who experienced carditis includes:
    1. Penicillin V 125–250 mg by mouth twice daily indefinitely.
    2. Erythromycin 800 mg by mouth twice daily.
    3. One-time dose of 2.0 million units of benzathine penicillin G, combined with penicillin G procaine (Bicillin C-R) intramuscularly.
    4. No medication prophylaxis is needed after a patient reaches the early 20s.

90. A patient has been prescribed lisinopril (Prinivil) 5 mg by mouth daily for hypertension. He has developed an intractable cough that is unrelated to heart failure (HF). Which of the following medications can be substituted for this medication?
    1. Calcium channel blocker.
    2. Digoxin.
    3. Angiotensin-converting enzyme (ACE) inhibitor.
    4. Angiotensin II receptor blocker (ARB).

91. A 60-year-old male with a history of unstable angina comes to the clinic complaining of increased pain that is not relieved by his nitroglycerin. During the assessment, the family nurse practitioner notes elevation of the ST segment on the patient's electrocardiogram. Oxygen therapy is administered, and an intravenous line is inserted. What other therapy should be initiated while arranging transfer to an acute care facility?
    1. Lidocaine drip at 2 mg/min.
    2. Metoprolol (Toprol) 100 mg by mouth.
    3. Morphine 2 mg intravenous push.
    4. Aspirin 162 mg chewed and swallowed.

92. A patient's blood pressure (BP) is within 4 mm Hg of the treatment goal after follow-ups at 1 and 4 weeks. What is the most appropriate strategy to take?
    1. Add new medication to get BP well within goal.
    2. Bring patient back in 1 month to see if at goal.
    3. BP is close enough to goal, so do not do anything.
    4. Discuss the risks and benefits of adding another medication with the patient.

93. A patient who is taking warfarin (Coumadin) has just vomited blood. The family nurse practitioner orders laboratory work revealing a protime of 42 seconds and an international normalized ratio of 4.5. What would the family nurse practitioner order?
    1. Phytonadione (vitamin K_1) 2.5 mg PO.
    2. Phytonadione (vitamin K_1) 1 mg IV over 1 hour.
    3. Protamine sulfate 20 mg PO.
    4. Protamine sulfate 20 mg slow IV push.

94. A 54-year-old patient with type 2 diabetes has been diagnosed with hypertension (HTN). Which antihypertensive drug is the recommended choice to treat HTN in patients with diabetes?
    1. Beta blocker.
    2. Diuretic.
    3. Calcium channel blocker.
    4. Angiotensin-converting enzyme (ACE) inhibitor.

95. A 68-year-old patient with a history of myocardial infarction who has experienced atrial fibrillation (AF) for 2 years comes to the clinic with a complaint of "increasing dyspnea with exertion and occasionally awakening at night with a feeling of smothering." The patient's heart rate is 110. Lung sounds are clear to auscultation. Which pharmacologic therapy would be most appropriate?
    1. Beta blocker and angiotensin-converting enzyme (ACE) inhibitor.
    2. Loop diuretic and beta blocker.
    3. Thiazide diuretic and calcium channel blocker.
    4. α_1-adrenergic blocker and nitrate.

96. A 70-year-old white female is a resident of a long-term care facility in which the family nurse practitioner makes rounds on a weekly basis. The nurse is reviewing recent laboratory results and notices the following: serum potassium of 5.9 mEq/L, serum sodium of 144 mEq/L, serum of chloride 111 mEq/L, blood urea nitrogen of 28 mg/dL, and creatinine of 1.8 mg/dL. Her current medications include furosemide (Lasix) 20 mg by mouth daily, potassium chloride (Klor-Con) 40 mEq by mouth daily, captopril (Capoten) 25 mg by mouth daily, and citalopram (Celexa) 10 mg by mouth daily. There have been no changes in her medications. What is the likely cause of her elevated serum potassium?
    1. Furosemide (Lasix).
    2. Potassium chloride.
    3. Captopril (Capoten).
    4. Citalopram (Celexa).

97. A 46-year-old female is being evaluated for Raynaud phenomenon (RP). Which of the following medications should the primary care nurse practitioner prescribe for symptomatic treatment in addition to lifestyle changes?
    1. Hydralazine.
    2. Amlodipine (Norvasc).
    3. Lisinopril (Zestril).
    4. Nitroglycerin.

98. Which of the following antihypertensive medications classes may cause ankle edema in older adults?
    1. A loop diuretic.
    2. An angiotensin-converting enzyme (ACE) inhibitor.
    3. A calcium channel blocker.
    4. A beta blocker.

99. The patient is instructed to take the lovastatin daily:
    1. In the morning with breakfast.
    2. 30 minutes before eating breakfast.
    3. In the evening.
    4. Around noon.

4 Cardiovascular Answers & Rationales

Physical Exam & Diagnostic Tests

1. Answer: 2

Rationale: With regard to gender, female patients may present with atypical findings associated with chest pain that may indicate a cardiac event. In this situation, the presence of adventitious lung sounds is a key indicator that the patient may be experiencing pulmonary edema, which would increase the likelihood of a cardiac event. Denial of drug use, absent T waves, and absence of jaw pain would be considered pertinent negative findings.

2. Answer: 3

Rationale: There are no specific preprocedure instructions for a TTE, because it is considered to be a noninvasive diagnostic test. Patients should be advised to wear comfortable clothing that can be removed easily and to take their regularly scheduled medications.

3. Answer: 1

Rationale: S_1 is heard loudest at the apex (characteristic "lub" sound) and S_2 at the base (characteristic "dub" sound). Each sound should be assessed carefully regarding the intensity of the sound in each area. The S_2 second heart sound has two components: A_2 is produced by aortic valve closure, and P_2 is produced by pulmonic valve closure.

4. Answer: 3

Rationale: The PMI represents the thrust and contraction of the left ventricle (LV). The LV lies behind the right ventricle and extends to the left, forming the left border of the heart.

5. Answer: 2

Rationale: The correct procedure is to listen for carotid bruits with the bell of the stethoscope, which brings out low-frequency sounds and filters out high-frequency sounds. The bell should be placed very lightly on the neck with just enough pressure to seal the edge.

6. Answer: 2

Rationale: The purpose of inspection and palpation of the precordium is to determine the presence and extent of normal and abnormal pulsations. A slight retraction of the chest wall just medial to the midclavicular line in the fifth interspace is a normal finding, whereas marked or active retraction of the rib is abnormal and may indicate pericardial disease. Pericardial friction rubs are heard by auscultation.

7. Answer: 1

Rationale: The splitting during inspiration refers to S_1 and S_2. The S_3 is usually normal (physiologic S_3) in children, young adults (but usually disappears by the age of 30), and pregnant women in the third trimester. It is also found in athletes and hyperkinetic states. In the older adult with heart disease, this sound is considered pathologic and often signifies heart failure, left ventricular enlargement, or cardiomyopathy.

8. Answer: 3

Rationale: The right side of the chest close to the sternal border at the second intercostal space is the correct area to auscultate the aortic valve. The mitral valve is auscultated at the fifth left intercostal space at the midclavicular line. The tricuspid valve is auscultated at the fourth left intercostal space at the sternal border. The pulmonic valve is auscultated at the second left intercostal space at the sternal border.

9. Answer: 2

Rationale: An 8- to 12-hour fast is recommended because of the influence of intake on cholesterol levels, which may increase. A normal diet for the 7 days before drawing the lipid profile is recommended so that an accurate picture of the patient's normal life is obtained. Alcohol should not be consumed for 48 hours before the test, because it may increase cholesterol, high-density lipoprotein, low-density lipoprotein, and triglyceride levels. If possible, all medications should be withheld until the blood test is drawn, especially corticosteroids, diuretics, beta blockers, oral contraceptives, and estrogens.

10. Answer: 1

Rationale: An S_4 may be a normal variant in people ages 65 years and older and may result from increased resistance to ventricular filling during atrial contraction. It may represent a decrease in ventricular compliance related to physiologic changes caused by aging.

11. Answer: 1

Rationale: Based on the Joint National Committee 8 report hypertension treatment guidelines, an appropriate BP goal for a patient aged 60 years or older is SBP <150 mm Hg/DBP <90 mm Hg. Patients younger than 60 years old, or patients at any age with diabetes or chronic kidney disease, should have BP goals set at SBP <140 mm Hg/DBP <90 mm Hg.

12. Answer: 2

Rationale: Acute rheumatic fever would most likely affect the aortic and mitral valves first; because these murmurs are difficult to auscultate, the mitral valve would be the best choice among the options given. The fifth intercostal space at the midclavicular line on the left side is the best place to auscultate the closure sounds of the mitral valve. Auscultating at the left sternal border, fourth left intercostal space describes the area of the tricuspid valve. Auscultating at the second or third intercostal space at the left of the sternal border describes the pulmonic valve area. The aortic valve area is auscultated at the second intercostal space on the right of the sternal border.

13. Answer: 3

Rationale: It is important to determine whether the coolness extends proximally from the hand, so feeling the forearms with the backs of the fingers is appropriate. Next, it would be important to palpate the radial pulses. The Allen test relates to arterial blood gas collection and is not indicated. Holding the hand in a dependent position would facilitate perfusion but would not help to determine bilateral comparison of extremities.

14. Answer: 1

Rationale: The mitral and tricuspid valves are considered AV valves. Closure of the AV valves produces the first heart sound (S_1). This marks the beginning of systole and emptying of both ventricles. The aortic and pulmonic valves are semilunar valves. At the end of systole, closure of the semilunar valves produces the second heart sound (S_2).

15. Answer: 4

Rationale: The apical and radial pulses must be evaluated simultaneously to determine whether all the apical beats are being reflected in the radial pulse. If there is an apical rate of 100 and a radial rate of 94, the patient is said to have a pulse deficit of 6. This is usually done with two people counting simultaneously over the same period.

16. Answer: 3

Rationale: A grade V heart murmur is very loud and can be heard with the stethoscope partly off the chest wall with a thrill that is easily palpable. A grade I murmur is barely audible in a quiet room or very faintly heard with the bell of the stethoscope. A grade II murmur is quiet but clearly audible. A grade III murmur is moderately loud. A grade IV murmur is loud and associated with thrill. A grade VI murmur is the loudest, is audible with the stethoscope removed from contact with the chest wall, and is accompanied by a thrill that is palpable and visible.

17. Answer: 4

Rationale: The normal aging process impairs automaticity, conductivity, and contractility. Ischemic changes and degeneration decrease sinus node automaticity and conduction velocity, resulting in bradycardic rhythms or atrial fibrillation. The poor myocardial contractility, usually related to hypertension or valvular disease, causes decreased ventricular emptying and increased filling pressures. These changes predispose the older adult patient to heart failure.

18. Answer: 4

Rationale: The most sensitive area for temperature on the examiner's hand is the back of the fingers. The fingertips should be used to assess texture and moisture.

19. Answer: 3

Rationale: The American College of Cardiology cholesterol guidelines no longer recommend treatment adjusted to a specific target lipid value. In a patient aged 40–75 without diabetes or clinical ASCVD, the patient's 10-year ASCVD risk should be calculated, and determination should be made whether the patient falls into a pharmacologic treatment benefit group. A heart-healthy diet, lifestyle modifications, and regular aerobic physical activity should always be included in the treatment regimen. Referral to a cardiologist is not appropriate at this time.

20. Answer: 3

Rationale: Dressler syndrome (post-MI syndrome) may develop 1–4 weeks post-MI and is characterized by pericarditis with effusion, fever, and markers of inflammation such as leukocytosis. Dressler syndrome is caused by antigen–antibody reactions. Laboratory findings include elevated white blood cell count and erythrocyte sedimentation rate. Treatment includes nonsteroidal antiinflammatory drugs and colchicine.

21. Answer: 1

Rationale: Jugular vein distention (JVD) is common in older adult patients. If JVD is present when the patient's head is elevated 45 degrees, further examination is necessary regarding the venous pressure, which reflects pressure in the right-side heart chambers. The supine position will increase venous pressure and does not provide valid information in this situation. Auscultation for carotid bruits is an important part of assessment but is not significant in evaluating JVD.

22. Answer: 1

Rationale: Mitral valve stenosis is a diastolic murmur of low intensity heard at the apex of the heart. Midsystolic ejection murmur heard loudest over the left lower sternal border describes characteristics of a murmur with aortic stenosis. A holosystolic murmur is characteristic of mitral valve regurgitation, which allows for backflow of blood from ventricles into the atrium and is heard loudest over the apex and left axillary area. A diastolic murmur heard loudest with the patient in a sitting position and leaning forward best describes aortic regurgitation.

23. Answer: 3

Rationale: The patient had a left ventricular MI. One of the most common complications is left-sided heart failure. This would manifest first as pulmonary congestion (crackles in lungs) and difficulty breathing.

24. Answer: 4

Rationale: Classically, intermittent claudication is described as pain in the lower extremity on activity that is relieved by stopping the activity. During exercise, there is an increased demand for blood supply to the extremity that cannot be met. Subsequently, there is a buildup of lactic acid and other metabolites in the muscle, which causes the tightening or cramping discomfort in the calf muscles.

25. Answer: 3

Rationale: A positive result on stress testing indicates the likelihood of coronary artery disease with 70%–77% sensitivity and specificity in males over age 50. Results are progressively lower in asymptomatic persons, with false-positive results increased in asymptomatic men under age 40, premenopausal women without risk factors, and patients taking digitalis. If nuclear imaging is combined with exercise, sensitivity and specificity rise to 90%.

26. Answer: 2

Rationale: A hyperkinetic impulse (increased amplitude) is caused by pressure overload of the left ventricle. Causes include hyperthyroidism, severe anemia, or mitral valve regurgitation. A pansystolic murmur is a classic finding of mitral valve regurgitation.

27. Answer: 2, 3, 4

Rationale: The TIMI risk score is a well-known tool used to identify risk for patients with unstable angina and non–ST-segment elevation myocardial infarction. Seven predictor variables are each given 1 point and include age ≥65, aspirin use in the last 7 days, at least three risk factors for coronary artery disease (CAD), severe symptoms of angina within the previous 24 hours, elevated cardiac markers (CK-MB or cardiac-specific troponin level), ST-segment elevation ≥0.5 mm, and prior CAD with ≥50% stenosis. Low risk is from 0–2 points, with 5–7 points considered as high risk. Warfarin use and a lipid profile are not part of the risk score. There are other risk scores using troponin-only levels (HEART [history, electrocardiogram, age, risk factors, and troponin], Global Registry of Acute Coronary Events, Emergency Department Assessment of Chest Pain Score) that provide better risk stratification.

28. Answer: 4

Rationale: Pulsus alternans (weak pulse alternating with strong pulse) is most often caused by left ventricular failure

(strong and weak ventricular contractions), is usually accompanied by an S_3 heart sound, and is seen in patients with left-sided HF. It may be present in severe acute aortic insufficiency (AI), but it is unusual in patients with chronic AI.

Disorders

29. Answer: 1

Rationale: This assessment reflects changes caused by chronic venous insufficiency, which includes edema, varicose veins, chronic skin changes, dependent cyanosis, and skin ulceration. The other assessment findings reflect chronic arterial insufficiency.

30. Answer: 1

Rationale: A diagnosis of HTN based on a single measurement of blood pressure (BP) elevation should not be done. A minimum of two readings on two or more separate occasions with an average greater than or equal to an SBP of 140 mm Hg and DBP of 90 mm Hg establishes the diagnosis. The 2017 American College of Cardiology guidelines recommended out-of-office BP measurements and ambulatory BP monitoring to assist diagnosis. An average of two or more readings taken at each of two or more visits should follow an initial screening. The patient should be seated with the arm at heart level. No caffeine or nicotine ingestion should be allowed for 30 minutes before the reading. The room should be quiet for at least 5 minutes, and an appropriate cuff should be used.

31. Answer: 3

Rationale: In the early stages of hypertensive heart disease, when there is an increased peripheral resistance to blood flow, the most significant change occurring in the heart is left ventricular hypertrophy. This is associated with an increase in the size of the myocardial cells without a corresponding increase in cell number (hyperplasia). Over time, all other options listed occur in the heart.

32. Answer: 2

Rationale: Clinical confirmation of nosebleeds in a patient who already has a diagnosis of HTN may be significant. As such, the family nurse practitioner should follow this physical symptom for its potential effect on the patient's vascular status. Both 20/20 vision screening and brisk capillary refill bilaterally are normal findings. An occasional nonproductive cough in response to the patient's self-identified seasonal allergies is considered a normal abnormal finding.

33. Answer: 1

Rationale: The classic chest pain associated with an MI may not be present in the older adult patient because of altered pain perception and diminished pain sensation.

34. Answer: 2

Rationale: Respiratory symptoms are predominant in patients with left-sided HF. Venous congestion and peripheral edema are associated with right-sided HF.

35. Answer: 1

Rationale: Cardiac tamponade occurs as a complication of pericarditis. An excessive accumulation of fluids between the pericardium and myocardium interferes with effective cardiac contraction and produces a paradoxical pulse. The triphasic friction rub is common to pericarditis but is not indicative of a complication of constrictive pericarditis. Jugular venous pressure is used to determine levels of venous distention.

36. Answer: 2

Rationale: Untreated HTN causes significant increased work of the left ventricle, eventually causing left-sided HF.

37. Answer: 2

Rationale: Palpable carotid pulse with each compression is the best sign of effective CPR. The other answers are appropriate but not the best indicators of effective resuscitation efforts.

38. Answer: 3

Rationale: A triphasic friction rub or pericardial rub occurs in the majority of patients with pericarditis. Paradoxical pulse may occur if constrictive pericarditis and cardiac tamponade are present. Pulse deficits and the presence of S_4 are not characteristic of problems with pericarditis.

39. Answer: 1

Rationale: Older adults experience atypical symptoms of MI, including dyspnea, diaphoresis, vomiting, syncope, confusion, and weakness.

40. Answer: 1

Rationale: Cardiovascular risk factors predisposing women to CVD include smaller body size, declining estrogen level, heart and thoracic cavity are smaller and lighter, coronary arteries are smaller in diameter, a shorter PR interval, and a higher resting ejection fraction. Increased body fat percentage and fat distributed in the abdomen may be mobilized more easily in response to stress. This may raise serum cholesterol and blood glucose levels. Females after menopause are more likely to develop microvascular disorders as well from the reduction of estrogen. Estrogen levels can also fall in younger women suffering from persistent stress. This may lead to increased risk of cardiovascular disease.

41. Answer: 4

Rationale: The family nurse practitioner must consider the geriatric patient's other medical problems and treatment along with race before prescribing medications for HTN. Frequently, geriatric patients cannot take beta blockers because of chronic pulmonary conditions; they may already be taking diuretics for problems of fluid retention. Therapy is individualized and should include consideration of existing comorbidities. Lifestyle changes should be initiated and medications adjusted as changes are made.

42. Answer: 2

Rationale: Hypertension is considered a major factor in the development of CAD in the geriatric patient. Female patients have an increased incidence of CAD after menopause; estrogen replacement therapy appears to have cardioprotective effects on the heart, thus decreasing the incidence of CAD. Although patients with diabetes have an increased incidence of CAD, most patients with CAD do not have diabetes.

43. Answer: 4

Rationale: Cor pulmonale is characterized by hypertrophy of the RV secondary to pulmonary hypertension (resistance) and central pulmonary artery enlargement noted on an x-ray. The increased P-wave amplitude (P pulmonale) occurs as the right atrium enlarges. The best method for identifying cor pulmonale is echocardiography.

44. Answer: 2

Rationale: The compensatory mechanism (activation of the renin-angiotensin-aldosterone system) causes excess secretion of aldosterone that predisposes to potassium excretion. Total body sodium content will be greater than normal, but the excessive secretion of antidiuretic hormone (ADH) causes greater retention of water, diluting the serum level. ADH is continually secreted because of the presence of low pressure at the carotid sinus baroreceptors, directly related to low cardiac output.

45. Answer: 1

Rationale: Water-hammer pulse, also known as Corrigan or hyperkinetic pulse (bounding pulse with a rapid rise and sudden collapse), results from an increase in pulse pressure and may be caused by increased stroke volume, decreased peripheral vascular resistance, or both. Because the family nurse practitioner suspects either aortic regurgitation or patent ductus arteriosus (primarily in children), auscultation for a diastolic murmur is indicated.

46. Answer: 2

Rationale: Occlusion of the coronary arteries deprives the myocardial cells of glucose needed for aerobic metabolism. Anaerobic metabolism occurs, which causes the accumulation of lactic acid. Lactic acid irritates the myocardial nerve fibers, sending pain messages to the cardiac nerves and upper thoracic posterior roots located in the left shoulder and arm.

47. Answer: 4

Rationale: Marked limitation in activity, feeling comfortable at rest, but ordinary activity leading to symptoms is noted as Functional Class III. Symptoms present at rest, with any activity leading to increased discomfort, characterizes Functional Class IV. Slight limitation in ordinary activity, resulting in fatigue, palpitations, dyspnea, or angina, is defined as Functional Class II. Functional Class I is characterized by no physical limitation in activity.

48. Answer: 1

Rationale: The moist crackles (rales) heard in the bases of the lung are the most prominent physical examination findings of early HF. They are caused by transudation of fluid into the alveoli and the airways. Later findings include distended neck veins, peripheral edema, hepatomegaly, and ascites (rather than weight loss).

49. Answer: 3

Rationale: Aortic dissection almost invariably begins with a sudden onset of severe chest pain that is tearing or ripping in quality and is accompanied by absent or decreased peripheral pulses and neurologic deficits. The pain of angina and AMI is usually described as "pressure." Pericarditis produces pain that is more gradual in onset.

50. Answer: 1

Rationale: The Adult Treatment Panel IV, the American College of Cardiology, and American Heart Association cholesterol guidelines recommend lifestyle modifications for patients with hyperlipidemia, including increasing vegetables, fruits, and whole grains and limiting sodium, sweets and sugar-sweetened drinks, red meats, and saturated fats, and should include <10% of unsaturated fat. The amount of fat in the average diet should be between 20% and 35% of the total calories. Daily protein intake should be between 10% and 35%. Carbohydrate intake should be monitored in the maintenance of a healthy weight.

51. Answer: 4

Rationale: Although the other dysrhythmias may occur after MI, the most life-threatening one is ventricular fibrillation.

The vast majority of deaths resulting from ventricular fibrillation occur within the first 24 hours, and more than half of these occur in the first hour. The majority of out-of-hospital deaths resulting from MI are caused by ventricular fibrillation.

52. Answer: 2

Rationale: Diet and exercise are the mainstays of any treatment program and would be used initially in all cases. First-line pharmacologic treatment is statin therapy, and the choice of a high-intensity or moderate-intensity statin is based on calculated cardiovascular risk. A bile acid sequestrant agent, ezetimibe, or PCSK9 inhibitors may be added if no improvement is seen with diet and exercise therapy plus statin therapy. Referral to a cardiologist is not necessary, unless the patient develops symptoms or shows resistance to treatment.

53. Answer: 2

Rationale: A stroke is often the outcome of chronic AF because of the blood pooling in the quivering atria. As a result, a blood clot can be formed in this pooling blood, which then travels to the brain and causes an ischemic stroke. For this reason, warfarin (Coumadin) should be maintained at an international normalized ratio of 2–3, or other anticoagulants, such as dabigatran (Pradaxa), rivaroxaban (Xarelto), and apixaban (Eliquis), may be prescribed.

54. Answer: 3

Rationale: Dyspnea is the most common symptom of HF. Initially, it is present only with moderate exertion, but as the severity of HF increases, dyspnea may occur on mild exertion or at rest. Fatigue is another common complaint. Right-sided HF is associated with weakness, anorexia, nausea, and dependent edema. Chronic left ventricular failure usually leads to right ventricular failure. Newer evidence suggests that 50% of patients with HF are not volume overloaded. The symptoms are the result of volume shifts from the splanchnic venous system (storage veins in the abdomen) into the cardiac and pulmonary system. Subsequently, weight gain may not be a symptom. If weight gain is present, it occurs 3–4 weeks after acute decompensation happens, making it a late symptom.

55. Answer: 3

Rationale: Palm and coconut oils, along with butter, are very high in saturated fats and should be avoided. The other selections are moderately high in fat content but are mainly unsaturated fats.

56. Answer: 3

Rationale: Anginal pain is difficult to differentiate from the pain of an infarction. One of the most characteristic symptoms of angina pain is relief with the administration of sublingual nitroglycerin.

57. Answer: 1

Rationale: Superficial inflammation of a vein may be caused by trauma (for example, blow to the arm or leg) or recent intravenous therapy with irritating fluids, or it may occur secondary to pregnancy, especially during the postpartum period, because of the increase in clotting factors (thromboplastin). Excessive use of oral anticoagulants can lead to bleeding but not to thrombophlebitis. Deep vein thrombosis associated with thrombophlebitis results from prolonged bed rest, major surgical procedures, injury to the blood vessel wall, and hypercoagulable states, such as use of oral contraceptives (especially in women who smoke or have cancer), cancer, and polycythemia vera.

58. Answer: 3

Rationale: Dizziness that improves when lying down and worsens when standing is symptomatic of cardiac involvement and may indicate serious cardiac dysrhythmias. If it occurs in certain positions, the dizziness suggests benign positional vertigo, which is common in older adults. Dizziness accompanied by tinnitus is common in acute labyrinthitis and, if preceded by rapid breathing, may be caused by hyperventilation.

59. Answer: 3

Rationale: The stated history of a recent coxsackievirus infection, pain that worsens when supine, and a friction rub is classic for viral pericarditis. The pain is often relieved by having the patient sit up and lean forward. Viral pericarditis can also cause significant pericardial effusions, which often present as dyspnea. The patient's age makes an AMI unlikely, and the pain is not typical for pleural effusion or esophageal reflux.

60. Answer: 1

Rationale: Signs and symptoms of hyperthyroidism in the older adult include progressive functional decline, AF, myocardial infarction, tachycardia, weakness, fatigue, weight loss, anorexia, diarrhea, nervousness, tremor, pruritus, memory loss, and heat intolerance. Symptoms of hypothyroidism include arthralgia; weakness; decreased mental function; depression; constipation; weight loss; dry, coarse skin with a yellowish cast; dry, sparse hair; and masklike puffy face with periorbital edema. Bradycardia would be assessed with sick sinus syndrome. Sick sinus syndrome is often associated with the "bradycardia–tachycardia" syndrome.

61. Answer: 4

Rationale: JVP of 14 cm H_2O is a sign of heart failure (normal JVP is 3–10 cm H_2O). Decreased exercise tolerance is a normal sign of aging. A grade II/VI systolic ejection murmur is a result of sclerosing of the aorta, which occurs with aging. Prolongation of PR intervals on an ECG is expected with the aging process.

62. Answer: 2

Rationale: This assessment is consistent with aortic stenosis. Aortic regurgitation is a diastolic murmur secondary to rheumatic heart disease, for which no history is given. Mitral valve disease is one of the most common valvular disorders. A small percentage of patients who have a mitral valve prolapse do experience autonomic dysfunction and complain of palpitations, atypical chest pain, orthostatic dizziness, near-syncope, cold extremities, throbbing headaches, and neurasthenia, and they manifest tachydysrhythmias. Patients who have mitral valve regurgitation may remain asymptomatic for many years because the left ventricle dilates and adjusts well to the increase in volume load. Onset of dyspnea and fatigue may not occur for decades.

63. Answer: 1

Rationale: Aortic stenosis is the most frequently diagnosed valvular heart problem and is caused by aortic valve thickening and calcification. The symptoms include syncope, angina, and dyspnea on exertion. Patients may develop aortic stenosis earlier in life if they have a congenital valve abnormality, such as a bicuspid valve, or if they have a history of rheumatic valve disease.

64. Answer: 3

Rationale: The talk test is one method to measure exercise intensity. Patients with HF should strive for an exercise intensity that permits carrying on a conversation (but not breathless conversation) with an exercise partner. Moderate- to high-intensity interval training consisting of aerobic exercise and resistance training is the ideal program for patients with HF. Current recommendations are 30–60 minutes of moderate intensity to high-intensity aerobic interval training (walking, cycling, or jogging), along with strength training of major muscle groups, at least three times per week.

65. Answer: 3

Rationale: The family nurse practitioner needs to repeat the cholesterol and obtain HDL and LDL values before initiating any treatment. The HDL and LDL will help stratify cardiovascular risk and aid in the determination of recommended management.

Pharmacology

66. Answer: 4

Rationale: Aspirin helps prevent the formation of platelet-aggregating substances and may help the occlusion of narrowed coronary arteries. Although furosemide and morphine have a role in treating acute myocardial infarction, aspirin can readily be given in the typical primary care office. Chewing the aspirin speeds absorption. Nitroglycerin should not be given, because the patient's systolic blood pressure is <90 mm Hg.

67. Answer: 4

Rationale: Niacin (Niaspan) is also known as vitamin B_3 and as such would be considered to be a natural medication approach. Niacin boosts high-density lipoprotein levels and modestly reduces low-density lipoprotein. It is generally only effective at higher doses. The other medications represent medication classes: a cholesterol absorption inhibitor (Zetia), a fibric acid derivative (Lopid), and a bile acid sequestrant (Welchol).

68. Answer: 3

Rationale: A female patient who is being treated with lisinopril (Prinivil) is being treated with an ACE inhibitor, which is contraindicated in pregnant women in the second and third trimesters. If a woman becomes pregnant on an ACE inhibitor, research has not shown adverse effects to the fetus in the first trimester but the medication should be discontinued. The family nurse practitioner should order an antihypertensive drug considered safe during pregnancy, such as methyldopa or labetalol. An immediate direct referral to a women's health care nurse practitioner is not indicated at this time because the patient is not pregnant but is discussing potential concerns at this time. A change in blood pressure medication is warranted at this time on the basis of the patient's voiced concerns.

69. Answer: 4

Rationale: Naproxen is associated with the fewest cardiovascular concerns. Dosage should be limited to the lowest effective dose as gastrointestinal and renal side effects are still possible. Diclofenac, ibuprofen, and celecoxib all have associated cardiovascular risks even with small doses and are associated with increased risk of coronary death or nonfatal myocardial infarction.

70. Answer: 1

Rationale: This patient is presenting with symptoms of digitalis toxicity—first-degree block and increasing cardiac irritability. If the patient's potassium level is low, it may be precipitating the toxicity. Also, it is important to determine that serum theophylline levels remain within the therapeutic range. No evidence indicates that the pulmonary disease is progressing. BP may be adequately controlled for this patient; further information should be obtained before adjusting the medications. On the basis of the information presented, referral to a cardiologist is not appropriate at this time.

71. Answer: 3

Rationale: The patient presents with the classic profile of digitalis toxicity, which is frequently related to hypokalemia, especially because the potassium replacement is rather low for an adult and the patient has a history of poor eating and nausea. The actions listed in the other options may be taken, but it is important to determine the presence of hypokalemia and digitalis toxicity so that these may be addressed immediately.

72. Answer: 1

Rationale: Angiotensin II receptor blockers (ARBs), such as losartan (Cozaar), block access of angiotensin II to its receptors in blood vessels, the adrenals, and all other tissues. By blocking the action of angiotensin II, losartan relaxes muscle cells and dilates blood vessels (arterioles and veins), reducing blood pressure. By blocking angiotensin II receptors in the adrenals, ARBs decrease release of aldosterone, which increases renal excretion of sodium and water. Sodium and water excretion are further increased through dilation of renal blood vessels.

73. Answer: 1

Rationale: Treatment regimens for patients with hypertension (HTN) should include initiation of statin therapy to decrease cardiovascular risk if three criteria are met according to the U.S. Preventive Services Task Force: (1) aged 40–75 years, (2) presence of one or more cardiovascular disease (CVD) risk factors (that is, dyslipidemia, diabetes, HTN, or smoking), and (3) calculated 10-year risk of a cardiovascular event of 10% or greater. Unless there is specific clinical evidence of fluid retention (or edema), a loop diuretic would not be indicated. Anticoagulation therapy would not be indicated because there is no clinical evidence to support increased cardiovascular risk. An antihistamine would not be indicated in this case, unless there is specific clinical evidence of seasonal allergies and/or nasal congestion.

74. Answer: 3

Rationale: Aldactone is a potassium-sparing diuretic. Patients should be instructed on the early signs of hyperkalemia, which include muscle twitching, numbness, tingling, and burning sensations of the limbs; diarrhea; palpitations; and skipped heartbeats. Hypokalemia symptoms are characterized by irritability; confusion followed by lethargy, abdominal cramping, distention, and constipation; and lower extremity weakness.

75. Answer: 1

Rationale: Beta blockers are myocardial depressants that suppress heart rate and contraction (negative inotropic). Calcium channel blockers decrease atrioventricular conduction, which suppresses heart rate. Initiation of other drugs are contraindicated with the acute onset of left ventricular dysfunction. Patients with heart failure (HF) should be maintained on beta blockers if currently prescribed but also should be prescribed diuretics. Only three beta blockers are approved for use in patients with left ventricular dysfunction, and these are carvedilol, sustained released metoprolol succinate, and bisoprolol. The increase in jugular vein distention and a 10-lb weight gain are associated with right-sided HF. The presence of S_3 indicates left ventricular dysfunction, especially when associated with signs and symptoms of right-sided HF.

76. Answer: 2

Rationale: The use of β-adrenergic blocking agents (for example, timolol), whether systemic or ophthalmic, may result in bradycardia and/or hypotension. Blood pressure, heart rate, and symptoms should be closely monitored.

77. Answer: 2

Rationale: Calcium channel blockers (1) depress the rate of discharge from the sinoatrial node and conduction velocity through the AV node, causing a decrease in heart rate; (2) relax the coronary and systemic arteries, producing vasodilation (decrease in afterload and BP); and (3) decrease myocardial contractility (negative inotropic effect).

78. Answer: 3

Rationale: According to the Joint National Committee 8 (JNC 8), African American males without diabetes or chronic kidney disease should be prescribed calcium channel blockers alone or in combination with a thiazide-type diuretic in the treatment of HTN. Enalapril and captopril are angiotensin-converting enzyme inhibitors, which should be used with caution in African Americans as they may be at increased risk for the development of angioedema. Metoprolol is a beta blocker and not recommended in the JNC 8 guidelines for the treatment of HTN unless comorbidities, such as atrial fibrillation exist.

79. Answer: 3

Rationale: All classes of antihypertensives should be used with caution in older adults. Older adults have decreased beta-receptor sensitivity. Consequently, normal doses of beta blockers may lead to significant bradycardia in this population. Larger doses may also result in depression, impotence, fatigue, and declining mental function. Older adult patients are especially likely to experience heart failure and peripheral vascular insufficiency resulting from β-adrenergic blocker toxicity. Blood pressure should be lowered cautiously by prescribing small doses of calcium channel blockers, ACE inhibitors, or diuretics in older adult patients and titrating slowly under close supervision.

80. Answer: 2

Rationale: Nitrates are venous and arterial dilators that decrease myocardial oxygen demand. Beta blockers have an antianginal effect and reduce myocardial oxygen demand. Calcium channel blockers relieve myocardial ischemia by reducing myocardial oxygen demand and dilate coronary arteries. Aspirin is effective for secondary prevention of myocardial infarction. Unless contraindicated, small doses of aspirin (81–325 mg daily) should be prescribed for patients with angina. Patients remaining symptomatic when treated with nitrates, beta blockers, or calcium channel blockers should be treated with a beta blocker plus another agent. Appropriate combinations are a nitrate or beta blocker plus a calcium channel blocker other than verapamil. Combination therapy does not include sedatives, vasoconstrictors, ACE inhibitors, or lipid-lowering drugs.

81. Answer: 3

Rationale: Adverse side effects of ACE inhibitors include cough (1%–30% of patients), headache, dizziness, and hyperkalemia. Patients who experience a cough side effect should be switched to a different medication. The cough will resolve within 10–14 days of discontinuation. Adverse effects of calcium channel blockers include peripheral edema, dizziness, headache, nausea, and tachycardia. Adverse effects of thiazide diuretics include nausea, vomiting, diarrhea, dizziness, and headache. Side effects of beta blockers include fatigue, bradycardia, impotence, depression, and shortness of breath.

82. Answer: 1

Rationale: Digoxin, once a first-line drug for all patients with HF, is now used in patients with AF, other tachycardias, and left ventricular dysfunction. By controlling the ventricular rate in the patient with AF or tachycardias, cardiac output increases. In cases of diastolic dysfunction with a sinus rhythm, digitalis is of no benefit. Digoxin is of relatively little value in most forms of cardiomyopathy, myocarditis, mitral valve stenosis, and chronic constrictive pericarditis.

83. Answer: 2

Rationale: Noncardiac adverse reactions include a change in mental status. Although visual disturbances, diarrhea, anorexia, nausea, and vomiting are also adverse reactions, they are not the most common in older adult patients.

84. Answer: 4

Rationale: The assessments indicate gout. A side effect of hydrochlorothiazide is hyperuricemia. Blood for a CBC should be drawn before therapy. The other options do not address the assessment of a tender and edematous right ankle. The cardiac assessments were benign. No evidence indicates a concern for hyponatremia, hypernatremia, hypokalemia, or hyperkalemia.

85. Answer: 2

Rationale: Beta blockers increase peripheral vascular resistance, a phenomenon that already occurs with normal aging, so these drugs can precipitate or worsen symptoms of asthma, COPD, peripheral vascular disease, sexual dysfunction, or heart failure. The other drug classes have no effect or decrease the effect on peripheral resistance.

86. Answer: 1

Rationale: ACE inhibitors have been shown to prolong life in patients with HF by improving overall cardiac function. Beta blockers and calcium channel blockers should be contraindicated in patients with new-onset decompensated HF. Three beta blockers, including carvedilol, metoprolol succinate, and bisoprolol, are approved for the treatment of HF after the patient is stabilized. Although the use of diuretics may be correct, diuretics are not a priority over ACE inhibitors.

87. Answer: 4

Rationale: The most likely precipitating cause of this patient's gout is the thiazide diuretic used to control his hypertension, because it blocks the excretion of uric acid, leading to hyperuricemia. Although gout may be more common in obese, alcoholic, and diabetic patients, these conditions are not indicated here.

88. Answer: 1

Rationale: The ACE inhibitor will preserve renal function, have less impact on sexual function, and is the first-line agent for patients with diabetes. The family nurse practitioner must monitor the patient's potassium and carefully follow renal status for change. The ACE inhibitor has fewer negative side effects or interactions with this patient's other medical conditions. In this case, if the BP remains high after the ACE inhibitor, the second-line option would be an α_1-adrenergic blocker as the patient also has benign prostatic hyperplasia. The medication would treat both HTN and this comorbidity.

89. Answer: 1

Rationale: Secondary prevention or preventing the recurrent attacks of acute rheumatic fever is controversial. Some authorities identify (1) reaching the early 20s and (2) 5 years since the last attack as the criteria for stopping the use of prophylactic penicillin, unless the patient is at increased risk of exposure to streptococcal infections, as are schoolteachers and health professionals. Other authorities recommend lifelong prophylactic drug therapy, depending on cardiac damage. Although erythromycin is an alternative medication for penicillin-sensitive individuals, the dose of 800 mg is for a patient having a dental or surgical procedure. The secondary prophylactic dose for erythromycin is 250 mg by mouth twice daily.

90. Answer: 4

Rationale: An annoying, untoward effect of ACE inhibitors is an intractable cough. Lisinopril is an ACE inhibitor. ARBs can be substituted as long as the cough is not related to HF. Antidysrhythmic agents, calcium channel blockers, and nonsteroidal antiinflammatory drugs should be avoided.

91. Answer: 4

Rationale: The American Heart Association recommends that aspirin (162–325 mg by mouth once) be administered as soon as possible whenever a patient is suspected of having a myocardial infarction. The decreased platelet aggregation effect of aspirin helps limit the size of the myocardial damage. Chewing the aspirin speeds absorption.

92. Answer: 4

Rationale: Follow-up visits should be performed in 1–4 weeks to assess BP results. If BP is not at target, discuss with the patient about either increasing the dose of the initial drug or the risks and benefits of adding a second drug. The family nurse practitioner should continue to follow BPs until at target and to uptitrate and/or add a third drug as needed.

93. Answer: 3

Rationale: Vitamin K_1 is given for warfarin overdose and may be given IV in an emergency. To reduce the incidence of an anaphylactic reaction, the medication should be infused slowly. In a nonemergency situation, it would be appropriate to give vitamin K_1 orally. Protamine sulfate is used for heparin overdose.

94. Answer: 4

Rationale: ACE inhibitors enhance renal function in patients with diabetes and slow the progression of kidney injury.

95. Answer: 1

Rationale: This patient with AF is exhibiting symptoms of left ventricular failure and poor rate control but does not appear to be in acute heart failure (HF). Treatment recommendations include beta blockers, ACE inhibitors, angiotensin II receptor blockers, and eplerenone, which reduce the rate and incidence of AF in patients who also have HF with reduced ejection fraction. A combination of beta blockers and ACE inhibitors remain the cornerstone of treatment for HF. A patient recently diagnosed with coronary artery disease is started on statin therapy with lovastatin (Mevacor) 20 mg.

96. Answer: 2

Rationale: The likely cause of the patient's elevated serum potassium is the potassium chloride. The family nurse practitioner should hold the potassium chloride (Klor-Con) and order daily serum potassium monitoring until the patient's serum potassium levels return to normal. The patient is taking furosemide, which is a potassium-wasting diuretic, and the amount of potassium given to compensate for the anticipated losses apparently was too much. This often occurs as a result of the changes of aging. Once serum potassium returns to normal, the level is monitored again at 1 week. With the low dose of furosemide and with captopril (an ACE inhibitor that may retain potassium), the patient may not need to have potassium chloride restarted.

97. Answer: 2

Rationale: Treatment for RP includes avoiding triggers, especially exposure to cold temperatures. Pharmacologic treatments for RP include the initial use of dihydropyridine calcium channel blockers, such as amlodipine and nifedipine.

98. Answer: 3

Rationale: Side effects of calcium channel blockers include swelling of feet, ankles, and legs; lightheadedness; low blood pressure; slower heart rate; drowsiness; constipation; increased appetite; gastroesophageal reflux disease; tenderness or bleeding of the gums; and sexual dysfunction. Beta blockers can cause cold hands and feet. ACE inhibitors can cause swelling of the neck, face, and tongue. Ankle edema is not associated with taking a loop diuretic.

99. Answer: 3

Rationale: Because most cholesterol is synthesized when the body is in a state of fasting (between midnight and 3:00 am), HMG-CoA reductase inhibitors (lovastatin) are best taken in the evening.

5

Respiratory

Physical Exam & Diagnostic Tests

1. The family nurse practitioner is assessing an adult patient who is complaining of shortness of breath and chest discomfort. His respirations are shallow at 26 breaths/min. When evaluating the diaphragmatic excursion, it is determined that the diaphragm on the right side is slightly higher than on the left side. What is the best interpretation of these findings?
   1. This is normal because the liver is located on the right side.
   2. There may be atelectasis in the right lower lobe.
   3. Consolidation is present in the right lower lobe.
   4. This indicates the presence of severe chronic obstructive lung disease.

2. The family nurse practitioner knows that normal breath sounds that have a low pitch, soft intensity, and are heard best on inspiration over the posterior lung fields are called:
   1. Bronchial.
   2. Vesicular.
   3. Bronchovesicular.
   4. Rhonchi.

3. When examining a patient, the family nurse practitioner suspects a small pleural effusion. What would be the most sensitive diagnostic test to determine a small effusion?
   1. Chest ultrasound.
   2. Chest radiograph.
   3. Spirometry testing.
   4. Ventilation/perfusion scan.

4. When auscultating for vocal resonance in a patient with possible consolidation of lung tissue, the family nurse practitioner tells the patient to say "ninety-nine," and the voice remains loud and distinct over the area of suspected consolidation. What is this called?
   1. Tactile fremitus.
   2. Bronchophony.
   3. Whispered pectoriloquy.
   4. Egophony.

5. The family nurse practitioner understands that in percussion of the lungs, hyperresonance is:
   1. A normal finding in the adult patient.
   2. Common when the lungs are hyperinflated, like with chronic emphysema.
   3. Characterized by soft intensity, high pitch, short duration, and extremely dull quality.
   4. Characterized by loud intensity, high pitch, medium duration, and dull quality.

6. What is the correct procedure when percussing the anterior and posterior chest?
   1. Percuss the entire right side of the anterior chest and move to the left side.
   2. Begin at the upper left side of the posterior chest and compare with the respective anterior side, moving from front to back.
   3. Percuss systematically and symmetrically the intercostal spaces of the posterior chest, moving from the left to the right side, and then percuss the anterior chest.
   4. Percuss the posterior chest, and then measure for diaphragmatic excursion on the anterior chest.

7. The family nurse practitioner understands that pleural friction rubs are:
   1. Auscultated best in the lower anterolateral chest.
   2. Heard best at the end of expiration.
   3. Characterized by a continuous, low-pitched, snoring sound that is heard early in inspiration.
   4. Noted when the patient says "e-e-e" and the examiner hears through the stethoscope "a-a-a."

8. What are normal physiologic changes in the respiratory system of the geriatric patient?
   1. Increased residual volume.
   2. Increased ciliary action, resulting in a more forceful and recurrent cough.
   3. Increase in number of smaller alveoli with decreased residual capacity.
   4. Decrease in anteroposterior (AP) diameter of the rib cage with decreased lung expansion.

9. An older adult patient who recently traveled outside the country is presenting to your office with significant dyspnea. The patient recently returned from Japan on a 12-hour flight. The patient's lungs are clear, heart rate and blood pressure are mildly elevated, and oxygen saturation is 88%. The patient has bilateral 1+ pedal edema. What is the most important diagnostic study to complete emergently?
   1. Electrocardiogram (ECG).
   2. Ventilation-perfusion (V/Q) scan.
   3. Chest radiograph.
   4. Computed tomography pulmonary angiogram (CTPA).

10. When assessing for tactile fremitus, the family nurse practitioner knows that increased fremitus:
    1. Occurs when there is an obstruction in the transmission of vibrations.
    2. Occurs with consolidation or compression of lung tissue.
    3. Is the symmetric transmission of vibration through the chest wall.
    4. Is found in emphysema.

11. On assessment of the patient's respiratory status, crepitation is felt over the third rib at the midaxillary line on the left side. What is the interpretation of this finding?
    1. There is consolidation of fluid in the left lower lobe of the lung.
    2. Severe inflammation is present on the visceral pleural surfaces of the left lung.
    3. An increase in pressure has occurred in the pleural cavity of the right lung.
    4. Air is present in the subcutaneous tissue.

12. An important anatomic landmark on the anterior thoracic wall is the angle of Louis. Where on the thorax is this landmark present?
    1. The midnipple line on either side of the manubrium.
    2. At the manubriosternal junction.
    3. Midline at the base of the suprasternal notch.
    4. Just below the clavicle, but above the manubrium.

13. During the assessment of an older adult patient's respiratory status, the family nurse practitioner determines increased tactile fremitus posteriorly at the second intercostal space. What is the best interpretation of this finding?
    1. Increased air trapping in the alveoli on the affected side.
    2. Presence of fluid or solid mass within the lungs.
    3. Increased pressure in the bronchial tree.
    4. Presence of reactive airway disease.

14. When the lateral diameter of the chest is the same size as the anteroposterior (AP) diameter, the family nurse practitioner correctly identifies this finding as:
    1. A normal finding in a younger adult.
    2. Pectus carinatum.
    3. Pectus excavatum.
    4. Suggestive of obstructive lung disease.

15. **QSEN** The family nurse practitioner is planning a community screening program for lung cancer in older adult patients. What does the current evidence-based practice suggest?
    1. Bronchoscopy with biopsy for cytology should be done every 2–3 years for smokers.
    2. Low-dose computed tomography (LDCT) should be used in high-risk individuals.
    3. Routine screening for lung cancer does not decrease mortality in high-risk populations.
    4. Chest x-ray with comparison of previous x-ray is a sensitive test for lung cancer.

16. An adult patient comes to the clinic with the chief complaint of "coughing up blood" and night sweats. The patient has no history of respiratory or cardiac problems. Their vital signs are pulse of 96 beats/min, respirations of 28 breaths/min, blood pressure of 140/92 mm Hg, and a temperature of 99°F (37.2°C) orally. The initial diagnostic evaluation of this patient includes:
    1. Electrocardiogram, pulmonary function studies, and sputum cytology.
    2. Complete blood count (CBC), chest x-ray, and sputum smear for acid-fast bacillus.
    3. Arterial blood gas (ABG) studies, CBC, and chest x-ray.
    4. Referral for direct bronchoscopy with biopsy and complement fixation antibody titer.

17. An adult patient comes into the clinic complaining of increased fatigue and irritability. The patient has gained approximately 20 pounds over the last year. Although the patient states sleeping through the night, the partner says the patient seems somewhat restless. Based on these symptoms, what else should be determined?
    1. Presence of ongoing daytime sleepiness.
    2. History of depression.
    3. Fluctuations in blood pressure (BP).
    4. Recent changes in medications.

18. When assessing the pulmonary function studies of a patient, which assessment finding is seen in chronic obstructive disease, such as in emphysema?
    1. Decreased forced vital capacity (FVC) and decreased forced expiratory volume in 1 second (FEV_1).
    2. Decreased functional residual capacity (FRC) and residual volume (RV).
    3. Decreased RV and increased total lung capacity (TLC).
    4. Increased FEV_1 and TLC.

19. When interpreting purified protein derivative (PPD) skin tests in patients at a long-term care facility, the family nurse practitioner identifies positive results in individuals with:
    1. Redness or erythema at the site.
    2. Induration reaction ≥5 mm.
    3. Induration reaction ≥10 mm.
    4. Induration reaction up to 15 mm.

20. A 65-year old obese patient presents to the clinic with difficulty breathing. On examination, there is a low suspicion of a pulmonary embolism. Which of the following should the family nurse practitioner use to rule out the likelihood of a pulmonary embolism?
    1. Decreased platelets.
    2. Normal fibrin D-dimer.
    3. Normal chest x-ray.
    4. Normal activated partial thromboplastin time.

21. The family nurse practitioner knows that screening for lung cancer includes:
    1. Sputum sample in those with a diagnosis of chronic bronchitis.
    2. Annual computed tomography scan of the chest in asymptomatic individuals between the ages of 55 and 80 who have a 30 pack-year smoking history or greater and continue to smoke or have quit less than 15 years ago.
    3. Chest x-ray in all current smokers.
    4. Pulmonary function testing in those exposed to second-hand smoke for more than 20 years and who have a 5 pack-year smoking history between the ages of 40 and 80 years.

22. A patient tested positive for latent tuberculosis (TB) infection from a tuberculin skin test. What should the family nurse practitioner do next?
    1. Order a chest computed tomography (CT).
    2. Start isoniazid after getting liver function tests.
    3. Repeat test in 3 months.
    4. Assess for signs or symptoms suggestive of infection.

23. A young adult patient is seeing the family nurse practitioner to obtain routine vaccine testing for a nursing program. This patient has had the bacilli Calmette-Guerin (BCG) vaccine administered in another country. The family nurse practitioner knows that:
    1. A tuberculin skin test is not sufficient to test for latent tuberculosis infection (LTBI).
    2. Ordering an interferon-gamma release assay is preferred because of the vaccine.
    3. The student does not need to be tested because they received the vaccine.
    4. A TB titer is the most accurate way of reviewing the effectiveness of immunity.

24. A family nurse practitioner performing a lung assessment using percussion is aware that:
    1. Percussion is best performed lateral to medial and inferior to superior beginning in the anterior chest.
    2. Percussion should start medial to lateral moving superior to inferior beginning in the posterior chest.
    3. Patient positioning is not important to the effectiveness of the assessment.
    4. Patients should not raise their arms while the nurse practitioner is percussing laterally because this causes movement of the rib cage.

25. The family nurse practitioner is auscultating a patient's chest and asks the patient to say "ninety-nine." With the stethoscope, a clear transmission of the words is heard indicating increased lung density. Which voice sound does this describe?
    1. Egophony.
    2. Pleural friction rub.
    3. Rhonchal fremitus.
    4. Bronchophony.

26. An adult patient with chronic asthma is seen in the clinic complaining of vomiting and stomach cramps. He is confused and unsure what medications he is currently taking. His vital signs are blood pressure of 158/92 mm Hg, pulse of 152 beats/min and irregular, and respirations of 28 breaths/min and shallow. What STAT diagnostic study should be obtained?
    1. Serum electrolytes.
    2. Digoxin level.
    3. Theophylline level.
    4. Arterial blood gases.

Disorders

27. A patient with severe chronic obstructive pulmonary disease (COPD) says he experiences fatigue and dyspnea with activity. In determining his activity level, the family nurse practitioner understands:
    1. Patients with moderate to severe COPD should avoid strenuous activity and conserve their energy.
    2. Pulmonary rehabilitation has been shown to improve symptoms and quality of life in everyday activities.
    3. It is important to first maximize pharmacologic therapy before increasing any type of activity level.
    4. Supplemental oxygen would be the best, most cost-effect choice for this patient.

28. In treating a patient with acute bronchitis, the family nurse practitioner understands:
    1. Most patients will need antibiotic therapy.
    2. There is strong evidence to support the use of over-the-counter (OTC) preparations.
    3. A β agonist should always be prescribed.
    4. Symptom management should be the primary focus of treatment.

29. A patient was hit in the chest. Which assessment finding would suggest a serious respiratory complication requiring immediate attention?
    1. Complaints of increased pain over the affected area.
    2. Oximetry readings consistently about 90%.
    3. Decreased breath sounds on the affected side.
    4. Fever of 102°F (38.9°C) and increased sputum production.

30. A patient with chronic obstructive pulmonary disease (COPD) smokes one pack of cigarettes daily. In approaching the patient about smoking cessation, the family nurse practitioner knows:
    1. Transitioning to e-cigarettes is a safe and effective alternative to smoking cessation.
    2. Smoking cessation does not significantly change the course of COPD.
    3. Counseling does not significantly increase quit rates over other strategies.
    4. Smoking cessation counseling should be done at every clinic visit.

31. The family nurse practitioner understands which of the following characteristics is more likely to occur when the adult patient has pneumonia (caused by *Streptococcus pneumoniae*) rather than bronchitis?
    1. Purulent sputum production.
    2. Nonproductive cough.
    3. Dyspnea.
    4. Wheezing.

32. **QSEN** A young adult is recovering from tuberculosis. What information should be included in a teaching plan for home care?
    1. It is critical for the young adult to take medications at the prescribed time; do not skip doses or allow the supply to run out.
    2. Respiratory isolation procedures need to be carried out at home; the young adult should avoid contact with immediate adult-gerontology primary care members.
    3. It will be necessary for the young adult to return to the clinic every week to have his or her sputum checked for viable bacteria.
    4. The young adult may experience a rash along with nausea and vomiting from the medications; if this occurs, he or she should decrease the dosage.

33. What would be a priority intervention for a patient experiencing respiratory arrest, who has a pulse?
    1. Starting chest compressions at 30 compressions followed by two breaths.
    2. Starting rescue breathing, which is one breath every 5–6 seconds or about 10–12 breaths/min.
    3. Giving oxygen using a rebreathing mask at 10 L/min.
    4. Pinching the nose and giving two breaths.

34. A patient comes to the primary care practice clinic complaining of difficulty breathing. What is most important to establish initially in this patient?
    1. Type of activity that produces the dyspnea.
    2. Presence of consolidation on chest x-ray.
    3. Arterial blood gases (ABGs) with respect to oxygen pressures.
    4. Presence of bilateral breath sounds over the lower lobes.

35. A patient's history strongly suggests the possibility of a foreign body in the bronchi. What assessment finding would support this diagnosis?
    1. Coughing and unilateral wheezing.
    2. Presence of crepitation on the anterior chest wall.
    3. Retraction of the lower chest wall with decreased breath sounds.
    4. A friction rub heard over the area of the bronchi.

36. A 22-year-old male comes to the office complaining of chest pain and shortness of breath. He states the problems started suddenly after running sprints in basketball practice. He states he has no past history of pulmonary problems. He is about 72 inches tall and 145 lb, with pulse rate of 118 beats/min, respiratory rate of 30 breaths/min, decreased breath sounds, and hyperresonance over the left lung. Based on these findings, what is the best diagnosis for the patient?
    1. Spontaneous pneumothorax.
    2. Exercise-induced asthma.
    3. Pulmonary edema.
    4. Acute bronchiectasis.

37. A young adult presents at the clinic with complaints of tingling in the face and hands, sudden shortness of breath, and vague chest discomfort. The patient appears very anxious and denies any history of respiratory problems. On examination, hands are cool to the touch; vital signs include respirations of 34 breaths/min, pulse regular at 100 beats/min, blood pressure 110/76 mm Hg, and normal temperature. Respiratory examination reveals bilateral breath sounds with tachypnea, no adventitious sounds, and normal percussion and visual examination of the chest. What is the best immediate treatment?
    1. Relaxation techniques and encouraging controlled diaphragmatic breathing.
    2. Two puffs of short-acting bronchodilator (albuterol) with metered-dose inhaler.
    3. Oxygen at 4 L and arterial blood gases (ABGs) after 30 minutes.
    4. Rebreathing into paper bag to increase $Paco_2$ levels.

38. A patient with newly diagnosed coronary obstructive pulmonary disease is being discharged from the hospital. What information is important to include in the home care teaching?
    1. Use the bronchodilator before exercising.
    2. Maintain bed rest for the first few days at home.
    3. Decrease the amount of fluid intake to prevent fluid overload.
    4. Use the inhaled corticosteroid inhaler only when significantly short of breath.

39. Age-associated changes that increase the risk for respiratory symptoms in the older adult patient include an increase in:
    1. Compliance of the chest wall.
    2. Diameter of the trachea and bronchi.
    3. Lung parenchymal elasticity.
    4. Force of cough.

40. An adult patient arrives at the family practice clinic complaining of difficulty breathing, a cough, and chest pain. History indicates that she was discharged from the hospital 2 days ago, after a cesarean section, and has a 15 pack-per year smoking history. What would be an appropriate action?
    1. Obtain a sputum specimen for culture and sensitivity.
    2. Order a chest x-ray, pulmonary computed tomography (CT) scan, and angiogram.
    3. Perform spirometry testing.
    4. Immediately transfer to the emergency department.

41. The family nurse practitioner is aware that the flu or influenza:
    1. Can be caused by receiving a live attenuated influenza vaccine when one's resistance is low.
    2. Is characterized by a slow, insidious onset of chills, fever, and muscle aches.
    3. In older adults, may persist for weeks and increase the prevalence of bacterial pneumonia.
    4. Is primarily contagious in the early autumn and spring.

42. An adult patient with a history of asthma calls to tell the family nurse practitioner that she is achieving 65% of her personal best on the peak flowmeter. She is talking in phrases and sounds calm. What advice would the family nurse practitioner give this patient?
    1. Call an ambulance immediately.
    2. Use a bronchodilator now and come in for evaluation in the office today.
    3. Use an inhaled corticosteroid inhaler now and every 4 hours as needed.
    4. Refer to a pulmonologist.

43. An older adult patient is evaluated by the family nurse practitioner for a complaint of cough, fever, pleuritic chest pain, and sputum production. In gathering a history on this patient, it is most important to know if the patient has:
    1. Received the pneumococcal vaccine.
    2. Traveled out of the country.
    3. Pets in the household.
    4. Recently changed or started new medications.

44. An older adult patient presents with signs and symptoms that suggest community-acquired pneumonia (CAP).

What assessment findings are specific to an older adult patient with this condition?
    1. Chest pain with inspiration.
    2. Confusion/disorientation with or without a low-grade fever.
    3. Productive cough.
    4. Fever with leukocytosis.

45. In developing a plan for a healthy older patient with typical pneumonia, the family nurse practitioner understands that 60%–65% of community-acquired pneumonia is caused by which organism?
    1. *Haemophilus influenzae.*
    2. *Klebsiella pneumoniae.*
    3. *Mycobacterium tuberculosis.*
    4. *Streptococcus pneumoniae.*

46. What would be most appropriate to include in the health promotion plan for an older adult patient who is at risk for developing pneumonia?
    1. Administer the pneumococcal vaccine annually.
    2. Administer the influenza vaccine annually.
    3. Perform sputum culture annually along with a chest x-ray.
    4. Perform purified protein derivative (PPD) skin test every 3–5 years.

47. The family nurse practitioner evaluates an older adult patient with a current history of alcoholism. The patient presents with an elevated temperature, congested cough with rusty sputum, and occasional chills. The suspected diagnosis is bacterial pneumonia. The Gram stain sputum smear would most likely reveal which organism?
    1. *Haemophilus influenzae.*
    2. *Klebsiella pneumoniae.*
    3. *Staphylococcus aureus.*
    4. *Pseudomonas aeruginosa.*

48. An older adult patient residing in a nursing home has recently been exposed to tuberculosis (TB). During the contact investigation, the family nurse practitioner interprets the initial purified protein derivative (PPD) skin test to be negative. Which plan would be most appropriate at this time?
    1. Evaluate the patient in another year.
    2. Repeat PPD test in 8–10 weeks.
    3. Immediately begin ethambutol.
    4. Evaluate the patient in 6 months because the patient is asymptomatic at this time.

49. Which two statements are accurate regarding sarcoidosis?
    1. Is a noninfectious, multisystem granulomatous disease.
    2. Affects only the lungs.
    3. May resolve spontaneously within 2 years.
    4. Commonly affects the older and frail adult.
    5. High-dose oral steroids are always prescribed.

50. The family nurse practitioner knows that Horner syndrome, a condition that can cause unilateral pupillary constriction and anhidrosis, is often associated with:
    1. Chronic bronchitis.
    2. Pulmonary tuberculosis.
    3. Pulmonary sulcus (Pancoast) tumor.
    4. Pulmonary embolism.

51. An adult patient who smokes presents with complaints of orthopnea. The family nurse practitioner notes on examination distention of chest wall veins, and mild edema of the head and neck. The family nurse practitioner recognizes this condition as:
    1. Thyroid abnormality.
    2. Chronic bronchitis with mild heart failure.
    3. Asthma with fluid retention.
    4. Superior vena cava syndrome (SVCS).

52. An older adult patient presents with postural hypotension, and laboratory studies reveal hyponatremia. The patient is currently not taking any medications that may cause this. Which condition is likely the cause of these findings?
    1. Respiratory acidosis.
    2. Blunt chest trauma.
    3. Bronchogenic carcinoma.
    4. Bronchitis.

53. During a routine follow-up visit for a patient with asthma, the patient states that she has been doing fine except that, when she goes out for dinner, she has increased bronchospasm and wheezing. Which of the following would be an appropriate response by the family nurse practitioner?
    1. "Have you been taking your medication?"
    2. "Do you usually have wine with dinner?"
    3. "I recommend you do not go out for dinner."
    4. "Does going out to dinner make you feel stressed?"

54. The family nurse practitioner is evaluating an adult with symptoms characteristic of obstructive sleep apnea. An overnight polysomnography is ordered. What is the characteristic result of this study that would be indicative of sleep apnea?
    1. Loud snoring all night long.
    2. Oxygen desaturation and 10-second periods of apnea.
    3. Frequent periods of brief arousal during sleep.
    4. Periods of 5-second apnea with brief arousal.

55. The family nurse practitioner is screening an older adult patient for problems related to obstructive sleep apnea (OSA). What risk factors are typically associated with this condition?
    1. Usage of sleep aids.
    2. Weight loss.
    3. Frequent nighttime sleep disturbance.
    4. Daytime hyperactivity.

56. A patient comes to the clinic complaining of difficulty breathing, lethargy, and coughing up blood in the sputum. They have no history of chronic illness or major health problems. The family nurse practitioner orders diagnostic tests to determine the problem. What diagnostic test results would require immediate treatment of this patient?
    1. Positive sputum smear for acid-fast bacillus.
    2. Sputum culture positive for *Pneumocystis carinii*.
    3. Presence of hemolysis on complement fixation test.
    4. Oxygen saturation 94%, leukocyte count >5000 WBCs/mm^3.

57. When determining the classification of asthma control in an adult patient with symptoms fewer than 2 days per week, no interference with normal activity, no reports of nighttime awakening, and use of a short-acting β_2 agonist two times per week, the family nurse practitioner would classify the patient as:
    1. Well controlled.
    2. Partly controlled.
    3. Uncontrolled.
    4. Out of control.

58. When examining the chest x-ray of a patient with an initial tuberculosis infection, you would expect to see changes most often in what part of the lung?
    1. Trachea.
    2. Upper lobes.
    3. Bronchi.
    4. Lower lobes.

59. A patient reports being exposed to secondhand smoke frequently at their place of employment. The family nurse practitioner knows that secondhand smoke exposure:
    1. Does not increase the patient's risk of cancer.
    2. Decreases with risk of stroke by approximately 10%.
    3. Could cause lung cancer even though the patient does not smoke.
    4. Does not increase the risk of heart disease.

60. How would an adult, who has an FEV$_1$ greater than 80%, has been experiencing nighttime awakenings (four to five times per week) and using a short-acting β_2 agonist three to four times per week, and reports minimal limitation to normal activity, be classified?
    1. Well controlled.
    2. Partly controlled.
    3. Uncontrolled.
    4. Severe persistent.

61. An adult female comes to the clinic with complaints of cough, clear rhinorrhea, and a low-grade fever for 2 days. The family nurse practitioner diagnoses acute bronchitis. The family nurse practitioner knows that with acute bronchitis:
    1. The patient will likely need antibiotics.
    2. A cough can last for 10–20 days.
    3. Routine sputum cultures are helpful because of nasopharyngeal colonization.
    4. Only 5%–10% of acute bronchitis cases have a viral etiology.

Pharmacology

62. An adult patient with asthma has had uncontrolled symptoms after starting treatment 3 months ago. Before considering any step up in treatment, the family nurse should consider that the current treatment may be ineffective because:
    1. The patient continues to use albuterol for shortness of breath.
    2. The patient is using inhaled corticosteroids only twice daily.
    3. The patient is using the inhaler incorrectly.
    4. The patient is taking montelukast concurrently for seasonal allergies.

63. **QSEN** The family nurse practitioner is following up on a patient who is experiencing acute asthma problems. Albuterol (Proventil) by metered-dose inhaler (MDI) (2 puffs) has been ordered as treatment. Which patient response would indicate to the family nurse practitioner that the patient understands how to take the medication?
    1. "I will take 1 puff of the medication, and then wait a minute before taking the second puff."
    2. "I will take 2 puffs of the medication every 4 hours, even if I am not short of breath."
    3. "It is important for me to take this medication on a regular cycle to prevent future attacks."
    4. "I will take 2 puffs, one right after the other, whenever I begin to get short of breath."

64. A patient with chronic obstructive pulmonary disease (COPD) complains of increased dyspnea and sputum volume over the last 2 days. The patient presents with a respiratory rate of 20 breaths/min, resting oxygen saturation of 88% on room air, and no cyanosis or peripheral edema. The patient is currently taking salmeterol (Serevent) 50 mcg Diskus one puff every 12 hours with tiotropium (Spiriva Handihaler) 18 mcg inhaled two puffs daily. What therapy should the nurse practitioner start to improve lung function and recovery time of the patient?
    1. Supplemental oxygen therapy.
    2. Azithromycin (Zithromax) 250 mg 2 tablets now and 1 tablet daily for 4 days.
    3. Prednisone 40 mg daily for 5 days.
    4. Theophylline 300 mg daily for 7 days.

65. A patient who was recently diagnosed with tuberculosis calls the clinic because her urine is reddish orange. The patient is taking isoniazid, rifampin (Rifadin), and pyrazinamide. What would be an appropriate response for the family nurse practitioner to make?
    1. "This is a urinary tract infection symptom; drink plenty of fluids."
    2. "This is a normal response to the rifampin."
    3. "This often is an indication of liver toxicity. Stop the medications."

4. "This is indicative of bleeding. You must see a physician immediately."

66. A patient with a history of bronchial asthma is seen in the clinic for increased episodes of difficulty breathing. He has been taking theophylline 100 mg PO tid. He is 40 years old and obese with an 18 pack-year history of cigarette smoking and excessive intake of coffee daily. He eats a low-carbohydrate, high-protein diet. Which identified factors decrease the therapeutic effects of the theophylline?
    1. Age and gender.
    2. Coffee intake and weight.
    3. Age and weight.
    4. Smoking history and diet.

67. **QSEN** An adult patient comes to the clinic with complaints of increased difficulty breathing over the past few days. Patient has a history of asthma, coronary artery disease, and recently diagnosed hypertension. Examination reveals no jugular vein distention and no productive cough. Breath sounds are present, but expiratory wheezes are noted bilaterally. Patient denies any chest pain. Vital signs include pulse of 72 beats/min, respirations of 34 breaths/min, and blood pressure of 170/100 mm Hg. Current medications are albuterol (Proventil) inhaler 2 puffs every 4 hours prn for wheezing, nitroglycerin transdermal patch for coronary artery disease, and propranolol (Inderal) 60 mg PO bid for hypertension. What is the best treatment for this patient?
    1. Discontinue propranolol (Inderal) and begin amlodipine (Norvasc) 5 mg PO daily.
    2. Start a prednisone burst with dosage taper over 1 week.
    3. Discontinue propranolol (Inderal) and begin atenolol (Tenormin) 50 mg PO daily.
    4. Start beclomethasone (Beclovent) inhaler 2 puffs three to four times daily.

68. What is the recommended range for maintaining serum theophylline levels?
    1. 0.05–2 mcg/mL.
    2. 10–20 mcg/mL.
    3. 20–25 mcg/mL.
    4. 30–40 mcg/mL.

69. An otherwise recently healthy nonsmoking patient presents with a dry cough for the past 5 months. She has a history of hypertension and gastroesophageal reflux disorder (GERD). She is on ranitidine (Zantac) 150 mg PO bid and lisinopril (Zestril) 20 mg PO daily. Which treatment would yield the highest probability of success?
    1. Switching from ranitidine to omeprazole.
    2. Starting albuterol (Proventil) inhaler, 90 mcg every 4–6 hours as needed.
    3. Starting dextromethorphan 20 mg every 4 hours as needed.
    4. Switching from lisinopril to amlodipine.

70. An immunocompromised patient in a long-term facility has a roommate who has been diagnosed with active tuberculosis. When should the patient be started on latent tuberculosis infection (LTBI) treatment?
    1. As soon as possible and initiated at the time of the tuberculosis skin testing (TST).
    2. In 72 hours after purified protein derivative (PPD) skin test results are obtained.
    3. Only if PPD skin test results are positive.
    4. In 3 months if the repeated skin test is positive.

71. In adults with asthma, the most common reason outpatient treatment fails, resulting in hospitalization, is:
    1. Exposure to allergens.
    2. Increased use of steroids.
    3. Improper inhaler technique.
    4. Use of cromolyn inhalers.

72. Which can elevate theophylline levels?
    1. Concomitant treatment with cimetidine (Tagamet).
    2. Intravenous ampicillin.
    3. Heavy smoking.
    4. History of seizure disorder.

73. A patient with a long history of chronic obstructive pulmonary disease (COPD) has noticed an increase in dyspnea and a change in sputum over the past few days, with increased amounts of thick, yellow-green mucus and congestion. What would be the appropriate therapy?
    1. Loratadine (Claritin) 10 mg PO daily.
    2. Amoxicillin/clavulanate (Augmentin) 500 mg/125 mg PO three times daily for 10 days.
    3. Acetaminophen with codeine 300 mg/30 mg PO every 6 hours as needed.
    4. Beclomethasone (Qvar) 40 mcg metered-dose inhaler 2 puffs every 4 hours as needed.

74. Which medication is most effective in promoting a decrease in airway inflammation and providing long-term medication coverage in a patient with asthma?
    1. Montelukast (Singulair).
    2. Beclomethasone (Vanceril; Beclovent).
    3. Albuterol (Proventil; Ventolin).
    4. Salmeterol (Serevent).

75. The family nurse practitioner is planning regular daily treatment for a patient with asthma. Which is the preferred medication for the asthmatic patient who is not currently experiencing an exacerbation?
    1. Antibiotic.
    2. Inhaled corticosteroid.
    3. β_2 agonist.
    4. Leukotriene receptor antagonist.

76. Patients with asthma need to be instructed to:
    1. Begin inhaled corticosteroids as soon as symptoms appear.
    2. Take 1–2 puffs of β_2 agonist as needed using metered-dose inhaler.
    3. Use inhaled corticosteroids when they experience bronchospasm.
    4. Start antibiotic regimen when they experience bronchospasm.

77. The family nurse practitioner understands that one of the following over-the-counter (OTC) preparations in high doses can cause euphoria, disorientation, paranoia, and hallucinations and has been known to be abused by adolescents. Which OTC preparation is it?
    1. Pseudoephedrine.
    2. Diphenhydramine.
    3. Guaifenesin.
    4. Dextromethorphan.

78. An adult patient is seen in the clinic complaining of increased difficulty breathing and an intermittent productive cough that worsens in the evening. The history reveals that the patient has a 20 pack-year history of smoking. Breath sounds are clear to auscultation, there is no evidence of fever, and chest radiography is within normal limits. The family nurse practitioner instructs the patient concerning the importance of smoking cessation and fluid therapy. After that, what does the nurse practitioner prescribe?
    1. Erythromycin 500 mg PO qid × 14 days.
    2. Albuterol 2 mg PO tid.
    3. Acetylcysteine (Mucomyst) 10 mL 10% solution nebulized q4h prn.
    4. Cough, cold, and antiinflammatories for symptom control.

79. When initiating preventive care to decrease the incidence of pneumonia in patients in an extended-care facility, the family nurse practitioner would identify high-risk patients as those who receive immunosuppressive therapy, use antibiotics frequently, have cognitive impairment, and those taking:
    1. β_1 adrenergic blockers.
    2. Calcium channel blockers.
    3. Diuretics.
    4. Histamine (H_2) antagonists.

80. An older adult patient presents with new complaints of dyspnea, cough, fatigue, and dependent edema that has been worsening over the past few days. What should the family nurse practitioner consider when planning treatment?
    1. Levofloxacin (Levaquin) 750 mg PO bid for 7 days.
    2. Referral for hospitalization for evaluation of heart function.
    3. Furosemide (Lasix) 40 mg PO daily.
    4. Addition of a calcium channel blocker to the patient's medications.

81. A patient with a history of Parkinson's disease has an initial positive tuberculosis (TB) skin test, and isoniazid (INH) is ordered for treatment of latent TB infection. Before beginning INH, it is important for the family nurse practitioner to determine:
    1. If the patient's Parkinson's condition is being treated with levodopa (Larodopa).
    2. How long the patient has been diagnosed with Parkinson's disease.
    3. How much respiratory compromise the patient is currently experiencing.
    4. The adequacy of urine output and renal function.

82. An adult patient with a history of chronic obstructive pulmonary disease presents to the clinic with increased dyspnea, temperature of 102°F (39°C), pulse of 104 beats/min, respirations of 44 breaths/min, and O_2 saturation of 84%. Physical exam reveals diffuse rales and rhonchi bilaterally. Medications include atenolol (Tenormin) 25 mg PO daily, prednisone (Deltasone) 10 mg PO daily, ipratropium bromide (Atrovent) 1–2 puffs 18 mcg qid prn, and fluticasone and salmeterol (Advair Diskus 100/50) 2 puffs bid. The family nurse practitioner's preliminary diagnosis is pneumonia, pending chest x-ray results. Which medication puts this patient at risk to become immunocompromised?
    1. Atenolol.
    2. Prednisone.
    3. Ipratropium.
    4. Fluticasone and salmeterol.

83. What is the pharmacologic treatment shown to be superior in multiple studies for the treatment of chronic obstructive pulmonary disease by reducing exacerbation, lowering cost, and improving lung function and quality of life?
    1. Albuterol (Proventil) metered dose inhaler.
    2. Theophylline (Theo-24).
    3. Ipratropium bromide (Atrovent) metered dose inhaler.
    4. Ipratropium bromide and albuterol (Proventil) combined.

84. The family nurse practitioner has diagnosed an adult patient with community-acquired pneumonia (CAP). What should the family nurse practitioner prescribe for this healthy patient with no comorbidities and no previous antibiotic use within the last 3 months?
    1. Doxycycline 100 mg PO bid for 10 days.
    2. Amoxicillin (Amoxil) 500 mg PO tid for 10 days.
    3. Azithromycin (Zithromax) 500 mg PO once, and then 250 mg daily for 4 days.
    4. Ciprofloxacin (Cipro) 500 mg PO daily for 7 days.

85. An adult male comes into the office with a complaint of a chronic cough. The cough has persisted for 6 weeks and continued following resolution of his upper respiratory infection. The family nurse practitioner understands that:
    1. This cough is chronic and is likely caused by cigarette use or exposure to secondhand smoke.
    2. This is a subacute cough and is likely postinfectious.
    3. The cough has lasted longer than 3 weeks, which means it is not related to past infection.
    4. The patient should be worked up for gastroesophageal reflux disease (GERD).

86. An adult male is started on ciprofloxacin (Cipro) 500 mg PO bid daily for 60 days for possible exposure to anthrax. Five days later, on return to the clinic, he notes increased pain in his posterior ankle. Understanding the potential complications with fluoroquinolone therapy, the family nurse practitioner knows:
    1. The posterior ankle pain is an unrelated condition.
    2. This is a known side effect and the ciprofloxacin (Cipro) should be continued as prescribed.
    3. This is a known adverse reaction and the ciprofloxacin (Cipro) should be discontinued.
    4. Ciprofloxacin (Cipro) should not be used empirically to treat anthrax exposure.

87. An adult teacher comes to the office with a loud cough starting 2 days before. She says that several children in her fourth-grade class have been out sick because of whooping cough. There is a high probability of exposure to *Bordetella pertussis*. Which treatment option does the family nurse practitioner think is the best?
    1. Watchful waiting to see if the cough clears up in the next few days.
    2. Doxycycline 100 mg PO bid daily for 7 days.
    3. Azithromycin (Zithromax) 500 mg PO once, and then 250 mg PO daily for 4 days.
    4. Oseltamivir (Tamiflu) 75 mg PO bid daily for 5 days.

88. During a first-time office visit, the family nurse practitioner sees an adult female with a history of asthma. She had been using albuterol (Proventil) metered-dose inhaler (MDI) one inhalation twice monthly over the last several years. More recently, she has been using her MDI inhaler five to seven times per week. Based on the Global Initiative for Asthma (GINA) guidelines, the family nurse practitioner diagnoses partly controlled asthma and starts her on "Step 2" therapy. What does Step 2 therapy include?
    1. Fluticasone and salmeterol (Advair) 250 mg/50 mg one inhalation bid.
    2. Fluticasone (Flovent) 44 mcg two inhalations daily.
    3. Fluticasone and salmeterol (Advair) 100 mg/50 mg one inhalation bid.
    4. Salmeterol (Serevent) 42 mcg one inhalation bid.

89. An older adult female comes in for a follow-up for chronic obstructive pulmonary disease (COPD). She notes an increased frequency of morning headaches and daytime somnolence. A complete blood count notes that her hematocrit is 52%. The family nurse practitioner understands that a common but not always recognized complication of COPD this patient could have is:
    1. Acute respiratory failure.
    2. Cor pulmonale.
    3. Depression.
    4. Nocturnal oxygen desaturation.

90. An adult patient in the family nurse practitioner's office has been diagnosed with community-acquired pneumonia (CAP). According to the Infectious Disease Society of America and American Thoracic Society (IDSA/ATS) joint guidelines for CAP, criteria indicating the probable need for immediate admission to an inpatient facility includes which three findings?
    1. White blood cell count (WBC) of 2500 cells/mm^3.
    2. Temperature of 96.2°F (36.8°C).
    3. Respiratory rate of 30 breaths/min.
    4. Platelet count of 165,000 cells/mm^3.
    5. Blood, urea, nitrogen (BUN) of 32 mg/dL.

91. The family nurse practitioner is teaching a patient about the role of medications in the treatment of asthma. Which statement by the patient would require further teaching?
    1. "My albuterol is my quick-relief medication."
    2. "The salmeterol that I take provides me with long-term control."
    3. "I do not need to use a spacer with my metered-dose inhaler (MDI)."
    4. "I need to use my peak flow meter to self-monitor how I am doing."

92. The family nurse practitioner is treating a patient with community-acquired pneumonia. There has been a high rate of macrolide-resistant *Streptococcus pneumoniae* in the area. What should the patient be started on?
    1. Clarithromycin 500 mg twice daily for 5 days.
    2. Doxycycline 100 mg twice daily for 5 days.
    3. Amoxicillin 1 g three times daily for 10 days.
    4. Levofloxacin 750 mg daily for 5 days.

93. The family nurse practitioner is treating a patient recently diagnosed with interstitial pneumonitis. The nurse practitioner knows that this was most likely caused by
    1. Methadone.
    2. Amiodarone.
    3. Propranolol.
    4. Amlodipine.

94. Which two medications are prescribed and used in smoking cessation?
    1. Cetirizine (Zyrtec).
    2. Valacyclovir (Valtrex).
    3. Varenicline (Chantix).
    4. Bupropion (Zyban).
    5. Lisinopril (Zestril).

5 Respiratory Answers & Rationales

Physical Exam & Diagnostic Tests

1. Answer: 1

Rationale: This is a normal finding because of the anatomic location of the bulk of the liver. Atelectasis and consolidation present with normal diaphragmatic movement, but with dullness to percussion over the affected area. Severe obstructive lung disease results in hyperinflation and limited diaphragmatic excursion but is bilateral.

2. Answer: 2

Rationale: Vesicular breath sounds are normal low-pitched, low-intensity sounds heard in the peripheral lung fields. Inspiration is 2.5 times longer than the expiratory phase. Bronchial breath sounds, normally heard over the trachea and larynx, are high-pitched loud sounds with a shortened inspiratory and lengthened expiratory phase. Bronchovesicular breath sounds that are heard mainly where fewer alveoli are located, which is over the second intercostal space anteriorly and between the scapulae posteriorly, have a moderate pitch and intensity with equal duration of expiratory and inspiratory sounds. Rhonchi are adventitious breath sounds that are usually not heard during normal respiration.

3. Answer: 1

Rationale: A pleural effusion should always be confirmed by ultrasonography because this will detect effusions as low as 5–50 mL, as will a CT scan. A chest radiograph does not always detect small effusions. Spirometry testing will suggest restrictive lung disease but will not identify the potential cause. A ventilation-perfusion scan will identify lung perfusion, but not lung effusion.

4. Answer: 2

Rationale: Greater clarity and increased loudness of spoken sounds are defined as bronchophony. If bronchophony is extreme (e.g., in the presence of consolidation of the lungs), even a whisper can be heard clearly and intelligibly through the stethoscope (whispered pectoriloquy). During auscultation, if the patient is speaking, their voice is normally heard as soft, muffled, and indistinct. When you ask the patient to say "ninety-nine," during auscultation, you will hear an abnormally clear distinct sound of ninety-nine, if there is lung consolidation. Whispered pectoriloquy is exaggerated bronchophony and is heard through a stethoscope when the patient whispers a series of words (e.g., "one-two-three"). In egophony, the spoken voice has a nasal or bleating quality when heard through a stethoscope, and the spoken "e-e-e" sounds like "a-a-a." Tactile fremitus is a palpable vibration of the thoracic wall that is produced when the patient speaks.

5. Answer: 2

Rationale: Hyperresonance is a percussion assessment finding suggestive of air trapping, which can be found in obstructive lung conditions like emphysema. It is characterized by very loud intensity, very low pitch, long duration, and a booming quality. It is not a normal finding.

6. Answer: 3

Rationale: Both the anterior and posterior chest should be percussed systematically and symmetrically at 4- to 5-cm intervals over the intercostal spaces, moving from left to right. Begin posteriorly with patient sitting with head bent forward and arms folded. As percussion moves laterally and anteriorly have the patient lift their arms up. Care is needed to ensure percussion is done in the intercostal spaces moving superior to inferior and medial to lateral. Diaphragmatic excursion is usually measured only on the posterior chest.

7. Answer: 1

Rationale: Pleural friction rubs are loud, dry, creaking, or grating sounds produced by the rubbing together of inflamed and roughened pleural surfaces. Rubs are heard best during the latter part of inspiration and the beginning of expiration, and in the lower anterolateral chest in which the lung expands the most. A continuous, low-pitched, snoring sound that is heard early in inspiration is characteristic of sonorous rhonchi. Egophony is noted when the patient says "e-e-e," and the examiner hears through the stethoscope "a-a-a," which is suggestive of lung consolidation.

8. Answer: 1

Rationale: With aging, the number of alveoli decreases. The alveoli become rigid and lose their recoil and elasticity, which affects the patient's ability to exhale effectively. This increases a patient's residual volume (the amount of air left in the chest after expiration). Residual volume increases, whereas basilar inflation and ability to expel foreign matter decrease. The AP diameter of the chest increases, as seen in patients with kyphosis.

9. Answer: 4

Rationale: Given the patient's recent 12-hour flight, the patient is at high risk for deep vein thrombosis and subsequent pulmonary embolism. The best test choice that would show a pulmonary embolism is the CTPA. A V/Q scan is useful only in hemodynamically stable patients with a normal chest x-ray, which would need to be completed before the V/Q scan. An ECG may have some nonspecific changes but is not diagnostic. A chest radiograph may likely be normal. Spirometry may be abnormal, but not specific. The patient will need emergent care.

10. Answer: 2

Rationale: Consolidation or compression of lung tissue will cause an increase in fremitus, which is noted with lobar pneumonia. Decreased fremitus occurs with obstruction of vibration, like in emphysema, pneumothorax, or obstructed bronchus. Symmetric transmission of vibration is a normal finding.

11. Answer: 4

Rationale: Crepitation or crepitus (also called subcutaneous emphysema) usually results from air bubbles under the skin caused by a leakage of air into the subcutaneous tissue. Infection by a gas-producing organism is a less common cause. Crepitation always requires attention. Severe inflammation of the pleural surface would not have a palpable abnormality. Fluid consolidation would cause an increased asymmetric fremitus on palpation.

12. Answer: 2

Rationale: This landmark can be used to determine the position of the second rib and intercostal space and corresponding spaces below that level. The angle of Louis (manubriosternal junction) is a visible and palpable angle of the sternum at the point in which the second rib attaches to the sternum.

13. Answer: 2

Rationale: Fluid or a solid mass will increase the transmission of vibration. Increased air trapping decreases or masks the transmission of vibration. A reactive airway results in wheezing because of mucous and inflamed airways. Increased pressure in the bronchial tree is not measurable and will not cause asymmetric vibratory changes.

14. Answer: 4

Rationale: The adult chest is usually symmetric and the AP diameter is often half the lateral diameter. Pigeon chest (pectus carinatum) is a forward protrusion of the sternum with the ribs sloping back. Funnel chest (pectus excavatum) is a depression of the sternum. Barrel chest occurs when the AP diameter equals the transverse diameter and is usually a sign of advancing obstructive lung disease.

15. Answer: 2

Rationale: According to 2013 guidelines, the U.S. Preventive Services Task Force recommends an annual screening for lung cancer with low-dose computed tomography in adults aged 55–80 years who have a calculated smoking history of 30 packs per year and currently smoke or have quit within the last 15 years. This should be discontinued after they have stopped smoking after 15 years. Current evidence-based research does support routine screening for lung cancer in the general population. There is insufficient evidence that lung cancer screening by x-ray or sputum cytology reduces mortality. Bronchoscopy with biopsy is a diagnostic test, not a screening test.

16. Answer: 2

Rationale: The patient should be initially evaluated for tuberculosis, which includes a chest x-ray, sputum smear for acid-fast bacillus, and a CBC. Pulmonary function studies, ABG studies, and bronchoscopy are not indicated initially. Complement fixation studies are done to diagnose atypical pneumonia.

17. Answer: 1

Rationale: A patient with recent weight gain and restless sleep is at risk for having obstructive sleep apnea (OSA). Ongoing daytime sleepiness is the hallmark sign of OSA. Although recurring depression could be a cause, a provider should consider physical causes of presenting symptoms first. Fluctuations in BP, including hypertension, can be seen in OSA, but they would not cause the fatigue and nighttime restlessness. Recent changes in medication should be evaluated but are unlikely to cause all his symptoms. Although men are two to three times as likely to have OSA at a younger age, the number of women with OSA is equal approaching menopause.

18. Answer: 1

Rationale: Hyperinflation caused by air trapping causes an increase in FRC, RV, and TLC, which may be twice normal. A corresponding decrease in FVC and FEV_1 occurs. This causes a flattening of the diaphragm, decreased inspiratory efficiency, and increased work of breathing.

19. Answer: 3

Rationale: Positive interpretation of PPD skin test results are as follows, based on the criteria from the Centers for Disease Control and Prevention:

Induration	Positive Purified Protein Derivative Skin Test Result
≥5 mm	Individuals with human immunodeficiency virus infection
	Individuals in recent close contact with persons who have active TB
	Individuals with chest x-ray indicating healed TB
≥10 mm	Medically underserved individuals
	Intravenous drug users
	Residents in long-term care facilities and health care workers
≥15 mm	All individuals

TB, Tuberculosis.

20. Answer: 2

Rationale: Fibrin D-dimer is normally <500 ng/mL and is elevated when plasmin cross-links fibrin and creates degradation products in the blood. Unless the suspicion of a pulmonary embolism is high, a D-dimer level of <500 can be used to rule out pulmonary embolism. D-dimer is sensitive but not specific and cannot be used to diagnose pulmonary embolism.

21. Answer: 2

Rationale: Current recommendations (December 2013) for lung cancer screening from the U.S. Preventative Services Task Force is for individuals (ages 55–80) to have a low-dose computed tomography who have a 30 pack-year smoking history and currently smoke or have quit within the last 15 years. This has proven to be the most effective in decreasing lung cancer–related deaths. Screening should be discontinued once a person has not smoked for 15 years or develops a health problem that substantially limits life expectancy or the ability or willingness to have curative lung surgery.

22. Answer: 4

Rationale: A chest CT is not indicated for initial assessment of active TB infection. Isoniazid is not indicated unless the patient is found to have active TB infection. If a positive skin test is found, the patient should be tested for active infection by assessing for signs and symptoms and obtaining a chest radiograph.

23. Answer: 2

Rationale: Although a tuberculin skin test is sufficient to test for LTBI, the interferon-gamma release assay is preferred when the patient has received the BCG vaccine. Nursing programs require proof of absence of infection regardless of vaccination, and there is no test available to measure a TB titer.

24. Answer: 2

Rationale: Percussion should start posteriorly and move from medial to lateral and superior to inferior. As the practitioner moves laterally, the patient is asked to raise his or her arms to make lateral access easier. The percussion assessment should start with the patient sitting with his or her head lowered and arms folded in front.

25. Answer: 4

Rationale: Bronchophony is the clear loud transmission of sound usually through abnormally consolidated lung tissue. Extreme bronchophony results in the ability to hear whispered words over the involved area (whispered pectoriloquy). With normal voice transmission, sound is soft, muffled, and indistinct; the sound can be heard through the stethoscope but cannot be distinguished as to what is being said. Egophony is a change to a more nasal quality of the sound best demonstrated by asking the patient to say a long set of "e-e-e" sounds. Normally these sounds are clearly heard through the stethoscope; with consolidation or compression, the e-e-e sounds change to a bleating long a-a-a sound (similar to a goat sound). A pleural friction rub is a dry, crackly, grating, low-pitched sound suggesting pleural inflammation. Rhonchal fremitus is vibration felt when inhaled air passes through thick secretions in the larger bronchi.

26. Answer: 3

Rationale: The drug therapy regimen for chronic asthma may include theophylline. Symptoms of toxicity include anorexia, nausea, vomiting, confusion, restlessness, tachycardia, dysrhythmias, and seizures.

Disorders

27. Answer: 2

Rationale: According to the 2019 Global Initiative for Obstructive Lung Disease standards, pulmonary rehabilitation has been shown to improve exercise capacity and quality of life across all levels of severity in COPD. It has shown to be the most cost-effective treatment strategy available. COPD patients should not avoid physical activity because this will only add additional immobility issues. Although it is important to optimize pharmacologic therapy, pulmonary rehabilitation is beneficial with any COPD patient. Supplemental oxygen should not be prescribed routinely even in patients who moderately desaturate with activity.

28. Answer: 4

Rationale: Most cases of acute bronchitis rely on symptom management as the primary treatment choice. In most cases, antibiotics are discouraged because of increased resistance and lack of evidence-based efficacy. There is no significant evidence for or against the usage of OTC preparations. Although a β agonist has been shown to resolve cough faster in those with underlying wheezing, there is nothing recommending wide use.

29. Answer: 3

Rationale: The most common respiratory complication after a traumatic injury to the chest is pneumothorax caused from a fractured rib. Oximetry readings less than 90% and increased pain are expected at this point and may not be indicative of a problem. Although fever and increased sputum are problems, they are not associated with early manifestations of blunt trauma chest injury.

30. Answer: 4

Rationale: According to the 2019 Global Initiative for Obstructive Lung Disease standards, there is no current research supporting the safe use of e-cigarettes in smoking cessation. Smoking cessation has the strongest ability to influence the natural course of COPD. There is a strong relationship between counseling by health care professionals, legislative smoking bans, and increased cessation success. Every tobacco user should be offered smoking cessation advice at every visit.

31. Answer: 1

Rationale: Community-acquired pneumonia caused by *S. pneumoniae* often presents abruptly with high fever, shaking chills (rigor), cough productive of purulent sputum, and pleuritic chest pain. In acute bronchitis, cough is the primary symptom and initially is dry and nonproductive. Fever, dyspnea, wheezing, and possible mucoid sputum production are also characteristic of acute bronchitis.

32. Answer: 1

Rationale: On discharge, a patient must understand the importance of taking medications as prescribed. Missed doses increase mutation of the tubercle bacillus and decrease the medication's effectiveness. Respiratory isolation at home is not necessary, and if the patient experiences problems of rash, nausea, and vomiting, he or she should contact the health care provider. A patient should never change a medication dosage without first consulting with a health care provider. Weekly sputum checks are not necessary.

33. Answer: 2

Rationale: According to the American Heart Association, the protocol for respiratory arrest (has a pulse) is rescue breathing, which is to give one breath every 5–6 seconds or about 10–12 breaths/min. Pulse should be checked every 2 minutes, if no pulse, then begin cardiopulmonary resuscitation with 30 chest compressions followed by 2 breaths.

34. Answer: 1

Rationale: It is most important to obtain more information about the dyspnea. This information is necessary to determine the severity of the patient's complaint. A chest x-ray gives only limited information and may be normal in conditions like asthma. An ABG result is abnormal when the symptoms are severe. Presence of bilateral breath sounds over the lower lobes is a normal finding.

35. Answer: 1

Rationale: The most common area for a foreign body obstruction is the right bronchus, which produces a unilateral retraction of the right chest wall and leads to cough and unilateral wheezing with diminished breath sounds to that area. Retraction of the lower chest occurs with lower respiratory problems, such as asthma. A pleural friction rub is heard when there is inflammation between the viscera and parietal pleura. Crepitation is present when air is leaking into the subcutaneous tissue.

36. Answer: 1

Rationale: Spontaneous pneumothorax occurs in healthy, thin young adults, especially after strenuous exercise; predominant symptoms include sudden pain, dyspnea, and asymmetric chest expansion. The clinical hallmark of asthma is wheezing; with pulmonary edema, there is frequently coughing, frothy sputum, and crackles heard on auscultation. Bronchiectasis is most often chronic and is characterized by moist crackles and wheezing on auscultation; cough is usually present.

37. Answer: 1

Rationale: The situation described is hyperventilation syndrome (HVS); treatment should be concentrated on patient education through reassurance and suggested breathing and relaxation techniques. Albuterol, oxygen, and ABGs are not appropriate initial treatments. Breathing into a paper bag is not recommended because significant hypoxemia and death has occurred in the past from this treatment.

38. Answer: 1

Rationale: To prevent dyspnea on activity, the bronchodilator should be used before walking or increased physical activity. The patient should not stay in bed and should be encouraged to increase activity gradually. Fluid intake of 2–3 L/day should be encouraged, unless there are cardiac problems. A corticosteroid inhaler should be used at regular intervals as ordered and is not meant for rescue during periods of acute dyspnea.

39. Answer: 2

Rationale: Age-associated physiologic changes include decreased compliance of the chest wall, making deep inspiration difficult. Increased trachea and bronchi diameters that increase dead space result in a decreased volume of air reaching the alveoli. An increase in small airway closure results in decreased vital capacity and increased residual volume. Less elastic lung parenchyma results in decreased function of the alveoli. Shallow breathing and less forceful cough occurs because respiratory muscles weaken.

40. Answer: 4

Rationale: The patient is at risk for a pulmonary embolism, as a result of hypercoagulation related to giving birth, smoking, and vascular injury (recent surgery). Immediate testing and treatment is critical to the survival of someone with a pulmonary embolism, so they should be referred or transferred to the highest level of care available. Assessment reveals common symptoms of a pulmonary embolism: dyspnea, cough, and pleuritic pain. Diagnostic tests include D-dimer test, chest x-ray, ventilation-perfusion (V/Q) scan, CT scan, and/or pulmonary angiogram, which would be ordered at the emergency department.

41. Answer: 3

Rationale: The flu or influenza is a highly contagious respiratory infection that occurs epidemically during the winter months and may increase the prevalence of bacterial pneumonia. It is characterized by a sudden onset of chills, elevated temperature (101°F–104°F [38.3°C–40°C]), headache, fatigue, muscle pain, dry cough, laryngitis, rhinorrhea, and red eyes occurring 24–48 hours after exposure directly through respiratory droplets from an infected person or indirectly by drinking from a contaminated glass. Flu vaccines do not cause the flu regardless of being manufactured with a live attenuated (nasal vaccine) or killed virus (injection).

42. Answer: 2

Rationale: According to the 2019 Global Initiative for Asthma guidelines, this patient does not need immediate transfer to an acute care facility because she is not achieving less than 60% of personal best on her peak flow meter, remains calm, and is speaking in phrases. The patient should use her bronchodilator immediately and be evaluated urgently. If she does not improve or becomes worse, she will need emergency intervention. Inhaled corticosteroids are used for maintenance therapy and are not for "rescue" symptoms. A referral to a pulmonologist may be necessary at some point, but not immediately.

43. Answer: 1

Rationale: The pneumococcal vaccine is recommended for older adult patients because their immune system is less efficient. The symptoms of fever, chest pain, and sputum production suggest pneumococcal pneumonia.

44. Answer: 2

Rationale: Confusion/disorientation with or without a low-grade temperature may be the first sign that the older adult patient has an infection. The older adult patient may not have a fever or leukocytosis; however, leukopenia may suggest severe CAP and require hospitalization. The older adult patient may not experience any discomfort or a cough with the onset of infection.

45. Answer: 4

Rationale: *S. pneumoniae* is the most common cause of community-acquired and nursing home-acquired bacterial pneumonia. *H. influenzae* is common in older adult patients with underlying chronic diseases (e.g., chronic obstructive pulmonary disease, diabetes). *K. pneumoniae* and other gram-negative bacteria are pathogens in patients with alcoholism, immunocompromised hosts, and hospitalized patients. *M. tuberculosis* is an infrequent cause of pneumonia.

46. Answer: 2

Rationale: The pneumococcal vaccination should be given to all adults 65 years or older but is not administered annually. The influenza immunization given annually will decrease complications and hospitalizations for the older adult patient. There is no evidence to support the use of an annual sputum culture or chest x-ray for pneumonia prevention. The PPD skin test should be done annually for high-risk patients and only detects exposure to tuberculosis.

47. Answer: 2

Rationale: *K. pneumoniae* is an important pathogen in patients with alcoholism. *S. aureus* generally affects older adult patients recovering from influenza and is also common in hospitalized patients with diabetes and in IV drug users. *P. aeruginosa* is most likely found in someone with structural lung disease (e.g., bronchiectasis).

48. Answer: 2

Rationale: If a person is infected, a delayed-type reaction may occur 2–8 weeks after infection. In a contact exposure, if the initial PPD skin test is negative, a repeat PPD test 8–10 weeks later is recommended in all patients. A patient should not be treated empirically for TB exposure. Six months is too long to wait for someone who could have active TB. A yearly evaluation should be reserved for those who work or live in high-risk environments but have not been exposed.

49. Answer: 1, 3

Rationale: Sarcoidosis is a noninfectious, multisystem granulomatous disease that may affect almost any organ system; however, 90% of affected individuals have pulmonary involvement. It most commonly affects young and middle-aged adults, with 80% of the presenting patients between age 20 and 45. The majority of patients have a spontaneous resolution within 2 years. Nonsteroidal antiinflammatory drugs and low-dose steroids are used to treat symptoms; however, many patients are asymptomatic and do not require medication. Higher dose steroids are prescribed when patients have acute respiratory failure or cardiac, neurologic, or ocular disease.

50. Answer: 3

Rationale: Horner syndrome, which is a paralysis of the cervical sympathetic nerves that results in ptosis, loss of sweating, pupillary constriction, and sometimes enophthalmos, is often associated with malignant tumors in the upper lung, leading to nerve compression (e.g., pulmonary sulcus [Pancoast] tumor or superior sulcus tumor found in smokers).

51. Answer: 4

Rationale: Over 70% of the cases of SVCS occur as a complication of lung malignancy involving the mediastinum. This is considered an oncologic emergency and requires immediate referral. Although chronic bronchitis or heart failure may cause orthopnea, upper extremity edema is usually not present. A thyroid abnormality usually results in unilateral or bilateral thyroid enlargement in the neck. Asthma does not cause fluid retention.

52. Answer: 3

Rationale: Hyponatremia results from the syndrome of inappropriate antidiuretic hormone secretion and can be caused by a bronchogenic tumor (e.g., small cell lung carcinoma). Blunt chest trauma could result in hemorrhage and fluid loss, causing hypernatremia. Bronchitis and respiratory acidosis do not usually cause sodium abnormalities.

53. Answer: 2

Rationale: Asking the patient about the consumption of wine with dinner is the most appropriate response. Many wines, especially white wines, contain sulfites, which can trigger a mild allergic response.

54. Answer: 2

Rationale: Desaturation and 10-second periods of apnea that occur 10—15 times per hour are considered clinically significant of obstructive sleep apnea. Loud snoring at night, frequent arousals during the night, and sleeping during the day are characteristic of the problem but are not diagnostic.

55. Answer: 1

Rationale: Frequent substance use, including alcohol, benzodiazepines, sleep aids, opiates, and muscle relaxants, can exacerbate OSA. Obesity, weight gain, nasal allergies, and polyps are common factors associated with this condition. Most patients with sleep apnea will not report nighttime sleep disturbances even though a spouse may witness nighttime restlessness. Snoring, daytime sleepiness, and fatigue are frequently reported symptoms. Men are more likely than premenopausal women to have OSA.

56. Answer: 1

Rationale: The positive sputum for acid-fast bacillus is indicative of active tuberculosis. *P. carinii* is a common organism in healthy respiratory tracts; it becomes a problem if the patient is immunocompromised. Hemolysis on a complement fixation test is a negative finding. When oxygen saturation is low and white blood cell count is within normal range, treatment is not as important as it is with tuberculosis.

57. Answer: 1

Rationale: According to the 2019 Global Initiative on Asthma, the level of control is based on the most severe impairment or risk category. This patient is well controlled. The components of well-controlled asthma are daytime symptoms ≤2 times/week, no nighttime awakening, no interference with normal activity, and using a short-acting β2 agonist ≤2 times/week.

58. Answer: 2

Rationale: Tuberculosis infection is seen most often in the upper lobes of the lung. In 13%–30% of the cases adults may have "atypical" radiographic patterns with infiltrates in the middle or lower lung zones. The local lymph nodes are infected and enlarged (hilar adenopathy). An asymptomatic period usually follows the primary infection and can last for years or decades before clinical symptoms develop. When there is a reactivation of the disease in a previously infected person, this scenario is more likely to occur in situations when defenses are lowered, such as with older adults and people with HIV disease. The apical posterior segments of the upper lobes are the most common site of reactivation.

59. Answer: 3

Rationale: Secondhand smoke is a known carcinogen and increases the patient's risk of lung cancer. In addition, there is a 20%–30% increase in stroke and heart disease when there is significant exposure to secondhand smoke.

60. Answer: 3

Rationale: According to the 2019 Global Initiative on Asthma, asthma control is evaluated based on the presence or absence of symptoms. Symptoms suggesting the asthma is not well controlled include daytime symptoms more than twice per week, night waking because of asthma, any activity limitation caused by asthma, and usage of an asthma reliever (i.e., short-acting β agonist) more than twice weekly. One to two of the criteria being true suggests the asthma is partly controlled, more than two being true suggests uncontrolled asthma.

61. Answer: 2

Rationale: Most cases of acute bronchitis are of viral etiology and do not require antibiotic therapy. Approximately 5%–10% of acute bronchitis is bacterial. A cough can last for at least 10–20 days, but routine sputum cultures are not helpful.

Pharmacology

62. Answer: 3

Rationale: When initiating pharmacologic therapy for asthma, patients should use a short-acting β agonist as needed for shortness of breath. Most inhaled corticosteroids should be taken only once or twice daily. Montelukast is indicated for the treatment of seasonal allergies and for the treatment of asthma. Up to 80% of patients use inhalers incorrectly.

63. Answer: 1

Rationale: A 1-minute lapse between the two puffs is necessary for the medication to be most effective. The first puff opens the upper airways, allowing more effective penetration of the lower tract with the second puff. Albuterol (Proventil) should not be used as maintenance therapy. Only inhaled corticosteroids should be taken on a regular schedule.

64. Answer: 3

Rationale: According to 2019 Global Initiative for Obstructive Lung Disease, 80% of COPD exacerbations are managed on an outpatient basis. Systemic corticosteroids (1 mg/kg/day commonly 40 mg daily for 5 days) are used for an acute exacerbation because they improve lung function, oxygenation, and short recovery time. Although oxygen is a key component of exacerbation treatment in the hospital, it is not an appropriate first choice in this patient. Antibiotics are recommended when a patient has increased dyspnea, increased sputum volume, and increased sputum purulence, which is not the case here. Methylxanthines such as theophylline are not recommended for exacerbations caused by an increased side effect profile.

65. Answer: 2

Rationale: Urine color change is a normal side effect of rifampin and is not a reason for the patient to stop taking their medication. Also, soft contact lenses may become discolored.

66. Answer: 4

Rationale: Because tobacco increases the metabolism of theophylline, a higher dose is required in smokers than in nonsmokers. A high-protein, low-carbohydrate diet increases the metabolism of theophylline and decreases serum concentrations. Coffee (and other xanthine-containing beverages) may increase the central nervous system effects of xanthine derivatives.

67. Answer: 1

Rationale: Beta blockers (propranolol, atenolol) are known to exacerbate chronic respiratory problems, especially reactive airway disease. Another antihypertensive, such as a calcium channel blocker (amlodipine), should be considered. The patient's pulse is 72 beats/min and blood pressure remains elevated, which indicates the beta blocker is probably not effective in decreasing blood pressure in this patient. Prednisone is not indicated unless other medications are not effective. Although beclomethasone may be appropriate to start, discontinuing the beta blocker, which is likely exacerbating the problem, is the better choice.

68. Answer: 2

Rationale: Therapeutic plasma levels range from 10–20 mcg/mL. Drug levels of ≥20 mcg/mL are associated with toxicity.

69. Answer: 4

Rationale: The most likely causes of subacute cough include postinfection, GERD, or asthma. This patient has been healthy and is currently being treated for GERD symptoms. A likely cause of this cough is lisinopril, an angiotensin-converting enzyme inhibitor. Albuterol and dextromethorphan may be good options if the cough does not clear within 4 weeks of discontinuing the lisinopril in favor of a different antihypertensive medication.

70. Answer: 1

Rationale: LTBI treatment is initiated at the time of the TST. TST testing should be repeated in 3 months if initial test results are negative. If the second TST is negative, LTBI treatment can be discontinued.

71. Answer: 3

Rationale: One of the most common causes of outpatient treatment failure is improper inhaler technique. Exposure to allergens may trigger an asthma attack, but proper use of inhalers will control the attacks in many cases. Use of both steroids and cromolyn inhalers have decreased the severity of asthma attacks.

72. Answer: 1

Rationale: Theophylline is used in the treatment of chronic lung disease and can accumulate in toxic levels. Cimetidine decreases the hepatic clearance of theophylline because it is a cytochrome P450 1A2 and 3A4 inhibitor. Nicotine and some antiseizure drugs may increase clearance, and ampicillin does not change the clearance.

73. Answer: 2

Rationale: In someone with COPD, antibiotic therapy is indicated when there is a change in color, consistency, or amount of sputum and increased symptoms of COPD exacerbation. Antitussives are not recommended in stable COPD. Inhaled corticosteroids should be taken on a schedule and not ordered as needed.

74. Answer: 2

Rationale: Beclomethasone is a long-acting corticosteroid that stabilizes mast cells and greatly reduces mast-cell degranulation when exposed to allergens. Albuterol is a short-acting bronchodilator used as a rescue medication. Salmeterol is a long-acting bronchodilator most useful in controlling nocturnal asthma symptoms. Montelukast, a leukotriene receptor antagonist, inhibits bronchoconstriction and is used as an adjunct to bronchodilators and corticosteroids.

75. Answer: 2

Rationale: Preferred, regular daily treatment (long-term treatment) of the patient with asthma includes inhaled corticosteroid for their antiinflammatory effects. Antibiotics are indicated if there is a concurrent infection, such as acute bronchitis. β2 agonists are used for their bronchodilator effects and rapid onset of action when a patient may need "rescue" or acute treatment of symptoms with quick-relief medications. Leukotriene receptor antagonist is another option, but it is not preferred to inhaled corticosteroid for regular daily treatment.

76. Answer: 2

Rationale: Patients with asthma should be instructed to keep their inhaled β2 agonists with them at all times in case of bronchospasm and use them prn. The β2 agonists are effective in reversing bronchospasm and should be used only for rescue symptoms. Inhaled corticosteroids are long acting and will not give immediate relief, so the patient should be instructed to use them as prescribed. Antibiotics are not indicated for acute bronchospasm.

77. Answer: 4

Rationale: Dextromethorphan is a widely used cough suppressant and is found in many cough and cold remedies. At low doses used for cough suppression, dextromethorphan lacks psychologic effects. However, at doses 5–10 times higher, dextromethorphan can cause euphoria, disorientation, paranoia, and altered sense of time, as well as visual, auditory, and tactile hallucinations. Guaifenesin is an expectorant, pseudoephedrine is a decongestant, and diphenhydramine is an antihistamine.

78. Answer: 4

Rationale: Most patients with acute bronchitis benefit from symptomatic treatment with antiinflammatory, cough, and cold preparations. Because underlying asthma and pneumonia differential diagnoses have been eliminated, current clinical guidelines do not support routine bronchodilator use or antibiotic therapy for acute bronchitis. Research has demonstrated that antibiotic-susceptible organisms rarely cause acute bronchitis.

79. Answer: 4

Rationale: Histamine H_2 antagonists neutralize the normal gastric acid barrier, allowing for an increased colonization of gram-negative bacilli and *Staphylococcus aureus*.

80. Answer: 2

Rationale: Worsening dyspnea and fatigue with increasing cough may indicate early pulmonary edema. Patients with pulmonary edema require hospitalization with oxygen therapy, IV furosemide (Lasix), and morphine. Patients suspected of having new-onset pulmonary edema should not be treated as outpatients. Calcium channel blockers are of little benefit in heart failure and can make dependent edema worse. Empirical antibiotics are not indicated in this situation and may delay proper diagnosis of a serious condition.

81. Answer: 1

Rationale: INH requires concurrent administration of vitamin B6 to prevent problems of optic neuritis. Vitamin B6 will decrease the effectiveness of levodopa. If the patient is to receive INH, his anti-Parkinson's medication needs to be reevaluated.

82. Answer: 2

Rationale: Prednisone is a corticosteroid that suppresses immune response and puts the patient in an immunocompromised state, increasing susceptibility to infections. Patients on prednisone therapy should be educated about the risk for developing infections and the need to seek medical attention if they suspect illness. Atenolol is a beta blocker used as an antihypertensive. Ipratropium is an anticholinergic used in the acute treatment of asthma. Fluticasone propionate and salmeterol is a combination of inhaled corticosteroid and a long-acting β agonist. Although inhaled corticosteroids can suppress immune response, absorption is considerably less than oral prednisone.

83. Answer: 4

Rationale: Multiple studies show that the combination of an anticholinergic and β agonist, particularly ipratropium bromide and albuterol, reduce exacerbation, lower cost, and improve lung function and quality of life.

84. Answer: 3

Rationale: In the absence of drug-resistant *Streptococcus pneumoniae* (DRSP) or other comorbidities, the Infectious Diseases Society of America guidelines suggest azithromycin (Zithromax) is the best choice with Level I Evidence, and doxycycline is a weak recommendation (Level III). If a β-lactam like amoxicillin is used, a macrolide should also be prescribed for better coverage. A respiratory fluoroquinolone is recommended in instances of comorbid conditions or the presence of additional risk factors for DRSP, and ciprofloxacin (Cipro) is not a respiratory fluoroquinolone. Moxifloxacin, levofloxacin, and gemifloxacin are respiratory fluoroquinolones.

85. Answer: 2

Rationale: The patient most likely has a subacute, postinfectious cough, which can last up to 8 weeks. After 8 weeks, it would more likely be a chronic cough related to environmental factors like smoking, asthma exacerbation, or GERD.

86. Answer: 3

Rationale: Posterior ankle pain is suggestive of Achilles tendonitis. Tendon ruptures are a known adverse reaction to fluoroquinolone therapy, and there have been a significant number of cases in the United States. If tendon inflammation or pain occurs, the fluoroquinolone should be discontinued immediately. Ciprofloxacin (Cipro) is recommended for 60 days as part of empiric treatment of anthrax, as postexposure prophylaxis.

87. Answer: 3

Rationale: In patients with high probability of exposure to *B. pertussis*, first-line therapy with a macrolide antibiotic will improve symptoms if started within 5–7 days of symptom onset. Doxycycline is not a first-line choice for *B. pertussis*. Waiting delays the possibility of limiting the spread and treatment of *B. pertussis*. Oseltamivir (Tamiflu) is an antiviral and will not be effective against *B. pertussis*.

88. Answer: 2

Rationale: According to GINA guidelines, Step 2 therapy should start with a low-dose inhaled corticosteroid (ICS). Flovent is an ICS and would be the most appropriate therapy to start, based on GINA guidelines. Fluticasone and salmeterol (Advair) is a combination ICS and long-acting β_2 agonist (LABA) used when reaching Step 3, and it should not be used for initial therapy. Salmeterol (Serevent) is a LABA and should not be used initially.

89. Answer: 4

Rationale: Although acute respiratory failure, cor pulmonale, and depression are common complications of COPD, they are less likely to cause the patient's current symptoms. Elevated hematocrit, morning headaches, and daytime somnolence are all potential signs of decreased oxygen saturation at night and would be an indication for home overnight oxygen monitoring or sleep disorder specialist referral.

90. Answer: 1, 3, 5

Rationale: Criteria for severe CAP includes WBC count less than 4000 cells/mm³, temperature less than 36°C, respiratory rate ≥30 breaths/min, arterial oxygen pressure/fraction of inspired oxygen (PaO_2/FiO_2) ratio less than 250, platelet count <100,000 cells/mm³, and uremia (BUN) >20 mg/dL.

91. Answer: 3

Rationale: It is important to emphasize how to take medications correctly. The MDI usually has three parts: mouthpiece, cap that goes over the mouthpiece, and a canister of medicine. A spacer device will help avoid getting less medication in mouth. The spacer connects to the mouthpiece. The inhaled medicine goes into the spacer tube first. The patient takes two deep breaths to get the medicine into the lungs, waiting a full minute between the two breaths. Using a spacer wastes a lot less medicine than spraying the medicine into the mouth. MDI technique is important, as well as understanding the use of the devices, such as the prescribed valved holding chamber, spacer, and nebulizer.

92. Answer: 2

Rationale: In the presence of macrolide resistance, clarithromycin (a macrolide) would not be a safe choice. Doxycycline is the best alternative. In cases in which the patient is unable to take doxycycline, a combination β-lactam and macrolide or a respiratory fluroquinolone should be considered.

93. Answer: 2

Rationale: Amiodarone can cause interstitial pneumonitis. All patients taking this medication should have yearly pulmonary function testing with diffuse lung capacity measurements to ensure early prevention and treatment. Methadone, propranolol, and amlodipine do not cause interstitial pneumonitis.

94. Answer: 3, 4

Rationale: Bupropion was originally marketed as an antidepressant, and later it was used for smoking cessation under the trade name of Zyban. It is thought to reduce cravings for nicotine and symptoms of withdrawal because of its capacity to block neural reuptake of the neurotransmitters, dopamine, and norepinephrine. Varenicline (Chantix) interferes with nicotine receptors in the brain, which decreases the pleasurable effects of the nicotine and reduces symptoms of nicotine withdrawal. Valacyclovir (Valtrex) is used in the treatment of herpes virus infections, including shingles, cold sores, and genital herpes. Lisinopril (Zestril) is an angiotensin-converting enzyme inhibitor used to treat high blood pressure and heart failure. Cetirizine (Zyrtec) is an antihistamine used to relieve allergy symptoms.

6

Immune & Allergy

Physical Exam & Diagnostic Tests

1. When taking the history of a patient with a suspected atopic disorder, what is the most important information to determine whether the reaction is immunoglobulin E mediated?
   1. Specific reaction.
   2. Duration of symptoms.
   3. Past history of similar reactions.
   4. Environmental exposure.

2. Which test is used to determine the concentration of gamma globulins that contain the majority of the immunoglobulins?
   1. C-reactive protein (CRP).
   2. Complement fixation.
   3. Protein electrophoresis.
   4. Antinuclear antibody (ANA).

3. Which diagnostic studies are typically abnormal when ruling in systemic lupus erythematosus (SLE) as a differential diagnosis?
   1. Complete blood count (CBC), comprehensive metabolic panel, and erythrocyte sedimentation rate (ESR).
   2. Chest radiograph and coagulation profile.
   3. Antinuclear antibody (ANA), ESR, and C-reactive protein (CRP).
   4. CBC, urinalysis, and chest radiograph.

4. Which tests are appropriate for the family nurse practitioner to order in an initial workup for asymptomatic patients at risk for HIV infection?
   1. CD4 count and HIV enzyme-linked immunosorbent assay.
   2. Serology for cytomegalovirus, herpes simplex virus, and Epstein-Barr virus.
   3. HIV-1/2 antigen (Ag)/antibody (Ab) combination immunoassay and HIV-1/HIV-2 antibody differentiation immunoassay.
   4. Hepatitis C virus screen and Western blot analysis.

5. The family nurse practitioner would identify which two laboratory findings as most significant in a patient with joint pain, malar rash, photosensitivity, weight loss, and fever?
   1. Presence of antinuclear antibodies (ANAs).
   2. Positive serum complement level.
   3. Decreased red blood cells.
   4. Thrombocytopenia.
   5. Glycosuria.
   6. Negative LE cell preparation.

6. When assessing a patient for angioedema, what would the family nurse practitioner examine?
   1. Neck and ears.
   2. Lower extremities.
   3. Torso.
   4. Eyes and mouth.

7. Which two tests are the most reliable for detecting the presence of specific immunoglobulin E (IgE) antibodies?
   1. IgE skin testing.
   2. Nasal smear for eosinophils.
   3. Complete blood count (CBC).
   4. Serum ImmunoCAP testing.
   5. Western blot analysis.

8. To diagnose allergic rhinitis and treat symptoms that do not respond to medical and environmental control treatments, which would the family nurse practitioner consider?
   1. Obtain a nasal smear for eosinophils.
   2. Order serum immunoglobulin E (IgE) level to environmentals.
   3. Refer for skin testing.
   4. Order a serum radioallergosorbent testing (RAST).

9. An adult patient presents to the clinic with fatigue, sore throat, and myalgia. On examination, the family nurse practitioner finds axillary lymphadenopathy and a slightly enlarged spleen. Based on the history, the nurse adds acute HIV infection to the differential diagnosis. Which STAT laboratory result increases concern about HIV infection?
   1. Hypochromic, normocytic anemia.
   2. Leukopenia and thrombocytopenia.
   3. Elevated lymphocyte count.
   4. Elevated neutrophil count.

Disorders

10. A young adult presents to the clinic with a 10-day history of fever, myalgia, sore throat, and measles-like rash. The patient is not taking any medications. Which viral syndrome is characterized by a measles-like rash?
    1. Influenza.
    2. Varicella.
    3. HIV.
    4. Mononucleosis.

11. A young woman presents to the urgent care center reporting that a male vaginally raped her last night. She is treated today for *Chlamydia* infection, gonorrhea, and syphilis and is started on a 28-day course of medications to prevent HIV. She wants to know why she needs the HIV therapy because no one she knows has AIDS. What is the basis for the family nurse practitioner's counseling?
    1. The patient should assume that the man was not HIV positive.
    2. She probably does not need the therapy, but it is a good idea to take the medications.
    3. More than 15% of HIV-infected individuals are unaware that they are infected.
    4. HIV is not easily transmitted.

12. A coworker has just stuck herself with a needle while performing a phlebotomy. She asks the family nurse practitioner for help and requests that the nurse manager not be informed about the incident. What should be the family nurse practitioner's initial response?
    1. Send the coworker to the nurse manager.
    2. Sit with her and calm her down.
    3. Have the coworker wash the needlestick area with soap and water.
    4. Put on gloves and pour povidone-iodine (Betadine) on the area.

13. Patient education regarding common antigens of anaphylaxis includes:
    1. Oats.
    2. Egg albumin.
    3. Dust mites.
    4. Animal dander.

14. Which assessment findings are typically associated with a diagnosis of systemic lupus erythematous (SLE)?
    1. Excitability, diarrhea, and vomiting.
    2. High fever, measles-like rash on limbs, and weight loss.
    3. Joint pain, malar rash, and photosensitivity.
    4. Weight loss, diarrhea, and generalized abdominal pain.

15. After a repeat HIV antibody test, a patient continues to test positive but is asymptomatic. Which is important for the family nurse practitioner to understand regarding the transmission of the virus by this patient?
    1. The patient is infectious when symptoms are active.
    2. The patient may remain infectious for life.
    3. The dormant virus is not infectious while the patient is asymptomatic and the T-cell count is high.
    4. Laboratory tests should be done every 4–6 weeks to identify the infectious periods of the disease process.

16. A young woman has just received news of a positive HIV test. She does not want her sexual partner to be informed. What is the family nurse practitioner's most appropriate response?
    1. Respect for her decision because she is the patient.
    2. Inform her that she has a legal responsibility to inform her partner and to notify the health department of her positive HIV test.
    3. Educate her about the importance of notifying all sexual partners and that it is the nurse's legal and ethical responsibility to report her case to the health department.
    4. Document her decision in the record for future reference.

17. A patient presenting with complaints of fatigue, malaise, arthralgias, oral ulcers, malar rash, and a positive antinuclear antibody (ANA) test would most likely be diagnosed as having:
    1. Chronic fatigue syndrome.
    2. Fibromyalgia.
    3. Scleroderma.
    4. Systemic lupus erythematosus (SLE).

18. What are the most common clinical manifestations of Sjögren syndrome?
    1. Corneal dryness and lack of saliva.
    2. Increased urination and hunger.
    3. Abdominal discomfort and thickening of the epidermis.
    4. Joint destruction and alopecia.

19. An older adult female patient presents to the family nurse practitioner with a low-grade temperature and a unilateral throbbing headache. She also reports scalp sensitivity and some visual disturbances. Laboratory results show a greatly elevated erythrocyte sedimentation rate (ESR) and anemia. She has been relatively healthy except for a recent history of polymyalgia rheumatica (PMR). Which condition should be diagnosed based on this clinical presentation?
    1. Bacterial meningitis.
    2. Primary angle closure glaucoma (PACG).
    3. Giant cell (temporal) arteritis.
    4. Subdural hematoma.

20. A middle-aged female patient presents with weight loss, heartburn, dysphagia, dry cough, pain, stiffness of the fingers and knees, and Raynaud phenomenon. The family nurse practitioner recognizes these as the symptoms of:
    1. Rheumatoid arthritis.
    2. Systemic lupus erythematosus (SLE).
    3. Barrett esophagus.
    4. Scleroderma.

21. The erythematous confluent macular eruption of the face known as the "butterfly rash" is characteristic of:
    1. Allergic drug eruption.
    2. Systemic lupus erythematosus (SLE).
    3. Acne rosacea.
    4. Seborrheic dermatitis.

22. The family nurse practitioner is discussing general health care with a female patient who has systemic lupus erythematosus (SLE) and is in remission. What are important points to include in the teaching?
    1. Check weight daily to assess for fluid retention.
    2. Decrease physical and psychologic stress.
    3. Avoid isometric exercise.
    4. Maintain diet low in fat and high in carbohydrates.

23. A 50-year-old male patient presents with complaints of frequent sinus infections, decrease in ability to hear, and arthralgia. Laboratory findings are mild normochromic/normocytic anemia, elevated ESR, mild hypergammaglobulinemia (elevated IgA), proteinuria, and hematuria with granular or cellular casts. Physical findings include mild conjunctivitis, vasculitis dermatitis, chronic cough, chest pain, dyspnea, paranasal sinus pain, occasional epistaxis, and imbalance of intake and output. What would be a tentative diagnosis?
    1. Connective tissue disease.
    2. Granulomatosis with polyangiitis (Wegener granulomatosis).

    3. Pulmonary neoplasm.
    4. Infectious granulomatous disease.

24. A patient presents with sneezing, watery eyes, postnasal drip, and sore throat. What diagnosis do these symptoms most likely suggest?
    1. Acute sinusitis.
    2. Allergic rhinitis.
    3. Vasomotor rhinitis.
    4. Influenza.

25. A 70-year-old woman presents with complaints of morning headache, malaise, and anorexia. What condition would the family nurse practitioner suspect?
    1. Pneumonia.
    2. Giant cell (temporal) arteritis.
    3. Anemia of chronic disease.
    4. Acute sinusitis.

26. When teaching a patient about risk factors and prevention of transmission of HIV, which statement is most appropriate?
    1. HIV can be transmitted by casual kissing.
    2. Unprotected oral sex with an infected partner may result in transmission.
    3. Sharing an office with an HIV-positive person increases the risk of HIV exposure.
    4. Using the same bathroom as an infected adult member puts one at risk of HIV exposure.

27. What are the signs and symptoms that alert the family nurse practitioner to identify a patient who is at an increased risk for HIV infection?
    1. Frequent emergency department visits for urinary tract infections (UTIs).
    2. Malaise and fatigue.
    3. Frequent sexually transmitted infections (STIs).
    4. Swollen glands and diarrhea.

28. What are the most frequently occurring symptoms of systemic lupus erythematous (SLE)?
    1. Splenomegaly and Raynaud syndrome.
    2. Pulmonary effusions and hepatomegaly.
    3. Butterfly rash on the face and lymphadenopathy.
    4. Fever, arthritis, arthralgia, and weight loss.

29. Which is an example of a systemic immunoglobulin E–mediated antigen–antibody response resulting in a life-threatening massive release of mediators?
    1. Recurrent urticaria.
    2. Allergic rhinitis.
    3. Anaphylaxis.
    4. Contact dermatitis.

30. During an immunoglobulin E–mediated allergic reaction, the release of histamine results in:
    1. Bronchoconstriction, vasodilation, and vascular permeability.
    2. Bronchodilation, vasodilation, and vascular permeability.
    3. Smooth muscle contraction and decreased vascular permeability.
    4. Increased vascular permeability and bronchodilation.

31. A patient who has a history of recent bone marrow transplant presents to the clinic. The family nurse practitioner identifies signs and symptoms of graft-versus-host disease (GVHD) that include:
    1. Fever, headache, and mental status changes.
    2. Chills, fever, and urticaria over the flank area.
    3. Increased serum bilirubin level and presence of maculopapular rash and abdominal cramping.
    4. Decreased red blood cells (RBCs), hematocrit, and hemoglobin, and the presence of petechiae.

32. The pathogenesis of systemic lupus erythematosus (SLE) is characterized by autoantibody development. This results in:
    1. Increased T-suppressor cells.
    2. B-cell increase.
    3. Polyclonal hypogammaglobulinemia.
    4. Decreased T-suppressor cells and inhibited cellular activity.

33. A 22-year-old male presents with breathlessness, weight loss, nonproductive cough, temperature of 100.4°F (38°C), pulse of 124 beats/min, respiration of 36 breaths/min, blood pressure of 120/78 mm Hg, and a history of positive HIV serum test. Based on this information, which is the most accurate diagnosis?
    1. *Klebsiella pneumoniae* infection.
    2. *Mycoplasma pneumoniae* infection.
    3. *Pneumocystis jirovecii* pneumonia.
    4. Community-acquired pneumonia.

34. A nurse who has never been vaccinated against hepatitis B virus (HBV) experiences a needlestick at the clinic from a patient with known hepatitis B. What postexposure prophylaxis (PEP) should be administered?
    1. IgE.
    2. IgA.
    3. Pegylated interferon (PEG-IFN).
    4. Hepatitis B immune globulin (HBIG).

35. Which sign/symptom is indicative of a type I hypersensitivity reaction?
    1. Contact dermatitis.
    2. Immediate wheal and flare reaction.
    3. Hematuria.
    4. High fever.

36. Which patient is at highest risk for developing HIV/AIDS?
    1. Immunocompromised patient.
    2. Sexually active teenager.
    3. Middle-aged adult.
    4. Marijuana user.

37. When assessing a patient for systemic lupus erythematous (SLE), what ophthalmologic findings would the family nurse practitioner determine to be consistent with this condition?
    1. Retinal hemorrhage.
    2. Conjunctivitis.
    3. Cotton-wool spots.
    4. Arteriovenous (AV) nicking.

38. What information does the family nurse practitioner include in the education for the patient with allergic rhinitis?
    1. Monitor air quality and the allergy index.
    2. Use a surgical-type mask when going outdoors.
    3. Remain inside during allergy season.
    4. Avoid working in the garden or yard.

39. A nurse from the operating room (OR) comes into the clinic with complaints of shortness of breath, itching, reddened hands, and wheezing. He says that he does not seem to have the symptoms when he is not working. Based on the history and symptoms, the family nurse practitioner would evaluate for:
    1. Indoor toxic mold exposure.
    2. Bronchitis.
    3. Latex allergy.
    4. Contact dermatitis.

40. Which statement is true regarding latex allergy?
    1. It usually produces symptoms of contact dermatitis and allergic rhinorrhea only.
    2. It is a progressive disorder that worsens with continued exposure.
    3. It affects less than 5% of the health care population.
    4. It is an autoimmune response.

Pharmacology

41. An adult patient comes to the urgent care clinic with nausea, vomiting, and acute abdominal pain. His history is significant for HIV infection, and for the last month, he has been taking didanosine (Videx) 400 mg daily, lopinavir/ritonavir (Kaletra) 400 mg/100 mg bid, and lamivudine (Epivir) 150 mg bid. After the examination, the family nurse practitioner determines that didanosine can cause pancreatitis and lactic acidosis. What laboratory tests would be ordered?
    1. Complete blood count (CBC), CD4 count, viral load, and electrolytes.
    2. CBC with differential, lipase, lactic acid, electrolytes, blood urea nitrogen (BUN), creatinine, and liver function tests (LFTs).
    3. Amylase, lipase, and lactic acid.
    4. Lipase, amylase, and LFTs.

42. A patient is asking about preexposure prophylaxis (PrEP) for HIV infection. The family nurse practitioner explains to the patient that the criteria for eligibility to take the PrEP medication includes all **except**:
    1. History of positive HIV infection.
    2. Documented negative HIV test before prescribing PrEP.
    3. No signs/symptoms of acute HIV infection.
    4. Normal renal function, no contraindicated medications.

43. Which drugs have been associated with a lupus-like syndrome?
    1. Sulfonamides (Septra DS) and penicillin (Pen-Vee K, Penicillin G).
    2. Progestin/estrogen oral contraceptives.
    3. Nonsteroidal antiinflammatory drugs (NSAIDs; ibuprofen [Motrin]).
    4. Procainamide (Pronestyl) and hydralazine (Apresoline).

44. A patient is diagnosed with giant cell (temporal) arteritis. What is the medication of choice?
    1. Prednisone (Deltasone).
    2. Ibuprofen (Motrin).
    3. Indomethacin (Indocin).
    4. Azathioprine (Imuran).

45. A patient with a bacterial infection that is susceptible only to meropenem (Merrem) requires treatment. The patient reports urticaria and pruritus when administered meropenem in the past. Which of the following is the best action by the family nurse practitioner when no other medications are available?
    1. Administer ciprofloxacin (Cipro).
    2. Inform the patient there is no medication available.
    3. Begin desensitization therapy.
    4. Administer normal-dose meropenem (Merrem).

46. The family nurse practitioner is selecting a preexposure prophylaxis (PrEP) medication for HIV infections. Which of the following has been approved for prophylaxis?
    1. Highly active antiretroviral therapy (HAART) therapy.
    2. Acyclovir.
    3. Tenofovir (TDF) plus emtricitabine (FTC).
    4. Corticosteroids.

47. Which four medications are used for malaria prophylaxis?
    1. Ampicillin (Omnipen).
    2. Doxycycline (Vibramycin).
    3. Ceftriaxone (Rocephin).
    4. Chloroquine phosphate (Aralen).
    5. Mefloquine (Lariam).
    6. Primaquine.

48. Which medications are used in the treatment of allergic rhinitis (AR)?
    1. Antihistamines, corticosteroids, and environmental control.
    2. Antihistamines, analgesics, and allergen control.
    3. Anticholinergics, antibiotics, and oral prednisone.
    4. Nasal saline rinses, corticosteroids, and antibiotics.

49. Development of an adverse drug reaction depends on which factors?
    1. Patient age, prior drug reactions, genetic factors, and degree of exposure.
    2. Patient gender, oral route of administration, and history of atrophic disease.
    3. Patient age, gender, and genetic factors.
    4. Genetic factors, prior drug reactions, and patient gender.

50. Treatment of a patient with chronic urticaria has failed with multiple antihistamine medications over the last 3 months. The patient has a history of tuberculosis (TB) and was compliant with all medical treatment 5 years ago. Which of the following medications is the most appropriate choice by the family nurse practitioner for long-term control of symptoms?
    1. Topical corticosteroids.
    2. Systemic corticosteroids.
    3. Omalizumab (XOLAIR).
    4. Adalimumab (HUMIRA).

51. Which is a medication frequently used for the prophylaxis and initial treatment of *Pneumocystis jirovecii* pneumonia?
    1. Fluconazole (Diflucan).
    2. Amphotericin B (Fungizone).
    3. Trimethoprim-sulfamethoxazole (TMP-SMX; Septra).
    4. Acyclovir (Zovirax).

52. The family nurse practitioner should advise an adult patient with idiopathic chronic urticaria controlled by cetirizine (Zyrtec) to avoid which of the following medications?
    1. Ibuprofen (Motrin).
    2. Celecoxib (Celebrex).
    3. Penicillin.
    4. Cephalexin (Keflex).

53. When instructing patients with allergic rhinitis about the use of topical nasal decongestants (nasal spray), it is important for them to understand:
    1. The condition is self-limiting and will resolve in a matter of weeks, regardless of whether the patient is reexposed to the allergen.
    2. A nasal decongestant used continuously for more than 3 days can result in rebound nasal turbinate swelling.
    3. It is not necessary to avoid exposure to the allergen once therapy has been initiated.
    4. Allergic rhinitis is seen only in the spring and fall; the condition requires treatment during these seasons only.

54. What is the major advantage of using second-generation antihistamines, such as cetirizine (Zyrtec) and loratadine (Claritin)?
    1. Decreased cost.
    2. Increased anticholinergic activity.
    3. Delayed absorption.
    4. Do not cross the blood-brain barrier.

55. What is the desired action of sympathomimetics (adrenergics) when used in the treatment of allergic rhinitis?
    1. Promote vasoconstriction in the nasal mucosa.
    2. Block mast cell degranulation.
    3. Decrease the effect of histamines.
    4. Increase mast cell degranulation.

56. In the older adult patient, histamine H1 blockers may cause which side effects?
    1. Ataxia.
    2. Nausea.
    3. Bradycardia.
    4. Gastrointestinal upset.

57. What information is important for the family nurse practitioner to include when teaching a patient about the use of antihistamines?
    1. Use of topical antihistamines is safe and has relatively few side effects.
    2. Do not use over-the-counter (OTC) medications without consulting the health care provider.
    3. Constipation and urinary retention are expected side effects and do not need to be reported.
    4. Once antihistamine therapy has been taken for 3 days, avoidance of allergens is not necessary.

58. A primary advantage of using loratadine (Claritin) in treating a patient with seasonal allergies is that it:
    1. Is prudent to take only as needed.
    2. Is used for once-a-day (daily) dosing.
    3. Costs considerably less than other medications.
    4. Effectively decreases nasal secretions.

59. What medications are drugs of choice for the secondary treatment of patients with an anaphylactic reaction?
    1. Antibiotics and anticholinergics.
    2. Nonsteroidal antiinflammatory drugs (NSAIDs) and decongestants.
    3. Decongestants and expectorants.
    4. Antihistamines and corticosteroids.

60. Patients newly presenting with signs and symptoms of systemic lupus erythematosus (SLE) should have their medication profile reviewed to determine whether they are taking any medication that may have caused drug-induced lupus. Which drug should the family nurse practitioner most suspect?
    1. Digoxin (Lanoxin).
    2. Procainamide (Pronestyl).
    3. Trimethoprim-sulfamethoxazole.
    4. Cimetidine (Tagamet).

61. An adult patient presents at the clinic and states that he has a history of anaphylactic reactions. What signs and symptoms indicate to the family nurse practitioner that the patient is experiencing another reaction?
    1. Cough, wheezing, and urticaria.
    2. Severe malaise, pallor, stridor, and dyspnea.
    3. Anxiety, nasal congestion, and tachycardia.
    4. Rhinorrhea, nausea, and gastrointestinal pain.

62. A 56-year-old female has been prescribed hydroxychloroquine (Plaquenil) to treat symptoms of Sjögren syndrome. Which of the following complications should the family nurse practitioner monitor during therapy?
    1. Hyperglycemia.
    2. Liver failure.
    3. Vision changes.
    4. Hypokalemia.

63. What are the sites of predilection for a patient presenting with atopic dermatitis?
    1. Dorsal surface of the forearms
    2. Anterior thighs
    3. Antecubital fossa
    4. Dorsum of the hands

64. Prior to starting a preexposure prophylaxis (PrEP), the family nurse practitioner would order which of the following laboratory tests? (Select 4 responses.)
    1. Hepatitis B surface antigen and surface antibody.
    2. Fourth generation HIV test.
    3. HIV viral load.
    4. Complete blood count.
    5. Creatinine.

65. An adult client reports having a wasp sting on her left arm and experiencing swelling, redness, and some itching. It has been 4 days since the wasp sting, and the symptoms persist. The patient requests an epinephrine autoinjector (EAI). The patient denied any trouble breathing, abdominal cramps, or other signs of a systemic anaphylactic reaction. What would be important teaching for the family nurse practitioner to provide to the patient?
    1. Use an oral second-generation H1-antihistamine (e.g., cetirizine [Zyrtec]) as soon as possible after an insect sting or bite.
    2. Immediately wash the sting area and apply a warm compress.
    3. Explain the importance of having allergy testing.
    4. Prescribe an EAI and demonstrate how to use the device.

6 Immune & Allergy Answers & Rationales

Physical Exam & Diagnostic Tests

1. Answer: 1

Rationale: The reaction to each allergen is most important to know. Often patients state that they have an "allergy" to a particular food or medication, such as symptoms of nausea, stomach pain, or diarrhea, which they regard as an allergy. The signs and symptoms of the reaction, speed of onset, duration, and successful treatments used in the past are also important information. Medication side effects must be distinguished from true allergic reactions to drugs, so patient statements of drug or food allergies should be thoroughly explored.

2. Answer: 3

Rationale: In protein electrophoresis, proteins are electrically separated on a strip. It is a screening test to measure various proteins in body fluids, usually serum or urine. It assists in screening for diseases characterized by an increase or decrease in immunoglobulins (Ig). Serum and urine protein electrophoresis are also used to identify occult malignancy in a patient with failing health when no cause can be found. Immunofixation electrophoresis determines the presence of a heavy-chain immunoglobulin (IgG, IgM, or IgA). Complement fixation and ANA are diagnostic studies for rheumatoid problems. CRP is a blood test used to diagnose bacterial infectious disease and inflammatory disorders.

3. Answer: 3

Rationale: Although all tests listed may be included in a complete physical examination, laboratory tests ordered related to the diagnosis of SLE include ANA, ESR, and CRP. The ANA has high sensitivity, but it has low specificity for SLE, and an elevation can indicate a number of disorders. The anti–double-stranded DNA and anti-Smith antibodies have high specificity for SLE and are usually ordered if there is suspicion of SLE. During flares, ESR and CRP are elevated.

4. Answer: 3

Rationale: Based on recommendations from the Centers for Disease Control and Prevention (2014), initial testing for HIV should be an antigen/antibody combination immunoassay to test for established HIV-1 or HIV-2 infection and for acute HIV-1 infection. No further testing is required for specimens that are nonreactive on the initial immunoassay. Specimens with a reactive Ag/Ab combination immunoassay result (or repeatedly reactive, if repeat testing is required by regulatory authorities) should be tested with an antibody immunoassay that differentiates HIV-1 antibodies from HIV-2 antibodies. Reactive results on the initial antigen/antibody combination immunoassay and the HIV-1/HIV-2 antibody differentiation immunoassay should be interpreted as positive for HIV-1 antibodies, HIV-2 antibodies, or HIV antibodies, undifferentiated.

5. Answer: 1, 4

Rationale: The majority of patients with systemic lupus erythematosus have ANAs present in their blood with leukopenia, thrombocytopenia, lymphopenia, anemia, positive LE cell preparation, elevated sedimentation rate, and positive C-reactive protein. Proteinuria with cellular casts is often noted.

6. Answer: 4

Rationale: Angioedema is edema of the mucous membrane tissue and is most easily seen in the eyes and mouth. It also affects the tongue, feet, hands, and genitalia. Diffuse erythema may be seen in the upper body parts. Gastrointestinal symptoms (e.g., vomiting, cramping, diarrhea) may occur. African American patients are more likely to experience angioedema when given angiotensin-converting enzyme inhibitors (e.g., lisinopril, captopril).

7. Answer: 1, 4

Rationale: The most reliable tests for the presence of the specific IgE antibody is the skin test and the serum ImmunoCAP test, which can provide quantitative measurement of IgE and accurately determine whether patients have allergies and determine what they are allergic to. The smear for eosinophils and CBC are not specific for IgE antibody. Western blot analysis is used as a follow-up test to confirm the presence of an antibody and to help diagnose a condition, such as HIV or Lyme disease.

8. Answer: 3

Rationale: A referral to an allergist for skin testing would be appropriate to identify the allergen for immunotherapy to treat the condition. A nasal smear for eosinophils is not recommended as routine practice to be performed in an office setting. Many patients who have uncomplicated allergic rhinitis have a normal serum IgE. Skin-prick testing should be performed by allergy-trained providers only. RAST determines serum levels of allergen-specific IgE titers, but skin testing is more sensitive and is the preferred diagnostic method.

9. Answer: 2

Rationale: Acute, primary HIV infection depletes the CD4 cells, which produces leukopenia and depletes platelets. A hypochromic, normocytic anemia is present more often in advanced HIV. Elevated lymphocyte counts are more likely in other viral illnesses, and elevated neutrophil counts are seen in bacterial infections.

Disorders

10. Answer: 3

Rationale: Acute HIV infection is characterized by a history of prolonged fever and a red, raised, discrete skin eruption described as morbilliform ("measles-like"). Neither influenza nor mononucleosis typically presents with a rash. Varicella (chickenpox) presents with a vesicular skin eruption.

11. Answer: 3

Rationale: Treating a woman who has been raped requires time for patient education, and postexposure prophylaxis (PEP) should be offered and recommended. The patient should not assume that the man was HIV negative. Evidence based on PEP in health care workers and infants supports its effectiveness. Traumatic sex increases the risk of sexually transmitted diseases, including HIV.

12. Answer: 3

Rationale: It is important after a needlestick injury that the person wash the area with soap and water and then report the incident to the immediate supervisor and immediately seek medical treatment for postexposure prophylaxis. Sending the coworker to the nurse manager does not address the medical need of washing the needlestick site. Talking with the coworker and providing support is necessary, but not until the family nurse practitioner addresses the need to wash the site immediately.

13. Answer: 2

Rationale: Egg albumin is one of many identified common antigens that may result in an anaphylactic reaction, most commonly in children. Other common antigens include vaccines, sulfonamides, penicillins, hormones, peanuts, berries, nuts, seafood, and venom stings (honey bees and vespids).

14. Answer: 3

Rationale: The symptoms most often experienced with SLE are arthritis, arthralgias, fatigue, Raynaud phenomenon, chronic low-grade or recurrent fever, sun sensitivity, hair loss, weakness, butterfly (malar) facial rash, and weight loss. Typically, the pulmonary, cardiac, renal, and central nervous systems are involved, which may cause multisystem failure and contribute to mortality in patients with SLE.

15. Answer: 2

Rationale: HIV infection creates a chronic infectious state in the body that is transmitted through blood or body fluids and transplacentally throughout the patient's life.

16. Answer: 3

Rationale: Educate the patient about the importance of notifying all sexual partners and that the family nurse practitioner is required by law to report the positive HIV test result to the health department. It is still up to the patient to give names of sexual partners to the health department, which the patient can refrain from doing. Only if the patient has been adequately counseled or the provider believes that the patient will not disclose the information and will place others at risk can the provider disclose the patient's HIV-positive status. Ethical response and behavior include notification of all persons at risk so that early intervention and treatment can be initiated.

17. Answer: 4

Rationale: The patient is presenting with 4 of the 11 criteria necessary for diagnosing SLE using the 1997 American College of Rheumatology classification for SLE. No single test exists for SLE, but these characteristics plus laboratory results (ANA, erythrocyte sedimentation rate [ESR], C-reactive protein) can differentiate the diagnosis.

18. Answer: 1

Rationale: Corneal dryness and lack of saliva are the most common clinical manifestations of Sjögren syndrome. Patients may also have joint inflammation, but this rarely leads to joint destruction.

19. Answer: 3

Rationale: About 40% of patients with giant cell (temporal) arteritis have a history of PMR. The other diagnoses may have some of these symptoms, but only arteritis has all symptoms listed for this patient. It is especially crucial to note visual disturbances because these patients can develop sudden blindness. Definitive diagnosis is confirmed by biopsy. Prior to confirmation of disease, immediate treatment is important for patients when there is any strong clinical suspicion. Treatment typically consists of increasing the patient's prednisone to 40–60 mg daily in single or divided doses for 4 weeks and then gradually tapering alongside ESR monitoring.

20. Answer: 4

Rationale: The symptom of Raynaud phenomenon differentiates this as scleroderma. Esophageal dysfunction is often an initial complaint in scleroderma, which affects women four times more often than men. Barrett esophagus is diagnosed in patients with long-term gastroesophageal reflux disease and is associated with an increased risk of developing esophageal cancer.

21. Answer: 2

Rationale: The butterfly (malar) rash is one of the characteristic symptoms of SLE. Allergic drug eruptions are characterized by an erythematous rash or hives. Acne rosacea is characterized by redness and small, red, fluid-filled papules. Seborrheic dermatitis is characterized by scaly patches and red skin, mainly on the scalp, eyebrows, and face with minimal pruritus.

22. Answer: 2

Rationale: Because SLE is considered an autoimmune disorder, psychologic and physical stress can exacerbate the condition. A balanced diet helps limit the side effects of some medications, and regular exercise helps reduce arthralgia and myalgia associated with SLE. It is not necessary to check weight daily.

23. Answer: 2

Rationale: Granulomatosis polyangiitis (Wegener granulomatosis) is a multisystem disorder that occurs more often in males. Peak occurrence is between 40 and 60 years of age. The disease usually targets the upper respiratory tract, lungs, and kidneys. Connective tissue disease, pulmonary neoplasm, and infectious granulomatous disease would be considered in the differential diagnosis.

24. Answer: 2

Rationale: The signs and symptoms presented are classic for allergic rhinitis. Acute sinusitis would present with sinus pressure and pain, perhaps with tooth pain and fever. Vasomotor rhinitis typically does not present with ocular symptoms and occurs in response to environmental triggers, such as cold air, strong smells, irritants, changes in weather, some medications (angiotensin-converting enzyme inhibitors, beta blockers), stress, exercise, and certain foods. Influenza presents with acute onset, fever, chills, and general malaise.

25. Answer: 2

Rationale: The family nurse practitioner should suspect giant cell (temporal) arteritis, an inflammatory disorder of unknown etiology that affects large- and medium-sized arteries. It occurs two times more frequently in women than in men and most frequently in older adults, but rarely in the African American population. The clinical findings would reveal temporal tenderness and temporal bruits. About 40% of the patients who have been diagnosed with polymyalgia rheumatica (PMR) also have temporal arteritis, and the older adult patient may be relating some of her arthralgia and myalgia to normal changes of aging rather than PMR. The family nurse practitioner should also check the patient's erythrocyte sedimentation rate and consider referring the patient to a rheumatologist.

26. Answer: 2

Rationale: Unprotected oral sex with an HIV-positive person puts one at risk for exposure to the virus. Human contact, such as casual kissing or sharing an office or bathroom, does not transmit the virus. The virus is transmitted in body fluids and secretions.

27. Answer: 3

Rationale: Frequent STIs would alert the family nurse practitioner to the patient's lack of protected sex and the possibility of multiple partners. Night sweats, malaise, fatigue, swollen glands, and diarrhea may be associated with many other illnesses. UTIs are not always diagnostic of frequent sexual activity.

28. Answer: 4

Rationale: Although any of the clinical symptoms listed may be present in patients with SLE, fever, weight loss, arthritis, and arthralgias occur most often. Butterfly rash of the face and lymphadenopathy occur in less than half the cases. Pulmonary effusion, hepatomegaly, splenomegaly, and Raynaud syndrome occur in less than one-third of patients with SLE.

29. Answer: 3

Rationale: The massive release of mediators triggers a series of events in target organs. Prior sensitization to the antigen must have occurred to trigger an anaphylactic reaction. Anaphylaxis may result from injection of an antigen, ingestion of food or drugs, or inhalation of antigens.

30. Answer: 1

Rationale: The release of histamine results in bronchospasm, vasodilation, and vascular permeability, leading to wheezing, increased mucus production in the lung, and edema of the airway.

31. Answer: 3

Rationale: The signs and symptoms of GVHD include maculopapular rash; generalized erythroderma with desquamation; increased bilirubin; increased aspartate aminotransferase (AST) and serum glutamic-oxaloacetic transaminase (SGOT); and/or increased alkaline phosphatase, abdominal cramping, and diarrhea. Infection is characterized by fever, mental status changes, and headaches. Decreased RBCs, hematocrit, and hemoglobin and the presence of petechiae are signs of anemia. Fever, chills, and urticaria are indications of a reaction to white blood cells in the bone marrow.

32. Answer: 4

Rationale: T lymphocytes are the white blood cells responsible for control of the immune response. In SLE, T-suppressor cells are decreased and cellular activity is inhibited, leading to hypergammaglobulinemia and B-cell proliferation. Patients with SLE often present with lymphopenia with a higher proportion of B cells to T cells. The overall count of B cells is decreased compared with that in a healthy individual.

33. Answer: 3

Rationale: Based on the history of an HIV-positive test and the symptoms presented, the patient is at risk for *P. jirovecii* pneumonia. Further examination would include chest radiography and pulse oximetry (for oxygen saturation). The lack of purplish lesions is considered in ruling out Kaposi sarcoma. *K. pneumoniae* is a nosocomial infection, not community acquired. *M. pneumoniae* infection is typically seen in teenagers and older adult patients with an insidious onset of symptoms.

34. Answer: 4

Rationale: HBIG alone has been demonstrated to be effective in preventing HBV transmission. There is no IgC antibody. IgA is the secretory immunoglobulin found in tears, saliva, and mucous secretions of the lung and gastrointestinal tract. IgE mediates allergic reactions. PEG-IFN is used for chronic HBV infection.

35. Answer: 2

Rationale: Type I hypersensitivity reaction causes an immediate wheal and flare reaction. Contact dermatitis is seen in type IV (delayed) reaction. Hematuria is seen in type II reaction that is caused by preformed circulating cytotoxic antibodies, such as in a blood transfusion reaction or autoimmune hemolytic anemia. High fever may be seen in type III hypersensitivity reaction when large quantities of antigen–antibody complexes are released in the body.

36. Answer: 2

Rationale: Sexually active teenagers are the fastest-growing group of HIV-positive patients because of unprotected sexual activity. Immunocompromised patients and elderly adults are at no greater risk for developing HIV than any other group. However, an increasing number of middle-aged males are becoming HIV positive from their association with prostitutes after the loss of their partners. Risk factors for HIV include unprotected sexual contact with persons of unknown HIV status, multiple sexual partners, intravenous drug use, hemophilia, and blood transfusions received before 1985.

37. Answer: 3

Rationale: Cotton-wool spots are the most common ophthalmologic problem associated with SLE, are signs of vascular insufficiency, and are described as edematous and ischemic neuronal tissues that appear as fluffy areas on a funduscopic exam. They are also a common symptom of amaurosis fugax (retinal artery occlusion). Retinal hemorrhages and AV nicking may be seen in patients with hypertension. Conjunctivitis is an infection of the conjunctiva.

38. Answer: 1

Rationale: Patients with allergic rhinitis should monitor the air quality and allergy index in their area and understand their allergy triggers. A surgical-type mask will not filter out small allergens. Remaining inside during allergy season is an unrealistic expectation and can lead to decreased socialization and increased depression for the patient. Patients can enjoy a summer garden if they are careful about the choice of plants and flowers. For example, the patient with an allergy to ragweed should avoid daisies, dahlias, and chrysanthemums.

39. Answer: 3

Rationale: The OR nurse likely has a latex allergy. The incidence of latex allergies has increased dramatically since the onset of standard precautions and increased use of latex gloves. In an effort to meet the increased demand for gloves, changes in the manufacturing process have resulted in a higher protein count in the gloves. The increased exposure to the protein has led to a proliferation of health care workers being diagnosed with a latex allergy.

40. Answer: 2

Rationale: Latex allergy is a progressive disorder that worsens with continual exposure. The symptoms range from contact dermatitis to anaphylaxis. Currently, latex allergy affects 17% of health care workers and 39% of dental professionals. Latex allergy is an acquired immune response to the latex protein allergen. No vaccine is available; the only defense is to avoid contact with latex.

Pharmacology

41. Answer: 2

Rationale: The laboratory tests ordered would be CBC with differential, lipase, lactic acid, electrolytes, BUN, creatinine, and LFTs. Assessment of immune function (CD4 count, viral load) is unnecessary at this point and would not change the management of the acute illness. Having the amylase, lipase, lactic acid, and LFTs would assist in the diagnosis of pancreatitis, but it would not provide information on the patient's hydration status, the status of the biliary system, or the presence of acute infection.

42. Answer: 1

Rationale: The only absolute contraindication to the initiation of PrEP is being HIV positive. In addition, it is important to have documented hepatitis B virus infection and vaccination status. PrEP is for prevention. If the patient has HIV infection, then they need to be monitored on a different medication regime versus a prophylaxis or preventive regime.

43. Answer: 4

Rationale: Procainamide, hydralazine, and isoniazid have been shown to induce a lupus-like syndrome. Discontinuation of the medication results in the disappearance of the clinical signs and symptoms. Antibiotics (e.g., sulfonamides, penicillin) have been associated with anaphylactic reactions in some patients. Oral contraceptives may increase blood pressure and the risk for thromboembolism. NSAIDs (e.g., ibuprofen) have been associated with gastrointestinal upset and gastric pain, especially when taken on an empty stomach, and are contraindicated in patients with renal disease.

44. Answer: 1

Rationale: Giant cell (temporal) arteritis, seen primarily in elderly patients, can lead to blindness if not treated immediately with corticosteroids. The usual daily dose of prednisone is 60 mg in divided doses initially and then in a single morning dose (every-other-day steroids are not used). A slow taper is initiated after 4 weeks if the patient is asymptomatic and the erythrocyte sedimentation rate is decreased. Tapering of the dose is individualized, and the patient may be on drug therapy for several months to years. The average time for disease remission is 3–4 years (range, 1–10 years).

45. Answer: 3

Rationale: Drug allergies, especially to antibiotics, are common in many patients. The goal of initial therapy should be to understand the type of reaction the patient had to the initial medication therapy. The best and safest option is to avoid any medications that cause allergies and choose a related medication. In many cases, bacterial sensitivities restrict the ability to choose different classes of antibiotics. When a medication causes an allergy in a patient and it is the only medication available, desensitization therapy should be initiated starting with the lowest possible dose along with close monitoring. Desensitization therapy should never be used in patients who experienced reactions such as Stevens-Johnson syndrome or erythema multiforme.

46. Answer: 3

Rationale: Two antiretroviral drugs, tenofovir disoproxil fumarate (also called TDF or tenofovir) and emtricitabine (also called FTC), taken in a single pill daily for HIV prevention are approved for PrEP. TDF/FTC is a combination pill manufactured under the brand name Truvada. The management of HIV infection includes HAART. A single antiretroviral medication, acyclovir, would not be used as a PrEP drug therapy. Corticosteroids are not indicated in the PrEP regime.

47. Answer: 2, 4, 5, 6

Rationale: Chloroquine phosphate, doxycycline, mefloquine, and primaquine are medications used for malaria prophylaxis. Ceftriaxone is used for bacterial septicemia and respiratory and urinary tract infections caused by gram-negative bacilli. Ampicillin is used to treat infections with a variety of organisms and as prophylaxis for bacterial endocarditis.

48. Answer: 1

Rationale: Unless there is a secondary bacterial infection, antibiotics are contraindicated. Antihistamines and reduction of exposure to the allergen will help reduce the symptoms. For continued control and stabilization of the mast cells, corticosteroids are indicated. Analgesics may treat any pain associated with AR but do not directly treat AR.

49. Answer: 1

Rationale: Adults are at greater risk for the development of adverse drug reactions, probably because of the increased number of medications used and the amount of exposure and effects of aging on the immune system. Patients with prior drug reactions are more likely to develop reactions to new drugs. The risk of an adverse drug reaction occurs in the first 2–3 weeks of therapy. Prolonged course of therapy, high dosage, and intermittent therapy increase the risk of an adverse reaction. Genetic factors may increase mediator and metabolic pathway activity. The patient's gender has no effect, except with muscle relaxants and chymopapain, where female patients are at greater risk of an adverse drug reaction. The route of drug administration contributes to the risk, with IV, IM, SC, PO, and topical ranked in the order of greatest to least risk.

50. Answer: 3

Rationale: Treatment of chronic urticaria involves initial treatment with second-generation antihistamines and leukotriene receptor antagonists (montelukast), followed by first-generation antihistamines and doxepin (SILENOR). Patients for whom these therapies fail require stronger systemic immunosuppressants, such as omalizumab, cyclosporine, or tacrolimus. Omalizumab is an IgG monoclonal antibody that inhibits IgE receptors. Adalimumab is contraindicated in this patient because of a risk of reactivation of TB. Corticosteroids are indicated only for short-term control of symptoms and are avoided for long-term use.

51. Answer: 3

Rationale: TMP-SMX is used to treat and prevent *P. jirovecii* pneumonia, usually with a 21-day course, with up to 7–10 days for a clinical response. Fluconazole and amphotericin B are antifungal drugs. Acyclovir is an antiviral used primarily to treat herpes simplex virus types 1 and 2 and herpes zoster (shingles).

52. Answer: 1

Rationale: Nonsteroidal antiinflammatory drugs that inhibit cyclooxygenase 1 (COX-1), such as aspirin and ibuprofen, often exacerbate symptoms in patients with urticaria and should be avoided. Selective COX-1 inhibitors such as celecoxib are generally well tolerated. Antibiotics and other medications should be restricted only for patients with known allergies to those medications.

53. Answer: 2

Rationale: The chronic use of nasal decongestants for more than 3 days can result in a rebound effect when discontinued, leading to increased nasal congestion from reflex vasodilation. The condition may take as long as 2–3 weeks to resolve. Allergic rhinitis is not a self-limiting illness associated only with spring and fall. Even though therapy is initiated, the patient should be instructed to avoid exposure to the allergen as much as possible.

54. Answer: 4

Rationale: The major advantage of the second-generation antihistamines is that they do not cross the blood-brain barrier and therefore do not cause sedation and psychomotor dysfunction. There is little anticholinergic activity and less dry mouth and constipation. The cost of these antihistamines is 15–30 times greater than for the first-generation antihistamines. The medications are rapidly absorbed within 1–2 hours of PO administration on an empty stomach.

55. Answer: 1

Rationale: Sympathomimetics (adrenergics) cause vasoconstriction, thereby reducing edema and secretions. Inhaled corticosteroids stabilize mast cells and block degranulation.

56. Answer: 1

Rationale: The use of H1 blockers can cause paradoxical central nervous system stimulation, resulting in ataxia in older adult patients. Antihistamines can cause many simultaneous side effects in older adults, such as impaired vision and gait, which can lead to falls, and impaired thinking, which can interfere with functional skills (cognition) and could necessitate an unnecessary hospitalization or nursing home stay. Antihistamines also may interact with the older adult patient's numerous medications and exacerbate the side effects (e.g., dry mouth, constipation).

57. Answer: 2

Rationale: The patient should be instructed not to use OTC medications without consulting the family nurse practitioner or pharmacist. The nurse should explain that OTC drugs and herbal supplements are considered medications and that they may interact with prescribed medications. To avoid possible interactions, the patient should inform the family nurse practitioner of all the OTC drugs and herbals the patient is taking. The patient should be cautioned on the extended use of topical antihistamines. Antihistamines do not affect circulating histamine, so the patient must avoid exposure to a known allergen. Constipation and urinary retention are adverse effects that should be reported to the family nurse practitioner.

58. Answer: 2

Rationale: An advantage of using loratadine is that the once-daily dosing helps with patient compliance. The cost is greater than for some first-generation antihistamines. Loratadine with pseudoephedrine (Claritin D) is an antihistamine/decongestant with twice-daily or extended-release (daily) dosing.

59. Answer: 4

Rationale: Medications such as antihistamines and corticosteroids are used to counter mediator release and block release of additional mediators. NSAIDs, antibiotics, and decongestants are contraindicated in the treatment of anaphylactic reaction.

60. Answer: 2

Rationale: Of patients receiving procainamide, 20% develop clinical drug-induced SLE. The other drugs listed have not been associated with an SLE-like syndrome.

61. Answer: 2

Rationale: Severe malaise, pallor, stridor, and dyspnea are signs and symptoms associated with a severe anaphylactic reaction. Symptoms may occur immediately or up to 2 hours after exposure to the allergen. Severe reactions require immediate intervention.

62. Answer: 3

Rationale: Hydroxychloroquine (HCQ) is an aminoquinoline derivative used to treat malaria, but it can also be used as an immunosuppressant for autoimmune disorders, such as rheumatoid arthritis, primary Sjögren syndrome, porphyria cutanea tarda, and systemic lupus erythematosus. The most common and severe side effect of taking this medication is ocular toxicity, which can occur in the form of a retinopathy or as corneal damage. Other side effects can include muscular damage to the heart, causing restrictive cardiomyopathy, renal failure, myelosuppression, and hypoglycemia. HCQ can exacerbate conditions such as G6PD deficiency, psoriasis, and porphyrias. Patients who begin HCQ should have a baseline eye examination and reexamination no less than every 5 years.

63. Answer: 3

Rationale: The antecubital fossa is the site of predilection for patients with atopic dermatitis in addition to the popliteal area. The other anatomic areas of the body listed have a variety of possible diagnoses excluding atopic dermatitis.

64. Answer: 1, 2, 3, 5

Rationale: All patients need to have a negative HIV antibody test (fourth generation preferred) before initiation of PrEP. An HIV viral load should be drawn on anyone who has had sex without a condom in the last 30 days or has symptoms of acute HIV infection. Test and monitor for chronic hepatitis B virus, and, if negative, consider vaccination. Hepatitis C screening should be included. In all patients, assess serum creatinine, estimated creatinine clearance (should be less than 60 mL/min), urine glucose, and urine protein. Conduct pregnancy testing in cisgender women and transgender men who are at risk of being pregnant. In addition, baseline screening for sexually transmitted diseases (syphilis, gonorrhea, and chlamydia) should be included. Assessment of a patient's osteoporosis risk should be reviewed, because the PrEP medication (tenofovir [TDF]/emtricitabine [FTC]) can reduce bone density, so ordering a dual-energy X-ray absorptiometry scan may be part of the screening tests.

65. Answer: 1

Rationale: It would be important to teach the patient to take an oral second-generation H1-antihistamine (e.g., cetirizine [Zyrtec]) as soon as possible after an insect sting or bite. The family nurse practitioner concludes the patient did not have a systemic anaphylactic reaction to the wasp sting based on the history. The patient had a large local reaction with a long onset of action. Therefore the risk of future anaphylaxis is thought to be minimal and an EAI would not be prescribed. Any evidence of a systemic reaction must be treated as anaphylaxis. Wash the area with soap and cool water and place a cold, damp washcloth on the area to reduce swelling and alleviate pain.

7

Head, Eyes, Ears, Nose, & Throat (HEENT)

Physical Exam & Diagnostic Tests

HEAD

1. The family nurse practitioner is examining lymph nodes in the neck. Which nodes are palpated in the anterior triangle of the neck?
   1. Posterior cervical chain.
   2. Anterior superficial chain.
   3. Periauricular lymph nodes.
   4. Supraclavicular lymph nodes.

EYES

2. When using an ophthalmoscope, the family nurse practitioner:
   1. Holds the ophthalmoscope in the right hand (uses right eye) while examining the patient's left eye.
   2. Starts the examination with the ophthalmic lens set at zero.
   3. Begins in a position 1 inch from the eye to check the red light reflex.
   4. Examines the anterior chamber in a well-lit room.

3. The family nurse practitioner checking for strabismus would use which test?
   1. Cover-uncover test.
   2. Vertical prism test.
   3. Ishihara plates test.
   4. Snellen eye chart test.

4. The family nurse practitioner observes lid lag in a patient with:
   1. Myasthenia gravis.
   2. Hyperthyroidism.
   3. Hordeolum.
   4. Chalazion.

5. The family nurse practitioner is examining an older adult patient. There is a glossy white circle around the pupils of the eyes with yellowing of the sclera, and the pupils have a decreased reaction to the direct light reflex. The patient has a history of presbyopia. What is the correct interpretation of these findings?
   1. Beginning development of cataracts with a significant decrease in visual acuity.
   2. Expected changes in the eyes as a result of the aging process.
   3. Decrease in depth perception and early eye changes associated with glaucoma.
   4. Visual changes secondary to long-term treatment with digoxin and corticosteroids.

6. The family nurse practitioner is preparing to examine the eyes of an adult patient. To examine the retinal vessels and assess for hemorrhages, the family nurse practitioner uses which aperture on the ophthalmoscope?
   1. Small aperture.
   2. Red-free filter.
   3. Slit.
   4. Grid.

7. When testing the eyes for the presence of a consensual response, the family nurse practitioner:
   1. Shines the light into the patient's pupil and observes the rate of pupillary constriction.
   2. Directs the light into one pupil and observes for the constriction or response of the other pupil.
   3. Holds a card in front of one eye and, while the patient focuses on a fixed object, removes the card and observes movement of the newly uncovered eye.
   4. Asks the patient to focus on an object, and then directs a light source to the bridge of the nose while observing for symmetric reflection in both eyes.

8. On ophthalmic examination, there appears to be a narrowing or blocking of the vein at the point at which an arteriole crosses over the vein. What is the significance of this finding?
   1. The need to evaluate the patient for chronic hypertension.
   2. The possibility of increased ocular pressure associated with glaucoma.
   3. Its association with papilledema, causing decreased venous drainage.
   4. It may represent a small embolus in the retinal vessels.

9. When examining the eyes, the family nurse practitioner determines that the pupils constrict when a patient shifts their gaze from a far object to a near one. This is interpreted as:
   1. Accommodation.
   2. Intact extraocular motor nerves.
   3. Appropriate consensual response.
   4. Visual acuity within normal limits.

10. During a physical exam, the family nurse practitioner notes xanthelasma. What laboratory test will the nurse order?
    1. Erythrocyte sedimentation rate.
    2. Complete blood count.
    3. Thyroid profile.
    4. Lipid profile.

EARS

11. When examining the ears of an adult patient, the family nurse practitioner determines that the tympanic membrane (TM) is pearl gray, shiny, and translucent. This is interpreted as:
    1. Scarring from previous infections.
    2. Decreased circulation to the membrane.
    3. Presence of serous fluid behind the membrane.
    4. Normal characteristics of the adult ear.

12. The Rinne test is performed to compare bone conduction (when the tuning fork is placed on the mastoid bone) with air conduction (when the tuning fork is held near the ear). A normal Rinne test is described as:
    1. Equal conduction through the mastoid bone and ear canal.
    2. Air conduction is greater than bone conduction.
    3. Bone conduction is twice as long as air conduction.
    4. Sound is clearer with bone conduction than with air conduction.

13. When assessing the tympanic membrane (TM), specific landmarks are determined and described according to the face of a clock. Where are the normal landmarks for the right TM located?
    1. Direct light reflex located at the 5- to 6-o'clock position and malleus at the 1- to 2-o'clock position, with the umbo in the center.
    2. Manubrium slanted to the left, with malleus at the 10-o'clock position.
    3. Direct light reflex in the center of membrane, with malleus at the 9-o'clock position.
    4. Umbo is to the left of the center, with anterior malleolar folds at the 10-o'clock position.

NOSE

14. During a routine physical examination, a family nurse practitioner notes three horizontal creases across the lower bridge of the nose in an adolescent patient. What should be the next appropriate response?
    1. Refer the patient to the dermatologist for further evaluation.

2. Assume that the finding is normal and continue with the examination.
3. Refer the patient to an allergist for skin prick testing.
4. Ask the patient about symptoms of sneezing, rhinorrhea, congestion, tearing, and itching of the nose/eyes/ears.

15. The family nurse practitioner understands that the nasal mucosa:
    1. Is dark pink, smooth, and moist.
    2. Is pale and translucent in appearance.
    3. Is pale and boggy.
    4. Is red and swollen.

THROAT

16. A bacterial throat culture is indicated for the following suspected cause of pharyngitis:
    1. Rhinovirus and coronavirus infection.
    2. Group A β-hemolytic streptococci (GABHS).
    3. Mononucleosis.
    4. *Candida albicans.*

Disorders

HEAD

17. The family nurse practitioner sees a 60-year-old white woman of Norwegian descent in her office for a 2-day complaint of pain in her right frontotemporal region and jaw claudication that is worse at night. She has had a low-grade fever of 100.1°F (38.3°C) and has felt tired for the last 2–3 days. She guards the area and asks you not to touch it because it hurts. What is the most likely differential diagnosis for this patient?
    1. Temporomandibular joint (TMJ) dysfunction.
    2. Trigeminal neuralgia.
    3. Giant cell (temporal) arteritis.
    4. Preherpetic neuralgia.

18. An adult patient presents to the office with a white plaque near the base of the tongue. The family nurse practitioner notes that the plaque does not wipe off and assesses it as:
    1. Hemangioma.
    2. Leukoplakia.
    3. Papilloma.
    4. Erythroplasia.

19. Which of the following are predominant risk factors for oral carcinoma?
    1. History of dental infections and age younger than 40 years.
    2. Tobacco use and alcohol use.
    3. Infection with human papillomavirus and tobacco use.
    4. Alcohol use and history of dental abscess.

20. The hallmark of early oral cancer is:
    1. Tissue retraction.
    2. Thickening oral tissues.
    3. Persistent red and/or white patch and nonhealing ulcer.
    4. Halitosis and cough.

21. An adult male patient is being evaluated for a complaint of a sore throat. He states that he has difficulty swallowing and has mild oral pain. On examination, the family nurse practitioner finds that the patient's mouth, tongue, and pharynx are coated with white, curdlike plaques that are difficult to remove and leave a red surface when scraped with a tongue blade. What would be the best next action for the family nurse practitioner to take at this time?
    1. Refer the patient to an ear, nose, and throat specialist for evaluation.
    2. Prescribe amoxicillin 500 mg PO tid for 10 days.
    3. Encourage the patient to have HIV screening.
    4. Recommend only clear liquids for the next few days.

22. The family nurse practitioner knows that the most common site for head and neck cancer is the:
    1. Sinuses.
    2. Oral cavity.
    3. Larynx.
    4. Nasal cavity.

23. What is the "rule of 80s" as related to neck masses in patients older than 40 years?
    1. 80% of all nonthyroid neck masses are malignant, and 80% of those are metastatic.
    2. 80% of neck masses are benign.
    3. 80% of neck masses are caused by goiter and Graves' disease.
    4. 80% of nonthyroid neck masses are always adenocarcinoma.

24. What are characteristics of a malignant mass in the neck? (Select 2 responses.)
    1. Fixed and soft.
    2. Firm and fixed.
    3. Pulsatile and warm to touch.
    4. Moves with swallowing.
    5. Mobile and soft.

EYES

25. A patient presents to an office of a family nurse practitioner complaining of acute-onset severe right eye pain with no precipitating injury. The patient has blurred vision and reports seeing halos around lights. On exam, the pupil is dilated and fixed. The family nurse practitioner recognizes that this is a condition that requires immediate evaluation by an ophthalmologist, and the patient is sent to the emergency department for further care. What is the most likely cause of the patient's symptoms?
    1. Open-angle glaucoma.
    2. Closed-angle glaucoma.
    3. Corneal abrasion.
    4. Iritis/uveitis.

26. A patient is being prepared for cataract surgery. What information is important for the family nurse practitioner to explain to the patient?
    1. The procedure is short, and the patient usually goes home the morning after the surgery.
    2. Both eyes will be patched for the first 24 hours, and it is important for the patient to stay in bed.
    3. The patient may have problems with headache and eye pain for the first 24 hours and should take the pain medication provided.
    4. Patients usually go home 2–3 hours after the surgery; the patient will have increased tearing, but it should not be painful.

27. A patient who is a sheet metal worker reports a foreign body sensation in his right eye that began shortly after working this morning. The initial assessment would most likely be to:
    1. Instill a topical anesthetic.
    2. Assess visual acuity.
    3. Examine the eye using a penlight.
    4. Examine the eye using fluorescein.

28. A patient works as a welder. He finished work about 8 hours ago and discovered that the protective glass on his welding hood was cracked. He is complaining of severe left eye pain and photophobia. What are the most likely diagnosis and next best action?
    1. Chemical keratitis; dilate with atropine twice daily.
    2. Viral conjunctivitis; supportive treatment with artificial tears.
    3. Corneal abrasion; oral analgesics and an ophthalmic antibiotic ointment.
    4. Ultraviolet keratitis; ophthalmic antibiotic.

29. An older adult patient presents to the clinic with complaints of bilateral blurred vision that has increasingly worsened over the last 2 years. The patient also has a problem with night driving but denies eye pain. The family nurse practitioner would first evaluate for the presence of:
    1. Glaucoma.
    2. Retinal detachment.
    3. Degeneration of the macula.
    4. Cataracts.

30. An adult patient presents to the family nurse practitioner for evaluation of a "red" right eye for 24 hours. The patient states that when he awoke, the eye was matted shut. The patient denies trauma to the eye, eye pain, and any changes in vision. During the exam, it is noted that the pupils are equal and reactive, and there is mild conjunctival hyperemia bilaterally and a significant amount of yellowish discharge. The family nurse practitioner treats this patient for:
    1. Allergic conjunctivitis.
    2. Corneal abrasion.
    3. Viral conjunctivitis.
    4. Bacterial conjunctivitis.

31. Which assessment of the eye is a deviation from common age-related physiologic changes?
    1. Arcus senilis.
    2. Presbyopia.
    3. Sensitivity to glare.
    4. Sustained nystagmus.

32. During a routine physical examination of a 30-year-old patient, the family nurse practitioner identifies arcus senilis. What is the significance of this disorder?
    1. High potential for future blindness.
    2. None because this is a normal variant of the aging process.
    3. Abnormal lipid metabolism requiring further evaluation.
    4. Hereditary variant of no consequence.

33. A 70-year-old patient comes to the clinic complaining of an increased sensitivity to glare, difficulty adapting to darkness, and altered depth perception. What should the family nurse practitioner suspect?
    1. Cataract.
    2. Macular degeneration.
    3. Glaucoma.
    4. Normal age-related physiologic changes.

EARS

34. A geriatric patient is complaining of difficulty hearing in both ears and states that the problem seems to have steadily worsened over the last few years. Which of the following would support a diagnosis of presbycusis?
    1. Complaint that they can hear voices but that everyone mumbles.
    2. Rinne test indicating air conduction greater than bone conduction.
    3. History of long-term tetracycline therapy for chronic infections.
    4. Weber test localizing increased tone in left ear versus right ear.

35. Which assessment finding of the ear would indicate a deviation from the normal aging process?
    1. A dull, retracted, and white tympanic membrane.

2. An elongated lobule.
    3. A sensorineural hearing loss.
    4. A bulging tympanic membrane with a distorted cone of light.

36. Which statement by the family nurse practitioner indicates an understanding of conductive hearing loss in the older patient?
    1. "This has occurred because of damage of the eighth cranial nerve from gentamicin."
    2. "This is a result of an inner ear infection."
    3. "This is a normal part of aging and is referred to as presbycusis."
    4. "This may be reversible after the cerumen is removed from the ear canal."

37. Sensorineural hearing loss is common in industrial settings and preventable with the use of adequate hearing protection. This type of hearing loss is usually first noted with changes at what level?
    1. 500 Hz.
    2. 200 Hz.
    3. 1000–2000 Hz.
    4. 3000–6000 Hz.

NOSE

38. A family nurse practitioner sees an older adult and diagnoses the patient with an idiopathic anterior epistaxis. The bleeding site was visualized and chemical cautery was successful at stopping the bleeding. Which of the following discharge instructions should be provided to the patient?
    1. Avoid touching or placing any lubricants, such as petroleum jelly or antibiotic ointment, into the nostrils.
    2. If the patient has the urge to sneeze, the patient should do so with the mouth closed.
    3. If bleeding recurs, the patient should perform digital compression of the nose with the patient's cervical spine hyperextended in a "sniffing" position for 5 minutes.
    4. Encourage the patient to use a humidifier at home and squirt nasal saline liberally.

39. An adult patient presents to the family nurse practitioner's office with the following complaints for the last 10 days: fever and complaints of right facial pain, copious yellow nasal discharge, and acute pain and headache, primarily when bending over. The physical examination is significant for right maxillary sinus tenderness on palpation. What is the most likely diagnosis?
    1. Chronic sinusitis.
    2. Acute sinusitis.
    3. Dental abscess.
    4. Giant cell (temporal) arteritis.

40. The family nurse practitioner notes a nasal septal perforation in a young adult. What does the family nurse practitioner suspect as the cause?
    1. Deviated nasal septum.
    2. Chronic epistaxis.
    3. Nose picking.
    4. Cocaine use.

THROAT

41. A potential complication of streptococcal pharyngitis that leads to contralateral uvular deviation, asymmetric tonsillar hypertrophy, muffled voice on exam but no stridor, drooling, or difficulty breathing or swallowing is recognized by family nurse practitioner as:
    1. Peritonsillar abscess.
    2. Peritonsillar cellulitis.
    3. Retropharyngeal abscess.
    4. Epiglottitis.

42. A 20-year-old patient presents to the family nurse practitioner's office with a chief complaint of "severe sore throat" for 3 days. The patient states that he also "ran a fever, but does not know how high it got," and has been very fatigued. Physical examination reveals enlarged tonsils with large, patchy exudate; erythematous pharynx; and nontender posterior cervical lymphadenopathy. The remainder of the examination is unremarkable. What diagnosis will the family nurse practitioner most likely make?
    1. Infectious mononucleosis.
    2. Leukoplakia.
    3. Scarlet fever.
    4. Oral candidiasis.

43. Which of the following clinical findings is most likely associated with bacterial streptococcal pharyngitis?
    1. Rhinorrhea.
    2. Cough.
    3. Enlarged erythematous tonsils with exudate.
    4. Small oral vesicles.

Pharmacology

44. An adult patient returns to the office of a family nurse practitioner 1 week after he was diagnosed with acute otitis externa and was started on otic ciprofloxacin/dexamethasone (Ciprodex). He explains that his symptoms of pain and itching of his left ear have worsened with the use of the medication. In addition, he now notes a white discharge from his left ear. Examination reveals a mildly edematous erythematous ear canal with white discharge and a normal tympanic membrane. What would be an appropriate treatment for this patient?
    1. Continue the current medication and prescribe antipyrine/benzocaine (Auralgan).
    2. Discontinue Ciprodex and prescribe carbamide peroxide (Debrox).
    3. Discontinue Ciprodex, irrigate the ear canal, and prescribe clotrimazole 1% (Canesten) solution.
    4. Continue the current medication and prescribe oral amoxicillin twice daily.

45. Mild circumoral swelling of the lips without airway obstruction in a 65-year-old male who is allergic to shellfish that started 12 hours ago after eating at a seafood restaurant should be treated with which of the following?
    1. Epinephrine (EpiPen), 0.3 mg injected subcutaneously.
    2. Diphenhydramine (Benadryl) 25 mg PO tid.
    3. Lisinopril (Zestril) 10 mg once daily.
    4. Montelukast sodium (Singulair) 10 mg daily at nighttime.

46. An adolescent who has a history of severe allergic rhinitis asks for a recommendation of a medication to try. What is the first-line agent for this condition?
    1. Fluticasone (Flonase) nasal spray, 2 sprays in each nostril daily.
    2. Azelastine (Astelin) nasal spray, 2 sprays in each nostril bid.
    3. Pseudoephedrine (Sudafed) 120 mg orally bid.
    4. Fexofenadine (Allegra) 180 mg orally daily.

47. When the family nurse practitioner decides to prescribe an antibiotic for the treatment of acute sinusitis, which antibiotic is recommended as first-line empiric therapy for nonpenicillin-allergic adults?
    1. Amoxicillin (Amoxil).
    2. Doxycycline (Vibramycin).
    3. Azithromycin (Zithromax).
    4. Amoxicillin-clavulanate (Augmentin).

48. A geriatric patient is diagnosed with chronic open-angle glaucoma. She has a past history of bradycardia and first-degree atrioventricular block. In consideration of her treatment, what medication is to be avoided?
    1. Pilocarpine (Isopto Carpine).
    2. Timolol (Timoptic).
    3. Hydrochlorothiazide (HydroDIURIL).
    4. Acetazolamide (Diamox).

49. The treatment plan for a patient diagnosed with infectious mononucleosis includes which of the following?
    1. Resting during the acute phase.
    2. Avoiding exercise during the acute phase.
    3. Corticosteroids during the acute phase.
    4. Ampicillin orally for 10 days.

7   Head, Eyes, Ears, Nose, & Throat (HEENT) Answers & Rationales

Physical Exam & Diagnostic Tests

HEAD

1. Answer: 2

Rationale: The conceptualization of triangles is useful in determining the location of palpable lymph nodes in the neck. The sternocleidomastoid muscle is the division between the anterior (containing the anterior superficial cervical chain) and the posterior (containing the posterior cervical chain) triangles. The trapezius muscle marks the posterior border of the posterior triangle. The supraclavicular nodes are palpated in the angle formed by the clavicle and the sternocleidomastoid muscle.

EYES

2. Answer: 2

Rationale: The correct use of the ophthalmoscope involves using the right hand and right eye to examine the patient's right eye. The room should be semidarkened for best visualization. The examiner initially inspects the lens and vitreous body from a distance of about 12 inches (at zero setting) and moves closer to the eye, usually rotating the lenses to the positive numbers (+15 to +20), which assists in focusing on near objects.

3. Answer: 1

Rationale: The cover-uncover test is used to detect latent strabismus. The vertical prism test is performed to assess for amblyopia. The Ishihara test is used to examine color perception. The Snellen test is done to assess visual acuity.

4. Answer: 2

Rationale: Lid lag occurs in patients with hyperthyroidism and is evaluated by having the patient follow the examiner's finger as it is slowly moved up and down. The patient has lid lag if sclera can be seen above the iris as the patient looks downward. Ptosis is a drooping lid margin that falls at the pupil or below and may indicate an oculomotor lesion or myasthenia gravis. A chalazion is a chronic, sterile, lipogranulomatous inflammatory lesion of the meibomian gland, whereas a hordeolum is an acute inflammation of one of the glands in the eyelid.

5. Answer: 2

Rationale: Yellowing of the sclera and arcus senilis (also known as corneal arcus) is a benign, yellow-whitish ring

around the limbus and is seen in the older adult because of age-related physiologic changes. Cataracts occur as a result of opacity of the lens of the eye that causes partial or total blindness. The visual acuity and depth perception of the patient cannot be determined from the information provided.

6. Answer: 2

Rationale: The red-free filter is used to visualize the vessels and hemorrhages in better detail by improving contrast. This setting will make the retina look black and white. The small aperture is used when the pupil is very constricted; the slit is used to examine contour abnormalities of the cornea, lens, and retina; and the grid is used for estimating the size of lesions found in the fundal area.

7. Answer: 2

Rationale: A light beam shining onto one retina causes pupillary constriction in both that eye, termed the *direct reaction* to light, and in the opposite eye, referred to as the *consensual reaction.*

8. Answer: 1

Rationale: Chronic hypertension stiffens and thickens arteries, resulting in arteriovenous nicking. Intraocular pressure cannot be determined from an ophthalmic examination. Papilledema is associated with swelling around the optic disc with blurred margins. Small emboli are represented by an abrupt impediment or severe narrowing of an arteriole not associated with where the retinal veins and arteries cross.

9. Answer: 1

Rationale: Accommodation is the ability of the lens to change shape. Changes in pupil size when focusing from near to distant objects (and vice versa) tests for accommodation. *Extraocular movements* refer to the ability to move the eye in six cardinal directions. Consensual response is constriction of the eye in response to light being shined in the opposite eye. The Snellen eye chart is used to determine visual acuity.

10. Answer: 4

Rationale: Xanthelasma is a soft or hard yellow plaque on the inside corners of the eyelids (near the inner canthus). It is made up of cholesterol and is found more often on the upper lid than the lower lid. Xanthelasma is a type of xanthoma and is associated with hyperlipidemias, so a lipid profile would be an appropriate test to order.

EARS

11. Answer: 4

Rationale: The normal TM is thin, translucent, shiny, and slightly concave with a pearl gray or pale pink appearance. This describes the normal characteristics of the TM. There is no evidence indicating scarring, presence of fluid, or decreased circulation to the membrane.

12. Answer: 2

Rationale: The Rinne test is positive (or normal) when air conduction (AC) is greater than bone conduction (BC) (AC > BC). If the patient hears the tuning fork better by bone conduction, the Rinne test is negative, which suggests a conductive hearing loss.

13. Answer: 1

Rationale: Direct light reflex located at the 5- to 6-o'clock position and malleus at the 1- to 2-o'clock position, with the umbo in the center, describes the correct position for the landmarks on the right ear. The manubrium slants to the right with the malleus at the 1- to 2-o'clock position for the right ear. The direct light reflex in the center of the membrane with the malleus at the 9-o'clock position describes the correct position for the left ear. The umbo is in the center with the anterior folds at the 1- to 2-o'clock position for the right ear.

NOSE

14. Answer: 4

Rationale: The family nurse practitioner recognizes the nasal crease to be a result of uncontrolled allergic rhinitis, which may be seasonal or perennial as the patient repeatedly wipes the nose with the palm. Dermatologic evaluation is not necessary. The finding is not normal. Before treatment is prescribed, a thorough history on allergic rhinitis should be obtained.

15. Answer: 1

Rationale: The nasal mucosa is normally dark pink, smooth, and moist. A pale, boggy mucosa suggests chronic allergy. A red and swollen mucosa suggests acute allergic rhinitis. The normal secretion is mucoid. Purulent, crusty, or bloody secretions are abnormal.

THROAT

16. Answer: 2

Rationale: Diagnostic studies used to detect GABHS (or GAS) infection include a throat culture and a RADT. Throat culture has been considered the gold standard method to establish the microbial cause of acute pharyngitis. RADT is often used because it is rapid and convenient; however, RADT is less sensitive (true positive) than a throat culture. A positive monospot test result reveals heterophile antibodies. The monospot test is highly specific and sensitive. *C. albicans* and rhinovirus are not diagnosed by bacterial cultures. Rhinovirus is one of the most common viral causes of pharyngitis. Oral candidiasis, a fungal infection, can be diagnosed with a potassium hydroxide smear showing mycelia (hyphae) or pseudomycelia (pseudohyphae) yeast forms.

Disorders

HEAD

17. Answer: 3

Rationale: Giant cell (temporal) arteritis is most commonly seen in women of Scandinavian descent and presents with pain in the frontotemporal region that is exquisitely tender. Trigeminal neuralgia typically presents as a sharp, shooting, momentary pain with radiation to the jaw or cheek. Preherpetic neuralgia is a preeruption phase of shingles that can present 2–3 days before the vesicular rash. It is a diagnosis of exclusion that is confirmed by a rash appearing 2–3 days after the onset of the discomfort. TMJ dysfunction presents as pain and tenderness over the TMJ joint, frequently associated with chewing and jaw movement.

18. Answer: 2

Rationale: Oral leukoplakia is a precancerous lesion that presents as white patches or plaques of the oral mucosa that cannot be rubbed off. Hemangiomas are usually benign tumors made up of blood vessels that typically appear as a purplish or reddish, slightly elevated area of skin that can include the lips, tongue, and buccal mucosa. Erythroplasia is an asymptomatic, red, velvety lesion on the oral or genital mucosa that is considered a precancerous lesion. Papillomas are benign verrucous lesions that are manifestations of human papillomavirus infection.

19. Answer: 2

Rationale: Tobacco and alcohol use are among the greatest risk factors for oral cavity and oropharyngeal cancers. Smokers are many times more likely than nonsmokers to develop these cancers. Tobacco smoke from cigarettes, cigars, or pipes can cause cancers anywhere in the mouth or throat. Drinking alcohol increases the risk of developing oral cavity and oropharyngeal cancers because about 7 of 10 patients with oral cancer are heavy drinkers. The disease is age related, occurring in those over 40 years of age and increasing with age. Infection with cancer-causing types of human papillomavirus (HPV), especially HPV-16, is a risk factor for some types of head and neck cancers, particularly oropharyngeal cancers that involve the tonsils or the base of the tongue.

20. Answer: 3

Rationale: Erythroplasia is accompanied by an inflammatory reaction in a patient with suspected oral cancer. Lesions persisting over 14 days strongly suggest early oral cancer. Tissue retraction and thickening of the oral tissues are later signs of oral cancer. Halitosis (odor) may be associated with dysfunction within the oral cavity (dental caries), nasal cavity, sinuses, or esophageal disorders. Cough is the primary symptom of respiratory disorders such as acute bronchitis or pneumonia.

21. Answer: 3

Rationale: Adults who present with thrush (oral candidiasis) may be immunologically impaired. It is important to screen these adults for HIV and diabetes mellitus because frequency of oral candidiasis increases with both of those illnesses. Treatment with amoxicillin is not the appropriate action because the presenting disorder describes a fungal infection.

22. Answer: 2

Rationale: The family nurse practitioner knows that the risk factors for head and neck cancer include tobacco and alcohol use; poor oral hygiene; and occupational exposure to asbestos, nickel, wood, or leather. The most common site is in the oral cavity, accounting for 48% of head and neck cancer diagnoses.

23. Answer: 1

Rationale: The "rule of 80s," often applied to adults over the age of 40, states that 80% of nonthyroid neck masses are neoplastic and that 80% of these masses are malignant. Eighty percent of malignancies in adults are squamous cell carcinomas, and 80% of metastatic lesions are from primaries above the level of clavicle. A neck mass in a child, on the other hand, has an 80%–90% probability of being benign.

24. Answer: 2, 3

Rationale: Firm and fixed neck masses are worrisome findings that are often associated with malignancy. Soft and mobile masses are less worrisome for a malignancy. A pulsatile mass may be a vascular tumor. A mass that is warm to touch has an infectious origin. A mass that moves with swallowing is often associated with the thyroid gland.

EYES

25. Answer: 2

Rationale: Closed-angle (acute) glaucoma is a medical emergency that requires immediate ophthalmologic evaluation. Corneal abrasion is commonly seen with contact lens wear or in the presence of ocular trauma. Open-angle glaucoma is most often an asymptomatic chronic condition. Iritis/uveitis is an infection/inflammation of the deeper structures of the eye and is most often associated with trauma or infection. Dilated, fixed pupils are not seen with iritis/uveitis.

26. Answer: 4

Rationale: Patients go home almost immediately after the procedure. The eye may be patched, depending on whether anesthesia was local or topical. The patient may experience some discomfort, but pain should not be a problem. The patient can be mobile and active as tolerated.

27. Answer: 2

Rationale: Initial assessment of visual acuity would provide the basis for comparison in the event of complications. Visual acuity should be measured before the instillation of a topical anesthetic or fluorescein. Following visual acuity assessment, an examination of the eye using a penlight is performed to evaluate for a penetrating foreign body.

28. Answer: 4

Rationale: Photokeratitis, also known as *ultraviolet (UV) keratitis*, is an acute syndrome that occurs after UV irradiation of the eyes and can be intensely painful. Although the exposure may not initially be apparent to the patient, there is a latency period of approximately 6–12 hours between exposure and onset of symptoms. Photokeratitis is generally a self-limited condition with complete resolution. Initial treatment consists of oral analgesics and lubricant antibiotic ointments. An eye injury resulting from a welder's arc is commonly known as *flash burn*, *welder's flash*, or *arc eye*.

29. Answer: 4

Rationale: A cataract is an opacity of the lens of the eye that causes partial or total blindness. Cataracts are characterized by painless loss of visual acuity over time. Retinal detachment most often occurs suddenly, with partial loss of the field of vision. Glaucoma results in the loss of peripheral vision, and macular degeneration involves primarily the central vision field.

30. Answer: 4

Rationale: Bacterial conjunctivitis presents with injection of the conjunctiva, no pain, and a history of purulent discharge. Bacterial conjunctivitis is usually in one eye, and viral conjunctivitis is more common in both eyes. Viral conjunctivitis will usually present with acute onset of a red eye with itching, photophobia, and excessive watery discharge. Unlike conjunctivitis with infectious causes, allergic conjunctivitis typically presents simultaneously in both eyes with the predominant feature of itching. The chief complaint of a corneal abrasion is pain.

31. Answer: 4

Rationale: Sustained nystagmus is indicative of a neurologic complication. The other options include normal age-related changes.

32. Answer: 3

Rationale: Arcus senilis is the deposit of lipids at the junction of the cornea and sclera that is present in many people over age 50 years. When identified in younger individuals, it may be related to a disorder of lipid metabolism. High cholesterol is more likely associated with a similar gray or white arc visible around the entire cornea (circumferential arcus) in younger adults.

33. Answer: 4

Rationale: These findings are normal age-related physiologic changes. Signs and symptoms of cataracts include reduced visual acuity; painless progressive loss of vision; and sensitivity to light, especially at night (night driving). Reduced color discrimination and presbyopia may also develop. Macular degeneration presents with a loss of central vision. Primary open-angle glaucoma presents with occasional headaches and seeing halos around lights but may be asymptomatic in its early stages. Primary angle-closure glaucoma can present with decreased vision, seeing halos around lights at night, and conjunctival redness.

EARS

34. Answer: 1

Rationale: In presbycusis, the ability to hear high-frequency sounds is diminished. These patients have difficulty distinguishing consonant sounds, so words such as "shoe" and "true" are heard as "oo." The Rinne test indicates that bone conduction is greater than air conduction. Tetracyclines are not ototoxic. The patient's family history may or may not contribute to the problem. If the hearing loss is sensorineural, the sound will be heard best in the normal ear when performing a Weber test. Normally, sound should be of equal intensity in both ears.

35. Answer: 4

Rationale: A bulging tympanic membrane with a distorted cone of light would be indicative of an inflammation of the middle ear (acute otitis media). The other options indicate age-related physiologic changes.

36. Answer: 4

Rationale: Conductive hearing loss may result from acute otitis media, perforation of the eardrum, and obstruction of the ear canal, as by cerumen. The other options result in sensorineural hearing loss.

37. Answer: 4

Rationale: Noise-induced hearing loss is a sensorineural hearing deficit that begins at the higher frequencies (3000–6000 Hz) and develops gradually as a result of chronic exposure to excessive sound levels.

NOSE

38. Answer: 4

Rationale: Idiopathic epistaxis is the most common type, and the majority of epistaxis events occurs in the anterior aspect. Although it is possible to eliminate bleeding with nasoconstricting agents and digital compression for at least 10—15 minutes with the cervical spine flexed "chin to the chest," some patients require chemical cauterization. Following a successful cauterization, the patient should be instructed to use a humidifier at home; squirt nasal saline liberally; and apply lubricants, such as petroleum jelly or antibiotic ointment, with a cotton swab intranasally because dry air contributes to bleeding and re-bleeding. The patient should not sneeze with the mouth closed because that increases intranasal pressure.

39. Answer: 2

Rationale: The patient is experiencing the classic characteristics of acute sinusitis. Viral causes of sinusitis show improvement by day 10, and bacterial sinus infections persist longer. A dental abscess can cause pain that radiates to the sinuses but more often causes constant, severe, tooth-associated pain and jaw tenderness. Giant cell (temporal) arteritis causes pain in the jaw and face but no nasal discharge.

40. Answer: 4

Rationale: Nasal snorting of cocaine results in nasal congestion and discharge. Because cocaine is a potent sympathomimetic, the nasal passages appear similar to what is found on physical exam of patients who abuse nasal decongestants (e.g., oxymetazoline [Afrin]). Chronic use of cocaine causes the nasal septal mucosa to become ischemic, which leads to tissue atrophy and eventual septal perforation, which is noted on physical exam and should be followed up with questions about snorting cocaine.

THROAT

41. Answer: 1

Rationale: Asymmetric tonsillar hypertrophy with contralateral uvular deviation are hallmark signs of peritonsillar abscess, whereas peritonsillar cellulitis is associated with deep erythema that extends beyond the tonsils and pharynx without structural changes. Retropharyngeal abscess is a deep soft tissue infection that is difficult to diagnose on examination but is frequently accompanied by stridor. Drooling, tripoding, and dysphagia are a classic clinical triad indicating epiglottitis.

42. Answer: 1

Rationale: Mononucleosis is often seen in adolescents and young adults. It often presents with sore throat, fever, tonsillar exudate, lymphadenopathy, and malaise. Oral leukoplakia is a white plaque or patches on the oral mucosa, generally precancerous. Scarlet fever, a complication of streptococcal pharyngitis, presents with sore throat, fever, abdominal pain, headache, erythematous fine rash, and strawberry tongue. Oral candidiasis presents with white, curdlike plaques on erythematous mucosa. The tongue is red with a white coat.

43. Answer: 3

Rationale: The clinical presentation of pharyngitis varies and depends on the causative agent. Characteristics of bacterial pharyngitis include sore throat, headache, erythema of the tonsils with white or yellow exudate, dysphagia, tender anterior cervical adenopathy, and fever. Small oral vesicles are seen with herpangina, an infection caused by the coxsackie virus. Cough is typically the primary symptom of acute bronchitis; the presence of cough decreases the likelihood of streptococcal pharyngitis. Rhinorrhea is associated with allergic rhinitis.

Pharmacology

44. Answer: 3

Rationale: The family nurse practitioner recognizes that the patient's condition is a result of otomycosis, a fungal infection of the external auditory canal that occurs either as a solitary infection or as a subsequent infection associated with use of antibiotic and steroidal otic therapy. The mainstay of treatment is meticulous cleaning of the ear canal and antifungal therapy. Otic antibiotics must be discontinued because they may be a causative agent and have no clinical benefit at this time. Carbamide peroxide (Debrox) is used to treat partial or complete earwax obstructions.

45. Answer: 2

Rationale: Mild allergic angioedema without airway obstruction should be treated with oral antihistamines and glucocorticoids. Lisinopril can be a causative agent of angiotensin-converting enzyme inhibitor–induced angioedema. An EpiPen is reserved for patients who are having anaphylaxis and should always be given intramuscularly.

46. Answer: 1

Rationale: Intranasal steroids (e.g., fluticasone) are most effective for moderate to severe allergic rhinitis, and they do not have any systemic side effects. Fexofenadine (Allegra) is a second-line choice for allergic rhinitis. The other medications listed are reasonable alternatives as they are effective, but they are not without side effects. Oral decongestants such as pseudoephedrine can cause insomnia, nervousness, or urinary retention. Azelastine (Astelin) can cause sedation and is expensive.

47. Answer: 4

Rationale: Amoxicillin has been recommended as a first-line agent in the past because of its narrow spectrum and relatively low cost. However, there is increasing emergence of antimicrobial resistance among respiratory pathogens, including pneumococci and *H. influenzae*. Amoxicillin-clavulanate rather than amoxicillin is recommended as empiric first-line therapy for nonpenicillin-allergic adults. Doxycycline is a reasonable alternative for first-line therapy and can be used in patients with a penicillin allergy. Azithromycin is not recommended for empiric therapy, because of its high rate of resistance of *S. pneumoniae*.

48. Answer: 2

Rationale: Topical beta blockers such as timolol lower intraocular pressure but can be absorbed systemically. The major side effects are similar to those associated with systemic beta blocker therapy, which can include a worsening of heart failure, bradycardia, and heart block. Topical beta blockers are contraindicated in some patients with cardiac or pulmonary disease.

49. Answer: 1

Rationale: Treatment of mononucleosis includes bed rest while the patient has fever and myalgia (10–14 days), supportive acetaminophen or ibuprofen, warm saline gargles, and throat lozenges or analgesic spray. The patient must avoid strenuous exercise and contact sports for 2 months because of the risk of splenic rupture. Splenomegaly is seen in 50%–60% of all patients with infectious mononucleosis. Corticosteroids are recommended only for patients with impending airway obstruction, and an immediate referral to an otolaryngologist is warranted. Ampicillin is not recommended, because of the viral etiology of this disease. Additionally, rashes are common in patients with infectious mononucleosis and are treated with amoxicillin or ampicillin. About 95% of patients with mononucleosis recover uneventfully with supportive treatment.

8

Integumentary

Physical Exam & Diagnostic Tests

1. The family nurse practitioner is performing a physical exam on a female patient as part of a scheduled office visit. Which finding, if noted, would represent a normal process associated with aging?
   1. Yellow-colored nails.
   2. Thinning of hair.
   3. Beau's lines.
   4. Absence of lesions.

2. The family nurse practitioner identifies clubbing on a male patient during an examination. Based on this finding, which three diagnostic tests/assessment techniques would be ordered?
   1. Imaging studies of the hands.
   2. Orthostatic blood pressures.
   3. Pulse oximetry reading.
   4. Electrocardiogram (ECG).
   5. Chest x-ray.

3. The family nurse practitioner describes an annular skin lesion as usually arranged in:
   1. Groups of vesicles erupting unilaterally.
   2. A line.
   3. A pattern of merging together, not discrete.
   4. A circle, or ring shaped.

4. A patient has pitting of the nails. Which condition does the family nurse practitioner understand this is associated with?
   1. Psoriasis.
   2. Iron-deficiency anemia.
   3. Malnutrition.
   4. Hyperthyroidism.

5. What diagnostic test would be appropriate to order for a patient who has acanthosis nigricans (AN)?
   1. Skin biopsy.
   2. Liver function tests (LFTs).
   3. Hemoglobin A1c (HbA1c).
   4. IgE electrophoresis.

6. The family nurse practitioner is inspecting a dark-skinned individual for signs of jaundice. Where is the best place to observe jaundice in dark-skinned individuals?
   1. Sclera of the opened eye.
   2. Palms and soles of the hands and feet.
   3. Oral mucosa.
   4. Nail beds.

7. When assessing an adult's hydration status, what is the best place to evaluate skin turgor?
   1. Just below the clavicle.
   2. Below the scapula on the back.
   3. On the inside of the forearm.
   4. On the back of the hand.

8. The Wood's lamp examination may be used to evaluate skin lesions. When the light is shone on the patient's skin, a bright-green fluorescence indicates:
   1. Presence of fungi.
   2. Lichenification.
   3. Keratinized cells.
   4. Bacterial colonies.

9. On examination of a patient's skin, the family nurse practitioner finds a lesion that is about 0.75 cm in diameter, brown, circumscribed, flat, and nonpalpable. What is the correct term for this lesion?
   1. Macule.
   2. Papule.
   3. Nodule.
   4. Wheal.

10. The history and physical of a patient indicate past occurrences of lichenification. The family nurse practitioner identifies the characteristics of this lesion as:
    1. Dried, crusty exudate, slightly elevated.
    2. Rough, thickened epidermis, accentuated skin markings.
    3. Keratinized cells shaped in an irregular pattern with exfoliation.
    4. Loss of epidermis with hollowed-out area and dermis exposed.

11. Clubbing of the nails commonly occurs in patients with chronic respiratory conditions. How does the family nurse practitioner assess for this condition?
    1. Evaluating the nail for transverse depressions and ridges.
    2. Placing the patient's hands together with palms inward and index fingers aligned.
    3. Placing nail beds of each index finger together to determine angle of nail plate.
    4. Determining whether there is diffuse discoloration of the nail bed from decreased oxygenation.

12. A circumscribed, elevated lesion >1 cm in diameter and containing clear serous fluid is best described as a:
    1. Papule.
    2. Vesicle.
    3. Bulla.
    4. Pustule.

13. In performing a skin assessment, which characteristic of a mole would necessitate immediate intervention?
    1. A 5-mm, symmetric, uniformly brown mole on the thigh that has not changed in appearance for more than 5 years.
    2. Multiple small (1–3 mm) flat moles across the upper back that are dark brown in color, round, and have smooth edges.
    3. A 3-cm, waxy papule with a "stuck-on" appearance, noted on the face.
    4. A new, 5- to 6-mm brown mole with an irregular red border that is occasionally pruritic.

14. Dermatophyte skin infections can be diagnosed from skin scrapings and prepared with which solution for microscopic exam?
    1. Hydrochloric acid.
    2. 10% or 20% potassium hydroxide (KOH) solution.
    3. Crystal violet.
    4. Distilled water.

Skin Disorders

15. A 65-year-old presents to the clinic for evaluation of small rough areas on his face that have increased in size over the past year. He states that he had several similar lesions on his neck removed a few years ago. Physical exam reveals 1 × 1-cm areas of erythematous, scaly sandpaper-like lesions that are yellow to light brown in color above his brow. No discharge is noted. Which of the following should the family nurse practitioner educate the patient regarding lesions of this type?
    1. Risk of squamous cell carcinoma.
    2. Risk of melanoma.
    3. Risk of infection.
    4. The lesions are benign.

16. A 34-year-old female patient presents with an erythematous area of skin on her left buttock. She states that it is painful because it is located along her bikini line. She is worried she may not be able to continue to relax in the hot tub at her apartment community in the evenings. She denies any recent injuries to the area. Which of the following should the family nurse practitioner suspect as the most likely cause?
    1. *Pseudomonas aeruginosa.*
    2. *Staphylococcus aureus.*
    3. *S. epidermidis.*
    4. Contact dermatitis.

17. A patient complains of intolerable itching in the pubic hair. On examination, the family nurse practitioner notes erythematous papules and tiny white specks in the pubic hair. The differential diagnosis includes all **except**:
    1. Pediculosis pubis.
    2. Scabies.
    3. Impetigo.
    4. Atopic dermatitis.

18. What finding would indicate to the family nurse practitioner that an immunoglobulin E (IgE)–mediated potential trigger was suspected in the presence of an adult patient who had acute urticaria?
    1. Increase in fluid intake in the last 24 hours.
    2. Body temperature of 101°F.
    3. Patient had eaten seafood salad that day.
    4. Patient also presented with flulike symptoms.

19. A 70-year-old female presents to the clinic complaining of pain on her left arm. Inspection of the extremity reveals no erythema. Her skin is intact with no evidence of lesions. The patient's past medical history includes herpes zoster. Which clinical diagnosis would the family nurse practitioner make as supported by this patient's presentation and past medical history?
    1. Phantom pain.
    2. Postherpetic neuralgia.
    3. Urinary tract infection.
    4. Tinea infection.

20. An older adult woman has an area of vesicles in clusters with an erythematous base that extend from her spine, around and under her arm and breast, to the sternum on her left side. She states that the area was very tender last week and that the vesicles started erupting yesterday. She is complaining of severe pain in the area. What is the probable diagnosis for this condition?
    1. Psoriasis.
    2. Herpes zoster.
    3. Contact dermatitis.
    4. Cellulitis.

21. What is a chronic skin condition that is sometimes associated with arthritis?
    1. Eczema.
    2. Psoriasis.
    3. Neurodermatitis.
    4. Pityriasis rosea.

22. What information should be provided to a patient with actinic keratosis?
    1. The affected areas are a normal part of aging and are benign.
    2. These lesions can develop into squamous cell carcinomas.
    3. This is part of an allergic reaction, and the offending allergen needs to be identified.
    4. This skin condition responds well to sunlight, which will help alleviate the symptoms.

23. A patient known to be positive for HIV presents with several painless, persistent, raised purple lesions on the lower arm. What is the most likely diagnosis of the lesions?
    1. Seborrheic dermatitis.
    2. Molluscum contagiosum.
    3. Kaposi's sarcoma.
    4. Fungal infection.

24. A middle-aged male patient presents to the clinic with a complaint of being bitten last night by another individual during a fight. He has a bite mark on his forearm, and the skin has been broken. He reports he does not remember any recent vaccinations for tetanus. Recommended treatment by the family nurse practitioner should include all the following **except**:
    1. Administer Tdap (Adacel).
    2. Instruct patient to watch for signs of infection.
    3. Initiate treatment with a β-lactam penicillin.
    4. Close the wound with sutures or Nexcare Steri-Strips.

25. What is the term for nail involvement secondary to primary foot-and-hand tinea, characterized by accumulation of subungual keratin that produces thickened, distorted, crumbling nails termed?
    1. Hippocratic nails.
    2. Onychomycosis.
    3. Koilonychia.
    4. Anonychia.

26. A middle-aged patient presents for an office visit with a complaint of a symmetric red rash on his trunk and spreading to his extremities. He was seen several days ago for bronchitis and started on trimethoprim-sulfamethoxazole (TMP-SMX; Septra) ds 1 tab PO bid. What is the recommended action for the family nurse practitioner?
    1. Instruct the patient to continue the medication and see if any change occurs in the rash.
    2. Discontinue TMP-SMX.
    3. Take the patient off medication for 3 days, then restart the drug.
    4. Decrease TMP-SMX to half-dose.

27. A patient complaining of hyperhidrosis should be counseled that:
    1. This is a normal occurrence.
    2. There are no therapies for this complaint.
    3. Bathing in 20% alcohol solution of aluminum chloride hexahydrate (Drysol) may be beneficial.
    4. A history and physical exam need to be completed to rule out any medical etiologies.

28. During the physical exam, the family nurse practitioner assesses a maculopapular skin lesion on a patient's back that is warty, scaly, greasy in appearance, and light tan in color. What would be the probable diagnosis?
    1. Actinic keratosis.
    2. Basal cell carcinoma.
    3. Seborrheic keratosis.
    4. Senile lentigines.

29. The family nurse practitioner is assessing an older patient diagnosed with herpes zoster (shingles) in the prodromal stage. What would the practitioner expect to find on the assessment of this patient?
    1. Erythematous lesions present over four different parts of the body.
    2. Red, pinpoint, painless rash.
    3. Burning pain in a line on only half the patient's chest that does not cross the midline.
    4. Painless purulent lesions for 2 days followed by complaints of itching, burning, and nausea.

30. A retired farmer presents with a dome-shaped, pearly, firm nodule with telangiectasia on his nose. In making a diagnosis, what does the family nurse practitioner recognize this to be?
    1. Compound nevus.
    2. Melanoma.
    3. Bullous pemphigoid.
    4. Basal cell carcinoma.

31. An adult female presents with an irregular, variegated nevus on her lower left back that has doubled in size in the last 3 months. What would be an appropriate action for the family nurse practitioner?
    1. Do a punch biopsy to confirm the diagnosis.
    2. Take a photograph of the lesion and recheck it in 1 month.
    3. Refer immediately to a dermatologist.
    4. Reassure the patient that these are normal changes related to hormone variations.

32. An older adult patient presents with pain over the right chest wall for the last 48 hours. On examination, the family nurse practitioner notices a vesicular eruption along the dermatome and identifies this as herpes zoster. The family nurse practitioner informs the patient that:
    1. All symptoms will disappear in 3 days.
    2. Oral medication can dramatically reduce the duration and intensity of symptoms.
    3. The patient has chickenpox, which may be contagious to grandchildren until the lesions are completely gone.
    4. The eruptions will recur at regular intervals.

33. A young adult female presents to the family nurse practitioner's office stating that she has had a red rash over her trunk for 2 weeks that does not itch. She has tried over-the-counter lotions and creams, but the rash is still there. The rash started as a small, round, red patch on her chest and has since spread across her chest, back, arms, and legs. A physical exam reveals a generalized distribution of erythematous and scaly macular lesions that run parallel to each other, creating a "Christmas tree" pattern. The family nurse practitioner should:
    1. Do a thorough medication history, investigate any potential allergens, and send the patient to an allergy specialist.
    2. Prescribe triamcinolone 0.025% cream (Aristocort A) bid for 2 weeks.
    3. Teach the patient the rash is self-limiting, lasting 2–8 weeks.
    4. Refer the patient to a dermatologist for a biopsy.

34. An adult male patient presents to the family nurse practitioner's office complaining of flulike symptoms, a large red spot in the right groin, headaches, and generalized muscle pain. These symptoms have persisted for about 4–5 weeks. In taking the history, it would be most important to determine whether the patient:
    1. Was using new skin care products.
    2. Was taking any new medications, such as vitamins or herbal therapies.
    3. Has had a recent insect bite or was potentially exposed to insects such as ticks.
    4. Has been exposed to a person with tuberculosis.

35. When do bites from insects, spiders, snakes, and bees most often occur?
    1. High humidity months.
    2. Spring to early fall.
    3. Winter.
    4. Any time of the year.

36. What does medical management for a brown recluse spider bite include?
    1. Warm moist soaks to the affected area.
    2. Ice pack and elevation and immobilization of the area.
    3. Active and passive range of motion to the area.
    4. Avoidance of antihistamines.

37. A scout leader is explaining about snakes and snake bites, and says to his group about the coral snake, "Red on yellow, kill a fellow; red on black, venom lack." Later, one of the boys is bitten by a snake described as having broad rings of red and black, separated by narrow rings of yellow. The family nurse practitioner understands that this patient will probably experience all the following **except**:
    1. Numbness and change in sensation.
    2. Local swelling at the fang mark site.
    3. Dizziness and diplopia.
    4. No symptoms, as the snake was not venomous.

38. How is psittacosis transmitted?
    1. Bats.
    2. Dogs.
    3. Birds.
    4. Cats.

39. The family nurse practitioner is examining a patient with a diagnosis of pityriasis rosea. Which three statements are correct about the condition?
    1. Pruritus is not present.
    2. Vesicles progressing to pustules occur within 2–3 days of eruption.
    3. Salmon-colored patch with fine scales is commonly noted on face, hands, and feet.
    4. Typical "Christmas tree" pattern of lesion distribution is observed.
    5. Presence of a herald patch before onset of generalized rash.

40. A young adult reports itching that seems to be worse at night. On examination, the family nurse practitioner notes a rash on the sides of the fingers and inner aspect of the elbows. The rash causes little bumps that often form a line that is approximately 2–3 mm long and the width of a hair. What does the family nurse practitioner suspect?
    1. Scabies.
    2. Hives.
    3. Fleas.
    4. Ticks.

41. What are common sites for atopic dermatitis (eczema) in adults?
    1. Cheeks, forehead, and scalp.
    2. Wrists, ankles, and antecubital fossae.
    3. Antecubital fossae, face, neck, and back.
    4. Hands and face.

42. The family nurse practitioner is presenting a community education program on rabies. Although most cases of rabies are found in developing countries, what is the primary source or reservoir of rabies in the United States?
    1. Dogs.
    2. Cats.
    3. Bats.
    4. Skunks.

43. An older adult presents with complaints of a red, greasy scaly rash on his scalp, forehead, and eyebrow. What is the most likely diagnosis?
    1. Seborrheic dermatitis.
    2. Atopic dermatitis.
    3. Psoriasis.
    4. Rosacea.

44. An 84-year-old female patient presents to the office with bilateral varicosities on her lower extremities noted in the calf area. Varicosities appear to be superficial, but the patient wants to know if there is any therapeutic option that may reduce their appearance. Detection of pulses is within normal limits. Based on the patient's stated concern, the family nurse practitioner would suggest which of the following therapies?
    1. Laser therapy.
    2. Debridement of varicosities.
    3. Use of supportive compression stockings.
    4. Hydrotherapy.

45. What is a recommended treatment option for actinic keratoses?
    1. Hydrotherapy.
    2. Observation as this is not considered to be a premalignant lesion.
    3. Topical chemotherapy.
    4. Systemic chemotherapy.

46. The family nurse practitioner understands that cat bites become infected more often than dog bites because:
    1. Dogs have a "cleaner mouth" than cats.
    2. Cat bites are often deep puncture wounds.
    3. Dog bites are usually on the face, which makes them less susceptible to infection.
    4. Cat bites are usually associated with clawing and spreading of microorganisms.

Pharmacology

47. An adult was bitten by a neighbor's dog 3 days ago. He has developed an infection in a large wound on his lower leg. What would be an appropriate management strategy for the patient?
    1. Prescribe amoxicillin-clavulanate (Augmentin).
    2. Approximate the edges of the wound together with suture.
    3. Prescribe cephalexin (Keflex).
    4. Have the patient return to the clinic for follow-up in 2 weeks.

48. An adult male patient presents for removal of a tick on his abdomen that he noticed 6 hours ago after he returned from hunting. He is sure it was not there this morning when he showered. He does not complain of any symptoms. A physical exam reveals an adult *Ixodes* tick attached just inferior to the left navel. No erythema or discoloration of the skin is noted. The patient inquires about prophylaxis for Lyme disease. Which of the following should the family nurse practitioner recommend?
    1. Doxycycline 200 mg PO bid for 7 days.
    2. Doxycycline 200 mg PO once.
    3. Reassurance.
    4. Serologic testing for Lyme disease.

49. What would be the appropriate management for a patient with herpes zoster (shingles)?
    1. Acyclovir (Zovirax).
    2. Miconazole (Monistat-Derm).
    3. Clotrimazole (Lotrimin).
    4. Corticosteroid (prednisone).

50. An adult male patient is diagnosed with seborrheic dermatitis of the face. Which of the following treatments should the family nurse practitioner choose as initial therapy? Select three appropriate therapeutic treatments for seborrheic dermatitis.
    1. Ketoconazole 2% topical.
    2. Chlorhexidine gluconate 4% topical.
    3. Betamethasone topical 0.1%.
    4. Hydrocortisone 2.5%.
    5. Clobetasol ointment 0.5% topical.

51. An obese woman presents to the clinic with complaints of tenderness and irritation under both of her breasts. An examination reveals a very irritated, moist, inflamed area with macules and papules present. What is the best treatment for the woman?
    1. Nystatin cream bid/tid for 10 days, with thorough drying of the area and exposure to light and air.
    2. Systemic antistaphylococcal antibiotics (dicloxacillin) and soaking with moist pads of normal saline three times daily.
    3. Gentle washing of the area and removal of crusts, then application of antibiotic ointment.
    4. Antiviral treatment (acyclovir) and topical ointment to prevent secondary infection.

52. Which three treatment options would the family nurse practitioner include in a plan of care for a patient presenting with scalp lesions attributable to psoriasis?
    1. Vigorous scalp massage every other day to facilitate plaque removal.
    2. Coal tar–based ointment.
    3. Topical vitamin D analog.
    4. Topical emollients.
    5. Fluid replacement.

53. Which classification of drugs has the potential to aggravate psoriasis?
    1. Beta blockers.
    2. Thiazide diuretics.
    3. Vasodilators.
    4. Tricyclic antidepressants.

54. All the following are true of postherpetic neuralgia, **except**:
    1. Capsaicin cream (Zostrix) may alleviate some of the discomfort.
    2. In most patients, the postherpetic pain gradually subsides over several weeks.
    3. Acyclovir (Zovirax) 200 mg 5 caps daily PO in divided doses is an effective therapy.
    4. It is more common in patients over age 60 years.

55. An older adult male patient presents to the outpatient health clinic with complaints of pruritus of both hands and axillae. On examination, multiple papules are visualized between the fingers and in both axilla. Small burrows can be appreciated proximal to the papules. Which of the following should the family nurse practitioner choose as treatment?
    1. Hydrocortisone.
    3. Permethrin.
    4. Diphenhydramine.
    5. Ketoconazole.

56. A family nurse practitioner is examining multiple geriatric patients with pediculosis in an assisted living facility. Which of the following treatments should be initiated first?
    1. Lindane shampoo.
    2. Ivermectin oral.
    3. Crisaborole oral.
    4. Pyrethrin shampoo.

57. When treating genital warts with topical podophyllin, it is important for the family nurse practitioner to:
    1. Apply the preparation directly to the wart and approximately 5 mm around the base.
    2. Cover with a dressing so that the solution remains moist and caution the patient not to remove the dressing for 24 hours.
    3. Instruct the patient to wash off the medication in 4–6 hours.
    4. Treat with liquid nitrogen before applying podophyllin.

58. An adult patient who is being treated for acne rosacea presents to the office complaining of continued facial redness despite topical treatments. Which three medications would the family nurse practitioner consider including in the treatment regimen that may also provide reduced facial flushing?
    1. Furosemide (Lasix).
    2. Clonidine (Catapres).
    3. Niacin.
    4. Ondansetron (Zofran).
    5. Propranolol (Inderal).

59. What is the recommended treatment of rosacea?
    1. Oral hydrocortisone.
    2. Oral ketoconazole.
    3. Low-dose oral tetracycline.
    4. Topical 5-fluorouracil.

60. An adult female patient presents to the health clinic complaining of a pruritic and uncomfortable area under her left arm for 2 days. She states that she has been unable to shave under her arm. Examination of the left axilla reveals multiple follicular pustules. The area is mildly erythematous and painful to touch. Which of the following interventions should the family nurse practitioner initially choose?
    1. Reassurance.
    2. Topical clindamycin.
    3. Penicillin PO.
    4. Trimethoprim-sulfamethoxazole PO.

61. An adult female patient presents with a pruritic rash on the extensor areas of her arms and legs for several months that is debilitating. She also complains of diarrhea and bloating for several years and is subsequently diagnosed with celiac disease. Which of the following medications would best be indicated for the cutaneous eruption of this syndrome?
    1. Corticosteroids PO.
    2. Tazarotene topical.
    3. 5-Fluorouracil topical.
    4. Dapsone PO.

62. When using lidocaine with epinephrine 1%–2% as a local anesthetic in the repair of an injury, it is essential to remember that the maximum allowable dose is:
    1. 4.5 mg/kg.
    2. 2.5 mg/kg.
    3. 10 mg/kg.
    4. 15 mg/kg.

63. An adult female patient presents to the health clinic complaining of excessive armpit sweating. She states that she has been "excessively sweaty" for as long as she can recall, but she inquires about treatment because a new job requires her to present publicly. She denies nervousness or anxiety and has no medical problems. Her only medication is oral contraceptives. She is prescribed aluminum chloride hexahydrate (Drysol) 20% to be applied to the underarms. Which three considerations should the family nurse practitioner educate the patient about regarding this medication?
    1. Avoid sunlight.
    2. Experience stinging sensation of affected area.
    3. Apply to wet skin.
    4. Avoid contact with broken or recently shaved skin.
    5. Use at bedtime.

64. A young adult female patient presents several days after being examined and treated for a localized skin infection for which she was prescribed oral antibiotics. Today she complains of a new-onset systemic maculopapular rash. She complains of intense pruritus but is in no acute distress. Her vital signs are within normal limits. A physical exam reveals diffuse small macules and papules. Which of the following should be the priority treatment in this patient?
    1. Prednisone 40 mg IV once, now.
    2. Topical corticosteroid cream.
    3. Diphenhydramine 50 mg IV once, now.
    4. Immediate cessation of antibiotic treatment.

65. The family nurse practitioner knows development of which of the following is possible regarding use of tacrolimus (Protopic) topically for treatment of recurrent psoriasis or atopic dermatitis?
    1. Lymphoma.
    2. Staphylococcal scalded skin syndrome.
    3. Seborrheic dermatitis.
    4. Bullous pemphigoid.

66. A patient reports a neighbor's cat scratched his arm about a week ago. The family nurse practitioner notes the following on physical exam: left forearm has a 2-cm, erythematous area around a red papule that is swollen with purulent drainage noted on the dressing. A swab of the wound drainage is collected for culture and sensitivity. The family nurse practitioner suspects cat scratch disease (CSD). What would be an appropriate antibiotic to prescribe?
    1. Azithromycin.
    2. Penicillin.
    3. Cefaclor.
    4. Corticosteroid.

67. On a return visit to the clinic, a patient receiving sulfonamide therapy exhibits generalized rash, mucous membrane lesions, skin sloughing on the palms and feet, high fever, and generalized malaise. What would these findings alert the family nurse practitioner to consider?
    1. Hepatitis B.
    2. Stevens-Johnson syndrome.
    3. HIV infection/AIDS.
    4. *Pneumocystis carinii* pneumonia.

68. What is the first-line treatment for tinea versicolor?
    1. Ketoconazole.
    2. Mupirocin.
    3. Prednisone.
    4. Tretinoin.

8 Integumentary Answers & Rationales

Physical Exam & Diagnostic Tests

1. Answer: 2

Rationale: Thinning of hair would be associated with normal age progression. Appearance of yellow nails would indicate a pathologic process, notably a fungal infection. Beau's lines would also indicate a pathologic process, notably related to systemic diseases. Absence of lesions does not correlate with the normal aging process. It is more likely that as a patient ages, lesions may become more prominent based on a combination of genetics, lifestyle, and environment.

2. Answer: 3, 4, 5

Rationale: The presence of clubbing is an abnormal finding indicating compromise in perfusion that can originate from the pulmonary or cardiovascular system. Therefore, obtaining a pulse oximetry reading would provide evidence of a patient's current perfusion. An ECG could provide evidence of cardiac status in terms of rate and rhythm. A chest x-ray would provide evidence of the cardiac silhouette and lung fields, allowing for an overview of the patient's cardiac and respiratory status. Imaging studies of the hands would not necessarily reveal pathology, unless the practitioner suspected structural deformities. There is no evidence to support ordering orthostatic blood pressures in a patient who presents with clubbing, unless there is evidence of dizziness or fainting episodes.

3. Answer: 4

Rationale: The term "annular" stems from the Latin word "annulus," meaning ringed. Lesions are circular or ovoid patches with a red periphery and central clearing (e.g., tinea corporis). Multiple groups of vesicles erupting unilaterally after the course of cutaneous nerves are described as herpetiform or zosteriform (herpes zoster). Linear lesions are arranged in a line (allergic contact dermatitis to poison ivy). Confluent lesions merge and are not discrete (scarlet fever rash).

4. Answer: 1

Rationale: Psoriasis, peripheral vascular disease, diabetes, tuberculosis, and other infectious diseases, such as syphilis, are associated with pitting deformities of the nail that may vary from pinpoint to pinhead size and may be linear or irregular in distribution. Iron-deficiency anemia, eczema, malnutrition, and pellagra are associated with koilonychia (spoon nails). Hyperthyroidism and hypothyroidism are associated with onycholysis, which is a separation of the nail from the nail bed starting at the free edge and progressing proximally.

5. Answer: 3

Rationale: AN typically occurs in patients who are obese or have diabetes and is a benign dermatosis characterized by velvety, hyperpigmented, hyperkeratotic plaques in body folds and creases (armpits, groin, and neck), which is associated with hyperinsulinemia and insulin resistance. A glycosylated hemoglobin (HbA1c) would be an appropriate diagnostic test to order.

6. Answer: 1

Rationale: The place to inspect for jaundice is in that portion of the sclera that is observed when the eye is open. If jaundice is suspected, the posterior portion of the hard palate should be examined for a yellowish cast. Pallor and cyanosis can be noted in the nail beds, palms, and soles. Oral mucosa may be affected by surface stains.

7. Answer: 1

Rationale: On an adult, the best place is just below the clavicle or on the abdomen. The best place to evaluate skin turgor for hydration status in children is the fleshy part of arms or legs because a child with a distended abdomen may have a tight abdomen, which appears to have adequate turgor, even though the child may actually be dehydrated.

8. Answer: 1

Rationale: Fungal lesions will be visualized as a bright-green or blue-green fluorescence when viewed with the Wood's lamp in a dimly lit room. Bacterial infections appear as coral-red or yellow-green (*Pseudomonas aeruginosa*).

9. Answer: 1

Rationale: A macule is less than 1 cm in diameter, nonpalpable, flat, and brown, red, purple, or tan (freckles, flat moles, rubella). A papule is elevated and palpable (warts, pigmented nevi). A nodule is 1–2 cm in diameter, solid, elevated, and deeper (lipoma). A wheal is elevated and irregular and has a variable diameter (insect bites, urticaria).

10. Answer: 2

Rationale: Lichenification occurs with chronic irritation, often of an exposed extremity (chronic dermatitis). Crusts are dried exudate (impetigo); scales are heaps of keratinized cells from exfoliation (psoriasis); and loss of epidermis is excoriation, as seen in an abrasion (repetitive scratching or picking).

11. Answer: 3

Rationale: The angle between the nail plate and the proximal nail fold when viewed from the side is >180 degrees and should form a diamond in clubbed nails. Normal nails form a 160-degree angle and should form a diamond shape between them when the nail beds of the index fingers are placed together. Transverse ridges and grooves may occur from trauma. Placing the palms together provides no assessment data. Diffuse discoloration may result from a fungal infection or an injury.

12. Answer: 3

Rationale: Bulla is the correct term. A papule is solid. A vesicle is <1 cm in diameter, and a pustule contains a purulent exudate.

13. Answer: 4

Rationale: The appearance of a new mole with high-risk features, including irregular border, color changes, and changes in sensation (e.g., pruritus), would necessitate immediate biopsy and/or referral to a dermatologist. Uniform moles, those that are symmetric and have smooth borders, and those not showing signs of change can be followed with annual skin assessments. Seborrheic keratosis is a benign skin growth, usually on sun-exposed areas, and appearing as waxy or "stuck-on" that requires no treatment.

14. Answer: 2

Rationale: Under microscopic exam, fungal scrapings in KOH solution will appear as threadlike hyphae crossing cell walls. The other solutions are not indicated to identify dermatophytes.

Skin Disorders

15. Answer: 1

Rationale: These lesions are most likely actinic keratosis. Actinic keratosis is a premalignant lesion at high risk of developing into squamous cell carcinoma of the skin. It is most likely seen in sun-exposed areas and is described as a scaly sandpaper-like lesion of a yellow to light brown coloration that may be erythematous.

16. Answer: 1

Rationale: Hot tub folliculitis caused by *Pseudomonas aeruginosa* is one of the most commonly considered gram-negative aerobic bacilli and should be suspected in any patient presenting with folliculitis and recent exposure to hot tubs. The infected area is most often in an area in which wet clothing causes extended close contact with infected water. *Staphylococcus* should be suspected in patients without a known exposure or risk factor because it is the most common cause of folliculitis overall.

17. Answer: 3

Rationale: Intense itching is characteristic of pediculosis pubis, scabies, and atopic dermatitis. Impetigo starts out as a tender erythematous papule and progresses through a vesicular to a honey-crusted stage with no itching.

18. Answer: 3

Rationale: Urticaria arising from IgE-mediated potential trigger could occur from food sensitivity/allergen exposure. Water intake and temperature elevations would be associated with nonimmunologically mediated causes. Flulike symptoms would be associated with non–IgE-mediated causes caused by the presence of a viral infection.

19. Answer: 2

Rationale: Postherpetic neuralgia refers to pain persisting beyond 4 months from the initial onset of the rash and is a potential complication that can occur after activation of herpes zoster virus. Unlike with acute presentations, there is no evidence of customary lesions associated with shingles leading patients to present with pain presentations classified as allodynia. Phantom pain presents in patients with an amputation. Although most elderly patients present with atypical symptoms in the presence of urinary tract infections, on the basis of this patient's past medical history, it is more likely that she is experiencing a complication of herpes zoster. Tinea infection would present with a skin lesion finding.

20. Answer: 2

Rationale: Herpes zoster typically presents with a history of tenderness followed by eruptions and vesicles that follow a dermatome on one side of the body. The condition is very painful. Other symptoms may include fever, headaches, and malaise. Psoriasis is characterized by thick, white, silvery, or red patches of skin. Contact dermatitis is a rash caused by touching something. Cellulitis is a skin infection characterized as red, hot, swollen, and tender skin.

21. Answer: 2

Rationale: Approximately 10%–30% of people with psoriasis develop an accompanying form of arthritis called psoriatic arthritis. Eczema (dermatitis), neurodermatitis (lichen simplex chronicus), and pityriasis rosea are dermatologic conditions that are not directly associated with arthritis.

22. Answer: 2

Rationale: Actinic keratoses are potentially precancerous lesions that are commonly found in areas of skin exposed to sunlight.

23. Answer: 3

Rationale: Although any of these conditions can affect the skin, particularly of a patient who is HIV positive, the description relates most closely to Kaposi's sarcoma and warrants a biopsy.

24. Answer: 4

Rationale: Delay wound closure until determination of no infection in approximately 24–48 hours. Mouth flora of humans is abundant, and a bite carries the risk of heavy bacterial inoculum and severe infection. Antibiotics are indicated. A Td booster should be given every 10 years. Tdap may be given as one of these boosters if the patient has never received Tdap before. Typically, one dose of Tdap is routinely given at age 11 or 12 years. People who did not get Tdap at that age should get it as soon as possible. Tdap may also be given after a severe cut or burn to prevent tetanus infection.

25. Answer: 2

Rationale: Onychomycosis is the correct term. Hippocratic nails are clubbed nails and fingers associated with chronic heart and lung disorders. Koilonychia is a concavity of the nail plate often associated with iron-deficiency anemia. Anonychia is a total congenital absence of the nail.

26. Answer: 2

Rationale: In case of suspected drug reactions, it is recommended that the drug be eliminated and documented in the patient's record so that it is not reintroduced.

27. Answer: 4

Rationale: Excessive sweating may be normal, but a history and physical exam are needed to rule out underlying causes. Therapies can be offered. Drysol is for use only on the feet and axilla.

28. Answer: 3

Rationale: The assessment describes a seborrheic keratosis. The actinic keratosis is an irregular, rough, scaly, white-to-erythematous macular lesion found most often on sun-exposed areas, such as on the dorsal surface of the hands, arms, neck, and face. It has malignant potential. The basal cell carcinoma is a smooth, round nodule with a pearly gray border and central induration. Senile lentigines are gray-brown, irregular, macular lesions on sun-exposed areas of the face, arms, and hands.

29. Answer: 3

Rationale: Herpes zoster (shingles) is a vesicular dermatomal eruption related to a reactivation of latent varicella virus. It increases with advanced age and is characterized by burning pain and paresthesia along one or two dermatomes, not crossing the midline, and may be accompanied by fever, malaise, or headache. The vesicular stage lasts 2–3 weeks. The vesicles are initially clear or blood filled and become purulent. The area along the dermatome is erythematous, and the vesicles crust and then scab, which may leave hypopigmented scars. The other options discuss painless lesions and are not specific to this prodromal stage.

30. Answer: 4

Rationale: These are classic signs of a basal cell carcinoma, also supported by the patient's employment history. Exposure to ultraviolet radiation from sunlight is the most important environmental cause of basal cell carcinoma. Melanoma would be pigmented, compound nevus would not be firm or have telangiectasia, and bullous pemphigoid results in bullous lesions.

31. Answer: 3

Rationale: Refer this patient immediately to a dermatologist because the findings are highly suspicious for a melanoma. A punch biopsy should never be done on a suspected melanoma, and any delay could be detrimental to the outcome.

32. Answer: 2

Rationale: The nucleoside analogs (acyclovir, valacyclovir, and famciclovir) are the preferred antivirals for treatment of acute herpes zoster infection and are very effective in reducing the intensity and duration of the symptoms if started early in the course (less than 3 days) of the disease. Herpes zoster does not usually recur at regular intervals but frequently lasts for several weeks. Once the rash has developed crusts, the person is no longer contagious. Shingles is less contagious than chickenpox, and the risk of a person with shingles spreading the virus is low if the rash is covered.

33. Answer: 3

Rationale: The patient presents with a classic case of pityriasis rosea, a benign, self-limiting skin eruption of unknown etiology. Although a medication/allergen history would be warranted, referral to an allergy specialist or dermatologist would not be necessary. Triamcinolone would not be indicated unless there is itching, because the treatment is mainly symptomatic. Sunlight in moderate amounts has been shown to hasten healing in some patients.

34. Answer: 3

Rationale: The signs and symptoms presented are classic for Lyme disease, which is transmitted by ticks. Therefore, it would be important to inquire about potential exposure to ticks before the signs and symptoms developed. Exposure to new skin care products would be important if the family nurse practitioner suspected an allergic reaction, which is not consistent with the signs and symptoms. Although always important, a thorough medication history probably will not reveal the cause of the signs and symptoms in this case. Tuberculosis does not present in this manner.

35. Answer: 2

Rationale: Insects reproduce, are more active, and are present in greater numbers in the warm months of spring to early fall.

36. Answer: 2

Rationale: Heat application is contraindicated; ice packs are preferred, as is elevation, to decrease the edema. The area should be immobilized. Tdap or Td may be given along with antihistamines to reduce swelling and relieve itching.

37. Answer: 4

Rationale: This was a venomous coral snake bite. The typical symptoms are those listed, as well as nausea, vomiting, and muscle fasciculations.

38. Answer: 3

Rationale: Psittacosis is a zoonotic disease caused by *Chlamydophila psittaci*, a bacteria, that is transmitted to humans by infected birds, such as cockatiels, parakeets, parrots, pigeons, doves, canaries, and macaws. Transmission occurs through exposure to the bird's feces and nasal secretions. Psittacosis is a systemic infectious disease of varying severity that initially causes influenza-like symptoms with a pronounced headache (most common symptom) and can affect the lungs, which can lead to an atypical pneumonia. Bats are the most frequent source for a rabies infection. Dog and cat bites can cause a variety of bacterial infections.

39. Answer: 3, 4, 5

Rationale: A herald patch usually appears on the skin first. This is usually an oval-shaped or round-shaped patch that can vary from 2–5 cm in diameter and is salmon-colored with fine scales. It is followed within days by a regional outbreak of numerous smaller erythematous patches, providing a key diagnostic clue with smaller lesions oriented along skin cleavage areas (Langer lines) in a Christmas tree pattern. It most commonly appears on the chest or upper back, although it can sometimes appear on the abdomen, neck, back, thigh, or upper arms. Mild pruritus occurs, which typically causes the patient to seek medical assistance.

40. Answer: 1

Rationale: The location and appearance of the lesions are typical of scabies. A rash causes little bumps that often form a line that is approximately 2–3 mm long and the width of a hair. The inflammatory lesions are erythematous and pruritic papules most commonly located in the finger webs, flexor surfaces of the wrists, elbows, axillae, buttocks, genitalia, feet, and ankles. The older adult may itch more severely with fewer cutaneous lesions and is at risk for extensive infestations, probably related to a decline in cell-mediated immunity. In addition, there may be back involvement in those who are bedridden.

41. Answer: 4

Rationale: Atopic dermatitis is a chronic, pruritic inflammatory skin disease that occurs most frequently in children but also affects adults. Atopic dermatitis in adults may be generalized; however, it frequently appears in the creases of the elbows or knees, dorsa of the feet, and nape of the neck in adults, and frequently the hands and face are involved in adults. The clinical presentation is typically on the face, scalp, and extensor limb surfaces of infants and toddlers; flexural areas are involved in older children and adolescents. Localized eczema (e.g., chronic hand or foot dermatitis, eyelid dermatitis, or lichen simplex chronicus) may continue throughout adulthood; typically, atopic dermatitis declines with increasing age.

42. Answer: 3

Rationale: Rabies is a viral zoonotic infection that is characterized as a rapidly progressive central nervous system infection caused by a ribonucleic acid rhabdovirus (Lyssavirus) affecting mammals. Although rabies is rare in the United States, bats are the most common reservoir. Transmission occurs via bites from infected animals or when saliva from an infected animal comes in contact with an open wound or mucous membranes. Throughout the world, rabies is widespread in both domestic and feral dogs.

43. Answer: 1

Rationale: Seborrheic dermatitis is usually salmon in color and has a red, greasy appearance with thick adherent crusts and indistinct margins. There is minimal pruritus. In adults, it is most commonly located in hairy skin areas: scalp and scalp margins, eyebrows and eyelid margins, nasolabial folds, ears and retroauricular folds, presternal area, middle to upper back, buttock crease, inguinal area, genitals, and armpits. Rashes in atopic dermatitis and eczema are pink, or red if inflamed, and have a whiter, nongreasy appearance. Scalp psoriasis is more sharply demarcated than seborrheic dermatitis and has crusted, infiltrated plaques rather than mild scaling and erythema. Rosacea is characterized by facial flushing, erythema, papules, pustules, and telangiectasia in a symmetric, central facial distribution and is uncommon in older adults (over 60 years of age).

44. Answer: 1

Rationale: With regard to appearance, use of laser or sclerotherapy is the best practice option to decrease the appearance of varicosities. Debridement is not recommended, because there is no indication of vascular compromise. The patient reports no clinical symptoms related to the varicosities, so the use of supportive compression stockings would not be indicated, as they would not reduce the patient's cosmetic concerns. Hydrotherapy is not an acceptable treatment for varicosities.

45. Answer: 3

Rationale: Actinic keratosis is considered to be a precancerous lesion, and topical chemotherapy is indicated for the affected areas. Hydrotherapy is not suggested as a treatment option. Cryotherapy can be used as a treatment option along with photodynamic therapy, scraping, or curettage.

46. Answer: 2

Rationale: Deep puncture wounds are more likely to become infected with anaerobic organisms. The narrow, sharp feline incisors deeply puncture tissue and may easily penetrate a bone or joint. Bites on the hand have the highest infection rate, whereas bites on the face have the lowest rate.

Pharmacology

47. Answer: 1

Rationale: Amoxicillin-clavulanate is an excellent choice for the empiric treatment of animal bites. Cephalexin is not indicated, because of resistant strains of *Pasteurella multocida*, an organism present in 25% of dog bites and 50% of cat bites. Avoid first-generation cephalosporins (e.g., cephalexin), penicillinase-resistant penicillins (e.g., dicloxacillin), macrolides (e.g., erythromycin), and clindamycin when it is not administered with another medication, as these medications are not effective against *P. multocida*. An infected bite should be followed daily until the infection clears. Open wound management is indicated, not suturing.

48. Answer: 3

Rationale: Lyme disease is caused by the spirochete *Borrelia* species and is transmitted by the *Ixodes* tick, endemic to the eastern United States. Nymphal (young) ticks more commonly transmit the disease than adults and are unlikely to transmit the bacteria until after 48–72 hours of attachment. Prophylactic one-time treatment with doxycycline 200 mg PO is indicated only if the tick is positively identified as an *Ixodes* tick, the tick has been attached for 36 hours or longer (or a known exposure within the same time), and the patient resides in an endemic area. Endemic areas include the eastern United States but specifically the northeastern states and

Great Lakes areas, including portions of Minnesota and Wisconsin. Serologic testing is not indicated, as early diagnostic indicators such as IgM antibodies to *Borrelia* will not begin appearing until 1–2 weeks after infection.

49. Answer: 1

Rationale: Antiviral therapy with acyclovir 800 mg 5 times daily for 7 days may expedite healing if started within 2–3 days of onset, especially in immunocompromised individuals. Miconazole and clotrimazole are antifungal creams. Prednisone would only be used to decrease the incidence of postherpetic neuralgia and may increase the incidence of disseminated infection, so it is not recommended during the acute phase.

50. Answer: 1, 3, 4

Rationale: Initial therapy in treatment of seborrheic dermatitis of the face includes topical low-potency corticosteroids, including hydrocortisone, and topical antifungals, including ketoconazole and ciclopirox. Systemic medications and higher potency topical corticosteroids, such as clobetasol, are not indicated for initial therapy or uncomplicated disease.

51. Answer: 1

Rationale: The description is consistent with intertriginous candidiasis, which is treated with an antifungal ointment or oral medication. It is not a staphylococcal infection; the area needs to be kept dry, not moist. An antibiotic ointment will not relieve the problem. Herpes zoster is treated with antiviral medications; this case is not described as particularly painful, and it is bilateral.

52. Answer: 2, 3, 4

Rationale: The presence of psoriasis on the scalp can be extensive, leading to scaling of the entire scalp. Included in the plan of care to treat scaling, one should use topical therapies such as coal tar ointment, emollients, and/or topical vitamin D analogs. Vigorous scalp massage would be contraindicated because that could lead to more discomfort and irritation. The process of removal of scales is done gently to facilitate response of medication to the surface area. Fluid replacement is not indicated in the treatment of psoriasis.

53. Answer: 1

Rationale: Beta blockers can exacerbate psoriasis. They are believed to decrease cAMP-dependent protein kinase, an inhibitor of cell proliferation. Drugs in the other classifications have no known effect on psoriasis.

54. Answer: 3

Rationale: Acyclovir treats the acute phase during initial eruption of vesicular lesions and offers no benefit for postherpetic pain.

55. Answer: 2

Rationale: The patient in this scenario likely has scabies, caused by the *Sarcoptes scabiei* mite. Treatment is aimed at both symptom relief and prevention of transmission. Treatment should include either permethrin 5% cream or oral ivermectin. For severe cases, combination treatment may be used. Other treatment choices include crotamiton, malathion, or lindane. Lindane is indicated only as an alternative therapy because of the risk of serious side effects.

56. Answer: 4

Rationale: Pediculosis is more common in children but can regularly be seen in long-term care facilities and older adults living in close quarters. Pediculosis is caused by the head louse (*Pediculus humanus capitis*). Initial treatments include over-the-counter pyrethrins, such as pyrethrin shampoo and permethrin lotion. Prescription medications include ivermectin lotion, benzyl alcohol lotion, malathion lotion, and spinosad topical suspension. The medication lindane has been restricted to use as a second-line agent because of the risk of serious side effects and has a U.S. Food and Drug Administration black box warning of severe neurologic toxicity and should only be used when first-line agents have failed. Additional care, including washing linens and clothing, should be instituted.

57. Answer: 3

Rationale: Patients need to be instructed to wash off podophyllin. It should be applied sparingly, only to the wart and avoiding normal skin, and allowed to dry thoroughly before the patient dresses. No rationale exists to treat with both liquid nitrogen and podophyllin.

58. Answer: 2, 4, 5

Rationale: Certain medications, such as clonidine (Catapres), ondansetron (Zofran), and beta blockers, such as propranolol (Inderal), can help decrease facial flushing. Furosemide (Lasix) does not have any reported effect on facial flushing. Niacin or vitamin B3 can cause facial flushing caused by vasodilation effects.

59. Answer: 3

Rationale: Systemic treatment with low-dose tetracycline is very effective for rosacea; topical treatment with metronidazole or low-dose hydrocortisone may also be useful. Oral cortisone and antifungal agents are not known to be effective. Topical 5-fluorouracil is used in the treatment of actinic keratosis, a precancerous skin condition.

60. Answer: 2

Rationale: Folliculitis of the axilla without other risk factors or exposures is most likely caused by *Staphylococcus*

aureus. Medical treatment is not usually indicated in singular eruptions of folliculitis. Patients with multiple sites or moderate skin involvement should first be treated with topical mupirocin and clindamycin. Oral antimicrobials are indicated for refractory or severe cases, including β-lactam antibiotics, TMP-SMX, clindamycin, or doxycycline for 7–10 days.

61. Answer: 4

Rationale: The mainstay of treatment of celiac disease is removal of gluten-containing products from the diet and oral dapsone (Aczone) for the treatment of dermatitis herpetiformis. Some patients may also be treated with topical corticosteroids as a secondary treatment or if intolerant to dapsone. Dapsone may cause hemolysis in patients with G6PD deficiency. Tazarotene is a topical retinoid indicated for treatment of acne and psoriasis.

62. Answer: 1

Rationale: The maximum allowable dose for adults is 4.5 mg/kg of lidocaine with epinephrine and 5 mg/kg of lidocaine without epinephrine. Although local anesthetics are often used, the maximum allowable doses are rarely emphasized, and overdose can result in anaphylactic shock.

63. Answer: 2, 4, 5

Rationale: Aluminum chloride hexahydrate (Drysol, Hypercare) is a common topical treatment for hyperhidrosis. It should be applied directly to the affected area at bedtime on only clean, dry skin and may be held in place with a snug-fitting shirt or plastic wrap for maximum effectiveness. This medication should not be applied to broken or recently shaved skin because of the risk of irritation. Common side effects include discomfort or a stinging sensation of the skin that may subside over time. Patients with skin irritation should discontinue treatment.

64. Answer: 4

Rationale: The patient most likely has experienced morbilliform (drug-induced) drug eruption, also commonly called an exanthematous drug eruption, which is a type IV hypersensitivity reaction that typically occurs 5–14 days after treatment. Many medications can cause reactions, but antibiotics like penicillin, cephalosporins, macrolides, quinolones, and trimethoprim-sulfamethoxazole are some of the most commonly implicated. Treatment priorities involve first stopping the offending agent followed by symptomatic treatment with corticosteroids and/or antihistamines. Immediate treatment with diphenhydramine or systemic corticosteroids would not be indicated because this patient is clearly not experiencing an acute reaction.

65. Answer: 1

Rationale: Tacrolimus is a calcineurin inhibitor that inhibits T-cell activation. Calcineurin inhibitors are second-line agents used as treatment for refractory psoriasis and atopic dermatitis. A black box warning was added in 2006 because of a possible risk of cutaneous malignancy development. For this reason, tacrolimus should be limited in treatment and used as a second-line agent. Systemic tacrolimus administration should be given only under the care of a provider familiar with immunosuppressive therapies because of significant risk of side effects, including neurotoxicity, renal toxicity, and increased infection risk.

66. Answer: 1

Rationale: The most common antibiotic treatment is the macrolide, azithromycin. Other medications that can be prescribed include rifampin, ciprofloxacin, doxycycline, gentamicin, or trimethoprim-sulfamethoxazole. Cat scratch disease (CSD) is a zoonotic infection caused by the bacteria *Bartonella henselae* and is most commonly transmitted by cats; however, a dog bite can also be a source of the infection.

67. Answer: 2

Rationale: Stevens-Johnson syndrome is a severe form of erythema multiforme that can be fatal. The clinical picture is mucous membrane lesions, conjunctival and corneal lesions, fever, malaise, arthralgia, and sloughing of the skin of the hands and feet. Distinguishing characteristics of the syndrome are eruption of vesicles, mucosal ulcerations, and sloughing skin.

68. Answer: 1

Rationale: Tinea versicolor (pityriasis versicolor) is a common skin infection caused by the fungal organism *Malassezia furfur*. First-line treatment involves topical antifungals (azoles, ciclopirox, terbinafine) and selenium sulfide. Patients should be educated that treatment may take several months to resolve symptoms. Treatment with corticosteroids or a retinoid would be ineffective. Mupirocin is indicated for bacterial infections.

9

Endocrine

Physical Exam & Diagnostic Tests

1. With nearly 70% of the adult population being overweight, including those who are obese, it is important to distinguish a bulge of subcutaneous fat at the base of the neck from a goiter. Which of the following statements is true regarding how to differentiate them?
   1. Swallowing cannot be relied on, as both tissues move up and down when drinking fluid.
   2. Fat layers remain in a fixed position, but a thyroid gland moves up and down while drinking.
   3. Goiters are typically visibly defined from the lateral position of observation.
   4. Fatty tissue appears to be less prominent when observed from the side compared with an enlarged thyroid.

2. What is the correct procedure for palpation of a patient's thyroid gland?
   1. Stand behind the patient, hyperextend the head, and palpate both sides simultaneously.
   2. Have the patient lower the chin and tilt the head slightly toward the side being evaluated.
   3. Hyperextend the head and have the patient lean away from the side being evaluated.
   4. Have the patient lean away from the side being examined and take a swallow of water.

3. When a patient sips water and swallows, the thyroid gland:
   1. Moves downward and slightly posterior and feels smooth on palpation.
   2. Elongates and enlarges during the swallow and immediately returns to a resting position.
   3. Moves slightly out during the sipping and backward during the swallowing.
   4. Moves upward during the swallow and feels symmetric and smooth to palpation.

4. Which characteristics of skin, hair, and nails are correctly listed for the thyroid condition?
   1. Thin nails and coarse and dry but warm skin are associated with hyperthyroidism.
   2. Thicker nails, coarse skin, and hair that breaks off easily are linked with hypothyroidism.
   3. Fine hair, coarse skin, and onycholysis of the nails are found with hyperthyroidism.
   4. Puffy facies, brittle nails, and hyperpigmented skin are associated with hypothyroidism.

5. Select the facial feature description linked with the correct endocrine pathology:
   1. Coarse facial features, heavier brow line, and prominent jaw: acromegaly.
   2. "Moon face," extra hair growth on the upper lip and chin with acne on the back and chest: acromegaly.
   3. Wide-eyed look with nervous tic and bulging eyes: hypothyroidism.
   4. Lid lag, moist skin, periorbital puffiness: hypothyroidism.

6. What blood test can be drawn to help identify whether the patient has type 1 or type 2 diabetes?
   1. Hemoglobin A1c.
   2. Glycosylated fructose.
   3. C-peptide level.
   4. Apo A versus Apo B.

7. What is the laboratory value that points most directly to parathyroid abnormality?
   1. Low thyroid-stimulating hormone.
   2. Elevated calcium.
   3. Elevated magnesium.
   4. Depressed phosphate.

8. While conducting the interview for a physical exam, the family nurse practitioner identifies which finding in the patient's history as being commonly associated with thyroid carcinoma?
   1. Family history of thyroid cancer.
   2. History of hyperthyroidism.
   3. Irradiation of the neck.
   4. Smoking for 15 years.

9. When doing a physical exam on a patient with hyperthyroidism, a common neurologic finding is:
   1. Memory, attention, and problem-solving deficits.
   2. Diminished deep tendon reflexes.
   3. Severe cognitive impairment.
   4. Delusions and psychosis.

10. The treatment goal for glycemic control in a person with type 2 diabetes is to achieve and maintain the hemoglobin A1c level (HgbA1c) of:
    1. <10%.
    2. 6%–9%.
    3. <7%.
    4. >8%.

11. The family nurse practitioner notes a solitary thyroid nodule on a patient during a routine physical exam. What is the next step for diagnostic testing?
    1. Thyroid scan and antibody level.
    2. Thyroid-stimulating hormone (TSH) level and ultrasound.
    3. X-ray film of the thyroid.
    4. Fine-needle aspiration (FNA) biopsy.

12. An adult female patient presents to the family nurse practitioner's office complaining of fatigue, weakness, and weight gain over the last 4 months. Physical exam reveals elevated blood pressure (BP), facial and supraclavicular fullness, hirsutism noted on the face, proximal muscle weakness, and facial and truncal distribution of acne. What are the appropriate laboratory tests the family nurse practitioner should order?
    1. Antinuclear antibody (ANA) and rheumatoid factor (RF).
    2. Three-hour glucose tolerance test and lipid profile.
    3. Red blood cell (RBC) count and a calcium level.
    4. Dexamethasone suppression test, urinary-free cortisol (UFC) level, and thyroid-stimulating hormone (TSH) and thyroxine (T_4).

13. The family nurse practitioner would anticipate which laboratory values in the patient with Graves' disease?
    1. Thyroid-stimulating hormone (TSH) levels to be increased.
    2. TSH levels to be decreased.
    3. TSH levels to be within normal limits.
    4. T_4 levels to be decreased.

14. Which information is correct regarding foot screening using a nylon filament (5.07-gauge Semmes-Weinstein)?
    1. Use a 25-gauge filament and apply along the perimeter of any scar or ulcer tissue.
    2. Apply the filament at a 45-degree angle to the skin surface.
    3. Apply sufficient force for approximately 1.5 seconds to cause the filament to bend.

4. Slide the filament across the skin and make repetitive contact with each of the 10 sites.

15. What two abnormal imaging studies should prompt the family nurse practitioner to perform an assessment for primary parathyroid dysfunction?
    1. Improving DEXA (bone density) scores in conjunction with bisphosphonate therapy.
    2. Early poor bone density scores in premenopausal women.
    3. Thyroid nodule scan that shows the nodule is not "hot" (is not actively producing thyroid hormone).
    4. Kidney stone noted on kidneys, ureter, bladder (KUB) film.
    5. X-ray of the pelvis showing "Brim sign."

16. An adult patient presents to the family nurse practitioner for evaluation of polyuria, polydipsia, and weight loss. Which laboratory result would require immediate intervention by the family nurse practitioner?
    1. A1c of 14%.
    2. Serum glucose of 150 mg/dL.
    3. A1c of 6.0%.
    4. Serum glucose of 65 mg/dL.

17. An adult patient is being evaluated for hypoglycemia because of a blood sugar level of 58 mg/dL. The family nurse practitioner would begin the differential diagnosis by:
    1. Deciding if the hypoglycemia is fasting or postprandial.
    2. Ascertaining if it is related to alcohol use.
    3. Deciding if the patient has other medical problems.
    4. Reassuring the patient that it is a benign problem.

18. An older adult male patient complains of lethargy, cold intolerance, weight gain, and yellowing of the palms. What would be the most important laboratory study ordered by the family nurse practitioner in diagnosing this condition?
    1. Complete blood count.
    2. Liver enzymes.
    3. Thyroid panel.
    4. Cardiac enzymes.

19. A middle-aged, normally healthy female presents for evaluation of intermittent palpitations. She also reports mood variability, tremulousness, difficulty falling asleep, and a 10-lb weight loss despite a normal appetite. She feels warm most of the time and wonders if she is perimenopausal. She has no history of heart disease. The objective data that would yield the most useful information would be:
    1. Electrocardiogram (ECG).
    2. Thyroid-stimulating hormone (TSH), free T_4.
    3. Electrolytes.
    4. Serum hormone level.

20. To make the diagnosis of diabetes, the patient must have two fasting plasma glucose levels documented on two occasions greater than or equal to:
    1. 200 mg/dL.
    2. 140 mg/dL.
    3. 126 mg/dL.
    4. 110 mg/dL.

21. A middle-aged woman presents with agitation, confusion, fever, tachycardia, and diaphoresis. Her daughter states that nausea, vomiting, and abdominal pain preceded these symptoms. The patient has no history of cardiac disease, diabetes, or substance abuse. She was started on some "anti-drug" 2 weeks ago and is scheduled for some form of throat surgery next week (per her daughter). Based on this history, what does the family nurse practitioner immediately order?
    1. Thyroid-stimulating hormone, T_4.
    2. Urinalysis.
    3. Spinal tap.
    4. Computed tomography of the head.

22. A patient with Graves' disease is to have radioactive iodine (I^{131}) therapy. Which information is important for the family nurse practitioner to include when teaching about this treatment?
    1. Patients are highly radioactive for approximately 7 days after treatment and need to be isolated.
    2. Patients should not become pregnant during or after receiving this therapy because of the teratogenic effects to the fetus that occur because of chromosomal abnormalities.
    3. Patients may become hypothyroid after this treatment and therefore need to have regular thyroid-stimulating (TSH) and T_4 levels drawn, with the potential for thyroid hormone replacement therapy.
    4. This therapy is contraindicated in patients with cardiac disease.

Disorders

23. The family nurse practitioner understands that acromegaly is typically caused by:
    1. Hypersecretion of benign pituitary tumors.
    2. Hyposecretion of pituitary hormones.
    3. Hypersecretion of adrenal cortex hormones.
    4. Metastatic tumors within the pituitary.

24. During a retrospective review of an established patient, the family nurse practitioner notes that the photographs of the person show more than just typical aging. They include increased spacing of teeth without loss of dentition, a deep furrowing of the brow, enlarging jaw, and a widening of the nose. What would be the initial intervention the family nurse practitioner should consider?
    1. Treat without intervention until the symptoms become of symptomatic concern.

2. Investigate with an oral glucose tolerance test (OGTT).
3. Test first to rule out a thyroid disorder.
4. Draw an insulin-like growth factor 1 (IGF-1) test.

25. Primary Cushing disease is linked to suppression of pituitary control over steroid homeostasis. Secondary Cushing syndrome must be considered in which of the following patient groups?
    1. Type 1 diabetes.
    2. Patients with chronic hypertension who respond to medications.
    3. Patients with cancers, especially of small cell variety.
    4. Any patient who is obese.

26. A patient has been diagnosed with diabetes for more than 5 years. To whom should the family nurse practitioner maintain an annual referral for this patient?
    1. Cardiologist.
    2. Dietitian.
    3. Vascular surgeon.
    4. Ophthalmologist.

27. Hirsutism presenting in a female with normal menstruation and normal plasma androgens is most likely:
    1. An ovarian tumor.
    2. Cushing syndrome.
    3. Idiopathic.
    4. Polycystic ovary disease.

28. An adult woman presents to the clinic complaining of fatigue, weakness, weight gain despite lack of appetite, and feelings of depression. Physical exam reveals an obese, alert patient with thinning hair, bilateral chest puffiness, increased facial hair, supraclavicular fat pad, thin arms and legs, purple striae on the abdomen, and multiple ecchymotic areas on the extremities. Her vital signs are blood pressure of 158/96 mm Hg, pulse of 88 beats/min, and respiration of 22 breaths/min. Laboratory results show fasting blood sugar of 200 mg/dL and an electrolyte panel within normal limits, except for potassium of 3.0 mEq/L, hemoglobin of 11.8 g, and hematocrit of 34%. This assessment information would support the family nurse practitioner's diagnosis of:
    1. Addison disease.
    2. Pheochromocytoma.
    3. Cushing syndrome.
    4. Hypoaldosteronism.

29. Because of its position in the base of the brain and its effect on the optic structures, tumors of the pituitary gland frequently manifest as:
    1. Exophthalmos.
    2. Loss of vision in half of the visual field.
    3. Ocular muscle disturbances.
    4. Loss of central vision.

30. What are the clinical findings in a patient with hypothyroidism?
    1. Hyperactive bowel sounds.
    2. Oily skin and acne.
    3. Postural tremors of the hands.
    4. Edema of the face and eyelids.

31. A young adult male reports anxiety, tremulousness, headaches, palpitations, and sweating 2–4 hours after eating. Physical exam is normal. No laboratory results are currently available. No medical conditions are noted in the history. What is the most likely diagnosis?
    1. Dumping syndrome.
    2. Hypoglycemia.
    3. Alcohol abuse.
    4. Hyperthyroidism.

32. A woman comes to your office complaining about adrenal fatigue because she has had continuous stress in the past year. What do you know about this condition?
    1. It is an "Internet diagnosis" not recognized by the scientific community as a formal syndrome.
    2. It is another term for laboratory-confirmed subclinical adrenal insufficiency.
    3. It is a constellation of symptoms commonly found in individuals who have adrenal gland secretion higher than usual levels.
    4. It is the most common complaint in persons seeking opiate drugs.

33. Which of the following is the most likely etiology for hypercalcemia in the medically well asymptomatic adult?
    1. Hyperthyroidism.
    2. Hyperparathyroidism.
    3. Hyperpituitarism.
    4. Hypothyroidism.

34. A middle-aged male with no previous medical history presents with a 30-lb weight gain in 2.5 months. He denies any medication use or allergies. He was recently laid off from a very active job and has been sedentary. Physical exam reveals blood pressure of 172/111 mm Hg, central obesity, and fasting blood sugar of 200 mg/dL. What is the most likely cause of the patient's weight gain?
    1. Cushing syndrome.
    2. Hypothyroidism.
    3. Depression.
    4. Diabetes.

35. A 45-year-old female patient presents to the office complaining of a 6-month history of fatigue, 15-lb weight gain, lethargy, an inability to tolerate cold temperatures, forgetfulness, hair loss, and constipation. Physical exam findings include dry, coarse skin; periorbital edema and puffy facies; bradycardia; hyporeflexia and muscle weakness; and a smooth, goitrous thyroid. What diagnosis would the family nurse practitioner make?
    1. Heart failure.
    2. Diabetes mellitus.
    3. Hypothyroidism.
    4. Thyroid cancer.

36. What does the role of the family nurse practitioner in the initial management of a patient with a thyroid nodule involve?
    1. Referring the patient to an endocrinologist for further evaluation.
    2. Obtaining fine-needle aspiration (FNA) biopsy of the nodule and sending it to cytology.
    3. Ordering an ultrasound and a thyroid panel.
    4. Ordering levothyroxine (Synthroid) to reduce the size of the nodule.

37. Once considered a "rare occurrence" or cause of hypertension, it is now recognized that what percentage of hypertensive patients have a component of adrenal gland disease?
    1. 5%.
    2. 10%–20%.
    3. 30%–50%.
    4. >50%.

38. When teaching a patient with diabetes about "sick day" guidelines, the family nurse practitioner explains that the patient should:
    1. Stop measuring blood glucose and only check urine for ketones.
    2. Not take the usual dose of insulin at the usual time.
    3. Be sure to take metformin (Glucophage) and acarbose (Precose), even if nausea and vomiting are present.
    4. Administer extra doses of regular insulin according to instructions for blood glucose levels above >240 mg/dL.

39. A young adult female patient presents to the clinic with complaints of nervousness, tremulousness, palpitations, heat intolerance, fatigue, weight loss, and polyphagia. After a complete history and physical, along with thyroid function tests, the family nurse practitioner makes the diagnosis of hyperthyroidism, recognizing that the most common cause of this condition is:
    1. Thyroid cancer.
    2. Graves' disease.
    3. Pituitary adenoma.
    4. Postpartum thyroiditis.

40. A young adult male patient presents to the office stating that he found a lump in his neck while shaving. Physical exam reveals a firm, 2-cm nodule that is fixed, nontender, and located on the right lobe of the thyroid gland. Right posterior cervical lymphadenopathy is also noted. The family nurse practitioner should:
    1. Order a thyroid-stimulating hormone (TSH) level and ultrasound and refer the patient to a surgeon for a possible fine-needle aspiration (FNA) biopsy of the nodule.
    2. No intervention is necessary at this time; schedule a follow-up visit in 6 months.
    3. Prescribe levothyroxine (Synthroid) 0.1 mg PO daily and schedule a 6-week follow-up visit.
    4. Immediately ablate the patient's thyroid with radioactive iodine and refer him to an endocrinologist.

41. During an evaluation of a patient with prediabetes (glucose intolerance), the family nurse practitioner identifies which finding in the patient's objective data is associated with the increasing insulin resistance?
    1. Triglycerides >150 mg/dL.
    2. High-density lipoprotein >40 mg/dL in men and >50 mg/dL in women.
    3. Blood pressure <130/85 mm Hg.
    4. Fasting blood sugar <110 mg/dL.

42. While taking a history on a patient, the family nurse practitioner identifies what finding that may be associated with osteopenia/osteoporosis?
    1. High calcium intake.
    2. Minimal alcohol intake.
    3. Smoking 1 pack/day for 20 years.
    4. Walking 30 minutes 4 days a week.

43. Of the following risk factors for osteoporosis, which would the family nurse practitioner see primarily with men?
    1. Smoking two packs of cigarettes a day.
    2. Excessive use of alcohol.
    3. Low testosterone level.
    4. Minimal exercise.

44. When prescribing a meal plan for a patient with type 2 diabetes, the family nurse practitioner tells the patient that the macronutrient with the most influence on postprandial glucose levels is:
    1. Fiber.
    2. Fat.
    3. Protein.
    4. Carbohydrate.

45. The family nurse practitioner understands the following about type 3c (pancreatic-disease related) diabetes:
    1. Caused by chronic pancreatitis.
    2. Diagnosed at age 25 or earlier.
    3. Increased insulin production.
    4. Diminished insulin sensitivity.

46. When does the family nurse practitioner suspect that undiagnosed primary hyperaldosteronism is at play in hypertension management?
    1. When the average blood pressure (BP) remains >140/80 mm Hg despite being on two antihypertensive medications.
    2. When BP readings consistently remain >160/100 mm Hg with three antihypertensive medications.
    3. When BP readings take more than 6 weeks to respond to initial treatment.
    4. When BP readings remain >150/100 mm Hg and are associated with hyperkalemia.

Pharmacology

47. Family nurse practitioners are very familiar with the precautions about tapering of steroid medications. Which of the following is a true statement about the actual need and/or process of doing so that the family nurse practitioner understands?
    1. All dosing regimens, no matter the dose and the duration of therapy, require tapering of doses.
    2. Patients who have had several steroid prescriptions in the past year are at lessened risk of sustaining a poor outcome if the doses are not tapered.
    3. Dosing regimens lasting longer than 2 weeks require consideration of a tapering schedule.
    4. Pulse doses of steroid (i.e., 3-day bursts) do not require tapering if they occur more than 6 months apart.

48. When prescribing oral medications for an overweight patient with type 2 diabetes who also has a voracious appetite, the family nurse practitioner is likely to prescribe which medication to encourage weight loss and reduce appetite, as an adjunct to improved diet and exercise?
    1. Exenatide (Byetta).
    2. Pioglitazone (Actos).
    3. Metformin (Glucophage).
    4. Glyburide (Micronase).

49. Timing of taking thyroid medication has traditionally been in the morning on an empty stomach. If the patient insists on taking thyroid medication with an evening meal, is this acceptable? What would be two appropriate responses?
    1. No, the circadian rhythm cycles are best supported with a.m. dosing.
    2. This is acceptable if there is a 2- to 4-hour separation from an ingested full evening meal.
    3. There is no difference between a.m. and p.m. dosing guidelines.
    4. This is a feasible option if there are no other medications taken at that time that would cause interactions or absorption issues.

50. Glargine (Lantus) is an insulin analog that essentially has no peak and is *usually* administered:
    1. Before meals.
    2. With lispro insulin (Humalog) in one injection.
    3. Before breakfast and dinner.
    4. Once daily.

51. Which of the following is the best alternative for treating hyperthyroidism diagnosed during the first trimester of pregnancy?
    1. Radioactive iodine in smaller than usual dose during first trimester.
    2. Propylthiouracil (PTU) during first trimester, subtotal thyroidectomy during second trimester, no thyroid replacement.
    3. PTU during first trimester, subtotal thyroidectomy during second trimester, thyroid replacement.
    4. No treatment until after delivery.

52. An adult male patient with type 2 diabetes has a creatinine level of 1.8 mg/dL. Which of the following drugs is contraindicated?
    1. Pioglitazone (Actos).
    2. Metformin (Glucophage).
    3. Repaglinide (Prandin).
    4. Acarbose (Precose).

53. Patients started on metformin (Glucophage) need to be monitored closely for what potential side effect?
    1. Significant increase in weight.
    2. Elevation of low-density lipoprotein (LDL) level.
    3. Lactic acidosis.
    4. Increase in insulin requirements.

54. A patient with type 2 diabetes is taking glipizide (Glucotrol) 10 mg PO bid. In evaluating the medication's effectiveness, the family nurse practitioner knows that glipizide reduces blood glucose by:
    1. Delaying the cellular uptake of potassium and insulin.
    2. Stimulating insulin release from the pancreas.
    3. Decreasing the body's need for and use of insulin at the cellular level.
    4. Interfering with the absorption and metabolism of fats and carbohydrates.

55. The family nurse practitioner would expect which symptom to be a side effect of metformin (Glucophage)?
    1. Gastrointestinal (GI) upset.
    2. Photophobia.
    3. Hypoglycemia.
    4. Skin eruptions.

56. The sodium-glucose cotransporter 2 (SGLT2) inhibitor medications are known to contribute to which of the two following outcomes in patients with type 2 diabetes:
    1. Reduced A1c level.

    2. Weight loss.
    3. Decreased issues of vaginal yeast infections.
    4. Decreased risk of breast and bladder cancers.
    5. Urinary retention.

57. A patient is receiving antithyroid medication. The family nurse practitioner understands that:
    1. Lifelong daily treatment is necessary to keep TSH levels within the normal range.
    2. Antithyroid medications do not cross the placenta.
    3. The drugs are somewhat expensive and have serious cardiac and hematologic side effects.
    4. Patients remain on drug therapy for 1–2 years, and then the medication is gradually withdrawn.

58. When prescribing an antihypertensive medication for a patient with type 2 diabetes, what are the drug classifications that would tend to reduce insulin sensitivity?
    1. Diuretics and calcium channel blockers.
    2. Diuretics and beta blockers.
    3. Calcium channel blockers and angiotensin-converting enzyme (ACE) inhibitors.
    4. Alpha blockers and ACE inhibitors.

59. A 35-year-old female sees the family nurse practitioner with a complaint of cold intolerance, fatigue, dry skin, weight gain, and heavy menstrual periods. Physical exam reveals a pulse of 58 beats/min; a "waxy," sallow complexion; and a firm goiter. Her thyroid-stimulating hormone (TSH) level is 176 mU/L. What is the best treatment choice for this patient?
    1. Begin levothyroxine (Synthroid) at 25 mcg (0.025 mg) PO daily and repeat TSH in 2 weeks.
    2. Administer loading dose of PO levothyroxine and start full replacement dose.
    3. Administer loading dose of IV levothyroxine and start on half replacement dose.
    4. Begin levothyroxine at 100 mcg (0.1 mg) PO daily and recheck TSH in 6 weeks.

60. The family nurse practitioner is performing a preoperative evaluation of a man scheduled to undergo coronary artery bypass grafting. Physical exam reveals mild facial puffiness, hoarse voice, and dry skin. The results of thyroid function tests show that the patient has a TSH level of 34 mU/L. What is the recommended treatment for the patient?
    1. Give loading IV bolus of levothyroxine (Synthroid) 500 mcg (0.5 mg) and proceed with surgery.
    2. Cancel surgery and send him home to begin levothyroxine PO 100 mcg (0.1 mg), then reschedule surgery.
    3. Begin PO levothyroxine and monitor the patient in the hospital until he is euthyroid.
    4. Proceed with surgery and treat the patient's hypothyroidism postoperatively.

61. What is associated with chronic overtreatment with levothyroxine (Synthroid)?
    1. Tachycardia.
    2. Osteoporosis.
    3. Insomnia.
    4. Sweating.

62. A middle-aged male presents for a diabetes follow-up examination. He has been in good health without identified complications of diabetes. His fasting blood sugar is 100 mg/dL, and his personal records indicate that he is taking insulin at the prescribed amounts and times. His vital signs are blood pressure (BP) 142/98 mm Hg, pulse 80 beats/min, and respiration 20 breaths/min. What actions would be included in today's plan? (Select 2 responses.)
    1. Begin diuretics and a beta blocker.
    2. Begin angiotensin-converting enzyme (ACE) inhibitor and consider a diuretic.
    3. Obtain electrocardiogram and chest x-ray.
    4. Return for BP check in 5–7 days.
    5. Order a serum creatinine and urine microalbuminuria test.

63. A patient on antithyroid drug therapy for hyperthyroidism presents with complaints of palpitations and dry mouth for the last 2 days. He has had a cough and cold symptoms for the last 3 days, which he has been treating with over-the-counter (OTC) medications. Which medication would the family nurse practitioner encourage the patient to avoid?
    1. Benzocaine (Chloraseptic) lozenges.
    2. Guaifenesin (Robitussin).
    3. Ibuprofen (Advil).
    4. Pseudoephedrine (Sudafed).

64. What is the most frequent complaint of patients who use insulin pumps?
    1. Problems with elevated glucose after changing the catheter-type (nonneedle) infusion set.
    2. Skin and site problems with dressing adhesive not sticking; redness and pain at infusion site.
    3. Mechanical problems with the pump's digital readout.
    4. Understanding "sick day" management modifications.

65. The family nurse practitioner understands that pioglitazone (Actos) or rosiglitazone (Avandia) is indicated for:
    1. Prenatal patients with gestational diabetes.
    2. "Brittle" patients with type 1 diabetes.
    3. Patients with type 2 diabetes requiring insulin who have poor glycemic control and insulin resistance.
    4. Patients with type 2 diabetes to prevent the rapid postprandial blood glucose surges by delaying carbohydrate absorption.

66. An older patient with a history of hypertension and coronary bypass surgery has been diagnosed with hypothyroidism. What is the appropriate medication management?
    1. Levothyroxine (Synthroid) 100 mcg (0.1 mg) daily and return in 6 weeks for follow-up.
    2. Desiccated thyroid extract 2 grains daily and return in 6 weeks for follow-up.
    3. Levothyroxine (Synthroid) 25 mcg (0.025 mg) daily for 6 weeks with a gradual increase in dosage every 4–6 weeks until a therapeutic level is obtained.
    4. Methimazole (Tapazole) 15 mg daily in three divided doses, gradually increasing the dose every 4 weeks until a therapeutic level is obtained.

67. A patient is newly diagnosed as being hypothyroid and is placed on levothyroxine (Synthroid) 100 mcg (0.1 mg) PO daily. What should be the family nurse practitioner's approach to follow-up?
    1. No follow-up visits are necessary.
    2. The patient should return to the clinic in 4–6 weeks for thyroid-stimulating hormone measurement (TSH) and determination of any symptomatic improvement.
    3. The patient should have weekly levothyroxine levels measured.
    4. The patient should have monthly complete blood count tests while on levothyroxine (Synthroid) because the medication has been found to be myelosuppressive.

68. What are the classes of medications typically used to treat hyperthyroid conditions?
    1. Antibiotics and corticosteroids.
    2. Angiotensin-converting enzyme (ACE) inhibitors, anxiolytics, and antithyroid medications.
    3. Beta blockers, nonsteroidal antiinflammatory drugs (NSAIDs), and antithyroid medications.
    4. Calcium channel blockers and corticosteroids.

69. A patient with hypothyroidism receiving daily levothyroxine (Synthroid) for 3 weeks presents to the clinic with complaints of intermittent chest pain. What is the appropriate therapeutic response?
    1. Discontinue levothyroxine because chest pain is a contraindication to its continuance.
    2. Schedule the patient for a stress test.
    3. Decrease dose of levothyroxine, order an electrocardiogram, and consult immediately with endocrine and/or cardiology health team members.
    4. Prescribe an anxiolytic agent for the patient.

70. When prescribing sulfonylureas, the family nurse practitioner educates the patient that the most common side effect of therapy is:
    1. Upset stomach.
    2. Diarrhea.
    3. Angina.
    4. Hypoglycemia.

71. What is the primary action of pioglitazone (Actos) and rosiglitazone (Avandia)?
    1. Decrease hepatic glucose output.
    2. Increase secretion of insulin from the pancreas.
    3. Increase glucose uptake into the muscle and fat.
    4. Increase postprandial uptake of glucose into the intestine.

72. A patient has been discharged to home on desmopressin acetate (DDAVP) for diabetes insipidus after removal of a pituitary tumor. On examination, the family nurse practitioner notes that the patient is lethargic but has 4+ deep tendon reflexes. What should the family nurse practitioner suspect?
    1. Noncompliance with therapy.
    2. Water intoxication.
    3. Increased vasopressor effect.
    4. Interaction with over-the-counter cough medicine products.

73. Some diabetic medication groups are being associated with a link to cancer. Which of the following drugs and links to possible cancer types is correct? (Select two responses.)
    1. The thiazolidinediones (TZD group) and bladder cancer.
    2. The biguanides and pancreatic cancer.
    3. The glucagon-like peptide agonists (GLP-1) and thyroid cancer.
    4. The sulfonylureas and prostate cancer.
    5. The incretin mimetics and stomach cancer.

74. Which of the following osteoporosis medications does not carry the critical warning that the patient must take the medication with a full glass of water and remain upright 30–60 minutes after dosing?
    1. Alendronate (Fosamax).
    2. Ibandronate (Boniva).
    3. Risedronate (Actonel).
    4. Zoledronic acid (Zometa).

75. A young adult is taking desmopressin acetate (DDAVP) nasally. The patient also has allergies to local plants, which creates a good amount of nasal congestion. What medication education is important to emphasize?
    1. If the patient is taking an antihistamine, the patient cannot take the DDAVP.
    2. If the patient's nasal passages are full of mucus, the patient should blow the nose to clear it before taking the DDAVP.
    3. The congestion makes the use of inhaled DDAVP ineffective, so the dose will have to be taken orally until the allergies diminish.

    4. The patient needs to take the DDAVP at least 1 hour apart from any oral antihistamine.

76. Education concerning home blood sugar testing with a personal glucometer includes the following key point:
    1. Use the matching test strips designed for the particular glucometer because different brands are not interchangeable.
    2. When opening a new canister of test strips, recalibration or setting control codes are no longer needed.
    3. The values obtained from self-monitoring glucometers match serum blood values.
    4. Remember to cleanse the fingertip or alternative testing site with alcohol before using the lancing-type device.

77. Which group of antihypertensive agents have some positive effect on the development of diabetic nephropathy?
    1. Alpha blockers.
    2. Beta blockers.
    3. Calcium channel blockers.
    4. Angiotensin-converting enzyme (ACE) inhibitors.

78. A patient with diabetes has been taking 6 U of regular insulin and 12 U of NPH insulin in the morning. In the evening, she has been taking 3 U of regular insulin and 8 U of NPH insulin. The patient has been monitoring her blood glucose levels (mg/dL) and shows the family nurse practitioner the following chart:

	7:00 AM	Noon	5:00 PM	Bedtime
Monday	100	76	98	109
Tuesday	119	75	88	110
Wednesday	119	66	86	100
Thursday	123	70	111	122
Friday	128	60	99	110

The family nurse practitioner adjusts the patient's insulin by:
    1. Increasing the a.m. regular insulin.
    2. Decreasing the a.m. regular insulin.
    3. Decreasing the a.m. NPH insulin.
    4. Increasing both p.m. insulins.

79. Which two of the following diabetic medication groups is linked with higher risks for hypoglycemia when given as monotherapy?
    1. Biguanides.
    2. Insulins.
    3. Sulfonylureas.
    4. Incretin mimetics.
    5. DDP-4 inhibitors (gliptins).

9 Endocrine Answers & Rationales

Physical Exam & Diagnostic Tests

1. Answer: 2

Rationale: Goiters are typically not visible from the lateral aspect in most patients without regard to weight. When examining, inspection from the side to identify any enlargement between the cricoid cartilage and the suprasternal notch is helpful. Any prominence noted in this area should be measured with a ruler and recorded. If the prominence is larger than 2 mm (0.08 inch), there is a high likelihood of goiter. A small goiter is one to two times the normal size of the thyroid, and a large goiter is more than twice normal size.

2. Answer: 2

Rationale: When examining the thyroid, it is important that the patient relax the sternocleidomastoid muscles, which is done by having the patient tilt toward the side being evaluated.

3. Answer: 4

Rationale: The thyroid gland is fixed to the cricoid cartilage and superior portion of the trachea and thus ascends during swallowing. This assists the family nurse practitioner to distinguish thyroid structures from other neck masses. The gland's size, degree of enlargement, consistency, surface characteristics, and the presence of nodules or bruits are noted during the examination.

4. Answer: 2

Rationale: Puffiness of the face and the skin around the eyes (periorbital) as well as dry, thickened skin, with coarse, breakable hair are linked with chronic low thyroid states. Classic signs of hyperthyroidism are onycholysis (brittle nails, Plummer's nails); warm, velvety skin; fine hair with hair loss; and pretibial edema. Onycholysis is the loosening or separation of a fingernail or toenail from its nail bed and is associated with fungal infections, trauma, and hyperthyroidism.

5. Answer: 1

Rationale: Coarse facial features, heavier brow line, and prominent jaw are associated with acromegaly. Other findings include frontal skull bossing (prominent, protruding forehead), mandibular overgrowth, maxillary widening, teeth separation, malocclusion, overbite, and skin thickening on the face (tongue, lips, and nose). Moon face and extra hair growth on the upper lip and chin with acne on the back and chest are typical Cushing characteristics. A wide-eyed look with nervous tic, bulging eyes (exophthalmos), lid lag, and warm, moist skin are associated with hyperthyroidism. Periorbital puffiness is associated with hypothyroidism.

6. Answer: 3

Rationale: Naturally occurring insulin has a C-peptide bond, which is removed during the processing of exogenous insulin as a drug. The level of C-peptide in the blood can show how much insulin is being made by the pancreas. Classically, a patient with type 1 diabetes has no C-peptide bonds because all circulating insulin is from exogenous sources. In comparison, a patient with type 2 diabetes is expected to have some innate insulin production, so C-peptides should be present. The hemoglobin A1c or glycosylated fructose can be used for either patient group. The Apo A and B levels deal with lipid values, not sugars. It should be noted that newer research shows that some patients with type 1 diabetes actually produce a bit of natural insulin, especially after the initial period, so the C-peptide laboratory value is not the absolute determinant of disease status.

7. Answer: 2

Rationale: The increased bone turnover related to abnormal parathyroid hormone levels is linked with increased calcium levels. Changes in other laboratory values can be associated with bone loss, but the link is stronger with calcium changes.

8. Answer: 3

Rationale: Papillary carcinoma, the most common form of thyroid cancer, is associated with a history of exposure to radiation. Family history, history of hyperthyroidism, and smoking are not considered significant risk factors for this malignancy.

9. Answer: 1

Rationale: Memory, attention, and problem-solving deficits are often-noted symptoms with hyperthyroidism. The high level of thyroid hormone affects the nervous system, causing sympathomimetic symptoms such as brisk deep tendon reflexes, fine rapid tremor of the hands, restlessness, irritability, insomnia, dreams, nightmares, and rarely severe cognitive impairment and psychosis.

10. Answer: 3

Rationale: The American Diabetes Association recommends an A1c level of <7% as an important treatment goal to decrease the risk of long-term complications. A laboratory test result of >6.5% A1c is an indication that action needs to be taken, either by a change in medication or a reinforcement of education. Counseling should be provided for prediabetes patients with A1c >5.7%. In some older patients, those with multiple comorbidities, or those with limited life expectancy, a goal of <8% may be used.

11. Answer: 2

Rationale: The primary care provider may obtain TSH, T_3, T_4, and T_7 levels and an ultrasound. Ordering antibody levels, thyroid scans, or FNA biopsy should be done after coordination with the endocrine team. The FNA aspirate is sent for cytology and interpretation.

12. Answer: 4

Rationale: The low-dose dexamethasone suppression test is the best screening test, and the 24-hour UFC is the best confirmatory test to use for Cushing disease. Late-night salivary cortisol is a screening test that would be elevated. TSH and T_4 may also be appropriate to rule out a thyroid condition because some of the patient's signs and symptoms are consistent with thyroid dysfunction. ANA and RF are ordered when rheumatoid arthritis or systemic lupus erythematosus is suspected; however, the patient's clinical picture is not consistent with these conditions. The RBC count would be done to rule out anemia, a potential problem for this patient based on the history of fatigue, but the rest of the clinical picture indicates more than anemia. No clinical findings support a calcium level being drawn.

13. Answer: 2

Rationale: TSH levels should be decreased in a patient with Graves' disease because thyroid-stimulating immunoglobulins bind to TSH receptors, which increase thyroxine and triiodothyronine synthesis and release, subsequently suppressing TSH levels.

14. Answer: 3

Rationale: The correct procedure is to use a 10-gauge (5.07-gauge Semmes-Weinstein) filament and apply it to 10 sites on the foot (one on the top of the foot and nine on the heel, sole, and toes). The filament is applied perpendicular (90-degree angle) to the skin surface with sufficient force for 1.5 seconds to cause the filament to bend. The filament should not be allowed to slide across the skin or make repetitive contact with each test site. Randomizing the selection of test sites (start with great toe → heel → instep area → fifth metatarsal) and the time between successive tests to reduce patient guessing and having the patient close the eyes are also helpful.

15. Answer: 2, 4

Rationale: Parathyroid dysfunction typically occurs in older age, but it is commonly the cause of unexplained osteoporosis in younger to middle-aged adults. The most frequent first presentation on imaging is kidney stones. The Brim sign (thickened iliopectineal line or pelvic brim) is noted on an x-ray in patients who have Paget disease.

16. Answer: 1

Rationale: An A1c of >8.0% indicates poor glucose control over the past few months. According to the American Diabetes

Association, an A1c of >8.0% is equal to an average daily blood glucose of 355 mg/dL. The normal serum glucose for adults ranges from 70–120 mg/dL. Diabetic acidosis is not of concern until the glucose level is >300 mg/dL.

17. Answer: 1

Rationale: True hypoglycemia can be organized around whether it is fasting or postprandial. Postprandial hypoglycemia may be caused by early adult-onset diabetes or postgastrectomy syndrome. Fasting hypoglycemia is most often caused by excessive doses of insulin, sulfonylureas alone, or with biguanides and thiazolidinediones.

18. Answer: 3

Rationale: The symptoms of lethargy, cold intolerance, weight gain, and yellowing of the palms suggest hypothyroidism, and thyroid studies (e.g., thyroid-stimulating hormone) would be most useful. A complete physical would be performed, and liver etiology is still a differential. Xanthoderma (yellowing of palms) typically occurs only because of a coexisting carotinemia. Thyroid etiology is the "most likely" choice because cold intolerance is given.

19. Answer: 2

Rationale: This middle-aged female patient presents with many of the classic symptoms of early hyperthyroidism (e.g., tremulousness, racing pulse, difficulty falling asleep, weight loss despite a normal appetite, and feeling warm). A suppressed TSH with an elevated free T4 establishes the diagnosis of hyperthyroidism.

20. Answer: 3

Rationale: The American Diabetes Association has defined the diagnostic criteria for diabetes to include any one of the three following methods, which must be confirmed on a subsequent day:

- Random plasma glucose ≥200 mg/dL and acute symptoms (polyuria, polydipsia, polyphagia).
- Fasting plasma glucose ≥126 mg/dL.
- Plasma glucose ≥200 mg/dL during an oral glucose tolerance test.
- Hemoglobin A1c >6.5%.

21. Answer: 1

Rationale: The woman is likely experiencing the life-threatening syndrome that can occur in decompensated hyperthyroidism. The clues are her symptom presentation and progression, the new "antidrug," and upcoming throat surgery, which suggest that the patient is likely on propylthiouracil or methimazole. Although other possible causes of delirium are eventually considered, the family nurse practitioner needs to go with the probabilities of occurrence within the given context.

22. Answer: 3

Rationale: Hypothyroidism often follows this treatment, with 50% of patients requiring replacement therapy in the first year and almost 100% requiring therapy in 10 years. For this reason, regular monitoring of TSH and T$_4$ levels should be performed. Patients emit a small amount of radioactivity after receiving the dose used to treat this condition and do not require isolation for 7 days. Radioactive iodine is perceived to be safe, without an increased risk of chromosomal abnormalities; therefore no contraindication exists to becoming pregnant after therapy, although patients are counseled to avoid pregnancy during treatment and to avoid children and pregnant women after receiving the oral ablation dose. This therapy is recommended for patients who have cardiac disease associated with their thyroid condition.

Disorders

23. Answer: 1

Rationale: Pituitary masses associated with acromegaly are usually benign tumors that create a disruption in normal feedback mechanisms. Symptoms noted on physical exam result from the effects of growth hormone excess or from the secreting tissue effect of the pituitary mass on surrounding brain structures. This is not typically an adrenal cortex dysfunction. Although tumors can cause acromegaly symptoms, pituitary masses associated with acromegaly are typically noncancerous lesions.

24. Answer: 4

Rationale: The earlier the intervention, the better the outcome for the patient with acromegaly. Initially, the common practice and best single test is to measure IGF-1, which, if normal, rules out acromegaly. Levels twice the upper limit suggest acromegaly. Although not a pancreas-centered disorder, the OGTT is performed as follow-up testing and is a sensitive diagnostic evaluation (done after checking the IGF-1 level), except in patients with known diabetes whose diabetes is uncontrolled. In normal patients, the values fall into normal ranges; in patients with acromegaly, growth hormone (GH) is suppressed by the blood sugar load. The GH level is measured before the OGTT is done and then again at 2 hours. GH levels may remain >2 ng/mL in patients with acromegaly. Although thyroid enlargement can be part of a general organomegaly presentation, it is not the typical cause of this clinical presentation.

25. Answer: 3

Rationale: Although abnormal glucose control is a hallmark of Cushing disease, it is typically in patients with diabetes who have a metabolic syndrome presentation, not in the type 1 diabetes group. Hypertension under good control is not linked to steroid overproduction; it is the patient who does not respond to medication who is evaluated for adrenal issues. Bronchogenic and other small cell types of cancers have been known to produce "ectopic" steroids. The "moon face" of Cushing syndrome is different from that of someone who is simply overweight.

26. Answer: 4

Rationale: An annual eye exam with the pupils dilated should be done by a specialist who can recognize subtle abnormalities. Diabetic retinopathy is the most common eye disease among people with diabetes. Although the other referrals can offer important contributions to diabetes care, these would be done on an as-needed basis rather than annually.

27. Answer: 3

Rationale: Because of the normal menstrual periods and androgen plasma level, hirsutism would be considered in a premenopausal woman. There are iatrogenic causes (i.e., medications). Diseases related to the ovaries would cause changes in the menstrual cycle and, with Cushing syndrome, would be associated with adrenal androgen overproduction.

28. Answer: 3

Rationale: The patient's physical findings and habitus, along with hypertension and hypokalemia, are associated with Cushing syndrome, which is a state of excessive cortisol production caused by a pituitary tumor. A Cushing-like syndrome is often associated with prolonged glucocorticoid administration. Obesity is the primary finding in Cushing syndrome, along with the "moon face," lipoma growths on the upper back, truncal obesity, hirsutism in women, and impotence and loss of body hair in men. Addison disease is characterized by hyperkalemia, hyponatremia, hypoglycemia, anemia, and hypercalcemia. Patients with hypoaldosteronism (impaired renin secretion) have hyperkalemia. Pheochromocytoma would be included in the differential diagnosis of this patient because of the hypertension; the other findings are not consistent with this diagnosis.

29. Answer: 2

Rationale: Hemianopia (also called hemianopsia) is loss of vision in half of the visual field and is a classic sign of pituitary enlargement. It can be unilateral or bilateral (bitemporal hemianopsia), depending on the extent of the lesion. Exophthalmos is associated with thyroid hyperactivity. Ocular muscle control is less likely with pituitary lesions. Central vision loss is most associated with diabetes mellitus and age-related macular degeneration.

30. Answer: 4

Rationale: Accumulation of hyaluronic acid in interstitial tissues increases capillary permeability to albumin and causes the interstitial edema of the face and eyelids in patients with hypothyroidism.

31. Answer: 2

Rationale: Although alcohol abuse may be a cause of hypoglycemia, the patient is presenting with classic symptoms of postprandial hypoglycemia. Assessment for alcohol abuse as the etiology of the hypoglycemia would be advisable. Increased circulating thyroid hormones increase beta-cell sensitivity and increase insulin release. This does not typically manifest as hypoglycemia; instead, most patients with hyperthyroidism develop glucose intolerance caused by an antagonism of the peripheral action of insulin on cells.

32. Answer: 1

Rationale: This "syndrome" of collective complaints has yet to be found to have a basis in actual physiologic laboratory values. It is not an established complaint in the endocrine community; however, patients presenting with these issues should have a laboratory workup done to establish other underlying causes with appropriate treatment plans.

33. Answer: 2

Rationale: Hyperparathyroidism accounts for more than 60% of patients with hypercalcemia and is likely to be the explanation for elevated serum calcium levels.

34. Answer: 1

Rationale: Although depression may explain the weight gain, Cushing syndrome is the correct diagnosis for the constellation of symptoms of rapid weight gain, hypertension, and elevated blood sugar. These symptoms suggest adrenal dysfunction. Serum cortisol and adrenocorticotropic hormone levels should be checked.

35. Answer: 3

Rationale: The symptoms (weight gain, lethargy, inability to tolerate cold temperatures, forgetfulness, hair loss, and constipation) describe the classic presentation of a patient with hypothyroidism. A patient with heart failure would have jugular venous distention, rales, and peripheral edema. The criteria for diagnosing diabetes mellitus are polydipsia, polyphagia, polyuria, and weight loss. Thyroid cancer typically presents without many physical symptoms other than hoarseness and dysphagia, and often the only physical finding is a hard, fixed nodule on the thyroid gland.

36. Answer: 3

Rationale: The family nurse practitioner's role in primary care for a patient with a thyroid nodule involves initially the early identification of the thyroid nodule on physical exam and ordering an ultrasound and thyroid panel, then referring the patient to an endocrinologist for further evaluation, and possibly obtaining some preliminary thyroid-stimulating hormone

(TSH) and antibody testing. The endocrinologist performs the FNA if the nodule is <1 cm with a normal TSH level. Levothyroxine may or may not be used to diminish the size of the nodule, based on the findings derived from the FNA and the endocrinologist's chosen treatment plan.

37. Answer: 2

Rationale: Primary aldosteronism is considered the most common cause of secondary hypertension. Approximately 10%–15% of all patients with hypertension are now considered to have "inappropriate aldosterone secretion" for a variety of reasons. Primary aldosteronism is particularly common in patients with resistant hypertension, with a prevalence of approximately 20%.

38. Answer: 4

Rationale: Patients with diabetes must understand that when they are sick, blood glucose levels will probably increase, even when they are not eating. They need to monitor blood glucose levels every 2–4 hours. The medications metformin and acarbose should not be given until the patient's nausea and vomiting have subsided and the patient has resumed a normal diet; blood glucose monitoring is important during this time. Dehydration will increase the risk of metabolic acidosis for patients on metformin.

39. Answer: 2

Rationale: Graves' disease, an autoimmune condition also known as "diffuse toxic goiter," is the most common cause of hyperthyroidism in this age group. Less common causes include cancer of the thyroid, adenoma of the pituitary gland, and postpartum (or silent) thyroiditis.

40. Answer: 1

Rationale: The TSH level should be ordered to determine whether the patient is euthyroid, hypothyroid, or hyperthyroid, along with an ultrasound. The patient should also be sent to an endocrinologist or surgeon because all nodules of the thyroid should be biopsied to rule out malignancy. "Watching and waiting" is inappropriate without having a biopsy performed. Thyroid hormone replacement therapy would be indicated only for patients found to be hypothyroid and in whom thyroid cancer has been ruled out. Thyroid ablation may be indicated in patients whose FNA biopsy results are positive for thyroid cancer, but this cannot be determined without an endocrinologist's intervention.

41. Answer: 1

Rationale: Improper use of glucose increases the release of free fatty acids, which elevates triglycerides. The other values are still within normal limits.

42. Answer: 3

Rationale: Smoking causes thinning of the bones and can lead to osteopenia/osteoporosis. A diet high in calcium with minimal alcohol intake and walking are all self-care practices that may prevent or delay the onset of osteopenia/osteoporosis.

43. Answer: 3

Rationale: Low testosterone levels may result from prostate cancer treatment and long-standing liver disease. Smoking, excessive use of alcohol, and minimal exercise are risk factors of osteoporosis that can occur in both men and women.

44. Answer: 4

Rationale: Carbohydrate is the macronutrient with the greatest impact on the postprandial glucose levels. Ingested protein has minimal effect on the blood glucose levels. A diet high in fat may be associated with cardiovascular disease. Fiber has little effect on the plasma glucose response, but it may result in decreased low-density lipoprotein cholesterol.

45. Answer 1:

Rationale: The most common cause of type 3c diabetes is chronic pancreatitis; however, other causes include pancreatic cancer, hemochromatosis, cystic fibrosis, or pancreatic surgery. It is characterized by deficient insulin production caused by impaired pancreatic function. There is normal insulin sensitivity. Type 2 diabetes has diminished insulin sensitivity. Age of diagnosis is adulthood, typically after age 50. Type 3c diabetes is most commonly misdiagnosed as type 2 diabetes.

46. Answer: 2

Rationale: Resistant hypertension needs a full workup to include adrenal impact, especially when BP readings remain >160/100 mm Hg despite the patient being on three antihypertensive medications. Aldosterone excess results in renin suppression via feedback mechanism, hypertension caused by volume expansion and sodium retention, and low potassium caused by increased renal losses. The risk is highest in those with familial early stroke and hypertension incidence and in those with hypokalemia, adrenal incidentaloma, and sleep apnea.

Pharmacology

47. Answer: 3

Rationale: Continuous dosing of steroid medication conditions the adrenal feedback system to become less sensitive to discontinuation of the exogenous hormone supply, which normally would trigger a natural ramp-up of innate steroid production. Duration longer than 2 or 3 weeks and moderate to high doses trigger the need to evaluate current values and prepare for a gradual reduction in dosage before the patient stops taking the steroid medication.

48. Answer: 1

Rationale: Incretin mimetic medications, such as exenatide, are associated with weight loss. Metformin is associated with weight neutrality and appetite suppression. Glyburide is considered a second-generation sulfonylurea, which tends to stimulate insulin secretion from the pancreas, causing a slight weight gain. Pioglitazone is an insulin sensitizer and increases glucose uptake in the muscle and fat. Common side effects include fluid retention and an increase in central adiposity.

49. Answer: 3, 4

Rationale: There is no change in thyroid function and hormone levels in patients who take evening doses, as long as there is a separation of meals and the other medications are not taken to avoid drug-to-drug interactions.

50. Answer: 4

Rationale: Glargine is a long-acting basal insulin usually given once daily and lasts almost 24 hours without a peak. This clear insulin must be given alone and not mixed with other insulins in the same syringe. Lispro insulin is a rapid-acting insulin usually given three times daily with meals. A basal insulin can be used at the same time with a different injection. In rare cases, basal insulins are given more than once per day, but this is not usual practice.

51. Answer: 3

Rationale: Low-dose antithyroid drugs are considered a good alternative to prevent the effects of hyperthyroidism on the mother and developing fetus until surgery can be performed. Another option is using an antithyroid drug until after delivery, and then having surgery. Removal of the thyroid during the second trimester can be performed safely and is the usual recommendation. Replacement is essential after removal of the gland.

52. Answer: 2

Rationale: Metformin should not be given to men with a serum creatinine level ≥1.5 mg/dL or to women with a serum creatinine level ≥1.4 mg/dL because it can predispose the patient to lactic acidosis. Pioglitazone and repaglinide are metabolized primarily in the liver and require monitoring of liver function tests. Acarbose is metabolized mainly in the gastrointestinal tract.

53. Answer: 3

Rationale: Lactic acidosis is a potentially severe and fatal reaction to metformin. Metformin does not contribute to weight gain; it often helps with weight loss and decreases LDL, triglyceride levels, and insulin requirements.

54. Answer: 2

Rationale: Sulfonylureas reduce blood glucose by stimulating insulin release from the pancreas. Over time, these drugs also may actually increase insulin effects at the cellular level and decrease glucose production by the liver, which is why sulfonylureas are used in patients with type 2 diabetes who still have a functioning pancreas.

55. Answer: 1

Rationale: Anorexia, nausea, and a metallic taste in the mouth are common side effects. Over time, GI symptoms subside and can be relieved by taking the medication with food or by starting at a lower dose. Metformin has a safety profile that does not include hypoglycemia unless mixed with other agents that trigger it.

56. Answer: 1, 2

Rationale: Positive outcomes include better glucose control over time and some potential weight loss. This SGLT2 medication class (e.g., canagliflozin, dapagliflozin) is linked to an increase in genital yeast infections, and some agents have been associated with increasing risks of cancer (though low on the basis of current information). A new black box warning was published in May 2017 to state that canagliflozin increases the risk of foot and leg amputations and should be used with caution. There is also the side of effect of an increased desire to urinate.

57. Answer: 4

Rationale: Antithyroid medications or thionamides (e.g., propylthiouracil, methimazole) are relatively inexpensive and do cross the placenta. The patient remains on the medications for 1–2 years with the hope of a permanent remission of symptoms when the medications are withdrawn.

58. Answer: 2

Rationale: Both of these drug classifications (diuretics and beta blockers) tend to reduce insulin sensitivity and can cause hyperglycemia. ACE inhibitors, calcium channel blockers, and selective alpha blockers are metabolically neutral; some may actually have a beneficial effect.

59. Answer: 4

Rationale: The patient's symptoms indicate hypothyroidism, as does the elevated TSH level (normal levels are 0.5–4.7 mU/L). A full replacement dose of levothyroxine should be the goal for the patient with a standard starting dose of 100–125 mcg (0.1–0.125 mg) for a 70-kg person. The TSH level should be checked in 6 weeks, which is the time it may take for a given dose to become effective. Loading doses should never be given, except in the case of coma, which is treated by IV medication in the hospital.

60. Answer: 4

Rationale: Patients with coronary disease who are found to be mildly to moderately hypothyroid can safely undergo urgent surgery (including bypass procedures) without prior replacement. The rate of complications is no greater than for nonhypothyroid patients, and the cardiac risks are less compared with initiating replacement therapy preoperatively.

61. Answer: 2

Rationale: Chronic overtreatment is associated with osteoporosis; the other options are related to acute overdose of levothyroxine and can be relieved by omitting the dose for 3 days and then starting on a lower dose.

62. Answer: 4, 5

Rationale: To initiate treatment for elevated BP, it is recommended that three elevated readings be recorded on three separate occasions. No evidence suggests that this patient had increased BP at prior visits. This patient should first be checked for microalbuminuria, which would indicate the immediate starting of an ACE inhibitor, especially because microalbuminuria is often the first sign of impending renal damage. The microalbuminuria test is typically performed in conjunction with a creatinine test to provide an albumin-to-creatinine ratio.

63. Answer: 4

Rationale: Pseudoephedrine and other decongestant medications that contain sympathomimetics lead to adverse reactions of central nervous system (CNS) overstimulation, palpitations, headache, hypertension, and nervousness. Guaifenesin in combination with dextromethorphan and phenylpropanolamine (Robitussin-CF) or pseudoephedrine (Robitussin-PE) can also cause palpitations and CNS overstimulation. Guaifenesin with dextromethorphan (Robitussin-DM) may cause gastrointestinal upset, drowsiness, headache, and rash. Many OTC medications also have an iodine component that may alter thyroid levels.

64. Answer: 2

Rationale: Infusion site problems and skin irritation are by far the most frequent complaints of patients who use an insulin pump and often are the reason why the pump is discontinued. Patients also find it is more time consuming and costly. However, the Diabetes Control and Complications Trial (DCCT) researchers reported a reduced risk of microvascular complications when insulin pumps and multiple daily injections were used.

65. Answer: 3

Rationale: Pioglitazone and rosiglitazone act by decreasing peripheral insulin resistance in skeletal muscle and adipose tissue without enhancing insulin secretion and improving glucose tolerance in patients with type 2 diabetes. Prenatal patients are managed with insulin or metformin, not an insulin sensitizer. The action of alpha-glucosidase inhibitors, such as acarbose (Precose) and miglitol (Glyset), prevents the rapid postprandial blood glucose surges by delaying carbohydrate absorption (known as "starch blockers").

66. Answer: 3

Rationale: Older patients, especially those with heart disease, need to be started on the smallest amount of thyroid medication replacement (between 12.5 and 25 mcg, not 100 mcg) followed by gradual increases until a therapeutic level is achieved. If thyroid replacement occurs too quickly, the heart may decompensate; 2 grains of thyroid extract is too much. Methimazole is an antithyroid medication used to treat hyperthyroidism.

67. Answer: 2

Rationale: The response to therapy is based on a clinical symptomatology and a TSH assay approximately 4–6 weeks after the initiation of therapy. This is continued until a stable dose is obtained. TSH and a free T_4 level are the two standard tests that can be used to monitor the status of the thyroid; a levothyroxine level cannot be measured. Levothyroxine is not a myelosuppressive.

68. Answer: 3

Rationale: Beta blockers are initially prescribed to reduce the signs and symptoms of the condition and to reduce the peripheral conversion of T_4 to T_3, NSAIDs are indicated for reducing inflammation associated with thyroiditis, and antithyroid medications (propylthiouracil, methimazole) are used to treat severe hyperthyroidism. Corticosteroids are sometimes used in the treatment of thyroiditis, but the remaining classes (antibiotics, ACE inhibitors, calcium channel blockers, and anxiolytics) are not routinely used in the management of hyperthyroidism.

69. Answer: 3

Rationale: Monitoring thyroid-stimulating hormone is the most accurate way to assess thyroid function in a patient taking levothyroxine. Decreasing the dose of levothyroxine and evaluating the patient's cardiac status are the appropriate interventions in this situation, in addition to quickly involving the other health care team members. Discontinuing the thyroid replacement would be inappropriate because the patient remains hypothyroid and requires therapy for life. An anxiolytic may be a helpful adjunct, but it is not appropriate as the sole intervention because it ignores the cardiac symptoms.

70. Answer: 4

Rationale: Hypoglycemia and weight gain are the most common side effects of sulfonylurea therapy.

71. Answer: 3

Rationale: Pioglitazone and rosiglitazone decrease insulin resistance, which increases the glucose uptake in the muscle and fat. Metformin decreases hepatic glucose output. Oral sulfonylureas increase insulin secretion in the pancreas. The alpha-glucosidase inhibitors increase postprandial glucose uptake in the intestine.

72. Answer: 2

Rationale: DDAVP promotes reabsorption of water in the renal tubules, which can lead to water intoxication. The signs of water intoxication are lethargy, behavioral changes, disorientation, and neuromuscular excitability.

73. Answer: 1, 3

Rationale: Bladder cancer, although rare, is linked with the selective sodium-glucose cotransporters (SGLT2) and the TZDs. Medullary cancer risk has prompted issuance of a black box warning for the GLP-1 medications. The biguanides, incretin mimetics, and sulfonylureas do not have these black box warnings.

74. Answer: 4

Rationale: Zoledronic acid (Zometa) is administered as an IV infusion. The others are all oral medications that carry the need to remain sitting upright to decrease the risk for esophageal irritation. The IV medication does require good hydration to decrease renal risks.

75. Answer: 2

Rationale: Nasally inhaled DDAVP must have direct contact with the nasal mucosa for absorption. Secretions, especially those that are thicker, prevent this, so clearing the nasal passages with an effective nasal-clearing blow will provide some additional time for "topical" absorption. There are no major problems with concurrent antihistamine use that would decrease the amount of secretions. The DDAVP is not taken orally, so the precaution about separation by 1 hour is not needed.

76. Answer: 1

Rationale: Test strips are proprietary to the specific monitor. Test strips are frequently not interchangeable, even in monitors from the same manufacturer. Similarly, lancets are specific to the device used to provide a skin puncture. Some newer monitors do not require frequent calibrations or a code number. Handwashing must be completed with soap and water. Alcohol is not used to cleanse the digits, unless medically indicated. Serum, capillary, and subcutaneous puncture glucose values do vary, especially over time.

77. Answer: 4

Rationale: Although the reduction of hypertension is important to renal health, the ACE inhibitors and some selected angiotensin II receptor blocker agents have a "renal protective" effect apart from the vascular tension issue. This does not extend to their direct renin inhibitor "cousins." There may be some positive effect from the sodium-glucose cotransporter group, but more research is needed.

78. Answer: 2

Rationale: The patient's blood sugar levels are low around lunchtime, which is when the a.m. regular insulin is peaking (3–4 hours), so a reduction in the a.m. regular insulin would address this problem.

79. Answer: 2, 3

Rationale: The risk of low blood sugar is greatest with the oldest of the diabetic remedies. This is especially true when insulins are mixed with sulfonylureas. The relative lack of hypoglycemic episodes with the other drug groups makes them a safer alternative.

Musculoskeletal

10

Physical Exam & Diagnostic Tests

1. The family nurse practitioner is performing a history and physical exam on a 72-year-old female patient who is complaining of slight pain in the left shoulder. Which observation would indicate that further testing should be initiated?
   1. Slight swelling is noted.
   2. Brisk capillary refill is noted in the fingers of the left hand.
   3. Bilateral comparison reveals similar pain in the right shoulder.
   4. Range of motion in the joint is limited.

2. Which diagnostic test provides a general indicator that inflammation is occurring within the musculoskeletal system?
   1. Serum amyloid A (SAA) proteins.
   2. Antinuclear antibodies.
   3. Erythrocyte sedimentation rate (ESR).
   4. HbA1c.

3. A goniometer is used in the musculoskeletal exam of a patient. What does the family nurse practitioner use this tool to determine?
   1. Strength of the muscles in the extremities.
   2. Degree of joint flexion and extension.
   3. Range of motion of the extremities.
   4. Point of joint flexion that is painful.

4. The family nurse practitioner places a patient in the prone position with the knee flexed 90 degrees. The tibia is firmly opposed to the femur by exerting downward pressure on the foot. The leg is rotated externally and internally. If locking of the knee occurs, this is accurately called a positive:
   1. Drawer sign.
   2. McMurray test.
   3. Apley test.
   4. Bulge sign.

5. A patient has numbness and tingling in the thumb and first two fingers when pressing the backs of the hands together (flexes wrists at 90 degrees) for 60 seconds. This is a positive:
   1. Tinel sign.
   2. Drawer sign.
   3. McMurray test.
   4. Phalen maneuver.

6. What is the sign that occurs when compressing the suprapatellar pouch back against the femur and feeling for fluid entering the spaces?
   1. Drawer sign.
   2. Kernig sign.
   3. Balloon sign.
   4. Bulge sign.

7. De Quervain's tenosynovitis can be diagnosed in part by a positive:
   1. Finkelstein test.
   2. Tinel sign.
   3. Phalen maneuver.
   4. Lachman test.

8. What are the primary exam techniques used for assessing the musculoskeletal system?
   1. Inspection and percussion.
   2. Auscultation and palpation.
   3. Inspection and palpation.
   4. Palpation and percussion.

9. What criteria can the family nurse practitioner use to suggest a diagnosis of polymyalgia rheumatica (PMR)?
   1. Chest radiograph showing pulmonary hyperinflation, asymmetric joint pain, and an elevated serum C-reactive protein (CRP).
   2. Serum protein electrophoresis, clonal bone marrow plasma cells $\geq$10% or biopsy-proven bony or soft tissue plasmacytoma, and presence of related organ or tissue impairment.
   3. Corticosteroid challenge, erythrocyte sedimentation rate (ESR) greater than 40 mm/h, proximally and bilaterally distributed aching, morning stiffness (lasting 30 minutes or more) persisting for at least 2 weeks, and age 50 years or older.
   4. ESR less than 40 mm/h, emitting seronegative symmetric synovitis with pitting edema and tremor with rigidity.

10. When performing an assessment, the family nurse practitioner understands that the metacarpophalangeal (MCP) joints are frequently involved with:
    1. Gout.
    2. Rheumatic fever.
    3. Rheumatoid arthritis (RA).
    4. Osteoarthritis.

11. To accurately assess a patient presenting with complaints of a back injury, it is critical to question:
    1. Family history of back problems.
    2. Previous injury.
    3. Personal history of chronic illness.
    4. Mechanism of injury.

12. The Tinel sign and Phalen maneuver are used in identifying a common workplace condition that the family nurse practitioner recognizes as:
    1. Lateral epicondylitis.
    2. Carpel tunnel syndrome.
    3. Dupuytren's disease.
    4. Thoracic outlet syndrome.

13. An older adult patient complains of fatigue, weakness, lightheadedness, and anorexia. He also complains of hot, swollen proximal interphalangeal (PIP) and metacarpophalangeal (MCP) joints. These symptoms occurred 5 months ago and recurred a few days ago. Which laboratory findings would be most conclusive of these assessments?
    1. High mean corpuscular volume (MCV), low serum ferritin.
    2. Normal MCV, high serum ferritin.
    3. Elevation in uric acid level.
    4. Elevation in white blood cell (WBC) count.

14. How is the talar tilt test conducted?
    1. The tibia is grasped with one hand, and backward pressure is applied to the heel.
    2. The talus is tilted into adduction and abduction and the laxity of the ligament is graded.
    3. The examiner passively inverts, everts, dorsiflexes, and plantar flexes the ankle.
    4. The patient actively inverts, everts, dorsiflexes, and plantar flexes the ankle.

15. A 66-year-old male patient presents with lower back pain, fatigue, and weight loss for the last 4 months. Five months ago, he had a right humeral fracture. Laboratory analysis reveals serum calcium 12.2 mg/dL, hemoglobin 9.2 g/dL, and hematocrit 27.1%. A lumbar x-ray is ordered and displays areas of hypodensity in the vertebral column and generalized osteopenia. Dipstick urinalysis reveals increased albumin. Which of the following tests would provide the most definitive diagnosis?
    1. Computed tomography (CT) of the lumbar spine.

2. Bone marrow aspiration and biopsy.
3. Digital rectal exam.
4. Prostate biopsy.

16. The family nurse practitioner understands that finding Heberden nodes in a physical exam of a patient is a cardinal sign of:
    1. Septic arthritis.
    2. Rheumatoid arthritis (RA).
    3. Gouty arthritis.
    4. Osteoarthritis (OA).

17. A young adult twisted his knee and comes to the clinic complaining of knee pain. He also states that in the past few weeks his knee has "locked up a couple of times." On physical exam, a positive McMurray test result is elicited. This is consistent with a diagnosis of:
    1. Anterior cruciate ligament tear.
    2. Dislocated patella.
    3. Medial meniscus tear.
    4. Chondromalacia patella.

18. Which **two** diagnostic tests are useful in assessing for anterior cruciate ligament (ACL) injury?
    1. Neer test.
    2. Lachman test.
    3. Phalen test.
    4. Anterior drawer test.
    5. Thomas test.

19. Bouchard's nodes are associated with which of the following conditions?
    1. Rheumatoid arthritis (RA).
    2. Osteoporosis.
    3. Osteoarthritis.
    4. Reiter's syndrome.

20. An older adult female complains of stiffness and pain in both her hands and left knee shortly after waking and worsens in the afternoon. She feels some relief with rest. On physical exam, the family nurse practitioner notices the presence of Heberden's nodes. Which of the following is most likely?
    1. Osteoporosis.
    2. Rheumatoid arthritis.
    3. Osteoarthritis (OA).
    4. Reiter's syndrome.

21. The result of a postmenopausal woman's dual-energy x-ray absorptiometry (DEXA) scan shows osteoporosis. Which of the following T-scores is indicative of osteoporosis?
    1. 0 to -1.0.
    2. -1.0 to -2.0.
    3. -2.5 or less.
    4. $+1.0$ or less.

Disorders

22. Which observation by the family nurse practitioner would lead to inclusion of a differential diagnosis of osteoporosis in a 78-year-old female patient who is complaining of bone and joint pain?
    1. Decrease in skin turgor.
    2. Low vitamin D level.
    3. Bilateral swelling of the feet.
    4. Temperature elevation.

23. A 45-year-old female complains of knee pain when kneeling and a "clicking" noise when walking up steps. The family nurse practitioner notes slight knee effusion and tenderness when palpating the patella against the condyles. What is the diagnosis for this patient?
    1. Anterior cruciate tear.
    2. Dislocated patella.
    3. Chondromalacia patella.
    4. Patellar tendonitis.

24. A patient has been diagnosed with a complete rotator cuff tear of the left shoulder. The nurse would expect the patient to have difficulty in:
    1. Abducting the left arm.
    2. Supinating the left forearm.
    3. Shrugging the shoulders.
    4. Touching the left hand to the right shoulder.

25. A patient has been diagnosed with polymyalgia rheumatica (PMR). The family nurse practitioner understands that this disorder is:
    1. An autoimmune, multisystem problem in which the body makes antibodies to its own proteins.
    2. A degenerative disorder with no inflammatory changes in which joint cartilage wears away with age and eventually causes bone spurs.
    3. An inflammatory disorder involving the axial skeleton and large peripheral joints.
    4. An inflammatory rheumatic condition that affects primarily older women and is associated with giant cell (temporal) arteritis.

26. A patient has a diagnosis of sarcopenia. The family nurse practitioner understands the following about sarcopenia:
    1. It is a progressive muscle wasting disorder in the young adult.
    2. Symptoms include a slow gait and patients having difficulty with balance or climbing stairs.
    3. It is screened in the outpatient setting by x-ray.
    4. Improvement is noted with increased physical activity, such as walking, dancing, or yard work.

27. The family nurse practitioner understands that chronic synovitis with pannus formation is the basic pathophysiologic finding in patients with:
    1. Systemic lupus erythematosus (SLE).
    2. Ankylosing spondylitis (AS).
    3. Rheumatoid arthritis (RA).
    4. Osteoarthritis (OA).

28. The family nurse practitioner is examining a patient who is complaining of pain in her hips and knees. She has a history of osteoarthritis. On physical exam, the joints are painful to movement and are warm to touch. What is the best immediate therapy for this patient?
    1. Physical therapy for range of motion of affected areas.
    2. Decreased physical activity and immobilizing splints for affected joints.
    3. Moist heat and/or cold therapy on painful joints.
    4. Erythrocyte sedimentation rate (ESR) to determine level of activity.

29. A 79-year-old female presents to the clinic for follow-up related to a recent fall (1 week ago) that took place in the home setting. No fractures were reported on the basis of prior imaging studies and/or physical exam. The patient had fallen on her right side, and there were several bruises noted on the right forearm that have resolved. Which physical finding, if noted by the family nurse practitioner, would warrant further inquiry?
    1. Brisk capillary refill of the fingers bilaterally is seen.
    2. Palpable nodule is located on the right forearm.
    3. Patient complains of feeling tired, but no more than usual.
    4. Patient has clear nasal discharge but no evidence of cough or respiratory compromise.

30. The history of a patient who may have contracted Lyme disease may include what characteristic?
    1. Erythematous rash on the bridge of the nose and on the cheeks with discoid patches on the trunk.
    2. Immediate development of arthritis symptoms, especially in the knees.
    3. Expanding rash with central clearing within 1 month of being bitten by a tick.
    4. Early symptoms of meningitis and myocarditis.

31. What are the competing diagnoses for an adult male patient who presents with acute onset of unilateral inflammation, pain, and erythema of the first metatarsophalangeal (MTP) joint?
    1. Gout, cellulitis, and osteoporosis.
    2. Cellulitis, rheumatoid arthritis, and gout.
    3. Osteoporosis, fibromyalgia, and cellulitis.
    4. Septic arthritis, rheumatoid arthritis, and osteoarthritis.

32. Which diseases often present as polyarthritic disorders?
    1. Lyme arthritis, rheumatic heart disease, ankylosing spondylitis, and psoriatic arthritis.
    2. Rheumatoid arthritis (RA), gout, Reiter's syndrome, and osteoarthritis (OA).
    3. Gonococcal arthritis, systemic lupus erythematosus (SLE), and septic arthritis.
    4. Pseudogout, gout, and psoriatic arthritis.

33. Pain in a lumbosacral strain typically begins:
    1. Immediately with the injury.
    2. 1–2 hours after injury.
    3. 6–8 hours after injury.
    4. 12–36 hours after injury.

34. An acute onset of pain that radiates to the lower leg and foot of a 25-year-old obese adult is likely to be a symptom of:
    1. Lumbosacral strain.
    2. Herniated intervertebral disk injury.
    3. Osteomyelitis.
    4. Osteoporosis.

35. The family nurse practitioner sees a patient with trauma to the knee that caused it to "give out," followed by severe pain and effusion. Later, he had "locking" of the knee with pivoting or turning. This patient has probably suffered:
    1. Patellofemoral stress syndrome.
    2. Growing pains.
    3. Shin splints.
    4. Patellar subluxation.

36. A patient with patellofemoral syndrome has quadriceps setting as a recommended exercise. The family nurse practitioner would teach the patient to:
    1. Lie supine on the floor with legs extended, dorsiflex the foot, and push the thigh into the floor.
    2. Sit on the floor, lean back on the elbows, flex one knee to 90 degrees, and extend the other completely and hold for 5 seconds.
    3. Lie on the floor and flex both knees to about 20 degrees with a rolled towel underneath them and extend one leg and hold for 5 seconds.
    4. Use resistive exercises with an elastic band.

37. Which risk factor is associated with gout?
    1. Female gender.
    2. Age 20 years.
    3. Ingestion of salicylate-containing medications.
    4. Overuse of extremity.

38. A patient with rheumatoid arthritis (RA) presents for follow-up. What is the best evaluative question the family nurse practitioner can ask that will help determine the severity of the disease?
    1. "Were you able to drive the car to your appointment today?"
    2. "Were you able to fix your dinner last night?"
    3. "How long does it take for your joints to loosen up after you get up in the morning?"
    4. "How many pounds can you carry?"

39. When counseling a postmenopausal 60-year-old female patient on prevention of osteoporosis, all of the following are therapeutic recommendations **except**:
    1. Cessation of smoking.

    2. Daily intake of 200 mg of calcium and 40 IU of vitamin D.
    3. Continue hormone replacement therapy.
    4. Monitor bone loss by dual-energy x-ray absorptiometry every 1–2 years.

40. A patient tells the family nurse practitioner that she has "whiplash." The family nurse practitioner understands that this is:
    1. Cervical facet joint dysfunction.
    2. Cervical disk injury.
    3. Zygapophyseal joint injury.
    4. Cervical strain.

41. A patient presents with a complaint of sudden pain and swelling in the knee unrelated to an injury. He also has chills and fever. On physical exam, the knee is warm, tender, and swollen with evidence of effusion. What action would the family nurse practitioner take first?
    1. Splint the affected joint.
    2. Obtain aspiration of synovial fluid from the affected joint.
    3. Initiate treatment with nonsteroidal antiinflammatory drugs.
    4. Recommend rest, ice, compression, and elevation of affected joint.

42. When determining the specific etiology of polyarticular complaints, which clinical clues are most helpful for diagnosis?
    1. Laboratory identification of antinuclear antibodies and ESR.
    2. Radiograph of the affected joints.
    3. Affected joint pattern and presence or lack of inflammation.
    4. Sexual history of the patient.

43. A patient with ankylosing spondylitis (AS) is receiving education on managing her disease. The family nurse practitioner would teach the patient all of the following **except**:
    1. Regular exercise program.
    2. Maintenance of systemic corticosteroid therapy.
    3. Use of indomethacin (Indocin) for discomfort.
    4. Observation for signs and symptoms of iritis.

44. An adult patient comes to the office complaining of foot pain. He can recall no specific injury, but he gives a history of being an occasional runner who drinks 6–10 beers on weekends. What physical findings would the family nurse practitioner expect to find?
    1. Redness, swelling, and warmth of first metatarsophalangeal joint.
    2. Swelling, ecchymosis, and decreased range of motion of ankle.
    3. Swelling of foot and decreased circulation.
    4. Decreased range of motion of ankle and obvious bone deformity.

45. Which of the diet selections indicate that the older patient understands health education regarding the prevention of osteoporosis?
    1. Chicken and baked potato.
    2. Glass of skim milk and toasted cheese sandwich.
    3. Hamburger and salad.
    4. Ice cream sundae with whipped cream.

46. What does the initial treatment of joint injury involve?
    1. Rest, ice, compression, and elevation.
    2. Narcotic pain control and radiograph.
    3. Specialist referral and magnetic resonance imaging.
    4. Nonsteroidal antiinflammatory drugs and exercise.

47. What is the most common complaint in a patient with back injury who has cauda equina syndrome?
    1. Urinary retention.
    2. Numbness below the level of injury.
    3. Weakness in the lower extremities.
    4. Leg pain.

48. Recognition of annular tears is important in the diagnosis of back pain because:
    1. They require immediate surgery.
    2. They are often misdiagnosed as strains or sprains, leading to herniation.
    3. They result in rapid paralysis.
    4. Radiography would reveal them, but x-rays are usually not ordered initially.

49. What chronic musculoskeletal problem may occur after an injury and is characterized by a 3-month history of widespread pain and tenderness on both sides of the body?
    1. Chronic osteoarthritis.
    2. Reflex sympathetic dystrophy.
    3. Tendinitis.
    4. Fibromyalgia.

50. Which patient is at highest risk for osteoporosis?
    1. A 55-year-old male smoker and retired athlete.
    2. A 60-year-old, 105-lb, postmenopausal white female switchboard operator.
    3. A 42-year-old black female intensive care unit nurse who is lactose intolerant.
    4. A 50-year-old obese white woman with three children living on a farm.

51. A patient, who has hypovitaminosis D, asks the family nurse practitioner if she should spend more time sunbathing without using sunscreen because she heard that your skin can manufacture vitamin D. What would be an appropriate response by the family nurse practitioner?
    1. Continue to use sunscreen, take vitamin D supplements, and choose foods high in vitamin D.
    2. The more ways to get vitamin D the better, so sunbathing is okay on a weekly basis.
    3. Avoid sunlight exposure and take vitamin D 50,000 IU supplements twice a day.
    4. Leave sunscreen off a sun-exposed area of the body and sunbathe for 20 minutes a day until the skin appears slightly red and tingles.

52. A 53-year-old woman presents with a complaint of 4 weeks of prolonged morning stiffness in the neck and back. She has pain in her pelvis and shoulder and fatigue. Her laboratory studies reveal elevated ESR (50 mm/hr), normal rheumatoid factor, normal creatine phosphokinase, and normochromic normocytic anemia. Her physical exam reveals an elevated temperature, bilateral pain, and stiffness of the pectoral and pelvic muscles. Based on this information, what is the most appropriate diagnosis?
    1. Polyarteritis nodosa.
    2. Wegener granulomatosis.
    3. Polymyalgia rheumatica (PMR).
    4. Rheumatoid arthritis.

53. A 55-year-old woman with a prior diagnosis of polymyalgia rheumatica (PMR) presents with headache, low-grade fever, aching, stiffness, fatigue, malaise, and anorexia. Based on the information, what preliminary diagnosis would the family nurse practitioner make?
    1. Influenza.
    2. Pneumonia.
    3. Temporal arteritis.
    4. Rheumatoid arthritis.

54. A man comes into the clinic complaining of low back pain that radiates down the lateral thigh. The pain began suddenly on the job after lifting a heavy object. The family nurse practitioner would further evaluate the patient for which **three** conditions:
    1. Compression fracture of lower lumbar vertebrae.
    2. Piriformis syndrome.
    3. Spinal cord injury.
    4. Compression of a lumbar disk.
    5. History of spinal cord injury.

55. What would be an appropriate schedule for the family nurse practitioner to teach the older adult patient about when to do strength training exercises?
    1. Every other week along with aerobic exercise.
    2. Every day for 20 minutes lift weights.
    3. Every other day walk or ride the bicycle for 30 minutes.
    4. Focus one day on upper-body exercises and the next day on lower-body exercises.

56. An 80-year-old resident of a long-term care facility, who has a history of multiinfarct dementia (MID), is alert but disoriented to person, place, and situation. His only health problems are MID and osteoarthritis. Over the last 2 weeks, he has become agitated and exit seeking and is constantly rubbing his knees. What does the family nurse practitioner suspect the patient is experiencing?
    1. Worsening dementia.
    2. Pain.
    3. Urinary tract infection (UTI).
    4. Acute cerebral infarct.

Pharmacology

57. A 65-year-old postmenopausal female has been treated with alendronate (Fosamax) for 6 years. Current screening indicates no increase in risk factors. Based on clinical guidelines, which treatment option would the family nurse practitioner suggest to the patient?
    1. Discontinue medication at this time.
    2. Switch medication from oral to intravenous route to maintain adequate coverage.
    3. Add vitamin D 500 IU/day to the treatment regimen.
    4. Increase calcium supplementation to 1500 mg/day.

58. The family nurse practitioner is seeing a middle-aged, severely arthritic woman who has been receiving maintenance therapy of prednisone 10 mg/day for the last 6 weeks. She now presents as acutely ill with signs and symptoms of acute pneumonia. She is fatigued and weak with loss of appetite, and her blood pressure (BP) is lower than at previous visits. Which action should be taken in regard to prednisone?
    1. Immediately discontinue the medication.
    2. Increase the dosage to 60 mg/day, then taper back to 10 mg/day.
    3. Gradually taper from 10 to 1 mg/day.
    4. Maintain the dosage at 10 mg/day.

59. An elderly patient is being treated with colchicine for prophylaxis related to an acute gout attack. Which of the following adverse reactions should the family nurse practitioner assess for?
    1. Constipation.
    2. Fluid retention.
    3. Fever.
    4. Dehydration.

60. What is the first line therapy for treating patients with newly diagnosed rheumatoid arthritis (RA)?
    1. Tramadol.
    2. Cyclobenzaprine.
    3. Methotrexate.
    4. Hydrocortisone.

61. A patient with rheumatoid arthritis (RA) is placed on prednisone 5 mg PO qd. In teaching the patient about her medication, it would be important for the family nurse practitioner to include what information?
    1. When the symptoms of arthritis subside, she will be able to quit taking her medication.
    2. It is important to take the medication as prescribed, even after the redness and swelling decrease.
    3. Increased fluid intake is important to prevent renal damage by the steroids.
    4. The medication should be taken about 30 minutes before eating.

62. Which of the following is most appropriate for the treatment of an acute episode of gout?
    1. Indomethacin (Indocin) 25 mg PO prn.
    2. Naproxen (Naprosyn) 100 mg PO bid.
    3. Colchicine 0.6 mg two tablets PO × 1, then repeat in 1 hour × 1.
    4. Indomethacin (Indocin) 50 mg q8h × 6–8 doses, then 25 mg q8h until resolution.

63. A family nurse practitioner is reviewing the medication profile of an older adult male patient with a history of renal failure who now presents with an acute exacerbation of gout. Which action should be taken by the family nurse practitioner at this time?
    1. Assess medications being taken for pain control.
    2. Monitor daily weight.
    3. Discontinue use of nonsteroidal antiinflammatory drugs (NSAIDS).
    4. Withhold dialysis treatments until gouty attack has subsided.

64. If a 24-hour urine test indicates that a patient is secreting too much uric acid (greater than 900 mg/day), what would the family nurse practitioner prescribe?
    1. Aspirin 325 mg PO daily.
    2. Tylenol 325 mg PO q4–6h prn.
    3. Indomethacin (Indocin) 25 mg PO q8h, then increase at weekly intervals by 25 mg daily.
    4. Allopurinol (Zyloprim) 100 mg PO qd × 1 week, then increase daily dose by 100 mg to a maximum of 300 mg/day.

65. What is the drug of choice for treatment of gout in the older adult patient?
    1. Xanthine oxidase inhibitor.
    2. Aromatase inhibitor.
    3. Angiotensin-converting enzyme (ACE) inhibitor.
    4. Beta blocker.

66. Which of the following is the most appropriate vitamin D dose for an elderly patient to prevent osteoporosis?
    1. 1500 mg of vitamin D every other day.
    2. 400 IU on a daily basis.
    3. 800–1000 IU on a daily basis.
    4. 600 mg of vitamin D on a daily basis.

67. What would be the most appropriate medication used to control pain for a patient with osteoarthritis?
    1. Acetaminophen.
    2. Systemic corticosteroids.
    3. Gold salts.
    4. Misoprostol.

68. What is a serious side effect of ibuprofen in the older adult patient?
    1. Rebound headaches.
    2. Impairment of renal function.
    3. Neuropathy.
    4. Pancreatic failure.

69. A patient has been on methotrexate (Rheumatrex) for 6 weeks. What parameters should the family nurse practitioner monitor?
    1. Monthly platelet count and complete blood count (CBC) with differential.
    2. Urinalysis, blood sugar, and electrocardiogram every 2 weeks.
    3. Monthly CBC, urinalysis, and electrolytes.
    4. Coagulation studies, electrolytes, and CBC every week.

70. A middle-aged male patient presents with a complaint of waking up yesterday morning with a swollen and painful big toe. The patient reports he has "never had anything like this before" and has not had previous health problems. On physical exam, the big toe is red, hot, and tender in the joint with inflammation extending into the surrounding tissue. His temperature is 99.8°F (37.7°C), and his white blood cell count is mildly elevated. Needle aspiration of joint fluid reveals urate crystals. Which of the following is the most appropriate treatment for this patient?
    1. Bed rest, very-low-calorie diet, and increased fluid intake.

2. Allopurinol (Zyloprim) 200 mg PO daily, continuing dose for maintenance therapy once symptoms resolve.
    3. Naproxen (Naprosyn) 500 mg PO tid, continuing full dose until symptoms resolve, then tapering and discontinuing over 72 hours.
    4. Injection of intraarticular corticosteroid to the affected joint.

71. What is the preferred medication used to treat chronic pain symptoms in elderly patients as a first-line therapy?
    1. Acetaminophen.
    2. Nonsteroidal antiinflammatory drugs.
    3. Opioid analgesics.
    4. Anticonvulsants.

72. An older adult woman comes into the clinic complaining of "sores" in her mouth. The family nurse practitioner observes several inflamed ulcers on her gums and lips. Which medication would the nurse identify as most likely to cause this problem?
    1. Propranolol (Inderal).
    2. Spironolactone (Aldactone).
    3. Fexofenadine (Allegra).
    4. Alendronate (Fosamax).

73. Glucosamine sulfate is a natural supplement that can be taken for which of the following conditions?
    1. Osteoarthritis.
    2. Cataracts.
    3. Rheumatoid arthritis.
    4. Osteoporosis.

10 Muscoloskeletal Answers & Rationales

Physical Exam & Diagnostic Tests

1. Answer: 4

Rationale: With regard to musculoskeletal system, limitation of range of motion of the joint indicates that further testing should be initiated. Slight swelling in the context of related pain may be caused by an injury, but unless swelling is pronounced, the area should just be monitored. Brisk capillary refill is a normal finding. The presence of pain in both shoulders may indicate osteoarthritic changes.

2. Answer: 3

Rationale: ESR provides a general indicator that inflammation is occurring within the musculoskeletal system. SAA proteins are apolipoproteins that are rapidly associated with high-density lipoprotein and can influence cholesterol metabolism. Antinuclear antibodies provide specific information related to immunologic diseases. HbA1c provides information related to glycemic control.

3. Answer: 2

Rationale: The goniometer is used to determine the degree of joint flexion and extension or joint range of motion.

4. Answer: 3

Rationale: A positive Apley test result, locking of the knee, or the sound of clicks and pain, may indicate a torn meniscus. The drawer sign tests the integrity of cruciate ligaments with the patient in a sitting and lying, not prone, position. The McMurray test assesses for medial meniscus injury when the knee is fully flexed and the tibia is externally rotated, with varus pressure applied to the knee while extended. For medial meniscus tears, the test is performed while applying valgus pressure to the knee.

5. Answer: 4

Rationale: The Phalen maneuver, when present, suggests carpal tunnel syndrome. The Tinel sign also tests for carpal tunnel syndrome, but it is performed by lightly percussing over the median nerve on the volar (palmar) side of the wrist, with characteristic tingling or shocklike sensations across the palm, thumb, and first two fingers. The drawer sign and McMurray test are used to assess the knee.

6. Answer: 3

Rationale: The balloon sign occurs when considerable fluid is in the suprapatellar pouch, with possible ballottement of the patella. The bulge sign is for testing fluid in the knee joint and is elicited with the knee extended by applying pressure to the medial aspect and watching for a bulge or fluid wave. A patellar tap suggests fluid in the knee as the patella clicks against the femur. The drawer sign tests the cruciate ligaments with the patient in a sitting and lying position. The Kernig sign for meningeal irritation is the inability to extend the lower leg when that leg is flexed at the hip, or there may be resistance or pain during elicitation of the sign.

7. Answer: 1

Rationale: Pain with gentle deviation of a fist (thumb tucked under the other four fingers) to the ulnar side is a positive Finkelstein test result and an indication of de Quervain disease, which is swelling and tenderness over the volar portion of the "snuffbox" resulting from chronic tenosynovitis. A positive Tinel sign (tapping gently over carpal tunnel causing tingling in thumb, index finger, and middle and radial half of ring finger) and a positive Phalen maneuver (holding dorsum of hands flexed 90 degrees back to back with the same distribution of tingling) are indicative of carpel tunnel syndrome. A positive Lachman test result indicates stability of the cruciate ligament of the knee.

8. Answer: 3

Rationale: The musculoskeletal system is examined by a visual inspection and palpation of the bones, joints, and surrounding musculoskeletal soft tissue. Percussion is generally not done, and auscultation is not appropriate to the system being examined.

9. Answer: 3

Rationale: Patients with PMR have a rapid, dramatic clinical response to corticosteroid therapy. Serum protein electrophoresis is used to rule out myeloma. The ESR is elevated in a number of diseases and is not specific to PMR. The chest radiograph is used to diagnose diseases affecting the lungs and thorax. The serum CRP would be elevated in PMR.

10. Answer: 3

Rationale: The wrist, MCP, and proximal interphalangeal joints, and other small joints of the hands and feet are involved with RA. The great toe is most often involved with gout. The large joints of the hip, knee, and shoulder, along with the distal interphalangeal joint and base of the thumb, are involved with degenerative joint disease (osteoarthritis).

11. Answer: 4

Rationale: A thorough history is very important in assessing any patient with an injury, but with a back injury the mechanism will provide the best indication of the extent of the injury and the proper diagnostic and treatment approaches. Determining loss of bowel or bladder control could indicate an emergent condition, cauda equina syndrome.

12. Answer: 2

Rationale: Carpel tunnel syndrome, a compression neuropathy of the median nerve at the wrist, is commonly caused by repetitive finger and wrist motion and results in a positive Tinel sign and Phalen maneuver. Tinel sign is considered positive when tapping over the nerve with a reflex hammer causes tingling in the distribution of the nerve. The Phalen maneuver is performed by fully flexing the wrist passively and noting tingling in the thumb or fingers.

13. Answer: 2

Rationale: The clinical assessments point to a chronic inflammatory process such as rheumatoid arthritis. The dizziness, fatigue, lightheadedness, and weakness may be a problem with anemia. The anemia of chronic disease is either a microcytic or normocytic anemia. The value that differentiates the anemia of chronic disease from other anemias is the serum ferritin (iron stores). The value will be either normal or high. An MCV of 104 indicates a macrocytic anemia, which would not include the anemia of chronic disease. Low serum ferritin would not be considered a possibility with this disorder. The uric acid level would be elevated in gout. The WBC count does not address the signs of anemia.

14. Answer: 2

Rationale: The talar tilt test is a ligamentous stress test that detects excessive ankle inversion by examining the integrity of the lateral ankle ligaments, particularly the calcaneofibular ligament. Anterior ankle stability is tested in the anterior drawer test, in which the tibia is grasped by the examiner's one hand while the heel is firmly grasped, and backward pressure is applied to the tibia with the examiner's other hand. In passive range of motion, the examiner inverts, everts, dorsiflexes, and plantar flexes the foot and ankle. The patient puts the foot and ankle through the complete range in active range of motion.

15. Answer: 2

Rationale: The patient most likely has multiple myeloma. This is best evidenced in this question as bone pain, hypercalcemia, and x-rays that show lytic bone lesions and osteopenia. In the absence of osteopenia or lytic bone lesions, a magnetic resonance imaging (MRI) scan may be ordered. Diagnosis of multiple myeloma requires greater than or equal to 10% clonal plasma cells found via bone marrow biopsy combined

with related organ damage or tissue impairment. End-organ damage often presents as renal insufficiency because of excess light chains and presents as albuminuria. Electrophoresis will reveal M proteins.

16. Answer: 4

Rationale: Deformities (bony protuberances) of the distal interphalangeal (DIP) joints are called Heberden nodes and are cardinal signs of OA. The DIP joints are seldom involved with RA. Gouty arthritis most often affects the great toe. Joints are warm, red, tender, and swollen with septic arthritis.

17. Answer: 3

Rationale: A positive McMurray test result (palpable click and pain when rotating the foot laterally and extending the leg) along with the symptoms is indicative of a medial meniscus tear. The drawer test is done to evaluate anterior cruciate ligament tears (knee flexed with foot on table; sit on foot and grasp both sides of tibia at knee; pull tibia forward; abnormal if movement of tibia is away from the joint).

18. Answer: 2, 4

Rationale: The Lachman test and anterior drawer tests are used to assess the ACL. The Neer test is used to assess the shoulder or rotator cuff impingement. The Thomas test is used to detect flexion contractures of the hip that may be masked by excessive lumbar lordosis. The Phalen maneuver or test is used to assess for carpal tunnel syndrome.

19. Answer: 3

Rationale: Bouchard's nodes are bony enlargements of the middle joints of the fingers and also the proximal interphalangeal joints on the hands. RA affects the small joints, metacarpophalangeal, leading to Boutonnière and swan-neck deformities, carpal bones of wrist, second to fifth metatarsophalangeal, and thumb interphalangeal joints. Reiter's syndrome, also known as reactive arthritis, is the classic triad of conjunctivitis, urethritis, and arthritis occurring after an infection, particularly those in the urogenital or gastrointestinal tract. Osteoporosis is characterized by low bone mass, deterioration of bone tissue, and disruption of bone architecture that leads to compromised bone strength and an increased risk of fracture.

20. Answer: 3

Rationale: Signs of OA include slowly developing joint pain, including stiffness of joints, typically worse in the afternoon and early evening. Usually, pain is typically worse with activity and improves with rest. A visible physical finding of OA are Heberden's nodes (bony overgrowths), which are found on the distal interphalangeal joint and are hard, nontender nodules usually 2–3 cm in diameter but sometimes encompass the entire joint.

21. Answer: 3

Rationale: The T-score is a comparison of a person's bone density with that of a healthy 30-year-old of the same sex. Osteoporosis is defined as having a T-score of −2.5 or less. The greater the negative number, the more severe the osteoporosis. Osteopenia (low bone density) is a T-score between −1.0 and −2.5. A T-score between +1 and −1 is considered normal or healthy.

Disorders

22. Answer: 2

Rationale: Low vitamin D level may be associated with a clinical diagnosis of osteoporosis. A decrease in skin turgor is a normal consequence of the aging process. Bilateral swelling of the feet may be caused by vascular insufficiency and/or a consequence of standing. An elevation in temperature is typically not associated with osteoporosis.

23. Answer: 3

Rationale: These are common symptoms of chondromalacia patella. With anterior cruciate tears, the patient generally cannot bear weight on the extremity without it buckling or giving way. With a dislocated patella, the patient would have severe pain associated with considerable effusion (loss of normal knee hollow on sides of patella) and possible patellofemoral compartment. Patellar tendonitis, or jumper's knee, causes pain, weakness, and swelling of the knee joint, but no "clicking" noises.

24. Answer: 1

Rationale: With a complete rotator cuff tear (most commonly a rupture of supraspinatus tendon), the patient would have difficulty abducting the arm and impaired internal/external rotation. Touching the hand to the opposite shoulder is adduction.

25. Answer: 4

Rationale: PMR is an inflammatory rheumatic condition that affects primarily older women and is associated with giant cell (temporal) arteritis. Anemia is common in PMR, along with an elevated ESR. There is a common complaint of morning stiffness; rheumatoid factor is negative. An autoimmune, multisystem disorder is characteristic of systemic lupus erythematosus. A degenerative joint disorder is characteristic of osteoarthritis. An inflammatory disorder involving the axial skeleton and large peripheral joints is characteristic of ankylosing spondylitis.

26. Answer: 2

Rationale: Sarcopenia is a complex geriatric condition that has become more prevalent and significant as the population ages. It is defined by low muscle mass and a decline in walking speed or grip strength. The family nurse practitioner would find during an assessment that patients who have a slow gait or are nonambulatory, cannot rise from a chair unassisted, and have difficulty with balance or stair climbing have consistent findings with a diagnosis of sarcopenia. Imaging techniques to assess lean body mass (muscle) and diagnose sarcopenia are computed tomography scan, magnetic resonance imaging, dual-energy X-ray absorptiometry (DXA), and bioimpedance analysis (BIA). The BIA is the most practical and inexpensive screening test; the other tests are more expensive. DXA does not provide accurate estimates of muscle quality. The key intervention for sarcopenia is resistance exercise training because muscle hypertrophy and strength development will occur only if there are progressive increases in the intensity and volume of resistance training over time.

27. Answer: 3

Rationale: The chronic inflammatory disorder RA involves synovial hypertrophy caused by chronic synovitis and pannus formation that results in progressive destruction of the cartilage, ligament, tendons, and bone. AS usually involves the large peripheral joints (e.g., sacroiliac) and is characterized by extreme kyphosis. There is no inflammation with OA. SLE has a distribution of symptoms similar to that of RA, but no pannus formation.

28. Answer: 3

Rationale: Moist heat or cold, whichever relieves the pain more effectively, is appropriate to use on acutely affected joints. Physical therapy is recommended after the acute involvement of the joint; care must be taken to decrease repetitive movements. Immobilization is avoided because it tends to increase the stiffness of the joint. The ESR is not an appropriate indicator to determine the level of activity in patients with osteoarthritis.

29. Answer: 2

Rationale: The patient has had a recent fall, so the appearance of a palpable nodule requires further inquiry as this can be indicative of further vascular damage. Brisk capillary refill is a normal finding. The fact that the patient complains of feeling tired, a fact that has not changed from previous reporting, is unremarkable. The fact that the patient has clear nasal discharge with no other contributory cold or flulike symptoms is unremarkable.

30. Answer: 3

Rationale: Expanding rash with central clearing may also be described as the "bull's-eye rash," which is associated with Lyme disease. An erythematous rash on the bridge of the nose and on the cheeks describes the malar or "butterfly" rash of systemic lupus erythematosus. The arthritis symptoms and other complications (meningitis and myocarditis) occur later in the disease process, especially if the patient is not treated with antibiotics, usually tetracycline, doxycycline, or amoxicillin.

31. Answer: 2

Rationale: Cellulitis usually presents with warm, erythematous, painful areas of the skin. Symptoms of erythema, edema, and pain of the first MTP joint are a common presentation for gout. Symptoms present in rheumatoid arthritis (RA) are similar: red, swollen, and painful joints. The inflammation of RA is usually symmetric but can present as erythematous, swollen joints. Systemic symptoms may also be present. Osteoporosis most often occurs in postmenopausal women because of bone loss that occurs with the decline of estrogen in the blood. Bone thinning leads to fractures, not inflammation of joints or skin. Osteoarthritis presents as pain and stiffness with decreased range of motion, stiffness in the morning for a few minutes that relieves with movement, and occasionally joint effusions. Chronic widespread pain present for at least 3 months is a symptom of fibromyalgia. Joint swelling and erythema are not present. In septic arthritis, joint pain, inflammation, and erythema would be accompanied by systemic symptoms of fever and chills. It would be considered in the differential diagnosis for this patient.

32. Answer: 1

Rationale: Lyme arthritis, rheumatic heart disease, ankylosing spondylitis, psoriatic arthritis, RA, Reiter's syndrome, osteoarthritis, gonococcal arthritis, SLE, and polymyalgia rheumatica typically occur as polyarthritic disease. Gout, septic arthritis, and pseudogout most often occur as monoarthritis.

33. Answer: 4

Rationale: As the soft tissue swells, pain onset occurs usually about 12–36 hours after injury.

34. Answer: 2

Rationale: Herniated intervertebral disk pain typically descends to the lower leg and foot. Lumbosacral strain causes pain in the back, buttock, and sometimes thigh. Osteomyelitis must be preceded by an event that permits an infectious agent to enter the bone. Osteoporosis occurs most often in postmenopausal women.

35. Answer: 4

Rationale: At the time a patellar subluxation occurs, a traumatic event causes the knee to give out, and the patella is usually laterally displaced; severe pain and an effusion result. Subsequent to the injury, the patient will notice a locking sensation in the knee with pivoting or turning. Patellofemoral stress syndrome is a form of overuse syndrome. Pain of a dull, aching quality is present in the knee, sometimes with clicking. Long periods of sitting or activities that involve knee flexion and compression of the patella in the groove cause increased pain. Growing pains usually occur at night and resolve by morning. The pain is deep and does not involve the joints. In shin splints, inflammation of muscles along the medial shaft of the tibia caused by overuse causes aching pain. Rest improves the pain.

36. Answer: 1

Rationale: In quadriceps setting, with the foot dorsiflexed, the thigh is pressed downward against the floor and held for 5 seconds. The straight leg raise involves lifting an extended leg while sitting on the floor and leaning back on the elbows with the opposite leg flexed to 90 degrees. A terminal arc extension requires that the patient lie on the floor supine with extended legs flexed to 20 degrees over a rolled towel. The patient then extends one leg and holds for 5 seconds. The exercise is repeated with the opposite leg. All of these exercises can be used to stretch and strengthen the quadriceps muscles in those with patellofemoral stress syndrome. Resistive exercises with an elastic band are general exercises that can be done with the extremities.

37. Answer: 3

Rationale: Gout generally affects men over age 30 and is associated with obesity; lead intoxication; starvation; and use of some medications, including salicylates (such as aspirin), diuretics, pyrazinamide, and alcohol.

38. Answer: 3

Rationale: Morning stiffness or activity and the length of time required for maximal improvement are American Rheumatism Association Classification criteria for RA and useful, measurable tools for effects of treatment. The other questions are good indicators of quality of activities of daily living but do not give a full, overall, measurable picture of the patient's joint discomfort.

39. Answer: 2

Rationale: This is a subtherapeutic amount of calcium and vitamin D. Recommended calcium for women ages 51 and older is 1200 mg daily, and recommended vitamin D is 800–1000 IU daily. The other choices are recommendations for prevention of osteoporosis.

40. Answer: 4

Rationale: Most whiplash injuries are associated with a cervical neck strain related to spasm of the cervical and upper back muscles from injury.

41. Answer: 2

Rationale: The patient's symptoms are indicative of septic arthritis, which is a medical emergency; if not treated promptly, the joint may be severely damaged or destroyed. Examination of the joint fluid is the most important diagnostic test. The other choices may provide some symptomatic relief, but the first goal of treatment is to determine whether the joint is septic.

42. Answer: 3

Rationale: When developing a differential diagnosis, the history and physical exam will help narrow the differentiation. Other procedures are important in completing the evaluation, but the most important information is the pattern of joints affected and whether it is inflammatory or noninflammatory disease.

43. Answer: 2

Rationale: Corticosteroids have limited value in treating AS, and long-term use is associated with many serious side effects. Important treatment includes regular exercise to strengthen supporting muscles and use of nonsteroidal anti-inflammatory drugs for pain. Approximately one-third of patients have recurrent attacks of acute iritis.

44. Answer: 1

Rationale: Trauma, increased alcohol intake on weekends, and physical stress have all been implicated in acute gout. Gout occurs primarily in adult men. Decreased circulation, ecchymosis, and bone deformity are not likely with acute gout.

45. Answer: 2

Rationale: Calcium intake is important in minimizing the development of osteoporosis. Both these foods contain calcium. The other options are not focused on calcium intake.

46. Answer: 1

Rationale: The RICE principle is used for initial treatment: **R**est, **I**ce, **C**ompression, and **E**levation. All other treatments mentioned may be appropriate, but not as the primary treatment.

47. Answer: 1

Rationale: Although all symptoms may be associated with cauda equina syndrome, urinary retention and loss of bowel or bladder control are important clues to the immediate need for surgery. Cauda equina syndrome is considered a surgical emergency.

48. Answer: 2

Rationale: Annular tears are tears of the annulus fibrosus of the intervertebral disk and are the first step toward herniation. Early recognition can help avoid the need for surgical repair of a subsequent herniation.

49. Answer: 4

Rationale: Fibromyalgia is a poorly understood condition that can prolong the normal treatment course of an injury considerably and is very difficult to treat. Osteoarthritis may follow an injury, as can reflex sympathetic dystrophy and tendinitis, but the patients do not have widespread pain and tenderness on both sides of the body.

50. Answer: 2

Rationale: The five risk factors for osteoporosis include being of female gender, white or Asian, over age 45, low body weight, postmenopausal, sedentary lifestyle, low calcium intake, and a smoker.

51. Answer: 1

Rationale: Although the skin can manufacture vitamin D from sunlight exposure, the majority of people can get their vitamin D from nutritional supplements and from vitamin D–fortified foods. Food sources include wild-caught salmon, mackerel, tuna and sardines, beef liver, eggs, cod liver oil, and mushrooms, along with fortified milk and foods, such as breakfast cereals, yogurt, and orange juice. Exposure to sunlight (UVB light) causes skin cancer, and it is important to teach patients to use sunscreen and protect their skin from excessive sunlight exposure. The American Cancer Society does not support sun exposure for increasing vitamin D. There are patients with specific issues who might need a prescription for high levels of vitamin D, but for most people, 50,000 IU daily will raise the vitamin D level too high. High levels of vitamin D can be toxic (signs of hypercalcemia), because it is stored in fat.

52. Answer: 3

Rationale: PMR is an inflammatory disorder of the proximal muscles presenting as described. Polyarteritis nodosa, an inflammatory disorder affecting the small arteries, presents with muscle weakness, myalgias, headache, and subcutaneous nodules along leg and arm arteries. Wegener disease presents with mild anemia, dyspnea, cough, chest pain, hemoptysis, and abnormal urinalysis.

53. Answer: 3

Rationale: Up to 40% of patients with temporal arteritis have a previous history of PMR. Presenting complaints include headache, low-grade fever, muscle aching and stiffness, fatigue, malaise, and anorexia.

54. Answer: 1, 2, 4

Rationale: The patient is presenting with the classic symptoms of nerve root compression secondary to pressure from a protruding lumbar disk. The sciatic stretch test (straight leg raise) maneuver will increase the radiation of pain down the hip. In piriformis syndrome, the piriformis muscle (a narrow muscle located in the buttocks) compresses or irritates the sciatic nerve. Spinal cord injury will result in focal pain or tenderness, bruising, hematoma, and palpable step-offs along the spine.

55. Answer: 4

Rationale: Different exercises should be performed at a minimum of two or more nonconsecutive days each week using major muscle groups. An easy schedule to explain to the patient is to make one day focused on upper-body muscles and the next day would focus on lower-body muscles. A third day could be rest to provide a sufficient recovery period from the strength training exercises and then repeat the schedule again.

56. Answer: 2

Rationale: This patient is likely experiencing an acute exacerbation of his osteoarthritis because he is constantly rubbing his knees. Because 85% of the residents of long-term care facilities have uncontrolled pain, he probably has uncontrolled pain. Starting him on routine acetaminophen (Tylenol) would be an excellent start to pain management. It is unlikely that the patient's dementia is worsening because this is an acute problem. Although a UTI is a good choice, the cues of rubbing the major joints would likely rule out a UTI as the problem. The patient is not exhibiting any neurologic symptoms, which would rule out an acute cerebral infarct.

Pharmacology

57. Answer: 1

Rationale: Patients who have low fracture risk after being treated with alendronate (Fosamax) for at least 5 years qualify for a drug holiday because the effects of the medication are still present. There is no need to switch the route of medication. Vitamin D supplementation should be within 800–1000 IU/day. Calcium supplementation greater than 1200 mg/day may be associated with an increased risk of complications ranging from kidney stones to cardiac events.

58. Answer: 2

Rationale: Patients on chronic steroid therapy should be evaluated for adrenal insufficiency during an acute illness, which increases stress. Signs and symptoms indicate subtle clinical manifestations of adrenal insufficiency. Recommended treatment is to treat the patient empirically with stress-dose corticosteroid during acute illness. Stopping the medication or maintaining the same dose may precipitate acute adrenal insufficiency.

59. Answer: 4

Rationale: The use of colchicine in the elderly patient can lead to the presence of nausea, vomiting, diarrhea, and dehydration. Constipation, fluid retention, and fever are not associated findings.

60. Answer: 3

Rationale: Methotrexate is the first-line DMARD in patients with active RA. Early disease-modifying antirheumatic drug (DMARD) therapy to slow disease progression and induce remission is the standard of care. Nonsteroidal antiinflammatory drugs can be used for symptomatic pain relief. Steroids (prednisone) may be given but are not the drug of choice and are administered when response is poor to other therapies. Tramadol is effective in RA pain but is not a first-line therapy. Cyclobenzaprine is a muscle relaxant.

61. Answer: 2

Rationale: The patient needs to understand the importance of maintaining the prescribed steroid dose. When symptoms decrease, the medication is effective. It is not influenced by fluids and should be taken with food.

62. Answer: 3

Rationale: This is the only effective dose listed for the treatment of an acute episode of gout. The other doses are incorrect and insufficient as dosed. The maximum dose of colchicine for an acute gout attack is 1.8 mg.

63. Answer: 3

Rationale: Patients with chronic renal disease should not be on NSAID therapy, as it relates to control of gout. The family nurse practitioner should be assessing pain medications for their effectiveness and monitoring the patient's weight as critical assessments. Withholding dialysis treatment would be against the standard of care.

64. Answer: 4

Rationale: Allopurinol reduces production of uric acid. The goal of therapy is a serum uric acid level less than 6.5 mg/dL. The other medications listed do not help lower serum uric acid levels, and aspirin can precipitate a gout attack.

65. Answer: 1

Rationale: Xanthine oxidase inhibitors are the drug of choice for the treatment of gout in the older adult patient. Aromatase inhibitors are used in the treatment of certain cancers. ACE inhibitors are used in the treatment of cardiac disease and hypertension. Beta blockers are used in the treatment of cardiac disease and migraine headaches.

66. Answer: 3

Rationale: Recommendations for vitamin D for patients ages 50 and older are 800–1000 IU on a daily basis. Vitamin D is measured in international units as opposed to the metric system of weights. For individuals who are below age 50, the recommendation is between 400 and 800 IU.

67. Answer: 1

Rationale: Acetaminophen or nonsteroidal antiinflammatory drugs (NSAIDs) are generally used for pain relief in patients with osteoarthritis. Systemic corticosteroids are not indicated in osteoarthritis. Gold salts may be one of several pharmacologic approaches to the treatment of rheumatoid arthritis. Misoprostol is used to minimize the development of NSAID-induced gastric ulcers.

68. Answer: 2

Rationale: Renal function may already be reduced in older adults, and ibuprofen can further impair renal function, which, in turn, can result in nephrosis, cirrhosis, and congestive heart failure.

69. Answer: 1

Rationale: The patient should be monitored for blood dyscrasias on a monthly basis, which would be a CBC with differential and platelet count. Women of child-bearing age should avoid pregnancy.

70. Answer: 3

Rationale: Nonsteroidal antiinflammatory drugs (NSAIDs; naproxen) are the recommended treatment for an acute gout attack in patients able to tolerate NSAID therapy. Allopurinol is contraindicated in an acute attack and can even precipitate an attack in the early stages of treatment. Low-calorie diets increase risks of gouty attacks. Joint injection would not be a first-line treatment choice, but for refractory cases in patients unable to take oral medication, it may be an option.

71. Answer: 1

Rationale: Acetaminophen is the preferred first-line therapy in treating pain in elderly patients because of its low profile for side effects if dosing regimens are followed according to therapeutic guidelines. The other medications can be used if acetaminophen dosing does not provide adequate relief, but these other drugs have a higher profile for side effects and as such should be used cautiously in the elderly patient.

72. Answer: 4

Rationale: Gastritis and oral ulcers are common complications of alendronate (Fosamax). Alendronate is used to increase calcium absorption in patients with osteoporosis. If these effects occur, the medication should be discontinued. The medications in the other options do not cause this problem.

73. Answer: 1

Glucosamine sulfate is a naturally occurring chemical (sugar) found in the human body. It is in the fluid that is around joints. Glucosamine sulfate is taken by mouth for the treatment of pain associated with osteoarthritis. It is also used by patients with glaucoma, interstitial cystitis, multiple sclerosis, and HIV/AIDS. Effects are not felt immediately after starting the medicine and may take up to 1–2 months for the patient to notice any change.

Neurology

11

Physical Exam & Diagnostic Tests

1. The family nurse practitioner is evaluating the mobility status of an older adult patient with the Timed "Up and Go" (TUG) test. The family nurse practitioner anticipates an adequate response by the patient performing the test within:
   1. 10 seconds.
   2. 30 seconds.
   3. 45 seconds.
   4. 60 seconds.

2. What would the family nurse practitioner perform to determine cerebellar functioning in the geriatric patient?
   1. Get up and go test.
   2. Tandem walk.
   3. Kinesthesia assessments.
   4. SPICES assessment.

3. Which image would provide the timeliest information to rule out a structural disorder in the brain?
   1. Computed tomography (CT) scan.
   2. Magnetic resonance imaging (MRI).
   3. Positron emission tomography (PET) scan.
   4. X-ray.

4. **QSEN** A 69-year-old patient presents with a headache. The laboratory workup indicates an elevated C-reactive protein. Which physical assessment would be a priority?
   1. Comparing blood pressure between the upper and lower extremities.
   2. Following up with laboratory tests for Lyme disease.
   3. Palpating the temporal arteries for tenderness.
   4. Referring to the emergency department for emergent lumbar puncture.

5. When assessing the neurologic status of an elder, what does the family nurse practitioner expects?
   1. Alcohol abuse is a rare cause of peripheral neuropathy in elders.
   2. It is a national recommendation to screen all elderly for dementia.
   3. Systemic medical illness should be a differential when any cognitive change is noted.
   4. Sensory testing is recommended in the lower extremities only.

6. What is considered a "soft" (or equivocal) neurologic sign?
   1. Positive Babinski reflex in an adult.
   2. Mirroring hand movements of the extremities.
   3. Brudzinski sign.
   4. Kernig sign.

7. A 60-year-old patient presents with new-onset seizures and his wife reports "he's just been different from himself" for the last 2 weeks. The patient is stable and sitting comfortably in the exam room. As the patient moves to the exam table you note slight ataxia. On neurologic assessment, he has a diminished pupillary response on the right. What imaging modality will you recommend?
   1. A computed tomography (CT) scan without contrast.
   2. A positron emission scan (PET) scan.
   3. An angiogram of the brain.
   4. Magnetic resonance imaging (MRI) with contrast.

8. A patient comes in with a family member who describes tonic-clonic seizure activity. The family nurse practitioner recommends an electroencephalogram (EEG). What is the diagnostic test of choice for new-onset seizures?
   1. A diurnal-cycle EEG.
   2. An EEG following high-sensory stimulation.
   3. A sleep-deprived EEG.
   4. A simple EEG as the initial study.

9. Which cranial nerve is being tested when the family nurse practitioner asks the patient to raise the eyebrows, smile, frown, or puff out the cheeks?
   1. Hypoglossal nerve.
   2. Acoustic nerve.
   3. Glossopharyngeal nerve.
   4. Facial nerve.

10. The family nurse practitioner notes an absent patellar reflex in a healthy patient. What might the practitioner ask the patient to do?
    1. Lift both arms above the head and count to five slowly as the reflex is tested.
    2. Raise both legs slowly and then lower and immediately test for the reflex.
    3. Clench both hands together and pull while the reflex is tested.
    4. Close eyes and hold breath while examiner tests for the reflex.

11. The family nurse practitioner is performing a vaginal exam on a patient with a history of spina bifida. With the insertion of the metal speculum, the patient suddenly feels nauseated and is sweating, and her skin turns blotchy. What is your most immediate reaction to this situation?
    1. Provide reassurance.
    2. Put a blanket over the patient's legs.
    3. Assess blood pressure.
    4. Remove the speculum.

12. With the patient in the supine position, the family nurse practitioner gently flexes the patient's neck in the direction of the chin touching the chest. If there is pain and resistance to the flexion, and if the hips and knees flex at the same time, the nurse accurately describes this finding as:
    1. Phalen sign.
    2. Romberg sign.
    3. Kernig sign.
    4. Brudzinski sign.

13. Which of the following differentials would be priority in a patient with new-onset syncope?
    1. Cardiac dysrhythmias.
    2. Postural hypotension.
    3. Symptomatic hypoglycemia.
    4. Vasovagal syncope.

14. **QSEN** A 46-year-old arrives at the clinic and is accompanied by his wife. His wife mentions his "personality is different than before, and we've been married for 27 years." Which assessment would be a priority?
    1. Assessing deep tendon reflexes (DTRs) and gait patterns.
    2. Analyzing judgment patterns.
    3. Completing a Mini-Mental State Exam (MMSE).
    4. Strength testing for neuromuscular weakness.

15. The family nurse practitioner is providing patient education about essential tremor. Which statement would be important to include?
    1. "Your tremor is noticed most often when you are at rest."
    2. "Your tremor will occur more often in your hands and arms."

3. "Your tremor will not stop you from doing your usual activities at home."
4. "Your tremor will not affect the sound of your voice."

Disorders

16. Which statement regarding meningitis in the older adult is correct?
    1. Symptoms are more pronounced in the older adult.
    2. *Neisseria meningitidis* is the most common bacterial cause.
    3. Outcomes are improved with use of systemic steroids.
    4. Neurosurgery does not affect risk of meningitis.

17. The family nurse practitioner is seeing a 65-year-old patient with a presenting complaint of headache. Which question would be most valuable in developing differentials for this patient?
    1. Do you have a family history of headaches?
    2. How old were you when the headaches began?
    3. When did this headache begin?
    4. Where is your headache located?

18. The family nurse practitioner understands that the most common form of facial paralysis in the adult patient is:
    1. Facial nerve fasciitis.
    2. Trigeminal neuralgia.
    3. Bell's palsy.
    4. Herpes zoster.

19. A patient has a history of injury at the fifth thoracic vertebra (T5) with full spinal cord compromise at that level. His condition has stabilized. The family nurse practitioner understands that, with this level of injury, the patient most likely will not be able to:
    1. Perform coordinated movements with his hands, such as writing.
    2. Achieve lower body strength and coordination for walking.
    3. Have adequate upper body strength to drive a car.
    4. Maintain the upper body coordination required for eating.

20. **QSEN** The family nurse practitioner is discussing safety measures for the home environment of a patient with Parkinson disease. It would be important for the family nurse practitioner to include what information?
    1. Sleep on a firm mattress that is high off the floor to facilitate getting into and out of bed.
    2. Pour hot liquids with the cup or container placed on the table to avoid spilling.
    3. Place a sheepskin pad on the bed to decrease the development of decubiti.
    4. Perform passive and active range of motion twice daily to prevent contracture.

21. A patient presents to a rural clinic after a diving accident. The family nurse practitioner suspects a spinal cord injury at the fifth cervical vertebra (C5). While awaiting emergency transport services, which assessment would be a priority in this level of injury?
    1. Checking for voluntary movement of extremities and sensation below the level of injury.
    2. Assessing breath sounds and evaluating movement of diaphragm with respiration.
    3. Maintaining cervical flexion to facilitate airway until cervical traction is initiated.
    4. Beginning neurologic checks with careful documentation of location of pain sensations.

22. Many patients who suffer from recurrent headaches have similar symptoms with each episode. Which is a sign that a headache may be from a more serious cause?
    1. It occurs on the right side.
    2. Rhinorrhea occurs with the headache.
    3. It becomes more and more painful.
    4. It increases when the patient bends over.

23. Which of the following are considered three risk factors for the development of Parkinson disease?
    1. Exposure to pesticides.
    2. History of concussion.
    3. Farming.
    4. Occupational exposure to rubber.
    5. Limited tobacco and caffeine use.

24. The family nurse practitioner understands that benign paroxysmal positional vertigo:
    1. Is described as vertigo and nystagmus with positional change and occurs most often in older adults.
    2. Is more common in young persons and occurs suddenly and in episodes that include vertigo, tinnitus, hearing loss, feeling of fullness in the ears, and nausea and vomiting.
    3. Follows a viral syndrome (upper respiratory or gastrointestinal) with exacerbation of the vertigo with position change without hearing loss or tinnitus.
    4. Involves gradual hearing loss and tinnitus along with vertigo, eventually with facial numbness and weakness.

25. A 52-year-old patient presents with "funny feeling in my feet and calves, like I can't feel them." The sensation has been continuous over the last 2 days and seems to be worsening. The patient is otherwise healthy except for a recent upper respiratory infection. What is the primary differential based on the patient's history?
    1. Amyotrophic lateral sclerosis.
    2. Guillain-Barré syndrome.
    3. Multiple sclerosis.
    4. Muscular dystrophy.

26. Which three of the following conditions are included in the differential diagnosis of a patient with facial paralysis?
    1. Herpes zoster.
    2. Bell's palsy.
    3. Trigeminal neuralgia.
    4. Otitis media.
    5. Myasthenia gravis.

27. What would be appropriate to include in the health promotion plan for a patient with a diagnosis of multiple sclerosis?
    1. Avoid aerobic exercise because of muscle weakness.
    2. Keep warm (especially extremities) to improve neurologic function.
    3. Avoid antioxidants (vitamins C and E, beta carotene); they contribute to loss of myelin sheath.
    4. Consume a low-fat, high-fiber diet with daily cranberry juice and calcium supplement.

28. A patient has had a stroke and is incontinent of urine. The family should be taught to:
    1. Restrict fluid intake.
    2. Insert a Foley catheter.
    3. Establish a scheduled voiding pattern.
    4. Reposition the patient often to reduce the discomfort of urgency.

29. What is the best approach to test the hearing of a patient with Bell's palsy?
    1. Stand out of sight of the patient and ask the patient to move or do something.
    2. Use a tuning fork to test for lateralization of sound.
    3. Stand in front of the patient and whisper "Raise your hand."
    4. Snap your fingers next to the patient's ear and ask if the sound was heard.

30. A patient presents to the clinic with symptoms of unilateral tremor, rigidity, flexed posture, bradykinesia, loss of postural reflexes, and freezing. The family nurse practitioner recognizes these symptoms as:
    1. Multiple sclerosis.
    2. Myasthenia gravis.
    3. Parkinson disease.
    4. Brain tumor.

31. What is the inflammation and swelling of the seventh cranial nerve with resultant unilateral facial muscle paralysis called?
    1. Bell's palsy.
    2. Temporal (giant cell) arteritis.
    3. Facial droop.
    4. Trigeminal neuralgia.

32. Which symptom(s) can occur in a patient who has experienced a transient ischemic attack (TIA) in the anterior cerebral circulation?
    1. Bilateral vision disturbance and diplopia.
    2. Dysarthria (speech disturbance).
    3. Disorders of behavior and cognition.
    4. Bilateral motor and sensory dysfunction.

33. Many visits to emergency departments by adults are prompted by headaches. Which symptom may help the family nurse practitioner differentiate a migraine headache from a headache that may indicate severe problems?
    1. It is preceded by an "aura."
    2. It occurs mainly behind one eye and tends to be grouped.
    3. Onset is sudden and accompanied by nuchal rigidity.
    4. It occurs mainly on awakening.

34. An adult patient presents with a complaint of facial paralysis that started suddenly. In making a diagnosis, the family nurse practitioner considers which of the following symptoms of Bell's palsy?
    1. Concurrent paralysis of the opposite arm and leg.
    2. Pain in the (ipsilateral) ear that accompanied or preceded the paralysis.
    3. Loss of bowel control.
    4. Loss of hearing on the opposite side.

35. An older adult woman is present when her husband is admitted for a myocardial infarction. She complains that she is having numbness and tingling in her hands and face. Her heart rate is 98 beats/min and her respiratory rate is 32 breaths/min. What is the best action for the family nurse practitioner to take?
    1. Administer oxygen per nasal cannula at 3 L/min.
    2. Schedule a magnetic resonance imaging appointment.
    3. Provide calming interventions by explaining the probable reason for the symptoms.
    4. Administer amitriptyline (Elavil) 25 mg PO.

36. The family nurse practitioner is evaluating an older adult's tremor. Which assessment finding would be characteristic of an essential tremor rather than a parkinsonian tremor?
    1. The handwriting is not affected.
    2. The tremor occurs with purposeful movements.
    3. The tremor occurs at rest.
    4. The tremor worsens with beta blockers or alcohol.

37. Which assessment may be evaluated in a patient with Parkinson disease?
    1. Macrographia.
    2. Micrographia.
    3. Exaggeration of rapid successive movements.
    4. Increased swinging of arms while walking.

38. A patient recently diagnosed with multiple sclerosis (MS) asks the family nurse practitioner about the disease process. The family nurse practitioner knows that:
    1. 90% of patients have a quickly progressive form of the disease.
    2. 90% of patients, after the first onset of symptoms, have relapses and remissions.
    3. 10% of patients will respond to corticosteroids.
    4. 10% of patients have problems with optic neuritis and sensory loss.

39. A 30-year-old female patient has had several episodes of incontinence, weakness, visual loss, and some ataxia. Physical exam reveals slight swelling of the optic disc on funduscopy, difficulty with heel-to-toe walking, lower extremity weakness, and 2+ deep tendon reflexes. Which condition does the family nurse practitioner suspect?
    1. Multiple sclerosis.
    2. Parkinson disease.
    3. Amyotrophic lateral sclerosis.
    4. Myasthenia gravis.

40. A patient presents to the emergency department, stating "this is the worst headache of my life." The patient reports that the headaches have not responded to the usual over-the-counter headache remedies. What is a priority differential?
    1. Brain tumor.
    2. Migraine.
    3. Onset of newly diagnosed seizure disorder.
    4. Subarachnoid hemorrhage.

41. A patient with a recent history of a left hemisphere stroke returns to the clinic for a checkup. What symptoms would the family nurse practitioner anticipate the patient to exhibit?
    1. Left-sided weakness.
    2. Bilateral weakness of lower extremities.
    3. Difficulty with speech.
    4. Left visual field deficit.

42. The family nurse practitioner is evaluating a group of older adult patients for risk factors of an embolic stroke. Which condition would be least likely to precipitate this type of stroke?
    1. Mitral valve disease.
    2. Atrial fibrillation.
    3. Endocarditis.
    4. Diabetes mellitus.

43. A patient returns to the clinic for a follow-up visit. She has a history of simple partial seizures. When questioning the patient, the family nurse practitioner would identify recurrence of this seizure activity if the patient reported:
    1. Short episodes when she loses consciousness but does not fall.
    2. No loss of consciousness, but jerking and tingling of her right leg, and then right hand.
    3. Auditory hallucinations, unconsciousness, and urinary incontinence.
    4. Short period of unconsciousness, followed by period of confusion.

44. An older adult woman comes to the clinic complaining of having difficulty when sewing. She states the shaking in her hands stops when she holds her hands in her lap. She walks straight, and no rigidity is noted with her movements. What tentative diagnosis would the family nurse practitioner make?
    1. Parkinson disease.
    2. Transient ischemic attack.
    3. Benign essential tremor.
    4. Resting tremor.

45. Which three exam findings would be associated with the diagnosis of Parkinson disease?
    1. Bradykinesia.
    2. Inappropriate affect.
    3. Rigidity.
    4. Tremor.

46. A patient with a history of myasthenia gravis presents with ptosis, facial weakness, dysphagia, and generalized weakness. What is important for the family nurse practitioner to ask on initial assessment?
    1. When did the symptoms first begin, and have they increased in severity?
    2. What medications is the patient taking, and when did he or she last take them?
    3. What activity was the patient participating in when the symptoms began?
    4. Has the patient experienced any seizure activity with the increase in symptoms?

47. A patient presents with miosis, ptosis, and anhidrosis of the ipsilateral face and neck. What would the initial diagnosis be?
    1. Horner syndrome.
    2. Damage to cranial nerves III and IV.
    3. Ménière syndrome.
    4. Mycotic aneurysm.

48. What are the initial symptoms of amyotrophic lateral sclerosis?:
    1. Weakness in the lower extremities and urinary incontinence.
    2. Weakness in the upper extremities and dysfunction in fine motor skills.
    3. Spasticity and hyperreflexia.
    4. Loss of continence and drooling.

49. Considering the risks for bacterial meningitis, which history question would **not** be helpful in refining your differential diagnoses?
    1. "Do you smoke now, or have you ever smoked?"
    2. "How much alcohol do you drink a day?"
    3. "Have you fallen in the past month?"
    4. "How are your blood sugars running?"

50. Which statement concerning movement disorders is correct?
    1. Essential tremor is most common in females.
    2. Medications can mask movement disorders.
    3. Movement disorders affect the central nervous system exclusively.
    4. Parkinson disease is a rare form of movement disorder.

51. Which two of the following are known risk factors for multiple sclerosis (MS)?
    1. Age.
    2. Black ethnicity.
    3. Male gender.
    4. Residency in a cold climate.
    5. Family history.

52. Which of the following three findings are associated with Guillain-Barré syndrome?
    1. A recent viral illness.
    2. Weakness more profound in the upper extremities.
    3. Headache and nuchal rigidity.
    4. Visual changes.
    5. Respiratory distress or failure.
    6. Protein in cerebral spinal fluid analysis.

53. The family nurse practitioner is seeing a patient for new-onset headaches. Which statement by the patient would cause the most concern?
    1. "This headache makes me sick to my stomach."
    2. "This headache is behind my right eye and is giving me stabbing pain."
    3. "This headache has awakened me from sleep for the past week."
    4. "I have needed to wear dark glasses for the last 3 days in a row."

54. The family nurse practitioner is treating a patient with Parkinson disease (PD). What finding should the family nurse practitioner anticipate?
    1. Visual hallucinations and paranoia.
    2. Bowel and bladder dysfunction.
    3. Disorders in extraocular movements.
    4. Pulmonary hypertension associated with left ventricular failure.

55. Which of the following statements is correct concerning brain tumors?
    1. Meningiomas are the most frequent type of primary malignant tumors.
    2. A history of breast cancer has no associated risk for brain tumor.
    3. New-onset seizures are a common clinical finding.
    4. Increased intracranial pressure is a classic early finding in meningioma.

56. A middle-aged, normotensive patient presents with asymmetric weakness of his right leg. The family nurse practitioner's primary diagnosis requiring urgent attention would be:
    1. Amyotrophic lateral sclerosis.
    2. Bell's palsy.
    3. Stroke.
    4. Guillain-Barré syndrome.

57. The family nurse practitioner recognizes that cerebral edema usually presents within what time frame following a head trauma?
    1. 24 hours.
    2. 48 hours.
    3. 72 hours.
    4. 1 week.

58. Bacterial meningitis is most common in which age group?
    1. Children younger than 2 years.
    2. Older adolescents.
    3. Middle-aged adults.
    4. Older adults over age 65.

59. What four symptoms are findings associated with post-concussion syndrome?
    1. Anxiety.
    2. Behavioral disturbances.
    3. Headaches.
    4. Fine tremors.
    5. Hallucinations.
    6. Sleep disturbances.

60. The family nurse practitioner recognizes which of the following two criteria as correct concerning multiple sclerosis (MS)?
    1. The onset is most likely between the ages of 20 and 50 years.
    2. It affects males and females equally.
    3. It is more commonly diagnosed in northern climates.
    4. Native Americans, Eskimos, and Asians are affected more than other ethnicities.
    5. MS is the result of exclusively an autoimmune disorder.

61. The family nurse practitioner suspects a patient has Parkinson disease. Which assessment would be least helpful in supporting this diagnosis?
    1. Observing the gait for center of gravity.

2. Performing passive flexion/extension of the forearm.
3. Pulling the patient's shoulders from behind.
4. Testing for hyperactive deep tendon reflexes.

62. The family nurse practitioner is reviewing the records of a patient who is recovering from a stroke. The records indicate the patient is experiencing homonymous hemianopia. This is interpreted as:
    1. Partial loss of visual acuity in the peripheral area of the visual field.
    2. Diplopia in the eye contralateral to the cerebral lesion.
    3. Nystagmus in both eyes, but movements are dissimilar.
    4. Loss of vision in both eyes in either the right or the left half of the visual field.

Pharmacology

63. **QSEN** Which product would be the safest choice for an 81-year-old patient with insomnia?
    1. Diphenhydramine (Benadryl).
    2. Doxepin (Silenor).
    3. Oxazepam (Serax).
    4. Ramelteon (Rozerem).

64. **QSEN** Which product would cause the family nurse practitioner the greatest concern based on review of a medication list belonging to a 68-year-old who fell from a ladder today and hit his right parietal region on asphalt?
    1. Metaxalone (Skelaxin).
    2. Ginseng (over the counter).
    3. Omeprazole (Prilosec).
    4. Acetaminophen (Tylenol).

65. A patient is taking an antiepileptic medication. The family nurse practitioner understands that the antiepileptic medication:
    1. Must be taken indefinitely.
    2. Is usually discontinued after 4 years of no seizure activity, and electroencephalogram (EEG) confirms lack of seizure activity.
    3. Is usually given in combination with other antiepileptics or sedatives to reduce the seizure threshold.
    4. Must be given to all patients who experience a seizure.

66. The family nurse practitioner is seeing a 33-year-old female with recurrent migraines. Which three medications would be reasonable selections for migraine prophylaxis?
    1. Amlodipine (Norvasc).
    2. Lisinopril (Prinivil).
    3. Labetalol (Normodyne).
    4. Methyldopa (Aldomet).
    5. Amitriptyline (Elavil)
    6. Sumatriptan (Imitrex).

67. A 67-year-old patient presents with the concern of right-sided facial pain. She describes the pain as burning and sharp. The pain has not awakened her from sleep. She explains she has to "press on it" when it starts, and she does not talk or move her mouth because it worsens the pain. What management will the family nurse practitioner consider based on these symptoms?
    1. Carbamazepine (Tegretol).
    2. Indomethacin (Indocin).
    3. Prednisone.
    4. Valacyclovir (Valtrex).

68. **QSEN** Which patient would be at lowest risk to use a cholinergic blocker to control Parkinson disease?
    1. A 65-year-old with chronic diarrhea.
    2. A 68-year-old patient with glaucoma.
    3. A 69-year-old patient with benign prostatic hypertrophy.
    4. A 72-year-old patient with atrial fibrillation.

69. Which product would reduce essential tremors?
    1. Alcohol.
    2. Caffeine (over-the-counter).
    3. Pseudoephedrine (Sudafed).
    4. Enalapril (Vasotec).

70. The family of a patient with Parkinson disease brings him to the clinic because he is experiencing increasing difficulty with ambulation. The family nurse practitioner increases the patient's dose of carbidopa (25 mg)/levodopa (100 mg) (Sinemet 25–100 mg) from three to four times daily. What is important for the family nurse practitioner to teach the family regarding the increase in the dose of this medication?
    1. Sleep disorders are common side effects of carbidopa/levodopa.
    2. Carbidopa/levodopa has shown efficacy in slowing disease progression.
    3. Orthostatic hypotension can be problematic at higher dosing ranges.
    4. The medication should be given on an empty stomach.

71. **QSEN** The family nurse practitioner is seeing a 56-year-old patient with a history of hypertension, dyslipidemia, and Barrett's esophagitis. The patient has experienced headaches since playing football in high school. Which product would you discourage the patient from continuing based on his chronic illnesses?
    1. Acetaminophen (Tylenol).
    2. Amlodipine (Norvasc).
    3. Sumatriptan (Imitrex).
    4. Prochlorperazine (Compazine).

72. Which medication class is recognized for the treatment of moderate to severe dementia?
    1. Cholinesterase inhibitors.
    2. N-methyl-D-aspartate (NMDA) receptor antagonists.
    3. Selective serotonin reuptake inhibitors (SSRIs).
    4. Central α_2 agonists.

73. **QSEN** Before prescribing an abortive agent for migraines, a priority question to ask the patient would be:
    1. "Do you have a history of gastric colic?"
    2. "Do you have a history of panic episodes?"
    3. "Do you have a history of cardiac disease?"
    4. "Do you have a history of seizure disorder?"

74. Which factor demonstrates the best evidence in patient outcomes when initially treating ischemic stroke?
    1. Cardiac rhythm control.
    2. Blood pressure control.
    3. Timely use of thrombolytics.
    4. Renal protection, including fluid support.

75. Which antibiotic class does the family nurse practitioner recognize can interfere with the metabolism of first-generation antiepileptic drugs, such as carbamazepine?
    1. Cephalosporins.
    2. Quinolones.
    3. Sulfonamides.
    4. Macrolides.

76. What information is important for the family nurse practitioner to teach the patient regarding the use of medications to treat trigeminal neuralgia?
    1. Medications may cause seizure-like activity.
    2. Therapeutic levels of the drug may take up to a month to be reached.
    3. Relief of the symptoms should occur within 24 hours of starting the medication.
    4. Permanent side effects are not a concern of this condition.

77. A patient arrives at the clinic having an acute attack of Ménière disease. Which three medications would the family nurse practitioner prescribe?
    1. Lorazepam (Ativan).
    2. Meclizine (Antivert).
    3. Atropine.
    4. Furosemide (Lasix).
    5. Nortriptyline (Pamelor).
    6. Penicillin.

11 Neurology Answers & Rationales

Physical Exam & Diagnostic Tests

1. Answer: 1

Rationale: To complete the TUG test (also referred to as the "get up and go" test), the patient is asked to stand up from a chair with arms, walk 10 feet, then turn around and return immediately to the chair. The complete test should be performed within 10 seconds or less and correlates with functional independence. Gait, balance, position change, and turning are evaluated. Additional testing is recommended if longer than 20 seconds are required to complete the test.

2. Answer: 2

Rationale: Asking the patient to tandem walk assesses cerebellar function, so it would be a reasonable method to evaluate an older adult's balance. The get up and go test assesses gait, balance, and position change and turning (also referred to as the Timed "Up and Go" test). Kinesthesia assessments determine proprioception ability. The SPICES assessment is an acronym of common older adult syndromes: **S** is for sleep disorders, **P** is for problems with eating or feeding, **I** is for incontinence, **C** is for confusion, **E** is for evidence of falls, and **S** is for skin breakdown.

3. Answer: 1

Rationale: A CT scan of the brain without contrast would be the preferred image if an emergent diagnosis was needed about a structural cranial disorder. No contrast should be given if bleeding is suspected because the contrast dye leaks from vessel walls and can obscure critical structures. Although CT scans have less resolution than MRI and therefore can miss small lesions, they can be performed within minutes, compared with an MRI that takes a minimum of 30 minutes. An x-ray provides information about bony structure and radiopaque foreign bodies. A PET scan, which is a nuclear study, provides information about active metabolic structures, which would not be a priority in initial diagnosis concerning a structural disorder.

4. Answer: 3

Rationale: Temporal arteritis presents clinically as a headache with associated tenderness over the affected temporal artery and elevated inflammatory serum markers (elevated sedimentation rate or C-reactive protein) with C-reactive protein having the highest sensitivity (95%–98%). A form of giant cell arteritis, temporal arteritis is associated with blindness if not diagnosed and treated with high-dose steroids as soon as possible after symptom onset. Patients over the age of 50 are at higher risk, with peak incidence between ages 70 and 79.

Temporal artery biopsy is the gold standard of diagnosis and, if suspicion is high, patients should be referred for temporal artery biopsy as quickly as possible. Comparison of blood pressures between the upper and lower extremities is helpful to rule out coarctation of the aorta. Lower extremity pressures should always be higher than upper extremity pressures. There is no indication for a high-risk procedure of lumbar puncture for the older adult. Laboratory tests for Lyme disease may be appropriate, but they are not a priority compared with recognition and emergent treatment of temporal arteritis.

5. Answer: 3

Rationale: Urinary tract infection, pneumonia, and other infections are common causes of confusion in the elderly. There is no national recommendation to screen an elderly patient for dementia unless there are signs of dementia. Alcohol abuse, diabetes, and vitamin B_{12} deficiency are common causes of peripheral neuropathy in elders. Sensory testing using light touch and pain is recommended in the distal upper and lower extremities.

6. Answer: 2

Rationale: Soft neurologic signs involve slight deviations of the central nervous system (CNS) that are present occasionally or inconsistently. Examples are short attention span; clumsiness; frequent falling (disturbances of gait); hyperkinesis; left-handed, but right-footed; anisocoria without altered mental status; and mirroring movements of the extremities (when one hand performs a movement, the other is also in motion). The other three options indicate a CNS problem that occurs consistently; Brudzinski and Kernig signs indicate meningeal irritation, and the presence of the Babinski reflex in an adult indicates an upper motor lesion in the corticospinal tract, but not the acuity of the lesion.

7. Answer: 4

Rationale: The MRI will provide the clearest image with the best resolution and has higher sensitivity to detect smaller lesions. Contrast will assist in visualizing blood vessels, including abnormal vessels. If the patient is unstable, a CT scan without contrast would be the image of choice for immediate diagnosis of intracerebral hemorrhage (e.g., from a bleeding vessel or hemorrhage into brain metastases) as the etiology of the new-onset seizures. A PET scan will provide information about highly active metabolic activity. This would be a secondary consideration following MRI findings if occult neoplasm is suspected or for staging purposes. An angiogram of the brain will limit findings to vascular structures (e.g., arteriovenous malformation) only.

8. Answer: 3

Rationale: A sleep-deprived EEG is a useful diagnostic tool because a baseline recording of background brain waves may reveal epileptic abnormalities. Generalized types of epilepsy (tonic-clonic activity) often produce abnormalities of spike and wave activity interictally that help diagnose epilepsy.

9. Answer: 4

Rationale: The facial nerve is tested by facial movement, taste in the anterior two-thirds of the tongue, sensation of a small area around the auricle, and motor to the stapedius bone in the inner ear, important for dampening of loud noises. The hypoglossal nerve is tested by the patient sticking out the tongue. The acoustic nerve is tested by a hearing test. The glossopharyngeal nerve is tested by taste, gag reflex, and having the patient drink and swallow.

10. Answer: 3

Rationale: Augmentation of the patellar reflex can be obtained by having the patient isometrically tense muscles not directly involved with the reflex arc being tested (the Jendrassik maneuver).

11. Answer: 4

Rationale: Patients with spina bifida can experience autonomic hyperreflexia as characterized by elevated blood pressure, sweating, blotchy skin, nausea, or goose bumps caused by stimulation of the bowel, bladder, or skin below the spinal lesion area. During a physical exam, the following can be causes of hyperreflexia: reactions to a cold, hard exam table or cold stirrups; insertion and manipulation of a vaginal speculum; pressure during the bimanual or rectal exam; or tactile contact with hypersensitive areas. The vaginal speculum should be removed, at which time the hyperreflexia ceases; the family nurse practitioner and the patient should mutually decide whether to continue the exam.

12. Answer: 4

Rationale: This describes Brudzinski sign. Phalen sign (maneuver) is elicited in carpal tunnel syndrome. The Romberg sign test is done to assess gross swaying by asking the patient to stand with feet together and eyes closed for 5 seconds. Kernig sign (inability to extend lower leg when leg is flexed at hip or when there is resistance or pain) along with Brudzinski sign indicate meningeal irritation and should be evaluated further.

13. Answer: 1

Rationale: Cardiac dysrhythmias or alterations in cardiac output are priority because of risk of sudden death from cardiac or cerebral ischemia. Syncope can be associated with metabolic concerns caused by electrolyte imbalance or alterations in glucose, and vagal sources from standing in one place or from straining/bearing down with bowel movement. Postural hypotension caused by medications, nausea, vomiting, dehydration, or anemia are differentials as well.

14. Answer: 2

Rationale: Analyzing the patient's judgments by speaking with him would be a priority to determine his risk of self-harm or harm to others. If self-harm or harm to others is identified, immediate evaluation by a mental health specialist is required. If the patient's judgments lead to potential unintentional harms (driving, cooking with a gas range, operation of machinery, etc.), this too would be a priority concern based on inadequate judgment. Although DTRs, gait patterns, and strength testing are components of a complete neurologic exam, they are not the priority of his assessment. An MMSE is a useful instrument in performing baseline and serial assessments of cognitive function, but it is not specifically useful for judgment.

15. Answer: 2

Rationale: Essential tremor is associated with action and is found more commonly in the upper extremities, head/neck, or voice. Essential tremor worsens with activity, causing impairment in fine motor activities, including dressing, sewing, writing, playing an instrument, or other hobbies a patient may enjoy.

Disorders

16. Answer: 3

Rationale: Corticosteroids improve outcomes in all adults, reducing long-term mortality. *Listeria monocytogenes* is more commonly associated with meningitis in the elderly. Atypical presentation is common in the older adult, and expected physical exam findings are not as pronounced. Basilar skull fracture, sickle cell disease, immunosuppression, alcoholism, and neurosurgery all increase risk for infections of the central nervous system.

17. Answer: 2

Rationale: Headaches should decrease in frequency and severity with age. New onset of headaches after age 50 can be a sign of increased intracranial pressure from either a space-occupying lesion or hemorrhage rather than a primary headache disorder and require urgent evaluation and treatment. Other dangerous signs include asymmetric responses to light in pupils, change in the patient's level of consciousness, headache described as "worst pain in my life," a "different" type of headache, headaches awakening the patient during sleep, painful temporal arteries, or behavioral changes.

18. Answer: 3

Rationale: The most common form of facial paralysis is Bell's palsy, a disorder affecting the facial nerve characterized by muscle flaccidity of the affected side of the face. Trigeminal neuralgia is a disorder of cranial nerve V that is characterized by an abrupt onset of pain in the lower and upper jaw, cheek, and lips. Herpes zoster affects the dermatomes and does not cause a paralysis, but rather pain, herpetic grouped skin vesicles, and possibly postherpetic neuralgia.

19. Answer: 2

Rationale: Fifth thoracic vertebra (T5) injuries do not affect the coordination or capacity of the upper body, arms, and hands; the lower body is paralyzed. The patient should be able to do all activities listed except walk, have full bowel and bladder control, and have normal parasympathetic regulation.

20. Answer: 2

Rationale: Pouring liquids is frequently a complicated task for this patient because of the tremors. If the cup or container to be filled is placed on the table, there is less chance of spilling the contents.

21. Answer: 2

Rationale: At this level of injury (C5), the intercostal muscles and diaphragm can be affected, and the patient may have respiratory compromise. Airway maintenance, cervical stabilization, and avoiding flexion of the neck are critical.

22. Answer: 3

Rationale: If a headache becomes more and more severe, if there is new onset of severe headache in a patient over 35 years old, if the headache's character or progression is different from other headaches, or if there is vomiting, but no nausea, there could be a new and serious cause for the headache. The side on which the headache occurs, and accompanying rhinorrhea, may or may not be significant. Increasing pain when bending over is characteristic of sinus pressure or infection.

23. Answer: 1, 2, 3

Rationale: Pesticide exposure, concussion, and farming/agricultural work are all risk factors to developing Parkinson disease. Rubber is an occupational concern to the development of cancers but is not associated with Parkinson disease. History of smoking and coffee and caffeine intake may reduce risk.

24. Answer: 1

Rationale: Benign paroxysmal positional vertigo usually occurs in older patients. Younger persons who experience a sudden episode of vertigo, tinnitus, hearing loss, sensation of fullness, and nausea and vomiting typically have Ménière disease.

Peripheral vestibulopathy usually follows upper respiratory or gastrointestinal viral illness and involves nearly incapacitating vertigo that increases with positional changes, but not hearing loss or tinnitus. The family nurse practitioner should suspect acoustic neuroma if gradual hearing loss, tinnitus, and vertigo occur before the development of facial numbness and weakness.

25. Answer: 2

Rationale: Guillain-Barré syndrome presents with progressive paresthesias and weakness most commonly in the lower extremities. It can occur following a recent illness. The symptoms are bilateral. Amyotrophic lateral sclerosis typically presents with unilateral paresthesias in one of the upper extremities, as does multiple sclerosis in a lower extremity. Muscular dystrophy commonly presents in younger patients and with pain and stiffness that gradually worsens over months to years, not days.

26. Answer: 1, 2, 4

Rationale: The differential diagnosis for facial paralysis includes bacterial ear infections, Lyme disease, herpes zoster, HIV, mumps, temporal bone fracture, acoustic neuroma, other tumors, and demyelinating diseases. Trigeminal neuralgia is associated with intense facial pain, not paralysis. Myasthenia gravis is characterized by fluctuating weakness and fatigability, often subtle, that worsens during the day and after prolonged use of affected muscles; it may improve with rest. Ptosis may be observed.

27. Answer: 4

Rationale: In addition to the factors listed, keeping cool, not warm, is associated with improvement of neurologic function. A regular exercise program is encouraged, along with daily intake of a multivitamin, antioxidants, and low-dose aspirin (81 mg). Maintaining ideal body weight, having rest periods or naps daily, and becoming informed about the disease process are important aspects of promoting health.

28. Answer: 3

Rationale: Reestablishing regularity will assist in maintaining bladder control. A catheter exposes the patient to infection. Fluids should not be restricted.

29. Answer: 1

Rationale: Bell's palsy can include a change in hearing, primarily hyperacusis, or the sensation that sounds are louder because of the loss of the loud noise–dampening effect of the stapedius muscle, which can be affected in Bell's palsy, depending on the location of the facial nerve dysfunction. In contrast to being able to read lips, this patient must be able to hear the direction of sound without any visual prompting. The tuning fork assists in differentiating between air and bone conduction of sound.

30. Answer: 3

Rationale: The clinical presentation of Parkinson disease is asymmetric or unilateral tremor, rigidity, bradykinesia with freezing, and flexed posture with loss of postural reflexes. The classic finding of myasthenia gravis is fatigability, which is also characterized by fluctuating weakness, often subtle, that worsens during the day and after prolonged use of affected muscles and may improve with rest and with ptosis of the eye that may shift from eye-to-eye. Patients with multiple sclerosis can present with a number of neurologic signs and symptoms depending on the locations of the lesions within the central nervous system. Typical symptoms include fatigue, depression, emotional instability, epilepsy, memory loss, diplopia, sudden vision loss, facial palsy, dysarthria, dysphagia, muscle weakness or spasms, ataxia, vertigo, falls, hyperesthesia or paresthesia, pain, bowel or bladder incontinence, urinary frequency or retention, or impotence. Brain tumor signs and symptoms may include new onset or change in pattern of headaches with the headache gradually becoming more frequent and more severe, unexplained nausea or vomiting, vision problems, such as blurred vision, double vision or loss of peripheral vision, gradual loss of sensation or movement in an arm or a leg, changes in personality, and other sensory issues.

31. Answer: 1

Rationale: The symptoms describe Bell's palsy, which is thought to be caused by a virus. This sudden onset of unilateral facial paralysis usually resolves within 2 weeks but can endure for months. A few patients may have residual problems. Temporal or giant cell arteritis is a generalized, large-vessel vasculitis commonly affecting the branches of the proximal aorta that supply the neck and the extracranial structures of the head. Facial droop occurs with Bell's palsy because of paralysis of the muscles innervated by the facial (seventh cranial) nerve. Trigeminal neuralgia is sudden pain along the fifth cranial nerve.

32. Answer: 3

Rationale: A wide variety of changes can occur in behavior and cognition after a TIA. Bilateral vision disturbance, diplopia, dysarthria (speech disturbance), and motor/sensory problems on both sides of the body are problems associated with TIA in the posterior cerebral circulation.

33. Answer: 3

Rationale: A sudden-onset headache associated with nuchal rigidity may indicate a subarachnoid hemorrhage. Migraine headache without aura is the most common; however, migraine with aura occurs before the onset of pain. Cluster headaches occur behind one eye and are grouped. Headaches associated with hypertension occur mainly on awakening.

34. Answer: 2

Rationale: Bell's palsy is typically preceded or accompanied by pain in the ear on the paralyzed side often 1–2 days before the onset of facial paralysis. The paralysis is confined to the face, and there is no bowel involvement. Postauricular pain, tinnitus, and a mild hearing deficit may occur on the affected side.

35. Answer: 3

Rationale: Patients who are under stress have periods of hyperventilation in which they "blow off" more carbon dioxide (CO_2) than necessary. They experience numbness and tingling in their hands and faces and may experience syncope. Reassurance and calming intervention techniques by explaining the voluntary component of the rapid breathing will often have dramatic results of correcting the symptoms. In the past, breathing into a paper bag was recommended because it was supposed to increase CO_2 level and relieve the symptoms of respiratory alkalosis; however, this is not supported in evidenced-based literature and may be dangerous in patients with hypoxia or other physiologic/pathologic causes for the hyperventilation.

36. Answer: 2

Rationale: The differentiating feature between the two tremors is that the essential tremor occurs with purposeful movements. Handwriting may be affected with both tremors. The tremor with Parkinson disease occurs at rest. Essential tremors improve with beta blockers and with alcohol.

37. Answer: 2

Rationale: Micrographia (small, cramped handwriting) is a classic manifestation of Parkinson disease. The patient has impairment of rapid successive movements and loss of automatic movements, such as swinging the arms while walking.

38. Answer: 2

Rationale: MS is characterized by exacerbations and remissions of the symptoms. Only 10% of MS patients have a progressive form of the disease from the onset. Many patients (35%–40%) have problems of optic neuritis, sensory loss, and weakness, and do respond to corticosteroids.

39. Answer: 1

Rationale: Involvement of more than one central nervous system area, age 15–60 years, two or more separate episodes of symptoms involving different sites, or gradual progression over at least 6 months all meet the criteria for multiple sclerosis.

40. Answer: 4

Rationale: This is a common patient complaint ("worst headache of my life") with a subarachnoid hemorrhage. This patient should have an emergent noncontrast computerized tomography scan of the brain and lumbar puncture with immediate referral to a neurologic surgeon, if either is positive.

41. Answer: 3

Rationale: The speech centers (e.g., Broca, Wernicke areas) are most often located in the left cerebral hemisphere. The patient may also experience weakness of the right side of the body and a right-sided visual deficit as well, depending on the size of the infarct.

42. Answer: 4

Rationale: Mitral valve disease, atrial fibrillation, and endocarditis all precipitate the development of an embolus that can result in an embolic stroke. Diabetes will precipitate occlusive disease of the cerebral arteries and the possible development of a thrombotic stroke, not an embolic stroke.

43. Answer: 2

Rationale: A simple partial seizure is characterized by unilateral paresthesia, numbness and tingling, and spastic movement of the extremities. The patient has no loss of consciousness or incontinence of the bowel or bladder.

44. Answer: 3

Rationale: The characteristics of a benign tremor are fine-to-coarse rhythmic tremors of the hands and feet that increase with activity and may be absent at rest. Frequently the voice is also involved. An ingestion of a small amount of alcohol may decrease symptoms.

45. Answer: 1, 3, 4

Rationale: Bradykinesia and rigidity are expected exam findings because of decreased dopamine resulting in increased inhibition of the thalamus and reduced excitatory input to the motor cortex. Resting tremor is also a result of dopamine depletion and initially is unilateral. Inappropriate affect is not an expected exam finding; however, hallucinations affect up to 40% of patients with Parkinson disease. Dementia and depression are also common psychiatric illnesses with Parkinson disease.

46. Answer: 2

Rationale: It is important to determine first whether the patient has stayed on the medication schedule. The symptoms may be the result of missed medication or overmedication,

especially with pyridostigmine (Mestinon). The symptoms may also be exacerbated by exercise and heat.

47. Answer: 1

Rationale: The clinical presentation is classic for Horner syndrome, especially the lack of sweating (anhidrosis) on the ipsilateral (same) side of the face and neck as the eye symptoms. The patient needs to be referred for further neurologic workup.

48. Answer: 2

Rationale: The upper extremities are affected initially in 40%–60% of cases. A frequent sign is low-amplitude fasciculations. Lower extremity weakness occurs in 20% of cases initially. Spasticity and hyperreflexia are other symptoms as the disorder progresses. Loss of continence is not a common concern. Drooling is one of the bulbar symptoms that can be present early in the disease. Additional bulbar symptoms include dysarthria and dysphagia.

49. Answer: 1

Rationale: Alcoholism, head injury or neurosurgery, and diabetes are all associated with risk of bacterial meningitis. Smoking has not been found to be an associated risk factor.

50. Answer: 2

Rationale: Medications and other types of chemicals (alcohol, illicit substances) can both mask and accentuate movement disorders. Essential tremor affects genders equally. Movement disorders are a concern of both the peripheral and central nervous systems. Parkinson disease is the most common form of movement disorder.

51. Answer: 1, 4

Rationale: MS has a predilection of onset between 20 and 50 years of age and is more common in northern climates. It affects more Caucasians, yet African Americans often have a more aggressive disease course. Women are affected three times more often than men. Several genes have been associated with MS, yet the etiology is still unknown.

52. Answer: 1, 5, 6

Rationale: Recent viral illnesses, respiratory dysfunction, and protein in cerebral fluid analysis are all findings in Guillain-Barré syndrome. Weakness is most profound in the lower extremities, progressing upward, leading to the risk of respiratory dysfunction. Headache and nuchal rigidity are associated with meningitis. Visual changes are associated with multiple sclerosis.

53. Answer: 3

Rationale: Headaches that awaken the patient from sleep can be associated with intracranial tumors. Although nausea can also be present with increased intracranial pressure, intracranial tumors are associated with vomiting. Headache behind one eye is associated with cluster headaches, and photosensitivity is a common finding in migraine headaches.

54. Answer: 1

Rationale: Psychosis is a common comorbidity of PD with up to 40% of patients experiencing hallucinations, especially during late stages. Bowel/bladder dysfunction, extraocular movement disorders, and cardiac complications, including left ventricular pathology, are not associated with PD.

55. Answer: 3

Rationale: Approximately one-half of patients with brain tumors have a seizure. A history of breast, lung, melanoma, renal, and colon cancer increases risk for brain metastases. Gliomas are the most common type of primary malignant brain tumors. Increased intracranial pressure is a late finding in slow-growing tumors.

56. Answer: 3

Rationale: Stroke would take priority over other diagnoses as emergent recognition and management is critical to optimal patient outcomes. Although the other neurologic disorders are important to recognize and treat in a timely manner, cerebrovascular accident would be the highest priority. Amyotrophic lateral sclerosis presents most commonly with unilateral weakness of an upper extremity. Bell's palsy presents most often with facial motor dysfunction. Guillain-Barré syndrome presents with bilateral paresthesia in the lower extremities that moves proximally.

57. Answer: 3

Rationale: Peak occurrence for cerebral edema usually is up to 72 hours after a neurologic insult. It gradually resolves over a 2- to 3-week period. Cerebral edema may be caused by either the initial injury to the neuronal tissue or secondarily in response to the biochemical cellular injury cascade, hypoxia, hypercarbia, or cerebral ischemia.

58. Answer: 1

Rationale: Children between the ages of 3 and 8 months have the highest incidence of bacterial meningitis. The second peak incidence is after age 60.

59. Answer: 1, 2, 3, 6

Rationale: Anxiety, behavioral changes, headaches, and sleep disturbances are associated with postconcussion syndrome. Hallucinations/psychosis and fine tremors are not associated with postconcussion syndrome.

60. Answer: 1, 3

Rationale: MS is most commonly diagnosed in northern Europe, North America, and Australia. It is uncommon around the equator. It affects whites more than other ethnicities, and females three times more often than males. MS is not a result of any one disorder, but it is felt to be caused by environmental, genetic, and autoimmune interactions.

61. Answer: 4

Rationale: Hyperactive deep tendon reflexes are not an expected finding of Parkinson disease. Asymmetric deep tendon reflexes may be present. Observing for flexed posture is a cardinal sign in the attempt to maintain a secure center of gravity with quick, short steps. Passive flexion/extension of the forearm with rigidity and cogwheeling is an expected finding, as is imbalance with sudden pulling of the shoulders from behind the patient.

62. Answer: 4

Rationale: Homonymous hemianopia is the loss of the vision in one-half of the visual field. Either the right or left field of vision may be affected. It is most often caused by a lesion or pathology in the optic tract or occipital lobe.

Pharmacology

63. Answer: 4

Rationale: Ramelteon (Rozerem) is a melatonin-receptor agonist, which has the lowest side-effect profile for the elderly. Ramelteon should be avoided in severe hepatic impairment. Diphenhydramine (first-generation antihistamine), doxepin (tricyclic antidepressant), and oxazepam (benzodiazepine) have anticholinergic properties including risk for sedation, confusion, falls, and urinary retention in the elderly patient.

64. Answer: 2

Rationale: Herbal products beginning with "G" are associated with anticoagulation. *Ginkgo biloba*, ginger, and garlic also contain similar properties. The patient's use of ginseng places him at higher risk for cerebral bleeding. Knowing prescribed medications and over-the-counter and herbal products is critical when developing differentials following an injury. Metaxalone, omeprazole, and acetaminophen are not recognized for anticoagulant/antiplatelet properties.

65. Answer: 2

Rationale: Although most medication is discontinued after 4 years of no seizure activity, a confirmatory EEG should be obtained. Not all seizure patients require medication; referral to and monitoring by a neurologist are appropriate.

66. Answer: 1, 3, 5

Rationale: Amlodipine, a calcium channel blocker, would be appropriate for prevention of migraines, as it will stabilize arteries reducing vasomotor dilation and constriction. Labetalol, a beta blocker, stabilizes blood pressure and pulse rate and reduces catecholamines, which are associated with anxiety. Beta blockers should be avoided in patients with unstable asthma. Sertraline (Zoloft) is a selective serotonin reuptake inhibitor, which assists in balance of neurochemicals. Weight gain and sexual side effects are potential side effects.

67. Answer: 1

Rationale: The patient's symptoms are diagnostic of trigeminal neuralgia. This disorder responds well to anticonvulsant therapy (carbamazepine). Indomethacin and prednisone reduce inflammation but are not considered first-line therapy in trigeminal neuralgia. Valacyclovir is an antiviral used to treat herpes zoster. This patient's pain has several similarities with herpes zoster, but herpes zoster is more continuous pain, including while trying to sleep.

68. Answer: 1

Rationale: The younger patient of the group even at age 65 would be at lowest risk for cholinergic side effects and may possibly benefit because of the problem of chronic diarrhea and the anticipated drying effects of these products (dry mouth, risk of urinary retention). Anticholinergics are associated with increasing intraocular pressure, making them a high-risk product for a patient with glaucoma. The associated urinary hesitancy and retention with anticholinergics will worsen the symptoms of benign prostatic hypertrophy. Anticholinergics are associated with tachycardia, making them a poor choice in either controlled or uncontrolled atrial fibrillation.

69. Answer: 1

Rationale: Patients with essential tremors are at higher risk for alcohol abuse as alcohol reduces the tremor. Caffeine products (tea, soda, coffee, chocolate) and over-the-counter cold/cough medications worsen tremor. Beta blockers are used to reduce tremors, not angiotensin-converting enzyme inhibitors.

70. Answer: 3

Rationale: Carbidopa/levodopa (Sinemet) induces a number of adverse reactions, including hypotension, gastrointestinal (GI) upset, psychosis, and motor complications. For best absorption, it should not be given around meals, despite GI side effects. It exerts no known effect on slowing disease progression.

71. Answer: 3

Rationale: Sumatriptan targets 5-hydroxytryptamine receptors in the brain that are associated with headaches. Triptans cause vasoconstriction, which can place patients at risk for cardiac and cerebral ischemia, especially with a medical history of preexisting cardiac and vascular disease. Acetaminophen, amlodipine, and prochlorperazine do not place the patient at risk for vasoconstriction.

72. Answer: 2

Rationale: NMDA receptor antagonists (e.g., memantine) are recognized as the class for management of moderate-to-severe Alzheimer dementia. This group of medications control the effects of glutamate (the major excitatory transmitter in the central nervous system) at NMDA receptors, which are believed to play a critical role in learning and memory. The NMDA receptor regulates calcium entry into the neuron. SSRIs are antidepressants used in the treatment of depression and anxiety. Central α_2 agonists are used in the treatment of hypertension.

73. Answer: 3

Rationale: Abortive medications for migraines cause cranial vasoconstriction, which will be generalized to all vessels, including cardiac. A history of cardiac disease, especially ischemia, increases risk for cardiac event.

74. Answer: 3

Rationale: Timely intervention with thrombolytics has the best evidence for patient outcomes. The goal from onset of symptoms to thrombolytics is 180 minutes. The risk of disability is greatly reduced with thrombolytic use, and the benefits outweigh the risk of a bleed.

75. Answer: 4

Rationale: Macrolide antibiotics, such as erythromycin and clarithromycin, can increase the plasma concentration of carbamazepine; therefore when these medications are used together, carbamazepine levels must be closely monitored.

76. Answer: 3

Rationale: Onset of drug action and relief of trigeminal neuralgia symptoms occur in 24 hours, usually in 4–6 hours. Laboratory tests are usually monitored based on the specific medication, not a peak and trough. These medications were first developed to treat epilepsy and fall in a class called antiepileptic drugs, although several have been found to be effective therapy for other, nonepileptic, neurologic disorders, including TN.

77. Answer: 1, 2, 3

Rationale: For symptom relief during an acute attack, benzodiazepines (diazepam or lorazepam) decrease vertigo and anxiety, antihistamines (meclizine/dimenhydrinate) decrease vertigo and nausea, anticholinergics (atropine) lessen abnormal sensations, and antiemetics (prochlorperazine) reduce nausea and motion sickness. Diuretics as a maintenance medication may assist in reducing acute attacks by decreasing endolymphatic pressure and volume; however, there is insufficient evidence to recommend routine use. Tricyclic antidepressants and antibiotics are not first-line medications for an acute attack.

12

Gastrointestinal & Liver

Physical Exam & Diagnostic Tests

1. The family nurse practitioner is preparing to examine the abdomen of a patient. What is the correct sequence in which to conduct the exam?
   1. Inspection, palpation, percussion, auscultation.
   2. Palpation, percussion, auscultation, inspection.
   3. Percussion, palpation, auscultation, inspection.
   4. Inspection, auscultation, percussion, palpation.

2. The family nurse practitioner is seeing a 22-year-old male who recently returned from Thailand on a 2-month mission trip. He had a sudden onset of five to seven loose, watery stools a day for the past month. He has had abdominal cramping, nausea, and stool urgency, but no blood. He has been taking bismuth subsalicylate (Pepto-Bismol) without any relief. He is unable to return to work. What would be the best course of action?
   1. Stool testing for culture and sensitivity, treatment with loperamide (Imodium), and ciprofloxacin (Cipro) 750 mg single dose.
   2. Stool testing for ova and parasites, treatment with bismuth subsalicylate, and levofloxacin (Levaquin) 500 mg single dose.
   3. Stool testing for fecal leukocytes, treatment with probiotics.
   4. Stool testing for culture and sensitivity, treatment with azithromycin (Zithromax) 1000 mg single dose.

3. When obtaining a history from a 21-year-old female adult patient with abdominal pain, which of the following should initially be assessed?
   1. Food effects on the pain.
   2. Location and onset of the pain.
   3. Change of pain with bowel movements.
   4. First day of last menstrual period.

4. To test for a positive obturator sign in a patient with abdominal pain, the family nurse practitioner:
   1. Passively flexes the right thigh at the hip, and medially rotates the leg from the 90-degree hip/knee flexion position.
   2. Asks the patient to take a deep breath while palpating in the abdominal right upper quadrant.
   3. Places his/her right hand above the patient's knee and has the patient raise the leg.
   4. Palpates the right abdomen one-third of the distance from the anterior superior iliac spine to the umbilicus.

5. The family nurse practitioner is performing the initial physical exam on a 51-year-old man. The history reveals that the patient's father died of colon cancer, but the patient is asymptomatic and has not had any screening for colon cancer. What are the first-line recommendations for screening this patient?
   1. Double contrast barium enema and flexible sigmoidoscopy.
   2. Computed tomography (CT) colonography and stool DNA testing.
   3. Colonoscopy and fecal immunochemical test (FIT).
   4. Fecal occult blood and capsule endoscopy.

6. A 76-year-old male patient has end-stage liver disease. Which of the following laboratory abnormalities is most likely to be seen?
   1. Sodium 145 mEq/L.
   2. Bilirubin, total serum 0.9 mg/dL.
   3. Albumin 5.0 g/dL.
   4. International normalized ratio (INR) 2.5.

7. The family nurse practitioner is obtaining recommended testing on patients born between 1945 and 1965 per the Centers for Disease Control and Prevention. Once a positive hepatitis C virus (HCV) Ab (hepatitis C antibody) test is found, what would the next step be?
   1. Call the patient and explain that hepatitis C is active and treatment is needed.
   2. Repeat the HCV Ab test to ensure it is positive.
   3. Test with a hepatitis B panel.
   4. Test for HCV ribonucleic acid (RNA).

8. A 25-year-old male patient comes in complaining that his girlfriend has been diagnosed with acute hepatitis B and he is afraid he may have it also. When testing the patient, the family nurse practitioner would determine a diagnosis of acute hepatitis B (HB) infection from which of the following blood test results:
   1. Negative HB surface antigen (HBsAg) and positive HB core antibody (HBcAb).
   2. Negative HBsAg and positive HB surface antibody (HBsAb).
   3. Positive HBsAg and positive HBcAb.
   4. Negative HBcAb and negative HBsAb.

9. The diagnosis of early acute pancreatitis would be considered by the family nurse practitioner based on a history of severe, constant, acute upper abdominal pain that radiates to the back and which of the following laboratory results?
   1. White blood cell (WBC) count of 10,300/mm³.
   2. Serum alanine aminotransferase of 60 IU/L.
   3. Serum amylase of 100 U/L.
   4. Serum lipase of 850 U/L.

10. A 74-year-old male complains of rectal bleeding for the past year. He has no change in bowel habits and denies abdominal pain, weight loss, and rectal pain. He has seen blood in the toilet water and when wiping approximately once every few weeks, but lately the bleeding has increased. He had a colonoscopy for colon cancer screening 5 years ago. The family nurse practitioner should:
    1. Send the patient home with a fecal occult blood test.
    2. Schedule colonoscopy.
    3. Schedule a flexible sigmoidoscopy.
    4. Schedule a double contrast barium enema.

11. An overweight, middle-aged woman has right upper quadrant pain that radiates to her right subscapular area and is severe and persistent. She is also experiencing anorexia, nausea, and a fever. Her most recent meal was a double quarter-pound hamburger with cheese, French fries, and a vanilla milkshake. Based on this information, the family nurse practitioner examines the abdomen and percusses for costovertebral angle tenderness. The abdomen is tender in the right upper quadrant. Which of the following signs, if positive, corresponds to the correct diagnosis?
    1. Obturator sign; patient has appendicitis.
    2. Costovertebral angle tenderness; patient has a urinary tract infection.
    3. Murphy's sign; patient has cholecystitis.
    4. McBurney's point sign; patient has acute appendicitis.

12. The family nurse practitioner is seeing a healthy 80-year-old male who has never had colon cancer screening. What is the most appropriate approach for him?
    1. Because he is over 75 years of age, he does not need any screening.
    2. Recommend screening with computed tomography (CT) colonography.
    3. Recommend testing with fecal occult blood and, if positive, then perform a colonoscopy.
    4. Recommend screening with a colonoscopy.

13. The family nurse practitioner reviews a patient's laboratory results that reveal a positive *Helicobacter pylori* stool antigen test. The family nurse practitioner would want to treat this if the patient complained of:
    1. Upper abdominal pain.
    2. Altered bowel habits.
    3. Dysphagia.
    4. Nausea.

14. While discussing colon cancer screening a patient whose mother had colon cancer asks the family nurse practitioner if she can have the new "blood test" instead of a colonoscopy. What would be the best response to the patient?
    1. The test can be used by anyone if they request.
    2. A colonoscopy is a high-risk procedure so we should consider alternatives.
    3. The test is not approved by the U.S. Food and Drug Administration (FDA) yet.
    4. The test is approved by the FDA and is recommended for average risk patients who decline first-line testing.

15. The family nurse practitioner knows that microbiologic testing is recommended for travelers' diarrhea when the:
    1. Diarrhea is severe or persistent or if anyone has failed empiric therapy.
    2. Diarrhea is bothersome to the patient and has not been treated.
    3. Diarrhea has lasted at least 4 days and has not responded to clear liquids.
    4. Patient has traveled outside the United States and is having moderate diarrhea.

16. Which of these symptoms is **not** considered an alarm symptom requiring upper endoscopy?
    1. Dysphagia.
    2. Bright red blood from the rectum.
    3. Weight loss.
    4. Odynophagia.

17. To assess for ascites in a patient with heart failure, the family nurse practitioner will test for shifting dullness. What result would indicate ascites is likely present?
    1. Dullness shifts to the more dependent side while tympany shifts to the top.
    2. Dullness shifts to the top and tympany disappears.
    3. This test does not indicate ascites.
    4. The border between tympany and dullness usually stays relatively constant.

18. Which hormone is responsible for stimulating the gallbladder contraction and secretion of enzyme-rich pancreatic fluid and is used to test gallbladder function in a hepatobiliary iminodiacetic scan (HIDA) scan?
    1. Gastrin.
    2. Gastric inhibitory peptides.
    3. Cholecystokinin.
    4. Secretin.

19. Which laboratory testing would not be useful when evaluating elevated liver function tests (LFTs) (transaminases)?
    1. Iron studies: ferritin and iron saturation.
    2. Chronic hepatitis panel for hepatitis B and C.
    3. Antinuclear antibodies (ANA) and smooth muscle antibodies (SMA).
    4. Vitamin D level.

20. The family nurse practitioner is explaining a patient's laboratory work following an acute hepatitis A (HAV) infection. What is the significance of a positive anti-HAV immunoglobulin (Ig)G?
    1. Indicates immunity to HAV.
    2. Indicates an acute HAV infection.
    3. Indicates patient needs HAV vaccine.
    4. Indicates patient has not had the HAV vaccine.

Disorders

21. A 20-year-old female patient in her third year of college presents with altered stool consistency and frequency for the last 6 months. She notes there is no pattern and she cannot predict when she will have diarrhea. She notes increased stress as she prepares for final exams. The family nurse practitioner suspects irritable bowel syndrome (IBS). What other history would assist in a diagnosis of IBS?
    1. Weight loss of 15 lbs.
    2. Lower abdominal cramping that is associated with a bowel movement.
    3. Symptoms occur frequently after she has cereal with milk in the morning.
    4. Stomach upsets in high school.

22. A sudden onset of diarrhea that consists of five to six loose stools a day and awakens the patient at night with cramping, but without blood in the stools, would most likely be caused by:
    1. Infection.
    2. Irritable bowel syndrome.
    3. Ischemic colitis.
    4. Lactose intolerance.

23. The family nurse practitioner is discussing *Clostridium difficile* (CD) infection with the family of a 68-year-old female who lives with them and who was recently diagnosed with CD infection. Which of the following statements would be the most important for the family to understand?
    1. CD infection has been reported to recur after an initial occurrence 50% of the time within 8 weeks.
    2. CD infection is the leading cause of health care–associated infections in hospitalized patients.
    3. Handwashing with alcohol-based hand sanitizer should be done in the home.
    4. Have the patient use a separate bathroom from the rest of the family.

24. The family nurse practitioner suspects peritonitis in a patient. What assessment finding is most indicative of peritonitis?
    1. Palpate and watch for a positive Murphy's sign.
    2. Perform a rectal exam and test the stool for blood.
    3. Auscultate the abdomen for increased bowel sounds.
    4. Palpate for rebound tenderness.

25. An older adult woman is noted to have iron-deficiency anemia. She has no pain or rectal bleeding. What history would raise the suspicion of a gastric ulcer?
    1. Symptoms of acid reflux for the last 2 years, occurring at least 3 times a week.
    2. Postmenopausal with no recent history of vaginal bleeding.
    3. Weight loss of 10 lb in the last 2 months.
    4. An ankle sprain requiring 800 mg of ibuprofen three times a day for the last 6 weeks.

26. A 45-year-old male is seen for anal itching and a rash. Symptoms have been present for 3 months and are worse after a bowel movement and at night. He uses medicated wipes to clean his perianal area several times a day. He notes intense itching, burning, and pain around the anus. He has no comorbidities and is otherwise healthy. He has tried hemorrhoid cream with no relief. The family nurse practitioner suspects pruritus ani. What would be the best treatment for him?
    1. Topical hydrocortisone cream applied to the perianal area three times a day for 6 weeks.
    2. Antifungal cream applied twice a day for 2 weeks.
    3. Keep the perianal skin dry and clean with water and avoid severe rubbing.
    4. Sitz baths four times a day and apply a moisture barrier cream such as zinc oxide daily for 3 weeks.

27. A patient with a chief complaint of diarrhea alternating with constipation, intermittent cramping, and bloating and relieved by a bowel movement is most likely:
    1. Antibiotic-induced diarrhea.
    2. Inflammatory bowel disease.
    3. Gastroenteritis.
    4. Irritable bowel syndrome (IBS).

28. Which patient presentation would most likely suggest dysphagia caused by esophageal spasm?
    1. They usually have more difficulty swallowing solids than liquids.
    2. There is a long history of gastroesophageal reflux.
    3. They have difficulty swallowing both solids and liquids.
    4. They have marked weight loss.

29. Which problem would most likely worsen the symptoms of gastroesophageal reflux disease?
    1. Small sliding hiatal hernia.
    2. An empty stomach when lying down.
    3. Gaining 10 lb over a period of months.
    4. Gastroparesis.

30. A patient comes to the emergency department concerned about pain and swelling in his groin. He tells the family nurse practitioner that his doctor said he has an incarcerated hernia. Which assessment finding correlates with an incarcerated hernia?
    1. Hernia that easily moves back and forth across the abdominal wall.
    2. Hernia that protrudes from the groin area and cannot be reduced into the abdomen.
    3. Hernia that is very painful to palpation with significant abdominal swelling.
    4. Hernia that decreases in size when the patient increases intraabdominal pressure.

31. Which finding most likely indicates a need for an endoscopy in patients with heartburn?
    1. Any new onset of heartburn.
    2. Symptoms persisting after 8–12 weeks of empiric therapy.
    3. Negative *Helicobacter pylori* test.
    4. Good response to empiric treatment after 7–10 days.

32. The family nurse practitioner has received a right upper quadrant ultrasound report that states: moderate hepatic steatosis, also known as nonalcoholic fatty liver disease (NAFLD). The 60-year-old male patient had elevated liver enzymes with an alanine transaminase (ALT) of 74 U/L and aspartate transaminase (AST) of 82 U/L. He has type 2 diabetes, hypertension, and a body mass index (BMI) of 36. Which statement below is most accurate concerning NAFLD?
    1. The most common cause of death in NAFLD is cardiovascular disease.
    2. He needs to consider bariatric surgery to improve his liver function.
    3. The most common cause of death in NAFLD is hepatocellular cancer.
    4. He has a 50% risk of developing cirrhosis.

33. The family nurse practitioner understands that hepatitis B can be transmitted through blood and blood products. What is another mode of transmission of hepatitis B?
    1. Respiratory contact.
    2. Arthropod vectors.
    3. Fecal-oral route.
    4. Perinatal exposure.

34. A 54-year-old female complains of intermittent crampy abdominal pain over the last 18 hours, loss of appetite, vomiting, abdominal bloating, and inability to have a bowel movement. She has a history of hysterectomy 20 years ago, cholecystectomy 5 years ago, and two laparoscopies for abdominal pain over the last 4 years. The family nurse practitioner sends her to the emergency room because the nurse practitioner suspects:
    1. Appendicitis.
    2. Small bowel obstruction (SBO).
    3. Biliary ductal obstruction.
    4. Gastroenteritis.

35. The family nurse practitioner sees a 65-year-old female with constipation. She reports a history of "slow bowels" for most of her life and has taken laxatives on a regular basis. She has had worsening symptoms requiring her to increase bisacodyl (Correctol) from every other day to daily over the last 3 months. She still has a stool every 3–4 days and can have no stool for 7 days or more at times. She has no abdominal pain and never feels that she has a "good bowel movement." What is her most likely diagnosis?
    1. Loss of bowel function related to chronic stimulant laxative use.
    2. Pelvic floor dyssynergia.
    3. Colonic inertia.
    4. Irritable bowel syndrome—constipation predominant.

36. Which is true about enterobiasis (pinworm infection)?
    1. The parasite is in the soil and enters the body through the feet. It can cause anemia.
    2. The parasite causes pruritus around the anus because the gravid females exit through the anus at night and lay eggs on the skin. The human is the only host of this parasite.
    3. The eggs of this parasite enter the body by ingestion of dirt (pica) or dirt on unwashed vegetables that contain the eggs, or through water containing the eggs.
    4. This parasite is a protozoan. The source is usually contaminated water, but it is spread from person to person by fecal-oral contamination.

37. Nonpharmacologic management of gastroesophageal reflux disease (GERD) includes which of the following?
    1. Weight reduction and sleep with head of bed elevated 4–6 inches with blocks.
    2. Lying down and resting after meals and weight reduction.
    3. Drinking large amounts of fluids with meals and avoiding alcohol.
    4. Avoiding mint, orange juice, and milk.

38. When a patient complains of chronic constipation with no alarm symptoms, what should be the first step?
    1. Colonoscopy to rule out blockage from colon cancer.
    2. Defecography to rule out rectocele.
    3. Increasing fiber intake to 30–35 g a day.
    4. Physical therapy to strengthen pelvic floor muscles.

39. What is an organism associated with the etiology of peptic ulcer disease?
    1. *Streptococcus pneumoniae*.
    2. *Helicobacter pylori*.
    3. *Moraxella catarrhalis*.
    4. *Staphylococcus aureus*.

40. What is a common cause of cirrhosis and need for liver transplantation in the United States?
    1. Hepatitis A.
    2. Nonalcoholic fatty liver disease (NALFD).
    3. Chronic hepatitis B.
    4. Alcohol ingestion.

41. What is the name of prolapse of the anal cushion, made up of vascular, connective, and muscular tissue, through the anal canal below the dentate line?
    1. Rectal prolapse.
    2. External hemorrhoid.
    3. Rectocele.
    4. Internal hemorrhoid.

42. Which of the following is an acute illness with jaundice, anorexia, malaise, arthralgias, an incubation period of 2–6 months, a chronic and acute form, and that is transmitted by parenteral, sexual, and perinatal routes?
    1. Hepatitis A.
    2. Hepatitis B.
    3. Hepatitis C.
    4. Hepatitis E.

43. A patient with a history of cholelithiasis presents to the office complaining of increased right upper quadrant (RUQ) abdominal pain. The family nurse practitioner would arrange immediate hospital admission for possible, prompt intervention if the history also showed that the patient is:
    1. 40 years old and having diarrhea.
    2. 75 years old and diabetic.
    3. 5 weeks pregnant.
    4. 23 years old and obese.

44. A 65-year-old male presents to the family nurse practitioner for evaluation of years of "heartburn" and recent significant weight loss (30 lb in 1 month). He has been taking antacids and an oral histamine 2 receptor antagonist (H_2 RA) for "years off and on," and has had some relief of his symptoms. He has a 60 pack-year history of cigarette smoking and drinks alcohol daily. What differential diagnosis must the family nurse practitioner consider first?
    1. Gastric ulcer.
    2. Gastroesophageal reflux disease (GERD).
    3. Esophageal cancer.
    4. Lung cancer.

45. A 70-year-old female complains of increased gas and bloating over the last 6 months. She has difficulty controlling the gas and expels it frequently. She also notes intermittent diarrhea after eating. The family nurse practitioner had seen the patient 6 months ago for bronchitis but had not treated her with antibiotics. She notes symptoms are worse when she has cheese and ice cream. She denies lactose intolerance. The following laboratory tests were normal: complete blood count, comprehensive metabolic panel, and urinalysis. Her thyroid-stimulating hormone (TSH) was 5.2, with upper limit of normal 4.5, and a *Helicobacter pylori* IgG antibody was elevated. What is the most likely cause of her symptoms?
    1. Lactose intolerance.
    2. Celiac disease.
    3. Hyperthyroidism.
    4. *H. pylori* infection.

46. An adult patient presents to the family nurse practitioner complaining of weakness and vomiting. He gives a history of "several" drinks per day for the last 22 years and cirrhosis, diagnosed 6 months ago. The family nurse practitioner questions the patient about excessive bleeding. The patient reports two episodes of hematemesis. What emergent condition is the family nurse practitioner most concerned about?
    1. Bleeding peptic ulcer.
    2. Excessive nosebleed.
    3. Hemoptysis.
    4. Esophageal varices.

47. A 66-year-old male was sent to the family nurse practitioner after an evaluation for a cough by pulmonary function test. His pulmonary function test was normal, and he is not responding to fluticasone propionate (Flovent) HFA or albuterol (Proventil HFA). He has had a dry cough for the past year that is worse after eating. Occasionally he wakens at night coughing. He denies chest pain, dyspnea, fever, or signs of an upper respiratory illness. He has type 2 diabetes and hyperlipidemia and is taking metformin and atorvastatin. He has no history of heart disease and had a negative ECG. He had gained 20 lb but his weight has been stable for the past year. What is the likely cause of his cough?
    1. Environmental allergies including pollen.
    2. Exposure to fumes at his job where he is an auto mechanic.
    3. Sinusitis and postnasal drainage.
    4. Gastroesophageal reflux disease (GERD).

48. A 19-year-old female presents to the family nurse practitioner for evaluation of 2 days of increasing crampy abdominal pain. She states that she also has some mild nausea, anorexia, and a low-grade fever. The patient states that the pain is periumbilical. Her STAT complete blood count reveals a slightly elevated white blood count but is otherwise normal. What is the family nurse practitioner's next step in the care of this patient?
    1. Refer to a gynecologist for evaluation of possible ectopic pregnancy.
    2. Order a computed tomography (CT) of the abdomen and refer to surgeon for evaluation of possible appendicitis.
    3. Observe overnight and reassess the next day.
    4. Place on a clear liquid diet and have patient watch for increasing symptoms.

49. A 54-year-old female has early alcoholic cirrhosis diagnosed by a liver biopsy. While teaching the patient to manage her symptoms, the family nurse practitioner instructs that it is most important that the patient:
    1. Take a daily vitamin E supplement.
    2. Decrease her alcohol intake to fewer than two drinks a day.
    3. Abstain from alcohol.
    4. Maintain a nutritious diet.

50. A 72-year-old female presents with fever, leukocytosis, and a sudden onset of lower left quadrant pain for the last 12 hours. She has not had a bowel movement since the pain began. What would be the family nurse practitioner's top differential diagnosis?
    1. Appendicitis.
    2. Diverticulitis.
    3. Irritable bowel syndrome.
    4. Ruptured ovarian cyst.

51. The family nurse practitioner knows that in patients with ulcerative colitis that involves the entire colon (universal or pancolitis), careful surveillance of the colon is required because of an increased risk of:
    1. Colon cancer.
    2. Diverticulosis.
    3. Ischemic colitis.
    4. Irritable bowel syndrome.

52. Which is true of peptic ulcer disease (PUD) in patients over the age of 65 years?
    1. Smoking does not increase the risk of PUD.
    2. Duodenal ulcers are more common in older adults.
    3. Perforation is a common complication.
    4. Weight loss and anorexia are often the only symptoms.

53. Which is true of early cancer of the esophagus in the older adult patient?
    1. Heavy alcohol intake and smoking increase the risk for adenocarcinoma of the esophagus.
    2. Esophageal cancer is associated with high caffeine use.
    3. Dysphagia for solids and cough may be the first symptoms.
    4. Boring-type midchest pain indicates mediastinal involvement and requires immediate surgery.

54. A 32-year-old patient presents with a complaint of intermittent diarrhea and cramping for the last 2 years. Screening blood tests reveal iron-deficiency anemia and elevated liver transaminases. What does the family nurse practitioner suspect?
    1. Hepatitis B.
    2. Celiac sprue.
    3. Salmonella infection.
    4. Bleeding peptic ulcer.

55. In a patient suspected of having celiac sprue with elevated tissue transglutaminase antibodies (tTG) but negative duodenal biopsy for villi blunting and celiac sprue, the family nurse practitioner knows:
    1. The patient may have a negative biopsy because of being on a gluten-free diet for 3 weeks.
    2. The positive antibodies are likely a false-positive result.
    3. The patient may have celiac disease.
    4. The biopsy may be a false-negative result.

56. A young female adult reports that she had the flu and recovered 2 weeks ago. She reports resolution of her symptoms, except she continues to have nausea, decreased appetite, and early satiety. What does the family nurse practitioner suspect?
    1. A relapse of the influenza infection.
    2. Postviral gastroparesis.
    3. Vertigo, causing nausea, related to a possible ear infection.
    4. Peptic ulcer from taking ibuprofen.

57. Irritable bowel syndrome (IBS) can produce which of the following symptoms?
    1. Abdominal cramping, rectal bleeding, and diarrhea.
    2. Diarrhea alternating with constipation, but no pain.
    3. Abdominal cramping, diarrhea, and fecal incontinence.
    4. Abdominal cramping, diarrhea, and bloating.

58. When discussing diet with a patient with irritable bowel syndrome (IBS), the family nurse practitioner tells the patient to avoid:
    1. Simple sugars.
    2. Dairy products.
    3. Red meat.
    4. Vegetables.

59. What should patient education for a patient with nonalcoholic fatty liver disease include?
    1. Working on lowering cholesterol intake.
    2. Discontinuing any statin medication.
    3. Beginning exercise and working on weight loss with diet.
    4. Taking vitamin A 15,000 IU daily.

60. This viral strain that can cause gastroenteritis is seen in adolescents and adults. It has a short incubation period (18–72 hours) and short duration of symptoms (24–48 hours). It is characterized by an abrupt onset of nausea and abdominal cramps, followed by vomiting and diarrhea, and is often accompanied by headache and myalgia. What is the most likely cause?
    1. *Campylobacter.*
    2. *Norovirus* (Norwalk).
    3. *Rotavirus.*
    4. *Cytomegalovirus.*

61. A family nurse practitioner is seeing a 20-year-old male who has returned from Ecuador after a 2-week trip. He is complaining of 10 days of diarrhea—three to four loose stools a day without blood that is not limiting his regular activities. It is important to recognize the severity of the symptoms. How would the family nurse practitioner classify his diarrhea?
    1. Mild.
    2. Moderate.
    3. Severe.
    4. Persistent.

62. What are the characteristics of visceral abdominal pain?
    1. Steady, aching pain more precisely localized over the involved structure.
    2. Felt in more distant sites, may be felt superficially or deeply, but it is localized.
    3. Gnawing, burning, cramping, difficult to localize.
    4. None of the above.

63. When evaluating acute abdominal pain, what characteristics would require emergent care?
    1. 3-week history of bloating, nausea, and upper abdominal fullness.
    2. 3-month history of nonspecific upper abdominal discomfort.
    3. 1-year history of worsening rising retrosternal burning pain occurring daily.
    4. Sudden knifelike epigastric pain.

64. A patient complains of melena—black, tarry stools. The family nurse practitioner knows that this:
    1. Has no pathologic significance.
    2. Involves a loss of blood less than 30 mL.
    3. Is likely bleeding from the colon.
    4. May likely be bleeding from the esophagus or stomach.

65. Management of nausea and vomiting is based on the underlying cause. Which of the causes listed below is the most common cause of nausea and vomiting in adults and children?
    1. Food poisoning.
    2. Peptic ulcer disease.
    3. Gastroenteritis.
    4. Cholecystitis.

66. A 54-year-old female complains of right upper quadrant (RUQ) abdominal pain, nausea, and vomiting that began last night about 4 hours after eating a rich, fatty meal. She has a temperature of 100°F and a palpable RUQ mass. What is the most likely diagnosis?
    1. Cholecystitis.
    2. Acute pancreatitis.
    3. Acute hepatitis A.
    4. Appendicitis.

67. A 21-year-old white college female complains of fatigue, RLQ abdominal pain, and diarrhea for the last 2 months. She has lost 10 lb and notes chills periodically. She denies rectal bleeding. She notes she is stressed about final exams. The family nurse practitioner would be most concerned about:
    1. Irritable bowel syndrome.
    2. Intestinal infection.
    3. Crohn's disease.
    4. Ulcerative colitis.

68. What would be two important teaching points to provide to a patient who has chronic pancreatitis?
    1. Take full course of antibiotics as prescribed to treat inflammation.
    2. Avoid alcohol consumption.
    3. Take enzyme supplements after meals.
    4. Discontinue tobacco use.
    5. Encourage a low-protein diet.

69. Which of the following three findings are associated with a diagnosis of acute hepatitis A (HAV)?
    1. Early appearance of anti-HAV immunoglobulin (Ig) M in blood work.
    2. Symptoms of jaundice, fever, malaise, bilirubinuria, right upper quadrant abdominal pain.
    3. Symptoms of rash, hematuria, hypotension, steatorrhea, fever, splenomegaly.
    4. Elevated bilirubin, alkaline phosphatase, and aspartate transaminase (AST)/alanine transaminase (ALT).
    5. Negative anti-HAV IgG serology.

Pharmacology

70. The family nurse practitioner is examining a 30-year-old obese man with a BMI of 35 who complains of almost daily indigestion and heartburn for the past year with a strong acid taste in the mouth about an hour after meals and frequent belching and awakening at night with choking. The history is negative for chronic illnesses and alarm symptoms. A diagnosis of gastroesophageal reflux disease (GERD) is made. What is the best initial treatment for the patient?
    1. Lansoprazole (Prevacid) 15 mg with breakfast daily.
    2. Hyoscyamine (Levsin) 0.125 mg tid 15 minutes before eating.
    3. Famotidine (Pepcid) 20 mg bid.
    4. Omeprazole (Prilosec) 20 mg every morning 30–60 minutes before breakfast.

71. A 42-year-old female complains of rectal pain after a bowel movement that persists for an hour. This began 10 weeks ago, after a particularly hard, large stool. Since then she has had pain with every stool and has noted a slight amount of bleeding on the tissue paper. The family nurse practitioner suspects an anal fissure. What would be the most appropriate treatment for a chronic anal fissure?
    1. Sitz baths, psyllium fiber, and bulking agents.
    2. Topical lidocaine gel.
    3. Pramoxine-hydrocortisone cream (Analpram-HC singles rectal).
    4. Topical nitrate ointment 0.2%.

72. Which of the following would be prescribed by the family nurse practitioner as initial treatment for a 72-year-old female with uncomplicated peptic ulcer disease (PUD) and negative *Helicobacter pylori* by stool antigen?
    1. Clarithromycin.
    2. Tetracycline and metronidazole and a histamine 2 receptor antagonist (H_2 RA).
    3. Pantoprazole (Protonix).
    4. Bismuth (Pepto-Bismol).

73. After percutaneous or permucosal exposure to a hepatitis B source, what is the appropriate treatment for the patient?
    1. In an unvaccinated patient, begin the hepatitis B series.
    2. In a person with a positive hepatitis B surface antibody, no treatment is necessary.
    3. In a vaccinated person with a negative antihepatitis B surface antigen, give hepatitis B immune globulin (HBIG), and initiate a new hepatitis B vaccine series.
    4. In a patient with a positive antihepatitis B surface antibody who completed the entire hepatitis B vaccine series, give a hepatitis B booster.

74. Successful treatment for an adult patient with *Helicobacter pylori*–induced peptic ulcer disease requires therapy with which regimen?
    1. Clarithromycin, amoxicillin, and omeprazole (Prilosec) for 14 days.
    2. Bismuth (Pepto-Bismol), cephalexin (Keflex), and metronidazole (Flagyl) for 10 days.
    3. Amoxicillin, bismuth (Pepto-Bismol), metronidazole (Flagyl), and cimetidine (Tagamet) for 10 days.
    4. Clarithromycin, tetracycline, cephalexin (Keflex), and lansoprazole for 14 days.

75. What is a primary therapy for patients with mild ulcerative colitis?
    1. Metronidazole (Flagyl).
    2. Mesalamine (Asacol).
    3. Ciprofloxacin (Cipro).
    4. Prednisone (Deltasone).

76. For a patient exposed to household or sexual contacts with hepatitis A, the family nurse practitioner would:
    1. Give immunoglobulin 0.02 mL/kg as soon as possible but no later than 2 weeks after exposure.
    2. Give one dose of hepatitis B immune globulin (HBIG) and immunoglobulin 0.02 mL/kg as soon as possible.
    3. Give immunoglobulin 0.02 mL/kg and two doses of HBIG.
    4. Understand that no injections are needed.

77. A young woman presents with a history of recent unprotected sexual activity (in the last 2 weeks) with a partner now diagnosed with hepatitis B. She is currently asymptomatic and does not recall having a vaccine in the past. What is the best action for the family nurse practitioner?
    1. Obtain a hepatitis B e antibody test (anti-HBe).
    2. Administer one dose of hepatitis B immune globulin (HBIG).
    3. Obtain a viral load for hepatitis B.
    4. Administer one dose of HBIG and initiate vaccination.

78. What condition is a contraindication for the administration of the hepatitis B vaccine?
    1. Pregnancy.
    2. Lactation.
    3. Severe hypersensitivity.
    4. Age greater than 60 years.

79. A 78-year-old patient was treated for community-acquired pneumonia with azithromycin and developed diarrhea 1 week after completing treatment. He is having six to seven loose watery stools a day. He is afebrile and his white blood cell count was 10.1 K/µL. He has tested positive for *Clostridium difficile* (CD) toxins A and B by stool enzyme immunoassay. The family nurse practitioner knows the first-line treatment should be:
    1. Probiotics (*Lactobacillus acidophilus* and *L. casei*) once a day for 4 weeks.
    2. Vancomycin (Vancocin) 125 mg PO qid for 10 days.
    3. Metronidazole 500 mg PO tid for 10 days.
    4. Vancomycin 500 mg PO qid for 4 days and metronidazole 500 mg IV tid for 3 days.

80. A patient takes bismuth subsalicylate (Pepto-Bismol). The patient calls the family nurse practitioner to report that his stools are unusually dark. He is not experiencing any gastric discomfort, orthostatic hypotension, or increased lethargy. How would the family nurse practitioner interpret the information?
    1. He is probably bleeding and should come in immediately.
    2. He ate something to affect the color of his stool.
    3. His stools are dark, secondary to Pepto-Bismol.
    4. The stool discoloration is caused by metronidazole.

81. In counseling a patient who is going to travel internationally and is worried about getting travelers' diarrhea, the family nurse practitioner knows that:
    1. Antimicrobial prophylaxis is recommended for all.
    2. Antimicrobial prophylaxis should be considered only for anyone at high risk of health-related complications of diarrhea.
    3. Bismuth subsalicylate is not recommended for prophylaxis.
    4. Fluoroquinolones are recommended for any prophylaxis.

82. A recently hospitalized 74-year-old male was treated for *Clostridium difficile* (CD) with oral metronidazole, and symptoms resolved 6 weeks ago. He now presents with a recurrence of diarrhea. Enzyme immunoassay (EIA) test results are positive for CD toxin. What is the best course of treatment at this point?
    1. Oral metronidazole 250 mg four times a day for 10 days.
    2. Vancomycin 125 mg four times a day for 10 days.
    3. Oral metronidazole 250 mg four times a day for 30 days.
    4. Vancomycin 125 mg two times a day for 2–8 weeks.

12 Gastrointestinal & Liver Answers & Rationales

Physical Exam & Diagnostic Tests

1. Answer: 4

Rationale: Inspection and auscultation should be conducted first to prevent eliciting pain and undue guarding. The family nurse practitioner should auscultate and listen to the abdomen before percussing and palpating it, because palpation may alter the frequency of bowel sounds. If the exam is painful initially, the patient will be uncomfortable, which will not allow the examiner to continue.

2. Answer: 4

Rationale: Acute diarrheal infections are common with travelers to developing countries. Diarrhea that lasts 14–30 days is classified as persistent and chronic if more than 30 days' duration. Guidelines recommend that stool be tested for culture and sensitivity if the symptoms are persistent or empiric therapy failed. It is important to know the most common organisms seen in the travel location to test appropriately. In Thailand, *Campylobacter* and *Salmonella* are two of the most common causes of infectious diarrhea. These organisms cause invasive diarrhea and should not be treated with rifaximin as that is an antibiotic that is not absorbed, working only in the intestines. Quinolone-resistant *Campylobacter* is common in Southeast Asia, but it is sensitive to macrolides, such as azithromycin (Zithromax), which is the preferred treatment if this organism is suspected. Concurrent treatment with loperamide may be used to provide symptom relief. Loperamide (Imodium) is an antiperistaltic, antidiarrheal medication that acts on opioid receptors in the gastrointestinal tract and does not enter the central nervous system. Bismuth subsalicylate (Pepto-Bismol) can be used for mild diarrheal illnesses but not concurrently with antibiotics. Bismuth has antiinflammatory, antacid, and antidiarrheal effects although the action is not well understood. Probiotics are not recommended for treatment of acute diarrhea. Azithromycin (Zithromax) is the preferred treatment for dysentery (bloody stools) or febrile diarrhea. Using single-dose regimens helps to minimize antibiotic exposure.

3. Answer: 4

Rationale: Although all the information is important in determining the cause of abdominal pain, for a young female patient of child-bearing age, ascertaining whether the patient is pregnant is a priority. A possibility of pregnancy would alter the testing that might need to be ordered, so a pregnancy test should be ordered. Additionally, abdominal pain may be from pelvic inflammatory disease or related gynecologic disorders. The family nurse practitioner should obtain a gynecologic, pregnancy, and recent sexual history, including dates of last two normal menstrual periods, condom use and other birth control use, and timing of last sexual intercourse. Food effects are important to ascertain because it may lead to a diagnosis of dietary intolerances. Location and associated symptoms are valuable to narrow down the differential diagnoses of the pain. Abrupt onset of pain has differential diagnoses that are different from pain that is recurrent/chronic, having occurred at least for 3 weeks. Acute pain can be visceral, parietal, or referred. Visceral pain originates in the hollow abdominal organs; is caused by contraction, distention, or stretching of the organ; and is usually felt along the midline of the abdomen. Parietal pain results from inflammation of the peritoneum, is usually severe, and is noted at the site of the originating disorder. Referred pain is usually noted distal to the site and is caused by innervation along the spinal level of the site. Referred pain may feel superficial or deep sensation. Change in bowel habits may indicate an intestinal origin if there is relief, even if only temporary. Pain not affected by a bowel movement or passing gas is not likely intestinal/colonic pain and may be related to other sources, such as kidney/bladder or the musculoskeletal system.

4. Answer: 1

Rationale: Passive flexion and medial rotation of the right leg cause right hypogastric pain, a positive obturator sign, which suggests an inflamed appendix. A positive Murphy's sign, severe pain, and a brief inspiratory arrest result when a patient takes a deep breath while the examiner applies pressure over the right upper quadrant, which is suggestive of cholecystitis. The psoas sign is positive with pain on pushing against the hand or with the patient on the left side extending and elevating of the right. When contraction or extension of the psoas muscle causes pain, it is a sign of inflammation of the psoas muscle and a sign of appendicitis. McBurney's point tenderness is in the right lower quadrant 2 inches from the anterior superior spinous process of ilium and is associated with acute appendicitis.

5. Answer: 3

Rationale: A colonoscopy is the most accurate and sensitive test to screen for colon cancer. Additionally, when polyps or cancers are found they usually can be completely removed at the time. The improved equipment, medication for sedation, and colon preparation have made this test safe and effective. Studies have found it to be the most effective screening in terms of cost, lives saved, and colon cancers prevented. Finding and removing colon polyps increases the prevention of colon cancer. FIT is recommended every 3 years as an alternative. A double-contrast barium enema has poor sensitivity and specificity for locating polyps and cancer and is not recommended. The test requires a bowel preparation and is uncomfortable for the patient. A flexible sigmoidoscopy is a limited exam of the lower portion of the colon. The CT colonography is performed by a CT scan, which adds the risk of radiation. It requires a bowel preparation and can be uncomfortable. It does not examine the rectum and can miss smaller polyps. Stool DNA testing is not considered a first-line screening. Fecal occult blood testing has low sensitivity and specificity and has limited use for screening. Capsule endoscopy has limitations and can detect polyps and cancers in the colon, but the sensitivity is lower than a colonoscopy and is a lengthy test.

6. Answer: 4

Rationale: Patients with end-stage liver disease are unable to form proteins and clotting factors and synthesize certain toxins. Although no single serologic test can diagnose liver disease, hyponatremia, hyperbilirubinemia, and hypoalbuminemia are often seen and used along with increased prothrombin/partial thromboplastin times and increased INR to monitor severity of end-stage liver disease.

7. Answer: 4

Rationale: Hepatitis C exposure will produce a positive HCV Ab test result; however, it is not necessarily indicative of active infection. Twenty percent of patients exposed to hepatitis C will clear the virus without treatment but will continue to have a positive antibody. Per guidelines from the American Association for the Study of Liver Diseases, to determine current infection with hepatitis C virus, testing with the sensitive HCV RNA test is recommended after a positive HCV Ab test result. This will show the presence of the virus. Repeating the antibody is not useful. Without confirmation, it is not appropriate to inform the patient of an active infection, but it should be explained that it is possible there is active infection. Testing for hepatitis B would be important because the risk factors are the same as for HCV but is not the initial action to take.

8. Answer: 3

Rationale: Positive HBsAg indicates active infection present. A positive core antibody can indicate infection, immunity, or an unclear interpretation, depending on other results. Negative surface antigen and positive core or surface antibody indicates immunity. Negative core and surface antibodies together indicate there is no immunity.

9. Answer: 4

Rationale: Serum lipase is thought to be more specific and remains elevated longer than amylase in acute pancreatitis.

It is the preferred marker but it can be elevated in other conditions as well. An upper limit of three to five times normal may be needed to consider pancreatitis, as diabetics tend to have higher than normal lipase levels, normally. Serum amylase and/or lipase elevated to three times normal or higher is one of the diagnostic criteria for acute pancreatitis. Amylase will elevate first, within 3–6 hours of onset, and normalize in 3–5 days. Lower sensitivity and specificity make it less reliable than lipase, and amylase can remain normal in up to one-fifth of patients with acute pancreatitis. In adults, the normal level for serum amylase is 30–110 IU/L and for serum lipase 13–141 IU/L. A mildly elevated serum transaminase may indicate chronic liver disease and if markedly elevated may be caused by biliary ductal dilation. A mildly elevated WBC is nonspecific.

10. Answer: 2

Rationale: Colonoscopy, which examines the entire 6 feet of the colon, should be performed to rule out colon polyps and cancer. Rectal bleeding should always be evaluated. Although the cause of bleeding may be hemorrhoids, colon polyps, cancer, and inflammation need to be considered. During a colonoscopy, any polyps seen can be removed at that time. A flexible sigmoidoscopy examines the lower 40–50 cm of the colon, needs a bowel cleansing, and is done without sedation. Polyps or cancer seen would warrant a more thorough exam with a colonoscopy. A barium enema is not a reliable test for colon polyps and cancer. It is uncomfortable for the patient and has a low yield. It is not recommended. A fecal occult blood test would not be warranted as the patient is having rectal bleeding and results would not change the course of action.

11. Answer: 3

Rationale: The history; right upper quadrant pain that radiates to the right subscapular area, especially after a fatty meal; and positive Murphy's sign are all associated with cholecystitis. A positive Murphy's sign is noted with severe pain with inspiratory arrest on palpation of the right upper quadrant.

12. Answer 4

Rationale: The current guidelines state that those who have had prior negative screening (especially with colonoscopy) may have screening discontinued when they reach age 75 years or have less than a 10-year life expectancy. However, if someone has not had prior screening then it is recommended that testing be considered up to age 85 years, depending on the age and comorbidities. Because this patient is healthy, a colonoscopy would be the most appropriate option. CT colonography is not recommended as a first-line screening. He needs a colonoscopy regardless of a fecal occult blood test, so this is not needed.

13. Answer: 1

Rationale: *H. pylori* is a bacterium that is common worldwide and is responsible for most gastric and duodenal ulcers (peptic ulcer disease) and gastric cancers. The most accurate noninvasive tests for active infection are the urea breath test and stool antigen test. Serum IgG and IgM antibody testing may not indicate a current infection, because the antibodies will be present even after the infection is eradicated. *H. pylori* causes gastric inflammation, which can present as upper abdominal pain. Altered bowel habits may be indicative of irritable bowel syndrome, which is not known to have an association to the bacterium. Dysphagia, or difficulty swallowing, is an esophageal disorder and is common with gastroesophageal reflux disease. Nausea is a nonspecific symptom with no strong correlation to the bacterial infection.

14. Answer: 4

Rationale: The septin 9 assay is the first FDA-approved serum test for colorectal cancer (CRC) screening. It detects septin 9 (m*SEPT9*) gene methylation, which has been associated with the pathogenesis of colorectal cancer (CRC) and is being considered as a biomarker for CRC. The sensitivity is 48% for detection of CRC but does not detect polyps. The test is new and there are limitations including expense, low sensitivity, and inability to detect advanced adenomas. It is not recommended for screening at this time. The test should not be used for anyone who has a family history of colon cancer, a positive fecal occult blood test, or a personal history of colon cancer or polyps. A colonoscopy is invasive, requires bowel cleansing, and has some risks (perforation 0.5/1000, bleeding 2.6/1000, and death 2.9/100,000), but it has high sensitivity for CRC and adenomas, which can be removed at the time. Colonoscopy is the preferred method for screening for CRC.

15. Answer: 1

Rationale: Current recommendation is to empirically treat mild-to-moderate diarrhea. Microbiologic testing with culture and sensitivity for ova and parasites is recommended only for severe or persistent diarrhea or have failed empiric treatment. Patients with persistent or chronic symptoms may need more complex diagnostics and should be referred to a specialist.

16. Answer: 2

Rationale: Bright red blood from the rectum indicates rectal outlet bleeding, not an upper gastrointestinal problem. It would warrant a colonoscopy, not an upper endoscopy. Dysphagia is difficulty swallowing and odynophagia is pain with swallowing. The other symptoms all warrant evaluation with upper endoscopy.

17. Answer: 1

Rationale: Assessing for ascites includes testing for shifting dullness and testing for a fluid wave. The border remains constant in a person without ascites.

18. Answer: 3

Rationale: Cholecystokinin is stimulated by fat and protein digestion products. It is injected during a HIDA scan to examine contraction and function of the gallbladder. Gastrin stimulates gastric section and motility. Gastric inhibitory peptides inhibit gastric secretion and motility. Secretin stimulates secretion of bile and alkaline pancreatic fluid.

19. Answer: 5

Rationale: Vitamin D level is not needed for a workup of elevated transaminases. Some of the differential diagnoses for elevated LFTs include hemochromatosis (iron studies), chronic hepatitis B and C (chronic hepatitis panel), and autoimmune hepatitis (ANA and SMA). Additional differentials to test for include thrombocytopenia indicative of cirrhosis, celiac sprue (celiac panel), and fatty liver disease (lipids and abdominal ultrasound).

20. Answer: 1

Rationale: The antibody test for total anti-HAV measures both IgG anti-HAV and IgM anti-HAV. The presence of IgM anti-HAV is found in the blood during an acute hepatitis A infection. Persons who are total anti-HAV positive and IgM anti-HAV negative have serologic markers indicating immunity consistent with either past infection or vaccination. IgG anti-HAV appears in the convalescent phase of HAV infection, remains present in serum for the lifetime of the person, and confers lifelong protection against disease.

Disorders

21. Answer: 2

Rationale: IBS is the most common disorder of gut–brain interaction, formerly known as a functional gastrointestinal disorder. Newly revised diagnostic criteria include abdominal pain at least 1 day a week for the last 3 months with onset at least 6 months prior, and/or associated with a change in stool frequency and/or stool appearance. An unexplained weight loss is an alarm symptom that requires further investigation and is not associated with IBS. Symptoms with dairy intake may be lactose intolerance in which the lack of the enzyme lactase inhibits the breakdown of mild sugar. A history of stomach upsets is nonspecific and could be related to gastroesophageal reflux, IBS, or other conditions.

22. Answer: 1

Rationale: Diarrhea is a common symptom with a wide differential. Clues include awakening at night and cramping without blood. A sudden onset that awakens a patient suggests pathology, which could be inflammation or infection. Obtaining a travel history, exposure to infection, and medication history may suggest infection. Irritable bowel syndrome is a functional disorder that does not awaken the patient. Ischemic colitis presents with rectal bleeding, and pain and diarrhea. Lactose intolerance and other dietary triggers cause functional diarrhea and cramping.

23. Answer: 4

Rationale: CD infection is highly transmissible, and precautions need to be taken to prevent spread to other household contacts. The patient should use a separate bathroom because of the possibility of contamination of CD spores on surfaces. Hand hygiene is extremely important to prevent transmission to others, but alcohol-based hand sanitizers are not effective against CD. These are nonsporicidal and do not remove CD from contaminated hands. Soap and water handwashing is necessary. CD infection can recur, but it is reported at 10%–20%, not 50%. CD infection is the leading cause of health care–associated infections worldwide, and elderly and hospitalized patients are particularly susceptible. However, CD infection can occur in the community as well. For the 2%–3% of healthy individuals who carry CD, the normal microbiome of the gut suppresses it. When antibiotics are taken, the balance of the microbiome is altered and CD can overgrow and produce toxins A, an enterotoxin, and B, a cytotoxin. Although CD infection usually is mild to moderate, it can be severe and develop into fulminant and life-threatening colitis.

24. Answer: 4

Rationale: Rebound tenderness is found with placing pressure on the abdomen and quickly lifting the hand. Patients will complain of more pain with release of the pressure on the abdomen rather than the pressure itself. This suggests parietal peritoneal irritation and inflammation. Other signs include a positive cough test, guarding, and rigidity. Murphy's sign is indicative of gallbladder inflammation and occurs with complaints of right upper quadrant pain and tenderness. Stool for occult blood is not a test for peritonitis because it would indicate gastrointestinal bleeding. Increased bowel sounds, also known as borborygmi, are more associated with the gastrocolic reflex and hyperactivity in intestines and would not be present with peritonitis. However, decreased bowel sounds may be present with peritonitis.

25. Answer: 4

Rationale: Nonsteroidal antiinflammatory drugs, such as ibuprofen, carry a high risk of gastrointestinal erosion and

ulcers. There may be no symptoms until anemia is noted. Gastroesophageal reflux does not contribute to anemia, unless there is gastritis with erosions or other signs of bleeding. Postmenopausal history is significant because it rules out a cause of anemia, but it is not a concern for ulcer development. Weight loss of 5 lb a month is a nonspecific symptom that needs further exploration.

26. Answer: 3

Rationale: Pruritus ani is an uncomfortable sensation around the anal orifice. It is common and may be associated with hemorrhoids. It affects men more than women and is more prevalent from ages 40–60 years. Idiopathic pruritus ani accounts for most of the cases, up to 75%, whereas secondary causes include proctitis, anal fistula, and psoriasis. The main symptom is intolerable impulse to scratch the perianal region, most often after a bowel movement and at bedtime. Hydrocortisone cream could relieve the symptoms but should be used for only a short period, such as 2 weeks or less. Long-term corticosteroid use can lead to atrophy, infections, and contact dermatitis. Antifungal cream would not be helpful unless there was secondary infection. The skin needs to be kept clean and dry and not vigorously rubbed. Moisture and creams are not helpful because the symptoms will continue. Some food and drink can exacerbate the symptoms and should be avoided, such as coffee, tea, cola, chocolate, and beer. Regular bowel habits are also important.

27. Answer: 4

Rationale: IBS presents with abdominal pain and altered bowel habits that can be erratic and unpredictable. The symptoms can be aggravated by stress and food triggers. Diarrhea should not occur during sleep, but abdominal pain can occur at any time. Antibiotic-induced diarrhea occurs in association with a recent course of antibiotics, especially in the previous 3 months. Antibiotics may trigger *Clostridium difficile* colitis. Bacterial or viral gastroenteritis presents with a sudden onset of diarrhea and does not alternate with constipation. Inflammatory bowel disease (IBD) presents with more consistent symptoms of diarrhea and pain and possibly rectal bleeding. In fact, the symptoms of IBD can be present for months to years before diagnosis. Extraintestinal manifestations, such as arthritis and skin lesions, may be present, and nocturnal diarrhea and fecal incontinence can be present if rectal inflammation is present.

28. Answer: 3

Rationale: Patients with dysphagia caused by an esophageal spasm may report difficulty with both liquids and solids because the spasm has closed the esophagus temporarily. Relaxation of the esophagus usually occurs within a minute and the food will pass down. This can cause choking with liquids as well. Spasm can occur for many reasons, one of which can be acid reflux. It is episodic, nonprogressive, and unpredictable. Difficulty swallowing solids and feeling that food is sticking is most likely because of an esophageal stricture or obstruction. Marked weight loss is not usually a symptom of dysphagia, unless is it related to esophageal cancer.

29. Answer: 4

Rationale: Gastroparesis can be a significant complication for patients with reflux. The lingering contents in the stomach contain acid and the frequency of reflux will be increased. Persons with a small sliding hiatal hernia are not likely to have a significant change in their symptoms. Reflux is less likely to occur after lying down with an empty stomach. Weight gain may worsen symptoms, but usually it is noted with a significant change in weight, not just 10 lb.

30. Answer: 2

Rationale: The most common hernia is an inguinal hernia, protruding at the inguinal canal. Incarceration means the hernia cannot be reduced or returned to the abdominal cavity. A reducible hernia easily moves across the abdominal wall. There should be no abdominal swelling, and if the hernia is particularly painful and associated with nausea and vomiting, strangulation/incarceration should be considered as a surgical emergency because there can be tissue necrosis.

31. Answer: 2

Rationale: An endoscopy is needed for patients with no/minimal response to therapy, indicated by persistent symptoms after 8–12 weeks of therapy. Heartburn may be characterized by burning substernal chest pain and may have gastroesophageal reflux. The factors that would raise a red flag would be long-term history of reflux, dysphagia, or weight loss. It is not recommended to test with endoscopy for all patients with heartburn. A negative *H. pylori* test lessens the chance of inflammation and ulceration. Response to treatment within 2 weeks is a positive indication that the patient has gastroesophageal reflux and can continue treatment and be followed in the office.

32. Answer: 1

Rationale: NAFLD is a primary cause of chronic liver disease and has a spectrum ranging from fatty liver (benign) to nonalcoholic steatohepatitis (NASH; inflammation and scarring). It is estimated that up to 25%–30% of the general population has NAFLD, with 6% affected with NASH, which can lead to cirrhosis and end-stage liver disease. Of patients with NAFLD, 30% will develop NASH. In Type 2 diabetes mellitus the estimated prevalence is 30%–60%. Major risk factors include obesity (82% of those with NASH), diabetes (30%–60% have NAFLD), and metabolic syndrome. Fifteen percent of non-obese patients have NAFLD. The most common cause of

death with NAFLD is cardiovascular disease with hepatocellular carcinoma and liver disease as the second and third most common causes, respectively. Bariatric surgery for morbid obesity, which includes gastric bypass, sleeve gastrectomy, and other options, has a goal of weight loss to improve the patient's health, including improving diabetes and hypertension. Rapid weight loss, which can occur after bariatric surgery, may improve liver function tests, but some studies demonstrate progression of liver disease and worsening liver fibrosis. Some studies indicate that cirrhosis develops in 4%–14% of patients with NASH over a 20-year period.

33. Answer: 4

Rationale: A means of hepatitis B virus (HBV) transmission is from an infected mother to baby, perinatally. Before the hepatitis B vaccine, it was estimated that 30%–40% of chronic HBV infections were transmitted perinatally. Since the widespread use of the vaccine and guidelines of vaccinating newborns, this rate has dropped dramatically. The main routes of transmission are contact with an infected person including sexually; by transfusions; sharing razors or toothbrushes; sharing needles, syringes, and other drug-injecting equipment; from blood and open sores; and from needlesticks or other sharp instruments. HBV is not spread by food, water, sharing eating utensils, breast-feeding, hugging, kissing, coughing, sneezing, or the fecal-oral route.

34. Answer: 2

Rationale: The patient's symptoms most likely represent an SBO. The history of multiple abdominal surgeries provides a possible cause because adhesions commonly develop after surgery and are one of the most common causes of SBO. Appendicitis would be documented on a computed tomography scan, which would likely be done at the emergency room. Appendicitis can present with these symptoms, but the pain is usually progressive and not intermittent. Biliary ductal obstruction is unlikely because the patient's gallbladder has been removed and although stones can reform it takes many years (usually more than 5 years). Another cause of biliary obstruction is a neoplasm, but patients usually do not have pain and bowels are not generally affected. Gastroenteritis usually is accompanied by diarrhea, not constipation.

35. Answer: 1

Rationale: Chronic long-term use of stimulant laxatives such as bisacodyl can worsen constipation because the bowels become dependent and develop a resistance to the stimulants. Pelvic floor dyssynergia can cause fecal incontinence, diarrhea, or constipation, but stimulant laxatives would cause diarrhea because colon motility is not the problem. Colonic inertia is an infrequent cause of constipation and can be severe; it may be a differential diagnosis, but not the most likely.

Irritable bowel syndrome has pain as a major symptom, which is not present with this patient's symptoms.

36. Answer: 2

Rationale: The pinworm parasites reside in the intestine. Females lay eggs on the skin outside the anus, resulting in extreme pruritus. The only host is humans and it is transmitted by the fecal-oral route, easily spreading among households, day cares, and schools. Hookworm larvae reside in the soil, enter the body through the feet, and can cause anemia. When dirt containing roundworm eggs are ingested through pica or unwashed vegetables, or if contaminated water is consumed, an intestinal infestation occurs. Giardiasis results from ingestion of the protozoan *Giardia lamblia* through contaminated water or oral-fecal transmission.

37. Answer: 1

Rationale: An important nonpharmacologic intervention for GERD is to advise the patient not to lie down within 2–3 hours after meals to allow the stomach to empty. Patients with GERD also should reduce weight, avoid large meals and exercise after meals, and elevate the head of the bed. Certain drinks (alcohol, mint, and orange juice) should be avoided because they can increase acid production and can relax the lower esophageal sphincter. Acidic foods (tomato products, spicy foods) may worsen symptoms of reflux and should be avoided. The patient should be taught to avoid bending after meals. Drinking large amounts of fluid with meals may affect GERD, depending on the volume of the fluids.

38. Answer: 3

Rationale: Lifestyle modifications should be the first step in managing constipation. Most patients do not have enough fiber in their diet. Thirty to 32g a day is recommended, most of which should come from the diet. Fiber supplements can help but do not add a significant amount of fiber. Patients need to read food labels to determine their fiber amount. Increasing fluids and exercise are also useful to maintain regular bowel function. In the absence of alarm symptoms such as weight loss, rectal bleeding, or significant abdominal pain, conservative therapy should be tried before considering testing. It is rare that colon cancer causes constipation and blockages because this would be an advanced cancer. Rectocele can be a cause of constipation and should be considered if lifestyle modifications are not improving bowel function.

39. Answer: 2

Rationale: *H. pylori* has been shown to be responsible for most duodenal and gastric ulcers. The other common cause of ulcers is from use of nonsteroidal antiinflammatory drugs at regular and/or high doses. The other organisms listed are implicated in other types of infections (e.g., acute otitis media; skin infections). *S. pneumoniae* and *M. catarrhalis* have been implicated as causative agents in pneumonia.

40. Answer: 2

Rationale: Hepatitis A never becomes chronic and is not a cause of cirrhosis. NAFLD is common, affecting 25%–30% of the general population, and it is related to metabolic syndrome. Excess fat deposits, partially caused by insulin resistance, can cause inflammation and scarring that lead to cirrhosis. NAFLD has been increasing in incidence and severity and is becoming the number one reason for liver transplant in the United States. Chronic hepatitis B is not a major cause of cirrhosis in the United States, but it is a worldwide epidemic and responsible for hepatocellular cancer. Alcohol in large and/or daily amounts can cause cirrhosis.

41. Answer: 2

Rationale: A hemorrhoid is a vascular anal cushion and can be internal (above the dentate line) or external (below the dentate line), which can enlarge and bleed. Everyone has internal hemorrhoids even though they may not have any symptoms. In a rectal mucosa prolapse, the wall of the rectum prolapses through the anal canal on straining. A rectocele is a herniation of the rectum into the vaginal wall and can cause constipation.

42. Answer: 2

Rationale: These characteristics describe hepatitis B, which affects less than 1% of the U.S. population and is a much less common cause of cirrhosis. Hepatitis A has symptoms of fever and jaundice (up to 50%), but the incubation period is 15–50 days (average 30 days) and does not have a chronic form. Hepatitis C infection causes jaundice up to 25% of the time and can cause arthralgia, but there is no fever. The incubation period is 14–18 days (average 42–49 days). Up to 75% of those infected with hepatitis C will develop chronic infection. Hepatitis E is characterized by oral-fecal transmission that is associated with contaminated food and water and has an incubation period of 14–60 days and no chronic disease state.

43. Answer: 2

Rationale: Although some patients need eventual intervention including a cholecystectomy, those who are older adults and diabetic are at increased risk for complications and should be hospitalized for prompt diagnosis, which could include a RUQ abdominal ultrasound, and possibly a magnetic resonance cholangiopancreatography (MRCP). The MRCP is very sensitive at documenting a gallstone lodged in the bile duct. Abnormally elevated transaminases and possibly pancreatic enzymes would be present with bile duct blockage, and the patient may have secondary pancreatitis.

Intravenous fluids, pain control, and surgical consultation would also be warranted.

44. Answer: 3

Rationale: Long-term GERD ("heartburn for years") without effective treatment (no complete relief of symptoms and no proton-pump inhibitor [PPI]) carries a risk of Barrett esophagus (a precursor to cancer) and esophageal adenocarcinoma, especially in a non-Hispanic white male smoker over the age of 50 years. Rapid weight loss is a concerning clinical finding that may indicate esophageal cancer or other cancer that had advanced to a hypermetabolic state. He also has a risk of squamous cell carcinoma of the esophagus because it is associated with cigarette smoking and alcohol use but is less common than adenocarcinoma (ratio 1:2). Adenocarcinoma of the esophagus most commonly develops in men (men/women ratio 6:1) age 65 years and older. The symptoms of heartburn caused by either gastric ulcer or long-term GERD will not likely be controlled with an H_2 RA/antacid and would require a PPI daily. A patient with a gastric ulcer should be tested for *Helicobacter pylori* and would be questioned about a history of nonsteroidal antiinflammatory drug use, and then treated appropriately. Clinical manifestations of lung cancer include cough, hemoptysis, dyspnea, chest pain, and weight loss, and the substantial pack-year history does place the patient at risk. This would be in the differential, but esophageal cancer would be the first diagnosis to rule out.

45. Answer: 1

Rationale: Intermittent diarrhea, gas, and bloating can occur after ingestion of dairy if the patient is lactose intolerant. This can occur at any time and can present after a viral illness. The decrease or loss of the enzyme lactase, which breaks down lactose in dairy, results in colonic bacteria breaking down the lactose and producing gas and diarrhea. Some patients can be extremely sensitive to all dairy, including butter. Patients with celiac disease are usually anemic and may have elevated liver enzymes. Hyperthyroidism can cause diarrhea, but the patient's TSH is high, meaning she has hypothyroidism. *H. pylori* infection can cause abdominal pain and bloating but would not necessarily cause diarrhea, and the elevated antibody is not confirmatory of infection.

46. Answer: 4

Rationale: Esophageal varices are dilated submucosal veins that are a late sign and complication of cirrhosis because of scarring of the liver and portal hypertension. The cirrhosis would likely be advanced for varices to develop, usually in the esophagus, but also can occur in the stomach. As these varices are under high pressure, the patient can have anything from a slow leak of blood to a major, life-threatening bleed. The varices should be diagnosed by endoscopy and treated with beta blockers to lower the blood pressure. Of patients

with cirrhosis, approximately 50% will develop gastroesophageal varices and will have a yearly rate of bleeding from 5%–15%. A history of heavy alcohol intake may be the cause of this patient's cirrhosis. These patients can present clinically with bleeding, spontaneous "coffee grounds" or bright-red blood, hypotension, and eventual shock. The other choices could all be associated with this patient. A bleeding peptic ulcer is possible but is not the first concern. An excessive nosebleed is possible because of thrombocytopenia from cirrhosis and would need to be explored. Hemoptysis implies lung disease.

47. Answer: 4

Rationale: GERD can present with a variety of symptoms including atypical extraesophageal symptoms such as cough. Acid in the esophagus can trigger a bronchospasm resulting in a cough and other pulmonary symptoms. The patient's weight gain coincides with the onset of the cough, which can worsen reflux. The timing of the cough, after meals and at night, correlates with when reflux is likely to be occurring. Not everyone who has GERD is aware of it and has no classic heartburn on regurgitation. Environmental allergies can contribute, but his symptoms would likely be more seasonal and not continuous the entire year, depending on his location. Exposure to fumes would trigger a cough, but pulmonary workup was negative, and he did not respond to treatment. Sinusitis and postnasal drainage can cause a cough, but likely would be seasonal and not necessarily occur after meals.

48. Answer: 2

Rationale: Increasing crampy abdominal pain that starts as periumbilical pain, anorexia, and fever are classic symptoms of appendicitis. A surgeon should evaluate the patient to decrease the risk of rupture. An abdominal CT scan has a high sensitivity to document appendicitis. Although ectopic pregnancy should always be a consideration in young females with abdominal pain, the characteristics of the pain and other symptoms are not typical of an ectopic pregnancy. However, a good gynecologic history would be needed. The patient should not be sent home unless the CT scan was negative, and then follow-up within 24 hours would be warranted.

49. Answer: 3

Rationale: Abstinence from alcohol, the most important treatment for cirrhosis, can halt progression of cirrhosis and reverse the damage, if the liver is minimally scarred. Continuing to drink even occasionally can be detrimental and rapidly increase the disease process. It is known that an average of one to two drinks a day for a woman raises her risk of cirrhosis up to four times the risk of the general population (two to three drinks for a man). A standard drink is considered 14 g of pure alcohol, which translates to 12 ounces of beer, 5 ounces of wine, or 1.5 ounces of distilled spirits.

Recent research shows that current drinking may be more of a factor than a lifetime amount. The patient's diet should be nutritious, and she should avoid herbal and other supplements because some have been known to cause liver toxicity. There is no recommendation for vitamin E supplementation.

50. Answer: 2

Rationale: Diverticulitis is defined as clinically evident macroscopic inflammation of a diverticulum or diverticula. It occurs in 4% of patients with diverticulosis. Patients usually present with a sudden onset of abdominal pain in the left lower quadrant. The patient may have a low-grade fever and leukocytosis. Patients with diverticulitis can have a range of mild to severe inflammation, and 15% will develop complications. Nausea and vomiting may accompany severe pain. Appendicitis may present with pain in the periumbilical region that eventually travels to the right lower quadrant and may not be severe for several hours after onset. Other signs, including nausea and vomiting, leukocytosis, and fever, may or may not be present. Irritable bowel syndrome (IBS) may present with aching or cramping in the periumbilical or lower abdominal regions, often precipitated by meals and relieved by defecation. The pain can be severe occasionally, and there is an altered frequency and consistency of the stools. Fever, leukocytosis, and awakening at night are not indicative of IBS. A ruptured ovarian cyst would not be a differential in an older adult woman as the ovaries shrink and stop functioning with menopause.

51. Answer: 1

Rationale: Colorectal cancer (CRC) risk in patients with left-sided and universal ulcerative colitis increases by 0.5%–1% per year after the eighth year of disease. Ulcerative colitis limited to the proctosigmoid region carries less of a risk. Crohn's disease, which can affect any part of the gastrointestinal tract from the mouth to the rectum, carries a higher risk if the colon is involved. Colonoscopy with random biopsies every 1–2 years is recommended beginning 8–10 years after the irritable bowel disease began. Diverticulosis is common in the general population but is less common in ulcerative colitis and is not a risk factor for CRC. Ischemic colitis occurs when a mesenteric artery is temporarily blocked and the colon at the splenic flexure develops ischemia from lack of blood flow. There is no higher risk of ischemic colitis for patients with ulcerative colitis. Irritable bowel syndrome is common in the general population and in patients with ulcerative colitis, but it is a disorder of brain–gut interaction and does not increase risk of colon cancer.

52. Answer: 4

Rationale: Patients with a gastric ulcer may not have any symptoms, especially the older adult. Weight loss and anorexia may be present, but the patient may attribute this to "getting older." The patient may not realize an ulcer is present until it bleeds and causes significant anemia. Smoking does increase the risk, and perforation can occur, but it is not common. Gastric ulcers are thought to be more common than duodenal ulcers in older adult patients.

53. Answer: 3

Rationale: Dysphagia and cough with solid and liquid intake may be the first indication that the patient has cancer, but this is usually late in development. Alcoholism and smoking are the primary risk factors for squamous cell esophageal cancer, which is not as common as adenocarcinoma, which is usually associated with chronic GERD and Barrett esophagus. Caffeine intake in one or more cups of coffee a day, specifically, may be protective against esophageal, oral, and pharyngeal cancer. Midchest pain indicates late disease, which does not usually respond to treatment including surgery.

54. Answer: 2

Rationale: Celiac sprue is a genetic disease of the small bowel that is caused by gluten intolerance. The diarrhea and cramping are related to the effects of malabsorption of gluten. Because of malabsorption, many patients have iron-deficiency anemia and can have elevated liver enzymes. Hepatitis B would produce elevated liver enzymes but not the other listed symptoms. *Salmonella* infection could produce diarrhea and cramping but not anemia. A bleeding ulcer could produce anemia but not the other symptoms.

55. Answer: 3

Rationale: Abnormal villi found on the duodenal biopsy are the gold standard for diagnosis. A negative biopsy could mean the disease has not manifested, but the patient has the potential to develop celiac disease. The tTG, IgA, and deamidated gliadin (DGP) are the most sensitive serologic tests for celiac disease. The antiendomysial antibody test (EMAIgA) is very specific for celiac disease; if it is positive then it is likely the patient has celiac disease. However, it is not as sensitive for celiac disease, and about 5%–10% will have a false-negative test for celiac. With this patient, an EMAIgA could be tested, and if positive, that might explain the patient's results as potential celiac disease. It is thought that a positive tTG does not cause nonceliac gluten sensitivity. Removing gluten from the diet may improve the patient's symptoms. A strict gluten-free diet will normalize the biopsy findings and convert the antibodies to negative, but both tests would be affected, and it could take 2–3 months or longer to have normal results. It is unlikely that a few weeks of a gluten-free diet would normalize the biopsy.

56. Answer: 2

Rationale: A common sequela of a viral infection is gastroparesis. The virus can affect the gastric pacer, causing it to malfunction and result in slow gastric emptying. Typical symptoms of nausea, decreased appetite, and early satiety occur because of the lingering of solid food in the stomach, which can be 4 hours or more. Typically, a stomach should empty in 1–2 hours for an average meal. Accumulation throughout the day can result in a full stomach that does not empty. These are not typical symptoms of an influenza infection. Vertigo causes nausea, but not the other symptoms. Although the patient may have taken ibuprofen for several days, it is less likely that an ulcer would have developed with a short course, but it should be in the differential.

57. Answer: 4

Rationale: The symptoms of cramping, diarrhea, and bloating are classic for IBS with diarrhea predominant. Abdominal pain is a symptom of IBS but is not associated with rectal bleeding or fecal incontinence.

58. Answer: 1

Rationale: People with IBS can have many food triggers. The challenge is to identify the foods without having them avoid entire food groups. Simple sugars, specifically fermentable oligo-, di-, and monosaccharides and polyols, can cause symptoms of cramping, gas, bloating, and diarrhea. Rather than avoiding all fruits and vegetables, patients need to be aware of the most offending foods and carefully avoid those that cause a problem. Dairy products have lactose, which is not able to be broken down when someone is lacking some or all lactase, the enzyme needed for digestion of lactose. Although people have IBS and lactose intolerance, it should not be assumed the patient has both. Red meat and saturated fat can cause some problems but are not prime offenders.

59. Answer: 3

Rationale: One of the ways patients can decrease the fat in the liver is to lose weight with exercise. It is important to treat hyperlipidemia because this is associated with fatty liver, and statins should not be discontinued. Lowering cholesterol is not as effective as lowering saturated fats in the diet. Adding vitamin A as a supplement is controversial, and excessive doses over 10,000 IU of vitamin A daily can cause or worsen liver damage.

60. Answer: 2

Rationale: *Norovirus* (Norwalk) can cause vomiting and diarrhea in adolescents and adults. The incubation period is short (18–72 hours) and the duration of symptoms is short, usually 24–48 hours. *Cytomegalovirus* rarely causes diarrhea and is commonly reactivated in patients after bone marrow transplant, late stages of HIV infection, and other immunocompromised situations. *Campylobacter* enteritis is the most common cause of bacterial diarrhea, especially in traveler's

diarrhea and food poisoning. *Rotavirus* mainly affects infants 3–15 months of age in the winter months, causing excessive watery diarrhea.

61. Answer: 1

Rationale: Mild diarrhea is tolerable, is not bothersome, and does not interfere with activities. Moderate diarrhea is bothersome or interferes with activities. Severe diarrhea is incapacitating or completely prevents activities; all dysentery (passage of grossly bloody stools) is considered severe. Persistent diarrhea lasts 2 or more weeks. Treatment is dependent on the classification. With mild acute diarrhea, the patient can use loperamide or bismuth subsalicylate. No testing is needed.

62. Answer: 3

Rationale: Visceral pain occurs when hollow abdominal organs contract forcefully or are distended or stretched. Parietal pain occurs because of inflammation in the parietal peritoneum and is more severe than visceral pain, steady and aching and localized. Referred pain occurs from innervation at approximately the same spinal level as the disordered structure, usually develops as the initial pain becomes more intense, and seems to radiate or travel from the initial site.

63. Answer: 4

Rationale: Sudden knifelike epigastric pain occurs with gallstone pancreatitis and would require immediate evaluation and intervention. Bloating, nausea, and abdominal fullness may be dyspepsia or gastroparesis. Nonspecific abdominal pain can be functional dyspepsia. Retrosternal burning pain is indicative of heartburn. However, all of the above can also represent more serious conditions and require further testing but not necessarily emergently. Keep in mind the duration can be a key to chronicity, but it is important to always consider what may be misleading when evaluating a history.

64. Answer: 4

Rationale: Black stools without a tarry, shiny, sticky appearance is likely of no concern. Tarry stools indicate passage of blood and usually from the upper gastrointestinal tract, involving a loss of at least 60 mL of blood.

65. Answer: 3

Rationale: All listed are common causes of nausea and vomiting, but gastroenteritis is the most common.

66. Answer: 1

Rationale: Patients with an acute attack of inflammation of the gallbladder usually have a gallstone obstructing the gallbladder–cystic duct junction. This is a typical presentation. Acute pancreatitis usually presents with a sudden onset of severe, deep epigastric pain that can radiate into the back. Acute hepatitis A will present with general symptoms of malaise, fever, jaundice, and fatigue. The patient with hepatitis can have RUQ pain and liver enlargement but not a defined mass. Appendicitis presents initially with abdominal pain, usually severe and throughout the entire abdomen before localizing to the RLQ. No mass is noted. All of these conditions can also present with fever and nausea and vomiting. The history of the onset after a high fatty meal is key to considering the top diagnosis of gallbladder origin. Laboratory testing and radiology can quickly differentiate the conditions.

67. Answer: 3

Rationale: Crohn's disease is a chronic, progressive inflammation of the intestinal tract, most commonly the small intestine. The peak age of onset is 15–25 years, with females and Caucasians more often affected. The patient's symptoms are a classic presentation. Irritable bowel syndrome is common, but there should not be weight loss or fever (chills). Infection should always be ruled out with chronic diarrhea, and a history of exposure to possible causes (travel, antibiotics, food poisoning) would increase suspicion. Ulcerative colitis usually presents with rectal bleeding and is less likely to have fever, and pain would more likely be in the RLQ.

68. Answer: 2, 4

Rationale: Avoiding alcohol consumption and smoking cessation are two important therapies for the patient with chronic pancreatitis. Enzyme supplements are given at the beginning of the meal, not afterward. It is recommended that the patient have small meals high in protein with approximately 20 g/day of fat. Patients with acute pancreatitis may be treated with antibiotics, if there is presence of an infection.

69. Answer: 1, 2, 4

Rationale: Symptoms of all types of viral hepatitis are similar and can include one or more of the following: fever, fatigue, anorexia, nausea, vomiting, right upper quadrant abdominal pain, gray-colored bowel movements, dark-colored urine (bilirubinuria), myalgias, and jaundice. Hepatomegaly is also common; splenomegaly is less common. The presence of IgM anti-HAV is found in the blood during an acute hepatitis A infection. Anti-HAV IgG appears soon after anti-HAV IgM and generally persists for the lifetime of the person and confers lifelong protection against disease. The AST/ALT is elevated with the value of the ALT usually greater than the AST. The alkaline phosphatase is mildly elevated. Both conjugated and unconjugated bilirubin are usually increased. Bilirubin rises typically follow rise in ALT/AST.

Pharmacology

70. Answer: 4

Rationale: Omeprazole is a proton-pump inhibitor (PPI) that blocks all three pathways of acid production: histamine, gastrin, and acetylcholine, for up to 24 hours. Treatment with a PPI is recommended for patients who have frequent symptoms, at least several times a week. It is important to take the PPI on an empty stomach, and then eat 30–60 minutes after for maximum pH control. PPIs need food to work, and, if a second dose is required, it should be taken before the evening dose. Anticholinergics (hyoscyamine and others) will likely increase his symptoms by lowering the lower esophageal sphincter pressure. Anticholinergics are effective for the cramping of irritable bowel syndrome. Famotidine is a histamine 2 receptor antagonist (H_2 RA) that blocks one pathway for acid secretion, histamine, but there are two other pathways that continue to secrete hydrochloric acid. An H_2 RA can be effective for occasional symptoms, a few times a week or less, or as a short trial for new onset of symptoms.

71. Answer: 4

Rationale: Topical nitrate ointment applied twice daily for 6–8 weeks has been associated with healing of chronic anal fissure at least 50% of the time. It can also decrease rectal pain. The most commonly occurring side effect is headache in 20%–30% of the patients. Topical calcium channel blockers are also used, but data are insufficient to conclude healing superior to placebo. Sitz baths, psyllium, and bulking agents are first-line therapy for acute anal fissure and can be helpful for symptomatic relief. Topical lidocaine gel can provide some relief of pain but not effect healing. Analpram-HC is used to treat symptoms of hemorrhoids, including pain, itching, and swelling. An anal fissure is a longitudinal tear in the midline of the anal canal, distal to the dentate line. An acute fissure looks like a simple tear in the anoderm, whereas a chronic fissure is defined as lasting 8–12 weeks and has edema and fibrosis associated with it.

72. Answer: 3

Rationale: Goals of PUD treatment include removal of the offending agent, relief of pain, healing of the ulcer, and cost-effectiveness. In this case the likely cause of her ulcer would be use of nonsteroidal antiinflammatory drugs (NSAIDS). It is estimated that up to 25% of patients taking NSAIDS chronically will develop ulcer disease and 2%–4% will develop bleeding or perforation. Risk factors for NSAID-induced ulcers include age greater than 65 years, high doses of NSAIDS, daily use, and use of aspirin or anticoagulants or antiplatelet medications. Proton pump inhibitors (PPIs) heal 90% of duodenal ulcers after 4 weeks and 90% of gastric ulcers after 8 weeks, if *H. pylori* is negative. PPIs, such as pantoprazole, are recommended for ulcers because these drugs provide faster pain relief and more rapid healing than H₂ RA because of their ability to decrease acid production. Clarithromycin, tetracycline, metronidazole, and bismuth (Pepto-Bismol) are some of the accepted treatments against active *H. pylori*–associated ulcers. Eradication of *H. pylori* requires a recommended regimen of acid blockers, antibiotics, and possibly bismuth in various combinations.

73. Answer: 2

Rationale: If a person exposed to a patient known to be positive for hepatitis B has sufficient immunity to hepatitis B, no treatment is necessary. If this same person had not been vaccinated, in addition to initiation of the hepatitis B vaccine series, HBIG 0.06 mL/kg IM is also administered. If an exposed person has had an inadequate immune response to the hepatitis B vaccine series (negative antihepatitis surface antibody), a hepatitis B booster should be given.

74. Answer: 1

Rationale: Patients with gastric or duodenal ulcers caused by *H. pylori* can be successfully treated with triple-drug therapy: a proton-pump inhibitor (PPI; bid for all except esomeprazole, which is qd), clarithromycin, and amoxicillin or metronidazole for 14 days (eradication rates 70%–85%). An alternative regimen approved by the U.S. Food and Drug Administration is a quadruple regimen with a (qd or bid) histamine 2 receptor antagonist (bid), metronidazole, bismuth, and tetracycline for 10–14 days (eradication rates 75%–90%). Treatment should continue with a PPI for at least 2–4 weeks after to promote healing of the ulcer. After completion of *H. pylori* therapy, it is recommended that testing is done with the stool antigen for *H. pylori* at 8 weeks to ensure eradication of the infection. The PPI would need to be stopped for 2 weeks before testing the stool because there can be false-negative results. Other treatment regimens have been suggested, but eradication rates can vary. Cephalosporins are not included in any recommended regimens for *H. pylori*.

75. Answer: 2

Rationale: Mesalamine (5-aminosalicylic acid) therapy for patients with mild ulcerative colitis has been shown to improve symptoms and induce and maintain remission. It is an antiinflammatory compound similar to aspirin, without the effects on platelets. There are several mesalamine products available, including rectal suspension and suppositories that can be very helpful for left-sided colitis. If no response is seen after 2–4 weeks, then the addition of corticosteroids (prednisone) can be helpful, but they are not first-line therapy. Ciprofloxacin and metronidazole are typically used for gastrointestinal infections,

including *Clostridium difficile*, which is common with ulcerative colitis.

76. Answer: 1

Rationale: To minimize the risk of a contact developing hepatitis A, which is spread by fecal-oral transmission, immunoglobulin 0.02 mL/kg should be given as soon as possible after exposure. It has not been shown to be effective if administered more than 2 weeks after exposure. HBIG is for hepatitis B.

77. Answer: 4

Rationale: For unvaccinated patients with exposure to hepatitis B, one dose of HBIG is administered and the hepatitis B virus series initiated. HBIG may be protective or may attenuate the severity of the illness if given within 7 days of exposure (adult dose of 0.06 mL/kg). If the patient thinks the individual may have been vaccinated but does not know whether there was a response, then the family nurse practitioner can test antihepatitis B surface antibody. Neither the HBe antibody nor the viral load would be a first-line test. Because of the timing of appearance of the antibodies to hepatitis B, testing would need to be delayed.

78. Answer: 3

Rationale: The only contraindication to the hepatitis B vaccine is prior anaphylaxis or severe hypersensitivity to the vaccine or components of the vaccine.

79. Answer: 3

Rationale: Metronidazole 500 mg PO tid for 10 days is the first-line treatment for mild to moderate CD infection. Vancomycin would be second-line treatment, if there is no improvement in 5–7 days. The patient has no symptoms indicating severe disease, which would include fever, abdominal tenderness, low albumin and creatinine, and leukocytosis greater than 15,000 with a left shift of greater than 20% neutrophils. For severe disease, vancomycin would be the drug of choice. The regimen of vancomycin and IV metronidazole is reserved for severe complicated disease that can include hypotension, ileus, mental status changes, and need for admission to intensive care. The probiotics *L. acidophilus* and *L. casei* have been suggested as helpful for infection and prevention control of CD infection, but the data on probiotics are insufficient at this time for a strong recommendation.

80. Answer: 3

Rationale: This is a common observation for a patient taking Pepto-Bismol. The patient also may experience a problem with discoloration of his tongue. The stool discoloration is not related to bleeding. Certain foods can affect the stool color, but bismuth is more likely the cause.

81. Answer: 2

Rationale: Prophylaxis is not recommended for all travelers but should be considered for those at high risk of complications. Bismuth subsalicylate can be considered for any traveler and is an inexpensive, safe treatment. Fluoroquinolones are not recommended as prophylaxis but are considered as treatment for moderate travelers' diarrhea. However, there is emergence of resistance to this drug class. When antibiotic prophylaxis is indicated it is recommended that rifaximin be used concurrently.

82. Answer: 2

Rationale: First-line therapy is appropriate with metronidazole. Recurrent CD infection is defined as complete resolution of presenting symptoms after therapy with return of symptoms within 8 weeks of the first episode. It is estimated that 10%–20% of cases recur after the first episode but can increase to 40%–65% after the first recurrence. Research indicates the recurrences are from the original strain, rather than reinfection. Testing should be accomplished before retreating with recurrence of diarrhea. The EIA can remain positive for up to 30 days even with symptom resolution. Multiple relapses may require 30 days of therapy or a taper pulse approach for up to 8 weeks.

Hematology

13

Physical Exam & Diagnostic Tests

1. A male patient with iron deficiency would most likely present with which of the following laboratory values?
   1. Hematocrit (Hct) 30%, serum Fe 18, mean corpuscular volume (MCV) 70, decreased transferrin, increased ferritin.
   2. Hct 22%, serum Fe 18, MCV 60, increased transferrin, increased ferritin.
   3. Hct 22%, serum Fe 18, MCV 70, increased transferrin, decreased ferritin.
   4. Hct 22%, serum Fe 18, MCV 90, decreased transferrin, increased ferritin.

2. Which test is most important for diagnosing iron-deficiency anemia?
   1. Direct Coombs.
   2. Serum folate level.
   3. Serum ferritin.
   4. Red blood cell (RBC) count.

3. The term *shotty* is often used to describe lymph nodes that are:
   1. Tender, mobile, and greater than 5 mm.
   2. Small and pellet-like.
   3. Discrete and cystic.
   4. Irregular, soft, and fixed to surrounding tissue.

4. A macrocytic, normochromic anemia is diagnosed in an older adult male patient. What should be the next test(s) ordered?
   1. Serum iron and total iron-binding capacity (TIBC) levels.
   2. Bone marrow biopsy.
   3. Colonoscopy.
   4. Vitamin B_{12} and red blood cell (RBC)/folate levels.

5. The family nurse practitioner would suspect disseminated intravascular coagulation (DIC) if the patient's laboratory results, including prothrombin time (PT), indicated:
   1. Increased PT, decreased platelet count, and decreased fibrinogen.
   2. Decreased PT, increased hematocrit, and increased fibrinogen.
   3. Increased platelet count, decreased hematocrit, and increased PT.
   4. Increased platelet count, increased hematocrit, and decreased PT.

6. When examining lymph nodes, what does the family nurse practitioner understand?
   1. Children are more likely to develop generalized lymphadenopathy than adults in response to a mild infection.
   2. Older adults frequently have enlarged, nontender supraclavicular and epitrochlear lymph nodes caused by aging.
   3. Lymphadenopathy in an adult indicates acute or chronic infection and rarely malignancy.
   4. Enlarged neck lymph nodes in children with no other physical findings are highly suspicious of Burkitt lymphoma.

7. After confirming the diagnosis of iron-deficiency anemia in an older adult male patient based on the complete blood count, peripheral smear, serum iron, total iron-binding capacity, and serum ferritin, what would be the next essential test for the family nurse practitioner to order?
   1. Fecal occult blood test (FOBT) $\times$ 3.
   2. Prothrombin time/partial thromboplastin time.
   3. Liver function tests.
   4. Endoscopy.

8. Evaluation of an older adult male patient reveals a macrocytic, normochromic anemia. Subsequent testing shows normal folate level and decreased vitamin B_{12} level. Further evaluation could include:
   1. Referral to a hematologist for a bone marrow biopsy.
   2. Assay for antiintrinsic factor (anti-IF) antibodies.
   3. Upper gastrointestinal (GI) series.
   4. No tests are indicated at this time.

9. The definitive test for the diagnosis of sickle cell anemia is:
   1. Complete blood count (CBC) with a peripheral smear.
   2. Bone marrow biopsy and aspiration.
   3. Hemoglobin electrophoresis.
   4. Hemoglobin and hematocrit.

10. An older adult male patient presents to the office with complaints of fatigue, dizziness, decreased activity tolerance, and occasional bounding heart rate. Physical exam reveals pallor (including mucous membranes), tachycardia, and general appearance of lethargy. The family nurse practitioner orders a complete blood count with differential, peripheral smear, serum iron, total iron-binding capacity (TIBC), and serum ferritin because there is a high index of suspicion for:
    1. Sideroblastic anemia.
    2. Pernicious anemia.
    3. Folic acid–deficiency anemia.
    4. Iron-deficiency anemia.

11. Anemia of chronic disease (ACD) reveals which of the following laboratory findings?
    1. Decreased iron, decreased total iron-binding capacity (TIBC), and decreased serum ferritin.
    2. Decreased iron, decreased TIBC, and increased serum ferritin.
    3. Decreased iron, increased TIBC, and decreased serum ferritin.
    4. Decreased iron, increased TIBC, and increased serum ferritin.

12. A patient is planning a trip to a malaria-endemic area and will be receiving prophylactic medications. Which of the following medical conditions would warrant additional considerations by the family nurse practitioner?
    1. Gilbert syndrome.
    2. Von Willebrand disease.
    3. Glucose-6-phosphate dehydrogenase (G6PD) deficiency.
    4. Bernard-Soulier syndrome.

13. A patient has a microcytic and hypochromic anemia and was placed on iron supplementation with no change in the anemia. Recent laboratory tests note normal ferritin and iron levels with continued microcytic and hypochromic anemia findings. What laboratory test will be used in the differential diagnosis to distinguish this anemia?
    1. Sickledex.
    2. Complete blood count.
    3. Reticulocyte count.
    4. Hemoglobin electrophoresis.

14. Which of the following would be a prudent decision by the family nurse practitioner?
    1. If the reticulocyte count is 100,000 mcg/L, then refer to a hematologist.

2. If the mean corpuscular volume (MCV) is above 100 fL, then order vitamin B_{12} and folate tests.
   3. If the MCV is below 50 fL, then order a platelet count.
   4. If the hemoglobin is less than 8 g/dL, then refer to a hematologist.

15. A patient has koilonychia. The family nurse practitioner understands this is associated with:
    1. Acute lymphocytic leukemia.
    2. Thrombocytopenia.
    3. Vitamin B_{12} and folate deficiency.
    4. Iron-deficiency anemia.

16. When reviewing the laboratory work of a patient diagnosed with thalassemia, the nurse practitioner expects which of the following? (Select 3 responses.)
    1. Microcytic anemia.
    2. Hyperchromic cells.
    3. Normocytic anemia.
    4. Macrocytic anemia.
    5. Elevated reticulocyte count.
    6. Normal red cell distribution width (RDW).

17. An older adult client is at the clinic for an annual exam. On physical exam, the family nurse practitioner notes nontender splenomegaly. The blood work findings are: white blood cells (WBCs) 30,000 cells/mm³, red blood cell count normal, hemoglobin 10.0 g/dL, presence of blast cells on complete blood count (CBC) differential, and elevated eosinophils and basophils. What would be an appropriate course of action?
    1. Monitor CBC and have patient return in 1 month for evaluation.
    2. Start patient on oral iron supplementation.
    3. Refer patient to a hematologist.
    4. Start patient on imatinib mesylate (Gleevec).

18. What tests are used to initially screen for sickle cell disease? (Select 2 responses.)
    1. Hemoglobin electrophoresis.
    2. Sickledex.
    3. Complete blood count (CBC).
    4. Bone marrow biopsy.
    5. Reticulocyte count.

Disorders

19. An older adult client is diagnosed with leukemia and has constitutional symptoms of night sweats, unintentional weight loss, and fatigue with painless lymphadenopathy. What type of leukemia does this older adult client have?
    1. Acute lymphocytic leukemia.
    2. Chronic lymphocytic leukemia.
    3. Acute myelogenous leukemia.
    4. Chronic myelogenous leukemia.

20. An adult patient presents to the family nurse practitioner with a history of erythrocytosis. What is one common complaint that could cause a serious complication for the patient?
    1. A laceration.
    2. Vomiting and diarrhea.
    3. Coughing.
    4. Dizziness.

21. After the loss of his wife 5 months ago, a 67-year-old male patient began abusing alcohol. He has no prior medical problems and no history of alcoholism. Which of the following would be the most likely cause of new-onset anemia development in this patient?
    1. Liver cirrhosis.
    2. Thiamine deficiency.
    3. Folate deficiency.
    4. Cyanocobalamin deficiency.

22. A patient has a folic acid–deficiency anemia. The family nurse practitioner teaches the patient to eat foods rich in folic acid, such as:
    1. Green leafy vegetables, nuts, and liver.
    2. Carrots, salmon, and avocados.
    3. Cottage cheese, yogurt, and skim milk.
    4. Lima beans, brussels sprouts, and potatoes.

23. Which three of the following statements are true about myelodysplastic syndromes (MDSs)?
    1. Affects predominantly older adults greater than 65 years of age.
    2. Is primarily one disease that has a variable clinical presentation.
    3. Symptoms relate to bone marrow failure.
    4. Patients often become dependent on red blood cell transfusion.
    5. Immunosuppressive drug therapy is rarely indicated.

24. Which of the following changes occurs in the RBC indices for pernicious anemia?
    1. Microcytic, normochromic.
    2. Microcytic, hypochromic.
    3. Normocytic, normochromic.
    4. Macrocytic, normochromic.

25. The family nurse practitioner knows which of the following is the most likely cause of acute hemolytic transfusion reactions?
    1. Contaminated blood products.
    2. ABO incompatibility.
    3. Immunoglobulin deficiency.
    4. Expired blood products.

26. Which statement is true concerning thalassemia?
    1. It is characterized by defective lymphocyte synthesis.
    2. Thalassemia minor does not require pharmacologic treatment.
    3. Thalassemia major is associated with high red blood cell (RBC) counts and elevated serum iron.
    4. It is characterized by an acute onset of symptoms leading to leukocytosis.

27. An older adult who has acute myelogenous leukemia (AML) is undergoing cytotoxic chemotherapy treatment and has the following laboratory reports: elevated serum uric acid, serum potassium, and serum phosphate and a low serum calcium level. The white blood cell (WBC) count is extremely elevated, and on physical exam, there is noted lymphadenopathy and splenomegaly. What is most likely the cause?
    1. Disseminated intravascular coagulation (DIC).
    2. Leukostasis.
    3. Pancytopenia.
    4. Tumor lysis syndrome.

28. Iron-deficiency anemia is an example of:
    1. Macrocytic, normochromic anemia.
    2. Macrocytic, hypochromic anemia.
    3. Microcytic, hypochromic anemia.
    4. Normocytic, normochromic anemia.

29. An adult patient with pernicious anemia may present with which signs and symptoms?
    1. Peripheral neuropathy, ataxia, lethargy, and fatigue.
    2. Hepatomegaly, jaundice, and right upper quadrant pain.
    3. Hypertension, angina, and peripheral edema.
    4. Blurred vision, diplopia, and decreased vibratory sensation.

30. Anemia of chronic disease is a:
    1. Normochromic, normocytic anemia.
    2. Normochromic, microcytic anemia.
    3. Hypochromic, microcytic anemia.
    4. Hypochromic, macrocytic anemia.

31. A young adult presents to the clinic for a routine checkup. History is unremarkable, but on physical exam, the family nurse practitioner palpates an enlarged (2 cm), mobile, nontender, rubbery lymph node on the left posterior cervical chain. What is the family nurse practitioner's next step?
    1. Order a throat culture and monospot test.
    2. Refer to a surgeon for a lymph node biopsy.
    3. Order a STAT chest x-ray.
    4. No intervention is necessary at this time.

32. The family nurse practitioner understands that "B" symptoms associated with non-Hodgkin lymphoma (NHL) include:
    1. Bruising and bleeding.
    2. Peripheral edema, shortness of breath, and ascites.
    3. Fever, night sweats, and unexplained weight loss.
    4. Headache, fatigue, and weakness.

33. In teaching a patient with anemia to include foods rich in iron in the diet, what does the family nurse practitioner encourage the patient to eat?
    1. Cheese, milk, and yogurt.
    2. Red beans, whole-grain bread, and bran cereal.
    3. Tomatoes, cabbage, and citrus fruits.
    4. Beef, spinach, and peanut butter.

34. Anemia of chronic disease is associated with:
    1. Malnutrition and vitamin B_{12} deficiency.
    2. Infections, inflammation, and neoplasms.
    3. Traumatic injuries and folate deficiency.
    4. Excessive menstrual flow, trauma, and heredity.

35. The family nurse practitioner understands that most adult patients with Hodgkin lymphoma present with:
    1. Nausea, vomiting, and diarrhea.
    2. Night sweats, weight loss, and fever.
    3. Painless, movable mass in the neck, axilla, or groin.
    4. Hepatosplenomegaly with a painful mass in the mediastinum.

36. What is the most common leukemia found in the older adult, typically asymptomatic and characterized by median survival of about 10 years?
    1. Acute myelogenous.
    2. Chronic myelogenous.
    3. Acute lymphocytic.
    4. Chronic lymphocytic.

37. A female patient tells the family nurse practitioner she has a diagnosis of hemophilia A. What is the family nurse practitioner's understanding of the condition?
    1. Her mother was a carrier for the disease and her father had the disease.
    2. Both mother and father have the disease.
    3. Her mother was a carrier.
    4. Both grandparents were carriers of the disease.

38. Folic-acid deficiency most often results from:
    1. Lead exposure.
    2. Poor dietary habits.
    3. Gastrointestinal bleeding.
    4. Genetic defect.

39. A client identifies that he has a deficiency of glucose-6-phosphate dehydrogenase (G6PD). What is the family nurse practitioner's understanding of the condition? (Select 2 responses.)
    1. Involves a reduction in platelet and coagulation factors leading to bleeding tendencies.
    2. It is considered a genetic X-linked condition that patient is born with.
    3. Deficiency of the enzyme, G6PD, leads to increased red blood cell (RBC) vulnerability caused by oxidative stress and can lead to hemolytic anemia.

    4. With mild forms of the deficiency, the prognosis is poor.
    5. Fava beans are known to reduce the symptoms associated with anemia and should be encouraged in the diet.

40. Which of the following three statements are accurate about sickle cell trait (SCT)?
    1. If an individual has SCT, they do not pass on the gene to their offspring.
    2. Acquiring two abnormal sickle genes from both parents leads to sickle cell disease.
    3. SCT is a common genetic mutation of white blood cells.
    4. In areas in which malaria occurs frequently, SCT offers some protection against infection caused by malaria parasites, especially by *Plasmodium falciparum*.
    5. Life expectancy is poor with SCT.
    6. SCT is a heterozygous carrier state, not a disease.

41. What are four common causes of megaloblastic anemia (macrocytic)?
    1. Acute alcohol intoxication.
    2. Lack of the intrinsic factor.
    3. Gastric surgery.
    4. Hyperthyroidism.
    5. Malabsorption syndrome.
    6. Chronic laxative use.

42. The family nurse practitioner teaches a client who has pernicious anemia to select which of the following foods?
    1. Rice, bread, and cereals.
    2. Green leafy vegetables.
    3. Beef, chicken, clams, oysters.
    4. Fresh citrus fruits.

43. What type of anemia is associated with lead poisoning?
    1. Normocytic anemia.
    2. Microcytic anemia.
    3. Macrocytic anemia.
    4. Aplastic anemia.

44. The family nurse practitioner understands the following about von Willebrand disease (vWD):
    1. Is a bleeding disorder caused by an excess of platelets.
    2. Common symptoms are ecchymosis and epistaxis.
    3. Has only one inherited type, unlike hemophilia, which has different types.
    4. Has a lowered life expectancy of all the coagulation disorders.

45. The family nurse practitioner suspects aplastic anemia in an adult patient with a long history of rheumatoid arthritis. What two findings are associated with this diagnosis?
    1. History of taking gold medications.
    2. Short stature with skeletal or nail changes.
    3. Lack of bruising and fever.
    4. Pancytopenia.
    5. History of taking immunosuppressive medications.

46. Which of the following findings are associated with heparin-induced thrombocytopenia (HIT)?
    1. Elevated platelet count.
    2. Paradoxical thrombotic state.
    3. Spontaneous bleeding episodes.
    4. Gastrointestinal upset.

Pharmacology

47. A 65-year-old female is being discharged after a successful hip replacement. What is the minimum duration of therapy the family nurse practitioner would expect for postoperative deep vein thrombosis (DVT) thromboprophylaxis with rivaroxaban (Xarelto)?
    1. 3–5 days.
    2. 5–7 days.
    3. 10–14 days.
    4. 14–21 days.

48. The family nurse practitioner determines that an adult male patient has an iron-deficiency anemia and has ruled out gastrointestinal (GI) bleeding as the cause. What does the family nurse practitioner do next?
    1. Refers the patient to a hematologist.
    2. Orders iron dextran 50 mg IM weekly for 4 weeks and schedules the patient for weekly office visits for the injection.
    3. Prescribes ferrous sulfate 325 mg PO tid and schedules the patient to return in 1 month for a repeat complete blood count, serum iron, and total iron-binding capacity (TIBC).
    4. Schedules the patient to return in 6 months for additional stool guaiac testing.

49. What information would the family nurse practitioner include in teaching a patient about the treatment of vitamin B_{12} deficiency following a total gastrectomy?
    1. The patient will be taking vitamin B_{12} tablets twice daily for 1 year.
    2. The patient will be taking oral folic acid supplements daily for life.
    3. The patient will receive monthly cyanocobalamin (vitamin B_{12}) injections for life (after being given daily weekly injections for the first month).
    4. The patient will require iron supplementation and monthly blood transfusions until the deficiency is corrected.

50. A 76-year-old female has been taking ciprofloxacin specifically because of a bacterial infection. She currently takes warfarin and has maintained therapeutic levels for the last 5 years. Her most recent international normalized ratio (INR) was 2.3. The family nurse practitioner would expect to do which of the following?
    1. Bridge to heparin.
    2. Check INR within 1 week.
    3. Withhold warfarin.
    4. Increase warfarin dosage.

51. Which of the following would most likely need to be given to a patient with sickle cell anemia?
    1. Cyanocobalamin.
    2. Niacin.
    3. Thiamine.
    4. Folate.

52. The family nurse practitioner has prescribed elemental iron 6 mg/kg/day in three divided doses for a toddler diagnosed with iron-deficiency anemia. What instructions would the family nurse practitioner include for the parents?
    1. Give the iron with food to increase the absorption of the medication.
    2. Give the medication through a straw to decrease the staining of the teeth.
    3. Avoid foods containing ascorbic acid, which decreases absorption of the medication.
    4. If a dose is missed, double up on the next two doses.

53. After initiating vitamin B_{12} therapy, the family nurse practitioner would expect which of the following at a 4-week follow-up visit to the clinic?
    1. Ferritin level of 40 ng/mL.
    2. Reduced red blood cells, white blood cells, and platelets.
    3. Increased macrocytosis and anisocytosis.
    4. Increased hemoglobin/hematocrit and reticulocyte count.

54. A patient has been prescribed trimethoprim-sulfamethoxazole (Bactrim). Which condition is contradicted for prescribing this medication?
    1. Iron-deficiency anemia.
    2. Thalassemia.
    3. B_{12} deficiency.
    4. Glucose-6-phosphate dehydrogenase (G6PD) deficiency.

55. Which of the following three medications have the adverse effect of causing aplastic anemia?
    1. Phenytoin (Dilantin).
    2. Chloramphenicol (Chloromycetin).
    3. Naltrexone (ReVia).
    4. Felbamate (Felbatol).
    5. Vitamin E.
    6. Indinavir (Crixivan).

56. A patient who has been prescribed oral ferrous sulfate reports taking extra doses for the past few months. The patient's serum iron level is 560 mcg/dL. What should the family nurse practitioner order for this patient?
    1. Parenteral deferoxamine (Desferal).
    2. Recheck the iron level in 2 weeks.
    3. Gastric lavage and treatment for acidosis and shock.
    4. Oral deferasirox (Exjade).

57. The family nurse practitioner understands that patients who take both folic acid and vitamin B_{12} can:
    1. Reverse the hematologic effects of vitamin B_{12} deficiency.
    2. Cause fetal malformation with high doses.
    3. Improve the neurologic effects of B_{12} deficiency.
    4. Cause a microcytic, normochromic anemia.

58. A patient is receiving oral ferrous sulfate (Feosol) for iron-deficiency anemia. The family nurse practitioner is considering placing the patient on an antibiotic drug. Which medication, if taken concurrently with iron, would decrease the absorption of the iron supplement?
    1. Cefixime.
    2. Metronidazole.
    3. Amoxicillin.
    4. Tetracycline.

59. The nurse practitioner understands that the therapeutic uses of erythropoietin (Epoetin alfa) are for patients with: (Select 4 responses.)
    1. Leukemia.
    2. Myeloid malignancies.
    3. Anemia of chronic renal failure.
    4. Chemotherapy-induced anemia in nonmyeloid malignancies.
    5. Anemia in patients who are preoperative.
    6. HIV taking zidovudine (AZT).

60. What is a potential side effect of filgrastim (granulocyte colony–stimulating factor) for a patient undergoing myelosuppressive chemotherapy?
    1. Infection.
    2. Headache.
    3. Thrombocytosis.
    4. Bone pain.

61. A patient presents at the clinic with complaints of shortness of breath with a pulse rate of 90. There is notable 3+ pitting edema bilaterally in the lower extremities. Which medication taken by the patient is most likely causing the patient's symptoms?
    1. Oprelvekin (Interleukin-11).
    2. Filgrastim (granulocyte colony–stimulating factor).
    3. Erythropoietin (Epoetin alfa).
    4. Sargramostim (granulocyte-macrophage colony–stimulating factor).

62. A patient with hemophilia A is undergoing a tooth extraction at the dentist's office. As an adjunct to factor VIII, what other drug would the family nurse practitioner order for the patient?
    1. Desmopressin (Stimate).
    2. Vitamin K.
    3. Tranexamic acid (Cyklokapron).
    4. Ibuprofen (Advil).

13 Hematology Answers & Rationales

Physical Exam & Diagnostic Tests

1. Answer: 3

Rationale: Iron-deficiency anemia is a hypochromic, microcytic anemia. Decreased iron stores (serum ferritin) are the hallmark of iron-deficiency anemia along with increased transferrin. The liver compensates by increasing production of transferrin, which also increases total iron-binding capacity (TIBC). Because iron stores are depleted, the percent of transferrin saturated with iron (% transferrin saturation) is decreased. Normal to increased iron stores (serum ferritin) with concurrent low-serum iron is the hallmark finding of anemia of chronic disease. Serum iron is decreased along with TIBC. Decreased iron, increased TIBC, and decreased serum ferritin contain the findings for iron-deficiency anemia.

2. Answer: 3

Rationale: The serum ferritin correlates with total body iron stores because it is the major iron storage protein. Its value is reduced in iron-deficiency anemia. Direct Coombs measures in vivo RBC coating by immunoglobulins and is positive in autoimmune hemolytic anemia, blood transfusion reactions, and drug-induced hemolysis. Serum folate measures the folic acid level in the blood. Ferritin levels less than 15 mcg/L are indicative of a diagnosis of iron-deficiency anemia (levels less than 30 mcg/L are a likely diagnosis of iron-deficiency anemia). Levels greater than 100 mcg/L rule out iron deficiency.

3. Answer: 2

Rationale: Shotty, or small and pellet-like, lymph nodes that are movable, cool, nontender, discrete, and less than 1 cm in diameter are usually considered normal and often represent enlargement of the lymph nodes after a viral infection. They feel like BBs or buckshot under the skin that move under the examiner's fingers when palpated. If shotty nodes are found in the epitrochlear or supraclavicular regions, they require additional evaluation. A fixed, or nonmovable, lymph node is cause for concern.

4. Answer: 4

Rationale: It is important to determine the type of macrocytic anemia so that the appropriate therapy can be ordered. Therefore, the vitamin B_{12} and RBC/folate levels would be ordered. These tests would determine whether the patient has a pernicious anemia (the most common type) or a folate deficiency (also common in older adult patients). Serum iron and TIBC would be ordered if an iron-deficiency anemia was suspected. There is no indication for a colonoscopy. It would be premature to order a bone marrow biopsy without performing initial testing and potentially overlooking an easily treated condition (e.g., pernicious anemia, folate-deficiency anemia). Measurement of certain metabolites of vitamin B_{12}, methylmalonic acid, and homocysteine provides additional information to help identify the cause of the anemia.

5. Answer: 1

Rationale: DIC is a complication of infection, malignancy, blood transfusions, liver disease, pregnancy, and sometimes trauma. DIC is the inappropriate accelerated systemic activation of the coagulation cascade, resulting in simultaneous hemorrhage and thrombosis. Laboratory results would show increased PT and decreased platelet count and fibrinogen in response to the hemorrhage and clotting. Fibrinolysis occurs as part of the DIC process, which results in increased fibrin degradation product and positive D-dimer.

6. Answer: 1

Rationale: Children often have generalized lymphadenopathy in response to mild infections of the skin or respiratory tract. Palpable lymph nodes are generally not present in healthy individuals, but some may have small, discrete, nontender nodes that are not clinically significant. Enlarged lymph nodes may indicate infection, inflammation, and malignancy in both children and adults. Tender lymph nodes are noted with inflammatory processes. Hard, fixed, and painless lymph nodes may indicate a malignant process. A painless, firm supraclavicular or cervical lymph node is a common sign of Hodgkin disease in children, not Burkitt lymphoma, in which the child has other associated symptoms depending on the system affected.

7. Answer: 1

Rationale: FOBT, or guaiac testing, would identify blood loss from the gastrointestinal tract—the most common cause of iron-deficiency anemia, along with menorrhagia in females. The other tests should be done if the FOBT results are positive. Finding the cause of the iron deficiency is paramount, and the FOBT is an easy, noninvasive method of ruling out gastrointestinal bleeding as the cause.

8. Answer: 2

Rationale: The anti-IF or antiparietal cell antibody assay test is the currently accepted method to verify the diagnosis of pernicious anemia. The presence of anti-IF antibodies is highly specific for pernicious anemia. In the past, the Schilling test was used to determine the cause of the vitamin B_{12} deficiency. In pernicious anemia, it will be important to distinguish between inadequate intake of B_{12} or a malabsorption problem (an intrinsic-factor deficiency). This will allow the practitioner to prescribe the most appropriate therapy for the patient. A bone marrow biopsy and an upper GI series are not indicated at this time.

9. Answer: 3

Rationale: Normal and abnormal hemoglobin can be detected by electrophoresis, which matches hemolyzed red blood cell material against standard bands for the various known hemoglobins, including hemoglobin S, the abnormal hemoglobin associated with sickle cell anemia. CBC with peripheral smear and hemoglobin/hematocrit would not yield enough information to diagnose sickle cell anemia. Low hemoglobin, normal to increased mean corpuscular volume, increased mean corpuscular hemoglobin, chronic reticulocytosis, mild-to-moderate anisocytosis, and poikilocytosis with numerous sickle cells and Howell-Jolly bodies would be noted on the CBC and differential. A bone marrow biopsy would not be necessary and would not indicate the presence of hemoglobin S.

10. Answer: 4

Rationale: This patient's clinical picture is a classic presentation for anemia. Further testing is needed to determine the type of anemia involved. The most common cause in older adult men is gastrointestinal bleeding, which would cause an iron-deficiency anemia. The tests that were ordered would confirm or rule out this diagnosis. The peripheral smear is especially important in diagnosing the specific type of anemia, for example, hypochromic and microcytic. TIBC would be increased, and serum ferritin and serum iron are decreased. If the smear ruled out the diagnosis of iron-deficiency anemia, it would lead the practitioner to other diagnoses (including the remaining choices) and the appropriate laboratory tests required for confirmation.

11. Answer: 2

Rationale: Normal to increased iron stores (serum ferritin) with concurrent low-serum iron is the hallmark finding of ACD. Serum iron is decreased along with TIBC. Decreased iron, increased TIBC, and decreased serum ferritin contain the findings for iron-deficiency anemia.

12. Answer: 3

Rationale: Malaria prophylaxis and treatment include medications that are high risk of causing hemolytic anemia in patients with X-linked G6PD. Patients who require primaquine for malaria prophylaxis must be screened for G6PD deficiency

before administration. Deficiency of G6PD can result in hemolysis and hemolytic anemia. Excessive oxidative stress on red blood cells by medications such as anti-malarials, aspirin, NSAIDS, and sulfonamides may induce hemolytic anemia.

13. Answer: 4

Rationale: The family nurse practitioner needs to distinguish iron-deficiency anemia from thalassemia in this patient. It is important to note that the anemia was not improved with iron supplementation. The gold standard diagnostic test is the hemoglobin electrophoresis. The test is normal with iron-deficiency anemia, and in beta-thalassemia it is abnormal, as noted by a variable increase in the amount of hemoglobin A2 and possibly increased hemoglobin F for beta-thalassemia and presence of hemoglobin H in hemoglobin H disease. The Sickledex is a screening blood test for sickle cell anemia.

14. Answer: 2

Rationale: Based on the MCV, anemias are classified as microcytic (MCV less than 80 fL), normocytic (MCV 80–99 fL), or macrocytic (MCV greater than 100 fL). If the MCV is greater than 100 fL, then order vitamin B_{12} and folate tests to evaluate for deficiencies. The tests should be ordered even if there are no neurologic signs (tingling, numbness). If the MCV is less than 80 fL, then a total iron-binding capacity, ferritin, and serum iron would be ordered, not a platelet count. The reticulocyte count evaluates bone marrow production of red blood cells (RBCs). Any value higher than $>100,000/\mu L$ is considered a marrow that is responding normally to anemic conditions. Reticulocyte count values less than $75,000/\mu L$ are considered consistent with impaired (decreased) RBC production and should be referred to a hematologist. Consultation with a physician (not necessarily a hematologist) is recommended for hemoglobin values less than 10 g/dL.

15. Answer: 4

Rationale: Koilonychia or spoon nails are characterized by a central depression of the nail with lateral elevation of the nail plate. The nails of the hand are most commonly affected and are abnormally thin with loss of their convexity, becoming flat or even concave in shape. Iron-deficiency anemia is the most frequent cause of koilonychia. The finding is also associated with syphilis, fungal dermatoses, and malnutrition.

16. Answer: 1, 5, 6

Rationale: Peripheral blood findings in patients with thalassemia include: microcytosis (mean corpuscular volume less than 70 fL), hypochromia (mean corpuscular hemoglobin less than 20 pg), high percentage of target cells, and elevated reticulocyte count. A normal RDW with a microcytic, hypochromic anemia is almost always thalassemia trait. The RDW can be elevated in approximately 60% of thalassemia trait patients. This is in contrast to iron deficiency anemia, where the RDW is almost always elevated (90%).

17. Answer: 3

Rationale: The family nurse practitioner suspects chronic lymphocytic leukemia based on the elevated WBC, splenomegaly, mild anemia, and presence of blast cells and elevated basophils and eosinophils on the differential. Referral to a hematologist is indicated for all suspected cases of leukemia. Chronic myelogenous leukemia is treated initially with imatinib mesylate (Gleevec) and is ordered by the hematologist.

18. Answer: 2, 3

Rationale: The Sickledex test is a blood test that is positive (turbid or cloudy test fluid) if greater than 10% of the hemoglobin is hemoglobin S. This is only a screening test and has variable sensitivity depending on the method used by the laboratory. Both sickle cell disease (homozygous for hemoglobin S) and sickle cell trait (heterozygous for hemoglobin S) can be detected by this screening study. For a definitive diagnosis of sickle cell disease, the next test ordered would be the hemoglobin electrophoresis to confirm the diagnosis. The CBC is an overall useful and initial test to determine status of anemia. A bone marrow biopsy is performed to diagnose, stage, and monitor for lymphoproliferative disorders, such as chronic lymphocytic leukemia, Hodgkin and non-Hodgkin lymphoma, hairy cell leukemia, myeloproliferative disorders, myelodysplastic syndrome, and multiple myeloma. The reticulocyte count is a test for determining bone marrow function and evaluating erythropoietic activity. It does not measure for hemoglobin S or sickling of red blood cells.

Disorders

19. Answer: 2

Rationale: Chronic lymphocytic leukemia (CLL) is the most common leukemia in older adults caused by proliferation of immature lymphocytes. Patients with CLL can have variable clinical presentations including constitutional "B" symptoms, including night sweats, unintentional weight loss, fever, and severe fatigue. Patients typically have painless lymphadenopathy and abnormal laboratory analysis with lymphocytosis, although neutropenia, anemia, and thrombocytopenia can be observed.

20. Answer: 2

Rationale: Erythrocytosis (or polycythemia) can be worsened by dehydration from any cause, for example, vomiting and diarrhea. Coughing and dizziness will have no effect on the condition, and a laceration may actually improve the symptoms because of the blood loss.

21. Answer: 3

Rationale: Patients who abuse alcohol often develop macrocytosis (mean corpuscular volume greater than 100 fL). Specifically, alcoholic patients often develop macrocytic anemia caused by folate (vitamin B_9) and cyanocobalamin (vitamin B_{12}) deficiencies. Folate deficiency manifests within a few months because of relatively lower stores in the liver compared with cyanocobalamin. Additionally, older adults are at a higher risk for development of folate and cyanocobalamin deficiency related to food malabsorption.

22. Answer: 1

Rationale: Green leafy vegetables, oranges and orange juice, and nuts are excellent sources of folic acid. Also, cereals and breads are now fortified with folic acid. Be sure to stress that folate is heat labile and rapidly destroyed by prolonged cooking or food processing. The other foods are not significant sources of folic acid.

23. Answer: 1, 3, 4

Rationale: Myelodysplastic syndromes (MDSs) are a heterogeneous group of bone marrow disorders characterized by symptoms related to bone marrow failure and/or specific symptoms related to cytopenias (anemia, thrombocytopenia, neutropenia, etc.) that affects primarily older adults (age greater than 65 years). MDS is not one disease but a diverse series of hematologic conditions that have variable clinical presentation. Immunosuppressive drug therapy is used for patients with MDS, with the primary goal of therapy being to improve quality of life. Patients often receive numerous red blood cell transfusions. When patients have received more than 20 red blood cell transfusions, patients become iron overloaded. With these patients, iron chelation becomes a consideration because iron overload may contribute to both increased mortality and morbidity in early-stage MDS.

24. Answer: 4

Rationale: A macrocytic (mean corpuscular volume greater than 100 fL), normochromic anemia resulting from atrophic gastric mucosa not secreting intrinsic factor is the definition of pernicious anemia. These indices could also include folic acid–deficiency anemia. Microcytic normochromic or hypochromic could include iron-deficiency anemia or anemia of chronic disease. Normocytic and normochromic could also include anemia of chronic disease.

25. Answer: 2

Rationale: Acute hemolytic transfusion reactions (AHTRs) most often occur within the first 24 hours of blood product administration. The most common cause is from clerical errors causing ABO incompatibility. Because of the serious risk of mortality associated with AHTRs, special attention to proper procedure, documentation, and communication should be observed.

26. Answer: 2

Rationale: Thalassemias are chronic, inherited anemias characterized by defective hemoglobin synthesis leading to a decreased RBC count, hypochromia (mean corpuscular hemoglobin less than 20 pg), microcytosis (mean corpuscular volume less than 70 fL), normal serum iron, and normal RBC distribution width (RDW) in thalassemia minor, which does not require pharmacologic treatment. It should be noted that although the RDW is usually normal, it can be elevated in about 50% of patients with thalassemia trait, which is in contrast to iron-deficiency anemia, in which the RDW is almost always elevated (90%). Patients with thalassemia minor should not be given iron supplements to resolve anemia. Patients with thalassemia major are usually managed by a hematologist.

27. Answer: 4

Rationale: Tumor lysis syndrome occurs when a patient has a high WBC count and is undergoing cytotoxic chemotherapy for the treatment of AML. It is characterized by the development of acute hyperuricemia, hyperkalemia, hyperphosphatemia, and hypocalcemia, with or without acute renal failure. It is the most common of all the oncologic emergencies. Other complications include leukostasis, DIC, and pancytopenia. Although AML is most often associated with DIC, it is characterized by a decreased platelet count, a prolonged prothrombin and partial thromboplastin time, and a decreased fibrinogen level with an elevation of fibrin degradation products. Leukostasis, blood sludging or stasis, occurs when the blood vessels become overcrowded with immature blast cells in patients with AML who have high WBC counts, which can lead to ischemia and infarcts in the pulmonary and cranial blood vessels. Pancytopenia is a drastic reduction in all types of blood cells (WBC, red blood cells, platelets) that can occur because of myelosuppression from cytotoxic chemotherapy.

28. Answer: 3

Rationale: Iron-deficiency anemia is a microcytic, hypochromic anemia. The red blood cells are smaller (microcytic) because of the decrease in hemoglobin production caused by inadequate amounts of iron, which also makes the cell appear pale (hypochromic). The other selections describe other types of anemia, which would be determined by the peripheral smear.

29. Answer: 1

Rationale: Vitamin B_{12} deficiency may result in neurologic signs and symptoms, including peripheral neuropathy, paresthesias, unsteady gait (ataxia), loss of proprioception, decreased vibratory sensation, lethargy, and fatigue. In the later stages of severe B_{12} deficiency, spasticity, hyperactive reflexes, and the presence of Romberg's sign are noted because of the formation of a demyelinating lesion of the neurons of the spinal cord and cerebral cortex and the presence of a beefy-red tongue. These findings are specific to pernicious anemia and must be assessed

in all patients who present with anemia. The other signs and symptoms are not characteristic of pernicious anemia.

30. Answer: 1

Rationale: Anemia of chronic disease is a chronic normochromic, normocytic, and hypoproliferative anemia. There is normal production of hemoglobin, along with normal maturation of red blood cells. The serum iron is low, and the ferritin level and total iron-binding capacity are elevated.

31. Answer: 2

Rationale: Lymphadenopathy as described, without evidence of infection, should always be referred to a surgeon for biopsy, the only definitive test to rule out a malignancy (a frequent cause of lymphadenopathy not caused by infectious processes). No signs or symptoms suggest the need for a throat culture, monospot test, or chest x-ray. Not intervening is inappropriate because the cause of lymphadenopathy needs to be determined.

32. Answer: 3

Rationale: This constellation of symptoms (fever, night sweats, and weight loss) is used in the staging of NHL, the presence of which is considered to be a poor prognostic indicator. The other symptoms may occur depending on the amount of disease involvement, but they are not considered "B" symptoms, also known as constitutional symptoms.

33. Answer: 4

Rationale: Beef, spinach, and peanut butter are iron-rich foods. The other options are examples of foods rich in calcium, fiber, and vitamin C, respectively.

34. Answer: 2

Rationale: Anemia or chronic disease is associated with infections (e.g., tuberculosis), chronic inflammatory conditions (e.g., systemic lupus erythematosus, rheumatoid arthritis), and malignancies. Excessive blood loss from menstrual flow or traumatic injuries would more likely cause an iron-deficiency anemia. Malnutrition can contribute to iron, vitamin B_{12}, and folate deficiencies.

35. Answer: 3

Rationale: Most patients with Hodgkin lymphoma present with a painless, movable mass in the neck, axilla, or groin. Constitutional symptoms may also occur, which include weight loss, persistent fever, and night sweats. Often the patient may experience pruritus and pain in the lymph node area after consuming alcohol (an unexplained finding). Hepatosplenomegaly presents with advanced disease.

36. Answer: 4

Rationale: Chronic lymphocytic leukemia (CLL) is found primarily in middle-aged and older adults (less than 10% of patients under age 50). Median age of diagnosis of CLL is 70 years, affecting more males than females. Acute myelogenous leukemia (AML) incidence increases with age, with median age greater than 70 years. Chronic myelogenous leukemia (CML) occurs between 50 and 60 years. Acute lymphocytic leukemia (ALL) is most common in children.

37. Answer: 1

Rationale: Hemophilia A is characterized by a deficiency of factor VIII and is caused by an X-linked chromosome recessive inheritance disorder. This means that males are almost exclusively affected with hemophilia and females are carriers. When a female has hemophilia, she is the offspring of a father with hemophilia and a mother who is a carrier. In the past, this rarely occurred because males with hemophilia rarely lived to adult reproductive age. Now with the availability of replacement factor VIII, male patients with hemophilia can live to reproductive age.

38. Answer: 2

Rationale: Folic-acid deficiency most often results from dietary deficits and frequently affects the older adult, chronically ill, alcoholic patients, and food faddists (poor food selections). Pregnancy requires an increase in folic acid, as do disease states such as cancer, chronic inflammation, Crohn's disease, rheumatoid arthritis, and malabsorption syndromes.

39. Answer: 2, 3

Rationale: Deficiency of the enzyme G6PD leads to increased RBC vulnerability caused by oxidative stress and can lead to hemolytic anemia. It is a genetic X-linked condition that the patient is born with, residing on the X chromosome (Xq28). Fava beans (favism) have triggered hemolysis, particularly in patients with the Mediterranean variant, and should be avoided. For those with the milder forms of the deficiency, the prognosis is excellent. The RBC is affected but not the platelet or coagulation factors.

40. Answer: 2, 4, 6

Rationale: SCT is the most common genetic mutation of hemoglobin. An individual with SCT inherits one mutated sickle β-chain hemoglobin gene from the mother or father, with a nonmutated gene from the other parent (heterozygous variant). SCT is a heterozygous carrier state, not a disease. Individuals with SCT are often from West Africa, the Middle East, the Mediterranean region, and India. These are areas in which malaria occurs frequently, and SCT offers some protection against malaria parasites, especially by *P. falciparum*, which is more than likely the major reason for the genetic continuation of the sickle hemoglobin mutation. Carrier status increases the risk of having an offspring with SCT, and if the partner also has SCT, then sickle cell disease is possible. The life expectancy of people with SCT is similar to the general population.

41. Answer: 2, 3, 4, 5

Rationale: Megaloblastic (macrocytic) anemias are associated with B_{12} deficiency and folate deficiency. Malabsorption can lead to vitamin B_{12} and folate acid deficiency—lack of intrinsic factor, gastric surgery, inflammatory bowel disease, sprue (tropical and nontropical), celiac disease, and hyperthyroidism. Inadequate intake from a vegetarian diet without meat food sources and chronic alcoholism can also lead to deficiencies. Medications, such as proton pump inhibitors, H2 antagonists, and antacids decrease gastric acidity, inhibiting B_{12} release from dietary protein; long-term metformin usage leads to B_{12} deficiency, not chronic laxative use.

42. Answer: 3

Rationale: The best food sources for vitamin B_{12} are of animal origin, including the following richest sources: beef and chicken liver, lean meat, clams, oysters, herring, and crab.

43. Answer: 2

Rationale: Lead poisoning can cause a microcytic anemia. Lead circulates through the body attached to erythrocytes. It affects heme production, competes with calcium in any calcium-mediated process, alters certain enzyme functions in the bone marrow, and damages the nervous system. Lead poisoning may be associated with a hypochromic, microcytic anemia because most patients have concomitant iron deficiency. Diseases included in the differential diagnoses of microcytic anemia include thalassemia, anemia of chronic disease, sideroblastic anemia, lead poisoning, and aluminium toxicity.

44. Answer: 2

Rationale: Epistaxis, menorrhagia, ecchymosis, and prolonged bleeding with cuts or dental extractions and in the intraoperative or immediate postoperative period are common symptoms of vWD. vWD is a bleeding disorder caused by deficiency or a defect of von Willebrand factor (vWF) protein and is the most common congenital bleeding disorder, occurring in up to 1% of the general population. There are three major types of vWD, all of which exhibit an autosomal inheritance pattern, affecting both males and females. vWF is critical to the initial stages of blood clotting, acting as a bridge for platelet adhesion; it also acts as a carrier for factor VIII. Life expectancy is not lower than other disorders of coagulation; actually, it is better with treatment.

45. Answer: 1, 4

Rationale: Aplastic anemia is a condition in which the bone marrow fails. The syndrome is characterized by immune-mediated bone marrow destruction and peripheral blood pancytopenia. Fatigue, pallor, exertional shortness of breath, or palpitations are seen secondary to anemia. Mucosal bleeding, easy bruising, petechiae, or heavy menstrual bleeding is seen secondary to thrombocytopenia. Infection is uncommon at clinical presentation, but severe neutropenia may lead to fever and sore throat. Short stature with skeletal or nail changes are associated with congenital acquired aplastic anemia. Drugs such as felbamate, cimetidine, non-steroidal antiinflammatory drugs, antiepileptics, gold salts, chloramphenicol, sulfonamides, trimethadione, quinacrine, and phenylbutazone are common etiologic factors in acquired aplastic anemia. The treatment for aplastic anemia includes hematopoietic stem cell transplantation and immunosuppressive therapy with antithymocyte globulin and cyclosporine or high-dose cyclophosphamide.

46. Answer: 2

Rationale: A sudden drop in the platelet count may be indicative of HIT requiring immediate cessation of any heparin infusion. HIT commonly does not induce bleeding but instead results in a paradoxical prothrombotic state. Gastrointestinal upset is not a common finding with HIT.

Pharmacology

47. Answer: 3

Rationale: The anticoagulant rivaroxaban (Xarelto) is a factor Xa inhibitor and is recommended for postoperative DVT thromboprophylaxis in hip and knee replacements. It should be started immediately after homeostasis has been achieved postoperatively for a minimum of 10–14 days. Therapy in some patients may be extended up to 35 days.

48. Answer: 3

Rationale: Treatment with iron orally for at least 6 months is necessary to correct both the anemia and the depleted body iron stores. Ferrous sulfate should be taken on an empty stomach 1 hour before meals. If the patient experiences GI symptoms, the dose can be reduced or the patient can take the iron with the meal; however, taking it with meals will reduce the delivery and absorption of the iron by 50%. Iron dextran (parenteral) may be used if the patient is unable to take PO medications or if the hemoglobin is less than 6 g/dL. The patient should have hemoglobin/hematocrit, iron, and TIBC rechecked after 1 month on iron supplementation. If there is no improvement in all parameters, most notably a rise in the hemoglobin by 1 g/dL, then the patient should be referred to a hematologist. Referral to a GI specialist or

repeat of stool guaiac testing is unnecessary because there is no indication that this patient's condition is caused by bleeding.

49. Answer: 3

Rationale: If the deficiency is not caused by inadequate intake, the patient will require lifetime supplementation of vitamin B_{12} (1000 mcg of cyanocobalamin) by intramuscular injection to ensure absorption. In patients with irreversible malabsorption (total gastrectomy) and severe neurologic symptoms, parenteral therapy is indicated: 1000 mcg/day for 7 days, and then 1000 mcg weekly for 4 weeks, followed by 1000 mcg monthly for life. The family nurse practitioner should keep in mind that high-dose, daily oral cyanocobalamin (1000–2000 mcg) is as effective as a monthly intramuscular injection and is the preferred route of initial therapy in most circumstances because it is cost-effective and convenient. Oral folic acid, iron, and blood transfusions would not treat the cause of the deficiency; therefore, the resulting anemia would not be corrected.

50. Answer: 2

Rationale: Warfarin is commonly affected by many medications including ciprofloxacin. Prothrombin time/INR levels should be checked within 1 week of administration of ciprofloxacin because of the possibility for increased effects of warfarin.

51. Answer: 4

Rationale: Because of increased red blood cell turnover, folate supplementation is often required in patients with sickle cell anemia because of their relatively low stores of the vitamin in the liver. Other supplementations may be indicated if dietary intake is insufficient, but they are given without iron. Deferoxamine or other iron chelators may be required in these patients because of a buildup of iron related to transfusions.

52. Answer: 2

Rationale: Iron medications can cause staining of the teeth, so it is a good practice to give the medication through a straw. It is best to give iron on an empty stomach (if tolerable) to increase absorption. Ascorbic acid increases absorption of iron. If a dose is missed, it is best to give the dose when it is remembered as long as it is not too close to the next dose. The next two doses would not be increased.

53. Answer: 4

Rationale: In addition to a sense of well-being, improved appetite, and decreased neurologic symptoms (gait disturbances, peripheral neuropathy, paresthesias [numbness/tingling in fingers], and extreme weakness), the hemoglobin/hematocrit and reticulocyte count should increase with vitamin B_{12} therapy.

54. Answer: 4

Rationale: G6PD deficiency is an inherited trait, which is most common among African Americans and people of Mediterranean origin. Deficiency of the enzyme G6PD leads to increased red blood cell (RBC) vulnerability related to oxidative stress and may cause hemolytic anemia. Following exposure to oxidative stress, G6PD-deficient RBCs are destroyed by intravascular hemolysis resulting in hemolytic anemia. Oxidant stressors include infections and chemicals (e.g., mothballs, antimalarials, some sulfonamides, rasburicase, methylene blue). In addition to hemolytic anemia, sulfonamides can cause agranulocytosis; leukopenia; thrombocytopenia; and, very rarely, aplastic anemia.

55. Answer: 1, 2, 4

Rationale: Aplastic anemia can occur in patients receiving phenytoin (Dilantin), felbamate (Felbatol), and chloramphenicol (Chloromycetin). Methyldopa can have hemolytic anemia as an adverse effect. Vitamin E is used in the treatment of hemolytic anemia. Naltrexone's serious effects are hepatotoxicity. Indinavir's major adverse effects are insulin-resistant hyperglycemia and ketoacidosis.

56. Answer: 1

Rationale: Iron is toxic in large amounts. If the plasma level of iron is elevated (greater than 500 mcg/dL), an iron-chelating agent, such as parenteral deferoxamine (Desferal), should be prescribed to immediately lower the iron level. Although gastric lavage may be ordered, it will only remove unabsorbed tablets that are present in the stomach. Oral deferasirox (Exjade) is used for chronic iron overload caused by blood transfusions.

57. Answer: 1

Rationale: Folic acid can reverse the hematologic effects of vitamin B_{12} deficiency, but it does not reverse the neurologic effects, so it is important to determine the degree of B_{12} deficiency to treat it. Folic acid does not cause fetal malformation, but it is administered prenatally to prevent neural tube defects. Folic acid causes a megaloblastic anemia.

58. Answer: 4

Rationale: Coadministration of tetracycline and iron reduces absorption of both iron and tetracycline. In addition, antacids reduce the absorption of iron. Cephalosporins (cefixime), metronidazole, and penicillin (amoxicillin) have no significant drug-to-drug interaction with iron.

59. Answer: 3, 4, 5, 6

Rationale: The therapeutic use for erythropoietin is indicated in nonmyeloid malignancy conditions requiring transfusions, when therapy is considered palliative, and with patients who have chemotherapy-induced anemia or anemia of chronic renal failure. Epoetin alfa may be given to increase erythrocyte levels in anemic patients scheduled for elective surgery. Epoetin alfa is approved for treating anemia caused by therapy with AZT in patients with AIDS. Epoetin alfa is not given to patients with leukemias or myeloid malignancies because the drugs can stimulate proliferation of these cancers.

60. Answer: 4

Rationale: Filgrastim stimulates the growth of white blood cells and is used to treat leukopenia. It causes bone pain in about 25% of patients. The pain is dose related and usually mild to moderate. Thrombocytopenia is a common side effect occurring quite often. Infection and headache are not common side effects of filgrastim.

61. Answer: 1

Rationale: Oprelvekin causes the kidneys to retain sodium and water, which causes peripheral edema and expansion of plasma volume. Some patients experience dyspnea caused by the fluid retention. Oprelvekin can cause tachycardia, atrial flutter, and atrial fibrillation. Fluid retention is not an adverse effect of epoetin alfa, filgrastim, or sargramostim.

62. Answer: 3

Rationale: Antifibrinolytic drugs (e.g., aminocaproic acid and tranexamic acid) can be used as adjuncts to factor VIII and factor IX in special situations, such as a tooth extraction. Nonsteroidal antiinflammatory drugs (ibuprofen) and aspirin should be avoided. Desmopressin is used as replacement therapy; it is not used specifically for tooth extractions, but it is indicated for minor procedures. Vitamin K is not indicated in this situation.

14

Urinary

Physical Exam & Diagnostic Tests

1. A basic urogenital evaluation in the older adult with complaints of new-onset incontinence should include:
   1. History, physical exam, postvoid residual, and urinalysis (UA).
   2. Postvoid residual, blood urea nitrogen (BUN), serum creatinine, and UA.
   3. History, physical exam, serum glucose, BUN, serum creatinine, and UA.
   4. Urodynamic/endoscopic/imaging tests, UA, and serum creatinine.

2. Differential diagnoses for a patient presenting with flank pain and hematuria include renal calculi, renal cell carcinoma, and hydronephrosis. Which one of the following diagnostic tools would be most useful in diagnosing this patient?
   1. Intravenous urography (IVU).
   2. Voiding cystourethrography.
   3. Intravenous pyelogram.
   4. Computed tomography (CT) urography.

3. A 39-year-old male bodybuilder is undergoing intense physical training. He tests his own urine using dipstick urinalysis in an attempt to measure his urinary ketones. He presents to the clinic inquiring about a single urinary analysis that indicated mild microscopic hematuria. Dipstick urinalysis today reveals no abnormalities other than ketones. What should the family nurse practitioner recommend?
   1. Reassurance.
   2. Evaluation for diabetes.
   3. Repeat urinalysis.
   4. Retrograde urethrogram.

4. Which of the following patients would be a good candidate for urodynamic studies (UDS)?
   1. Patient with history of stress incontinence and urge incontinence.
   2. Patient with recent surgery for bladder suspension.
   3. Patient with initial incontinence episode after total knee replacement.
   4. Older adult male with postvoid residual catheterization findings of 45 mL after 250-mL voiding.

5. The family nurse practitioner is evaluating blood chemistries on a patient who is experiencing an increase in blood pressure. She has no previous history of hypertension or other chronic disease. Which serum laboratory value would be most concerning?
   1. Serum creatinine 4.2 mg/dL.
   2. Blood urea nitrogen 30 mg/dL.
   3. Serum potassium 4.5 mEq/L.
   4. Serum osmolarity 290 mOsm/kg.

6. When taking a history of voiding patterns in adults, what should the family nurse practitioner consider?
   1. Adults normally void q2–3h in a 24-hour period (8–12 times a day).
   2. Urge sensation to void occurs when the bladder fills to 200–300 mL.
   3. Normally, 15–20 minutes pass between first urge to void and reaching functional capacity.
   4. Adults typically reach functional (comfortable) capacity at 200–300 mL and normally experience some leakage if voiding is delayed.

7. The family nurse practitioner understands the following about urine culture and sensitivity testing: (Select 2 responses.)
   1. The isolation of two or more bacterial species from a urine culture signifies a contaminated specimen unless the patient is being managed with an indwelling catheter or urinary diversion or has a chronic complicated infection.
   2. A conventional threshold is growth of greater than 100,000 colony-forming units (CFU/mL) from a midstream-catch urine sample.
   3. In symptomatic patients, a smaller number of bacteria (between 5 and 10 CFU/mL of midstream urine) are recognized as an infection.
   4. Immediately place the urine culture and sensitivity specimen on ice after patient clean catch collection.
   5. A negative urine culture result is typically greater than 100,000 CFU/mL.

8. The family nurse practitioner is evaluating a urinalysis report. Which findings are considered normal? (Select 4 responses.)
   1. Specific gravity 1.015.
   2. Large numbers of epithelial cells and casts.
   3. White blood cells (WBCs) ($\leq$5).
   4. Leukocyte esterase negative.
   5. Hyaline casts too numerous to count (TNTC).
   6. Few red blood cells (RBCs) ($\leq$2).

Disorders

9. A 68-year-old female returns for ongoing evaluation of *stress* incontinence that was thought to be associated with chronic urinary tract infections. She has been on low-dose trimethoprim-sulfamethoxazole (Bactrim) 40/200 mg for 6 months without resolution of her symptoms. What should this patient be evaluated for?
   1. Pelvic organ prolapse.
   2. Dementia or a neuromuscular disorder.
   3. Environmental barriers in the home.
   4. Addition of a tricyclic antidepressant.

10. A 65-year-old female explains to the family nurse practitioner that she has been having frequent and painful urination. A clean-catch urine specimen for routine urinalysis (UA) with culture and sensitivity (C&S) is ordered. Laboratory results show 10^5 colony-forming units (CFU)/mL of *Escherichia coli* and 10^4 CFU/mL of *Staphylococcus epidermidis*. What would be the family nurse practitioner's next step?
    1. Treat the *E. coli*.
    2. Order amoxicillin.
    3. Treat the *S. epidermidis*.
    4. Encourage citric fruit juices.

11. Which plan would be most appropriate for an older patient with functional incontinence?
    1. Evaluate need for incontinence pads.
    2. Limit fluid intake in the evenings.
    3. Perform the Credé maneuver.
    4. Provide a bedside commode.

12. A 60-year-old man presents with recurrent urinary tract infections and low-grade fever. What is the most likely cause?
    1. Balanitis.
    2. Epididymitis.
    3. Chronic bacterial prostatitis.
    4. Benign prostatic hypertrophy.

13. Which statement characterizes functional incontinence?
    1. Leakage of urine during activities that increase abdominal pressure, such as coughing, sneezing, and laughing.
    2. Mainly caused by factors outside the urinary tract, especially immobility, that prohibit proper toileting habits.

3. Characterized by the inability to delay urination, with an abrupt and strong desire to void.
4. Occurrence of incontinence with overdistention of bladder.

14. What are the two most common pathogens in community-acquired urinary tract infections (UTIs)?
    1. *Klebsiella pneumoniae.*
    2. *Proteus mirabilis.*
    3. *Staphylococcus saprophyticus.*
    4. *Escherichia coli.*
    5. *Staphylococcus aureus.*
    6. *Streptococcus pyogenes.*

15. A healthy adult female presents with cystitis. The family nurse practitioner would expect which of the following findings?
    1. No symptoms noted.
    2. Acute onset of chills, fever, flank pain, headache, malaise, and costovertebral angle tenderness.
    3. Complaints of dysuria, urgency, frequency, nocturia, and suprapubic heaviness.
    4. Signs and symptoms of fever, irritability, decreased appetite, vomiting, diarrhea, constipation, dehydration, and jaundice.

16. Fifteen days after completion of a course of antibiotics for a urinary tract infection (UTI), a 66-year-old female returns to the clinic with recurring symptoms. Recurrent UTIs in women are caused by relapse or reinfection. The family nurse practitioner understands the following about relapse:
    1. It is less common than reinfection and occurs within 2 weeks of completing drug therapy for the infection.
    2. It is responsible for most recurrent UTIs in women.
    3. It may result from residual urine after voiding caused by prolapsed uterus or bladder or lack of estrogen.
    4. It can be treated with the same medication regimen used for the original infection.

17. The family nurse practitioner understands the following about pyelonephritis:
    1. Young adults with severe illness may present with altered mental state and absence of fever.
    2. Patients complain of localized flank/back pain combined with systemic symptoms, such as fever, chills, and nausea.
    3. Requires hospitalization for most cases including parenteral antibiotic therapy.
    4. Requires no follow-up.

18. What is the term given to the type of urinary incontinence associated with conditions such as Parkinson disease or Alzheimer disease?
    1. Stress incontinence.
    2. Urge incontinence.
    3. Functional incontinence.
    4. Overflow incontinence.

19. A 60-year-old male patient presents with complaints of blood in his urine; he denies dysuria or abdominal pain. The family nurse practitioner obtains a urinalysis to confirm hematuria. There is no evidence of infection. What is the priority diagnosis in the list of differentials?
    1. Cancer of the prostate.
    2. Prerenal failure.
    3. Renal calculi.
    4. Renal cell carcinoma.

20. An older adult patient is diagnosed with renal failure. Lipid panel is noted to be within normal limits, as is the patient's glycosylated hemoglobin. Which one of the following is most likely the cause of his renal failure?
    1. History of myocardial infarction (MI) with severe hypotensive episode.
    2. Advanced prostatic hypertrophy with hematuria.
    3. Renal vascular changes secondary to long history of diabetes.
    4. Exposure to carbon tetrachloride at the job site.

21. A family nurse practitioner recognizes which factor as contributing to the development of prerenal azotemia?
    1. History of a hypovolemic shock.
    2. Extended treatment of an infection with gentamicin (Garamycin).
    3. Acute pyelonephritis with subsequent glomerulonephritis.
    4. Renal vascular changes secondary to atherosclerotic disease.

22. A family nurse practitioner teaching a female patient about bladder health would include which three of the following guidelines:
    1. Drink at least six to eight glasses of water per day.
    2. Avoid doing Kegel exercises.
    3. Avoid constipation.
    4. Consider weight loss, if incontinence occurs.
    5. Have at least one cup of coffee or tea daily.

23. Early signs of renal damage in patients with diabetes mellitus and hypertension include which two of the following?
    1. Increased blood urea nitrogen (BUN).
    2. Increase in serum creatinine.
    3. Presence of proteinuria.
    4. Decrease in glomerular filtration rate (GFR).
    5. Hematuria.
    6. Elevated A1c.

24. A 75-year-old white female patient presents to the clinic with her husband, her primary caregiver. She has a history of multiinfarct dementia, likely from a long history of untreated hypertension. Her husband reports that for the last 2 days she has been agitated and increasingly confused, and he has not been able to redirect her. He denies the addition of new medications or over-the-counter herbal supplements. What would the family nurse practitioner suspect?
    1. New infarct.
    2. Worsening of dementia.
    3. Urinary tract infection (UTI).
    4. Underlying stress to caregiver.

25. A patient presents to the clinic with complaints of chills, severe flank pain, dysuria, and urinary frequency. Vital signs are temperature of 102.9°F (39.4°C), pulse of 98 beats/min, respirations of 24 breaths/min, and a blood pressure of 120/68 mm Hg. Urinalysis reveals pyuria with leukocyte casts, mild proteinuria, and urine leukocyte esterase positive. What is the probable diagnosis?
    1. Urethritis.
    2. Acute prostatitis.
    3. Interstitial cystitis.
    4. Pyelonephritis.

26. Which of the following would **not** be a primary consideration in a differential diagnosis of hematuria?
    1. Urinary tract infection (UTI).
    2. Renal calculi.
    3. Renal carcinoma.
    4. Warfarin medication.

27. A patient is diagnosed with interstitial cystitis. What would be the clinical findings?
    1. Bladder pain that lessens as the bladder fills.
    2. Pyuria with urine culture sensitivity of *Escherichia coli* greater than 100,000 colony-forming units per milliliter from a midstream-catch urine sample.
    3. Urinary frequency or urgency, hematuria, and nocturia.
    4. Elevated temperature and severe flank pain.

28. Which patient with a urinary tract infection will require hospitalization and intravenous antibiotics?
    1. A newly pregnant woman with bacteriuria, urgency, and frequency.
    2. A young man with dysuria, suprapubic pain, and recurrent urinary tract infection.
    3. An older adult man with a low-grade fever, flank pain, and an indwelling catheter.
    4. A preschool age child with a slight fever, dysuria, and bacteriuria.

29. When should the family nurse refer a patient with renal calculi to a urologist?
    1. Signs of urosepsis.
    2. Dysuria and urgency.
    3. Sudden onset of severe colicky pain.
    4. Appearance of gross hematuria.

30. What are important teaching points the family nurse practitioner should include when discussing urolithiasis in a client with a history of calcium oxalate stones?
    1. Encourage 2–3 L/day intake; advise patient to have clear urine rather than yellow.
    2. Have at least four to five servings a week of green leafy vegetables, rhubarb, nuts, chocolate, and beer.
    3. Increase protein and salt intake.
    4. Decrease calcium intake by not ingesting dairy products.

31. A patient has been diagnosed with an acute lower urinary tract infection (UTI) and prescribed 160 mg trimethoprim (TMP)/800 mg sulfamethoxazole (SMX) twice daily for 3 days. The patient calls the clinic stating that it is still painful to urinate and the frequency and urgency have only slightly diminished. What would be a priority in this patient's plan of care?
    1. Renew the 160 mg TMP/800 mg SMX antibiotic for 14 days.
    2. Change the medication to Ciprofloxacin 250 mg twice daily for 3 days.
    3. Obtain a urinalysis and urine for culture and sensitivity.
    4. Have the patient increase fluids and encourage more frequent urination.

Pharmacology

32. A 69-year-old male patient with renal failure receives dialysis once per week. Results from his most recent laboratory results include phosphorus 6.6 mg/dL, potassium 5.0 mEq/L, and sodium 133 mEq/L. Which of the following medications should be administered to control the imbalance?
    1. Insulin.
    2. Sevelamer (Renagel).
    3. Magnesium citrate.
    4. Sodium bicarbonate.

33. A 67-year-old female patient presents with weakness. Available laboratory results include leukocytes 5200/mm³, hemoglobin of 7.6 g/dL, and hematocrit of 22.7%. She has a history of nondialysis-dependent chronic kidney disease (CKD). Which of the following medications would the family nurse practitioner expect to be administered?
    1. Epoetin alfa (Procrit).
    2. Filgrastim (Neupogen).
    3. Sargramostim (Leukine).
    4. Sevelamer (Renvela).

34. A 69-year-old female patient reports worsening stress incontinence. Which one of the following agents would be useful in treating her symptoms?
    1. Propantheline (Pro-Banthine) 15 mg before meals; 30 mg at bedtime.

2. Oxybutynin 2.5 mg three to four times a day.
3. Doxepin (Sinequan) 10–25 mg once a day initially to maximum total daily dose of 25–100 mg.
4. Conjugated estrogen (Premarin) 0.3–1.25 mg/day orally or vaginally and medroxyprogesterone (progestin) 2.5–10 mg/day continuously or intermittently.

35. A 56-year-old female patient presents to the outpatient health clinic with complaints of urgency and vaginal pruritis. A urinalysis reveals 100,000 colony-forming units/mL gram-negative rods. The patient history includes no prior urinary tract infections (UTIs), but that she has multiple allergies including sulfa and penicillin medications. Which of the following three medications would be best indicated for this patient?
    1. Nitrofurantoin (Macrodantin) 100 mg PO once.
    2. Nitrofurantoin (Macrodantin) 100 mg PO bid for 5 days.
    3. Trimethoprim-sulfamethoxazole (TMP-SMZ) 160/800 mg PO daily for 3 days.
    4. TMP-SMZ 160/800 mg PO daily for 7 days.
    5. Ciprofloxacin (Cipro) 500 mg PO bid for 7 days.
    6. Fosfomycin (Monurol) 3000 mg PO once.

36. To decrease the production of uric acid kidney stones, the family nurse practitioner orders which medication?
    1. Allopurinol (Zyloprim).
    2. Indomethacin (Indocin).
    3. Bethanechol (Urecholine).
    4. Colchicine (Colcrys).

37. A 70-year-old woman is treated with oxybutynin (Ditropan XL) for her urinary frequency and urgency. The family nurse practitioner would explain to the patient she will probably experience:
    1. Increased sensitivity to sunlight.
    2. Dizziness on standing.
    3. Dry mouth and increased thirst.
    4. Increased bruising.

38. An older adult male in an assisted living facility begins to experience urinary incontinence. The family nurse practitioner is reviewing his medication list and finds that the following three medications may be responsible for this new onset:
    1. Temazepam (Restoril) 30 mg PO at bedtime.
    2. Nitrofurantoin (Macrodantin) 150 mg PO at bedtime.
    3. Diazepam (Valium) 5 mg PO prior to magnetic resonance imaging (MRI).
    4. Polyethylene glycol 3350 (MiraLax) 1 capful in water or juice daily as needed.
    5. Amitriptyline (Elavil) 75 mg PO at bedtime for postherpetic neuralgia.
    6. Tramadol (Ultram) 50 mg PO every 8 hours as needed for pain.

39. The family nurse practitioner has selected low-dose trimethoprim-sulfamethoxazole (TMP-SMZ) for treatment of chronic urinary tract infection (UTI) in an adult female patient. Which two parameters should be evaluated before administration of TMP-SMZ?
    1. Creatinine clearance (greater than 50 mL/min).
    2. Levels of serum alanine aminotransferase.
    3. Current medications that include anticoagulants.
    4. History of allergic reactions to sulfa-based medications.
    5. Serum blood urea nitrogen (BUN).

40. A patient with recurrent calcium oxalate renal calculi can be treated with which of the following medications to aid in the prevention of stone formation?
    1. Triamterene (Dyrenium).
    2. Furosemide (Lasix).
    3. Hydrochlorothiazide (HCTZ).
    4. Acetazolamide (Diamox).

41. A 72-year-old man with a history of renal calculi presents with complaints of severe flank pain radiating to his groin area. He is also experiencing nausea and vomiting, and his temperature is 99°F (37.2°C). What is the best initial therapy that the family nurse practitioner can provide?
    1. Ketorolac 30 mg IM.
    2. Ibuprofen (Advil) 600 mg PO q6h.
    3. Increase fluid intake and strain all urine.
    4. Trimethobenzamide (Tigan) 250 mg PO.

42. The family nurse practitioner is prescribing nitrofurantoin (Macrodantin) for a young woman who is experiencing problems with urinary tract infections. What specific directions should be given to the patient regarding administration of nitrofurantoin?
    1. Take with food and expect brownish discoloration of urine.
    2. Do not take with milk products; take on an empty stomach for better absorption.
    3. Take four times a day until symptoms have subsided for at least 24 hours.
    4. Do not take acetaminophen (Tylenol) or ibuprofen (Advil) with nitrofurantoin.

43. An adult woman presents with complaints of burning on urination, frequency, and urgency. Phenazopyridine (Pyridium) is prescribed. What specific directions should the family nurse practitioner provide for the patient regarding phenazopyridine?
    1. May discolor contact lenses; if sclerae begin to turn yellow, return to the office.
    2. Always take on an empty stomach to increase absorption.
    3. Do not take any medication containing aspirin or salicylate.

4. May interfere with effectiveness of minipill for birth control.

44. When prescribing oxybutynin for the patient with stress incontinence symptoms, which disorder in the patient's medical history must the family nurse practitioner consider before prescribing?
    1. Diabetes.
    2. Cough.
    3. Narrow-angle glaucoma.
    4. Gallstones.

45. A 65-year-old female patient visits the clinic for urinary incontinence. She complains that she has been frequently losing small volumes of urine with no urge for micturition. She also confirms nocturnal wetting. She has a history of uncontrolled diabetes and peripheral neuropathy. Which of the following medications would the family nurse practitioner select for this patient's symptoms?
    1. Bethanechol (Urecholine).
    2. Atropine.
    3. Hyoscyamine (Levsin).
    4. Mirtazapine (Remeron).
    5. Dicyclomine (Bentyl).

46. A patient with no history of allergies presents with an uncomplicated urinary tract infection. When considering fluoroquinolones for the treatment, the family nurse practitioner correctly understands that:
    1. A fluoroquinolone, such as ciprofloxacin, is the drug of choice for urinary tract infections.
    2. Fluoroquinolones are preferable to both nitrofurantoin and trimethoprim-sulfamethoxazole because of high levels of antibiotic resistance.
    3. Fluoroquinolones are considered safe in pregnancy.
    4. Fluoroquinolones should be used cautiously because of potential serious side effects.

47. A frail older adult female presents for her annual physical exam. Her comprehensive metabolic panel (CMP) reveals a glomerular filtration rate (GFR) of 38; the previous year her GFR was 64. Which one of the following medications should be eliminated from her profile?
    1. Ibuprofen (Motrin).
    2. Levothyroxine (Synthroid).
    3. Metoprolol tartrate (Lopressor).
    4. Clopidogrel (Plavix).

48. A 72-year-old male patient is scheduled for a renal angiogram. His list of medications is as follows. Which should the family nurse practitioner be concerned about?
    1. Glyburide (DiaBeta).
    2. Metformin (Glucophage).
    3. Captopril (Capoten).
    4. Temazepam (Restoril).

49. The family nurse practitioner is prescribing nitrofurantoin for a patient's recurrent lower urinary tract infection. If the patient reported having side effects, which one would require discontinuation of the medication?
    1. Fatigue and drowsiness.
    2. Gastrointestinal upset.
    3. Tingling of the fingers.
    4. Dark, amber-colored urine.

50. What is important for the family nurse practitioner to know before prescribing methenamine (Hiprex) to a patient?
    1. Prescribe a sulfonamide to enhance the absorption of methenamine.
    2. Check patient's renal function.
    3. Medication is useful in prevention of catheter-induced urinary tract infections (UTIs).
    4. Medication is indicated for acute upper urinary tract infections only.

51. After completing a 3-day course of trimethoprim-sulfamethoxazole (TMP-SMX 160/800 mg 2 times per day) for a urinary tract infection (UTI), the patient continues to have a positive urine culture 1 week after completion of the treatment. Which of the following is an appropriate action for the family nurse practitioner?
    1. Order a one-time IV dose of ceftriaxone 1 g.
    2. Start a 2-week course of TMP-SMX 160/800 mg 2 times per day.
    3. Initiate long-term prophylaxis with TMP-SMX 40/200 mg 3 times per week at bedtime for 6 months.
    4. Order a voiding cystourethrogram to evaluate for a structural abnormality of the urinary tract.

52. A young adult female patient has suprapubic discomfort, pyuria, dysuria, and bacteriuria greater than 100,000/mL of urine for the last 24 hours. Which is the most likely diagnosis and treatment?
    1. Uncomplicated upper urinary tract infection (UTI) requiring 14 days of oral antibiotics.

    2. Uncomplicated lower UTI treatable with short-course therapy.
    3. Complicated lower UTI treatable with single-dose therapy.
    4. Complicated upper UTI requiring hospitalization and IV antibiotics.

53. A young adult male patient reports having two to four urinary tract infections (UTIs) over a 6-month period. What would be important for the family nurse practitioner to do?
    1. Refer to a urologist.
    2. Start patient on a 7-day antibiotic regime of trimethoprim-sulfamethoxazole.
    3. Obtain a urine for culture and sensitivity.
    4. Discontinue patient's long-term nitrofurantoin (Macrodantin) medication.

54. Which medication is a urinary analgesic?
    1. Nitrofurantoin (Macrodantin).
    2. Phenazopyridine (Pyridium).
    3. Trimethoprim (Primsol).
    4. Methenamine (Hiprex).

55. What is important for the family nurse practitioner to know before prescribing nitrofurantoin (Macrodantin) to a young adult patient?
    1. Used in the long-term treatment of chronic pyelonephritis.
    2. Determine whether the patient is pregnant.
    3. Can be administered parenterally for acute urinary infections.
    4. Should not be given with milk.

14 | Urinary Answers & Rationales

Physical Exam & Diagnostic Tests

1. Answer: 1

Rationale: A basic evaluation of urinary incontinence should include a history and physical; there are systemic reasons for incontinence, which include neurologic, gastrointestinal, and genitourinary/reproductive organ impairments. Measurement of postvoid residual by either pelvic ultrasound (bladder scan) or catheterization is done to determine retention and potential overflow incontinence. UA may indicate urinary tract infection as the cause of incontinence. The other tests may be performed based on the findings from the initial evaluation including the 3-incontinence questionnaire and voiding diaries.

2. Answer: 4

Rationale: CT urography has become the most useful diagnostic tool in different urinary tract abnormalities, such as complex congenital anomalies, trauma, infection, and tumors. The use of CT urography in different anomalies including vascular, parenchymal, and urothelial evaluation has a great impact in the management of patients. CT urography has many disadvantages over IVU, including its high cost and the higher radiation dose, but it is more effective than IVU at visualizing the structures of the kidney.

3. Answer: 1

Rationale: Transient microscopic hematuria on dipstick analysis is a common finding and does not warrant further investigation unless significant risk factors are present. False-positive results on urinary dipstick analysis are commonly caused by exercise, contaminated samples, or menstruation. Significant or nontransient hematuria would warrant laboratory microscopic urinalysis for evaluation of myoglobinuria and other disorders.

4. Answer: 1

Rationale: The optimal patients for UDS include those who have not had prior incontinence surgery or who have clear symptoms of stress or urge incontinence. Urodynamic testing is a group of tests that examine how well the bladder, sphincters, and urethra are storing and releasing urine. Most urodynamic tests focus on the bladder's ability to hold urine and empty steadily and completely. Urodynamic tests also can show whether the bladder is having involuntary contractions that cause urine leakage. Postvoid residual volume may be seen in an older adult male patient.

5. Answer: 1

Rationale: The primary concern in the patient is the elevated serum creatinine level of 4.2 mg/dL. All the other blood chemistry values are within normal limits. The patient should be referred to a nephrologist immediately because of the elevated creatinine level. The family nurse practitioner, in addition to completing a history and physical, should order a parathyroid hormone level, liver function tests, lipid and renal panels, complete blood count, and magnesium/calcium levels. Having these laboratory tests completed will assist the nephrologist in determining the cause of the patient's renal failure. A review of the patient's medications should be initiated to determine whether she is taking any medications that are nephrotoxic, including angiotensin-converting enzyme inhibitors. Nephrotoxic medications should be discontinued. The patient's family history may be reviewed to rule out familial kidney disorders (e.g., Alport syndrome, polycystic kidney disease).

6. Answer: 2

Rationale: Adults normally void four to six times in a 24-hour period (q4–6h). Most adults usually do not awaken to void at night unless they have a medical problem (e.g., benign prostatic hypertrophy, urge incontinence, or diuretic therapy). The feeling of the bladder filling occurs at about 90–150 mL, with the first urge sensation at 200–300 mL. Normally, 1–2 hours pass between the first urge to void and reaching functional capacity. Adults typically reach functional (comfortable) capacity at 300–600 mL and should *never* experience leakage if voiding is delayed.

7. Answer: 1, 2

Rationale: Clinically significant polymicrobial infections are uncommon (less than 5%). Interpret mixed bacterial cultures with caution—they most likely indicate contaminated specimens. The findings of a urine specimen for culture and sensitivity are as follows: negative reports less than 10,000 CFU/mL and positive reports are greater than 100,000 CFU/mL. Transport the specimen to the laboratory immediately (within 30 minutes). If this is not possible, the specimen may be refrigerated for up to 2 hours; however, it is preferable to not refrigerate the specimen. In symptomatic patients, a smaller number of bacteria (between 100 and 10,000 CFU/mL of midstream urine) are recognized as an infection.

8. Answer: 1, 3, 4, 6

Rationale: Normal specific gravity for an adult is 1.005–1.030, usually with a range of 1.010–1.025. Leukocyte esterase is a screening test used to detect leukocytes in the urine and should be negative because positive results indicate urinary tract infection (UTI). A few hyaline casts are normally present, especially after strenuous exercise. TNTC numbers of hyaline casts are associated with proteinuria. The presence of occasional epithelial cells is not remarkable; however, large numbers are abnormal. Tubular (epithelial) casts are often seen with renal tubular disease or toxicity. A few WBCs (5 or fewer) and RBCs (2 or fewer) are considered normal. The presence of five or more WBCs in the urine indicates a UTI involving the bladder or kidneys, or both. Patients with more than three RBCs per high-power field in two out of three properly collected urine specimens should be considered to have microhematuria; hence they should be evaluated for possible pathologic causes.

Disorders

9. Answer: 1

Rationale: Stress incontinence in postmenopausal women is associated with weakness in the pelvic floor that can lead to pelvic organ prolapse; multiparity is a key factor. Dementia is associated with overflow incontinence. Environmental barriers put one at risk for functional incontinence, and the addition of tricyclic antidepressants or any hypnotic or sedative can cause retention leading to overflow incontinence.

10. Answer: 1

Rationale: *E. coli* is the most common organism causing urinary tract infections (UTIs) in women. Counts of 10^5 CFU/mL are diagnostic. Counts of 10^2–10^3 CFU/mL should be considered positive and indicate treatment when it is *E. coli*. *E. coli* will likely respond to trimethoprim-sulfamethoxazole (Septra DS) or any suitable, sensitive antiinfective agent, and the patient should also be treated for the UTI. *S. epidermidis* is normal skin flora and is likely a contaminant because of an inappropriate clean-catch specimen collection technique.

11. Answer: 4

Rationale: Functional incontinence is the inability to toilet appropriately because of impaired mobility or deficits in cognition. Ensuring that the patient has the appropriate equipment in the home (bedside commode, walker, wheelchair, accessible bathroom, and clothing that is easily removed) will assist the patient in maintaining independence. The patient may also benefit from scheduled toileting every 2 hours to reduce "accidents." Often these patients become socially isolated and depressed because of their concern about an accident in public. The family nurse practitioner should explore all options available. Evaluating the need for incontinence pads is effective with stress incontinence. Limiting fluid intake in the evenings to reduce nocturnal incontinence is appropriate for urge incontinence. Performing the Credé maneuver is appropriate for overflow incontinence.

12. Answer: 3

Rationale: The patient likely has chronic bacterial prostatitis, which is difficult to treat because the bacteria reside in prostatic calculi and corpora amylacea. Chronic bacterial prostatitis requires 3–4 months of therapy with trimethoprim-sulfamethoxazole (Septra DS) or a quinolone (e.g., ciprofloxacin) to prevent urinary symptoms, although care should be taken when prescribing quinolones in patients because of risks of Achilles tendon rupture and other potential side effects.

13. Answer: 2

Rationale: Functional incontinence is the inability to toilet appropriately because of impaired mobility or deficits in cognition. Stress incontinence is leakage from the bladder during activities that increase intraabdominal pressure and, therefore, pressure on the bladder, forcing urine leakage. Urge incontinence is an inability to delay urination, with a strong, abrupt urge to void, caused by bladder hyperactivity or hypersensitive bladder. The patient often has little warning before urine passes out of the bladder. Incontinence with overdistention of the bladder is called overflow incontinence, caused by an underactive or noncontracting detrusor muscle or by bladder outlet or urethral obstruction. It is characterized by frequent urination in small amounts.

14. Answer: 3, 4

Rationale: *E. coli* is the pathogen in 80% of community-acquired UTIs. Gram-positive *S. saprophyticus* is the second most common pathogen in 15% of community-acquired UTIs. *K. pneumoniae* and *P. mirabilis* are also possible pathogens. In hospital settings, *E. coli* is less prevalent. *S. aureus* infections typically are not associated with UTIs but are found more often with skin (impetigo; mastitis), lung (pneumonia), bone (osteomyelitis), and blood vessel (thrombophlebitis) infections. Enterococci and group B streptococci rarely cause cystitis.

15. Answer: 3

Rationale: Cystitis in adults usually presents with dysuria, urgency, frequency, nocturia, and suprapubic heaviness. Acute onset of chills, fever, flank pain, headache, malaise, and costovertebral angle tenderness are common in pyelonephritis in adults.

16. Answer: 1

Rationale: Relapse is an uncommon cause of recurrent UTIs in women and occurs within 2 weeks of completion of antibiotic therapy. It may need to be treated for 2–12 weeks. Reinfection is the cause of most UTIs in women and may be caused by residual urine resulting from a prolapsed uterus or bladder or by lack of estrogen in perimenopausal women. If the patient has up to two UTIs a year, single-dose or 3-day antibiotic therapy may be used.

17. Answer: 2

Rationale: Pyelonephritis is characterized by localized flank/back pain, costovertebral angle tenderness, combined with systemic symptoms, such as fever (100.4°F [38°C]), chills, and nausea. In older adults, mental status changes and absence of fever is noted. Suggested follow-up is by telephone contact within 12–24 hours of initiation of antibiotic therapy and at 2 weeks and 3 months for posttreatment urine cultures. Outpatient therapy is usually how the patient is followed for mild to moderate illness (not pregnant, no nausea/vomiting; fever and pain not severe), uncomplicated, and tolerating oral hydration and medications. Most patients can be treated as outpatients. With extremes of age (older adult) and severe illness, inpatient treatment is indicated.

18. Answer: 2

Rationale: Urge incontinence, an established incontinence versus transient incontinence, is associated with conditions such as Parkinson disease or Alzheimer disease and involves the central nervous system causing detrusor motor and/or sensory instability. Urge incontinence is the involuntary leakage accompanied by or immediately preceded by urgency.

19. Answer: 4

Rationale: Painless hematuria, flank pain, and a palpable abdominal renal mass are the classic triad of symptoms in the patient with renal cell carcinoma. Men over the age of 50 with a history of smoking who have painless hematuria almost always have a diagnosis of renal cell carcinoma. There is no evidence of renal failure (oliguria; edema). Renal calculi would be characterized by both hematuria and flank pain, but no abdominal mass. Prostate cancer often presents with the other symptoms of benign prostatic hypertrophy, along with anorexia and bone pain (occurs with metastasis).

20. Answer: 2

Rationale: Postrenal azotemia results from development of an obstructive problem distal to the kidney, as seen in advanced prostatic hypertrophy with hematuria, bladder tumor, or pelvic mass. A severe hypotensive episode, often seen after acute MI, is considered prerenal. The vascular changes resulting from diabetes and the exposure to nephrotoxic chemicals are considered intrarenal disease.

21. Answer: 1

Rationale: The precipitating factor in prerenal failure is most often an incident that precipitated renal ischemia, such as hypovolemic shock. Treatment with nephrotoxic medications such as gentamicin (Garamycin), pyelonephritis, and renal vascular changes are causes of intrarenal failure or intrinsic renal disease.

22. Answer: 1, 3, 4

Rationale: Routinely performing Kegel (pelvic floor) exercises should be taught because they assist in maintaining strong pelvic floor musculature. Weak pelvic floor musculature may contribute to urinary incontinence, especially with activity. Recommend weight loss if patient is overweight and incontinence occurs. The family nurse practitioner should include teaching about avoiding dietary substances that can irritate the bladder, such as caffeine, alcohol, and spicy foods.

23. Answers: 3, 4

Rationale: The earliest indication of renal damage from diabetes is the presence of microalbuminuria; because of this all patients with diabetes should have this tested annually, beginning at the time of diagnosis of type 2 diabetes and 5 years after diagnosis of type 1 diabetes. A decrease in GFR is also noted. Diabetic nephropathy is characterized by proteinuria, hypertension, edema, and renal insufficiency. BUN and serum creatinine may not elevate until 50% of renal function is lost. Hematuria is not usually found. Elevated A1c is related to diabetic control and not specifically indicative of renal damage, although consistently high levels do correlate with the long-term complication of nephropathy.

24. Answer: 3

Rationale: Acute onset of increased confusion, inability to redirect, and increased agitation indicate an infection, likely a UTI, in the older adult patient with dementia. The family nurse practitioner should obtain a urinalysis (UA) and empirically treat for UTI until the UA results are received. Because the patient has no neurologic symptoms (e.g., weakness; flaccidity), a new infarct is unlikely. Acute confusion is not a sign of worsening dementia because dementia is a gradual process. The caregiver bringing the patient with this acute problem would not indicate underlying caregiver stress, which usually presents when persons complain of stress to their own primary care provider.

25. Answer: 4

Rationale: Pyelonephritis is characterized by fever (100.4°F [38°C] or greater); costovertebral angle tenderness with patient complaints of chills, severe flank pain, dysuria, urinary urgency and frequency with urinalysis findings revealing pyuria with leukocyte casts; mild proteinuria; and urine leukocyte esterase positive. Interstitial cystitis is characterized by frequent, urgent, relentless urination day and night with more than eight voids in 24 hours. Patients with urethritis typically have the following complaints of urethral discharge, dysuria, and erythema of the urethral meatus. Acute prostatitis is characterized by high fever, chills, malaise, myalgia, dysuria, frequency, urgency, and nocturia but not by severe flank pain. It also is characterized by perineal pain that may radiate to the back, rectum, or penis.

26. Answer: 4

Rationale: Routine use of anticoagulants should not cause hematuria unless there is an underlying urologic abnormality. Hematuria is the most common sign of bladder cancer. A urinalysis with red blood cell (RBC) casts indicates hematuria originating from the renal parenchyma. The presence of intact RBCs, white blood cells, and bacteria suggests hematuria resulting from a UTI. Patients with renal calculi most commonly have hematuria and renal colic or severe flank pain.

27. Answer: 3

Rationale: Interstitial cystitis (urethral syndrome, bladder pain syndrome) is a chronic bladder condition that causes pain, pressure, and discomfort in the bladder and surrounding structures. It is characterized by urinary frequency or urge to urinate. Bladder pain worsening as the bladder fills and then resolves with bladder emptying is a symptom of interstitial cystitis. Acute pyelonephritis is characterized by fever, chills, and localized flank or back pain. Pyuria with a positive urine culture is associated with a UTI.

28. Answer: 3

Rationale: The patient with an indwelling catheter and signs of acute pyelonephritis requires hospitalization and IV antibiotics. The other three patients show signs of uncomplicated urinary tract infections that are not severe and can be treated with oral antibiotics. The family nurse practitioner should consider hospitalization for a urinary tract infection if a patient is pregnant, if there is severe nausea/vomiting with dehydration, and any child aged less than 2 years.

29. Answer: 1

Rationale: Urgent referral to a urologist is indicated if the pain is uncontrollable, urosepsis is present, patient is unable to keep fluids down, or oliguria/anuria is present. A patient with renal calculi has a history of sudden onset of severe pain in the costovertebral angle, flank, and/or lateral abdomen; colicky or constant pain with patient unable to find a comfortable position (often may pace to relieve the pain); hematuria with gross hematuria noted in one-third of patients; nausea; and vomiting. Most patients can be conservatively managed with pain medications (opioids and nonsteroidal antiinflammatory drugs) and increased fluids. The majority of patients pass the stone within 48 hours.

30. Answer: 1

Rationale: Increased fluid intake for life cannot be overemphasized for decreasing recurrence of renal calculi. The family nurse practitioner should encourage 2–3 L/day intake and advise patient to have clear urine rather than yellow. When patients form calcium oxalate stones, they should minimize high-oxalate foods such as green leafy vegetables, rhubarb, peanuts, chocolate, and beans. Other diet considerations are to decrease protein and salt intake and increase phytate-rich foods, such as natural dietary bran, legumes and beans, and whole cereal. It is not advisable to lower calcium intake, because it may increase urine calcium excretion. Patients should avoid excessive vitamin C and/or vitamin D supplements.

31. Answer: 3

Rationale: If UTI symptoms persist after 2–3 days of medication therapy, obtain a urinalysis and urine culture/sensitivity and change antibiotic accordingly. Switch to another antibiotic drug class and treat for 7–10 days. It would not be prudent to order an additional course of medication without first collecting a urinalysis and culture and sensitivity. Increasing fluids and promoting frequent urination are good bladder health teaching points but do not address the current infection not responding to the prescribed antibiotic.

Pharmacology

32. Answer: 2

Rationale: Hyperphosphatemia is often seen in patients with chronic kidney disease (CKD) as glomerular filtration rate (GFR) declines below 25–40 mL/min. In addition to dietary restriction of phosphates, phosphate binders such as sevelamer (Renagel) and calcium carbonate are routinely administered. Controlling hyperphosphatemia in CKD has been associated with decreased mortality. Because patients with CKD have a further decline of GFR with associated hyperphosphatemia, increasing frequency or duration of dialysis is also indicated.

33. Answer: 1

Rationale: CKD is often the result of a loss of erythropoietin as the glomerular filtration rate decreases. This increases the risk of anemia. After evaluating and ensuring iron levels are appropriate, initiation of therapy with an erythropoiesis-stimulating agent (ESA) is appropriate. Initiation of therapy is typically considered at hemoglobin levels less than 9 g/dL for nondialysis-dependent patients (less than 10 g/dL if dialysis dependent), especially if the patient is near transfusion levels. Treatment is at 4-week intervals and should be reduced or stopped if hemoglobin is greater than 11 g/dL because of adverse side effects.

34. Answer: 4

Rationale: Combination hormone replacement therapy using conjugated estrogen (Premarin) 0.3–1.25 mg/day orally or vaginally and medroxyprogesterone (progestin) 2.5–10 mg/day continuously or intermittently can be useful for management of stress incontinence. Propantheline and oxybutynin may be useful in urge incontinence; research is limited on their use for stress incontinence. Doxepin (Sinequan) is a tricyclic antidepressant and is used infrequently.

35. Answer: 2, 5, 6

Rationale: First-line treatment options for uncomplicated cystitis or UTIs without recent or recurrent infections include TMP-SMX, nitrofurantoin, and fosfomycin. There are other outpatient treatment options including fluoroquinolones, like ciprofloxacin, and β-lactam antibiotics. These should only be selected if known contraindications exist such as allergy, renal failure, known antibiotic resistance, or suspicion of pyelonephritis. Nitrofurantoin is administered for a minimum of 5 days but is avoided in renal failure (glomerular filtration rate less than 30). TMP-SMX is contraindicated in this patient because of sulfa allergy but is normally indicated at 160/800 mg (double strength) PO bid for 3 days. TMP-SMX should be avoided if a patient has recurrent UTIs or has taken TMP-SMX within the last 3 months. Ciprofloxacin is acceptable, but in 2016 the U.S. Food and Drug Administration advised against first-line systemic use in uncomplicated UTIs for patients with other treatment options. Fosfomycin is acceptable as a one-time treatment but is contraindicated in patients with suspicion of pyelonephritis.

36. Answer: 1

Rationale: To decrease the formation of uric acid kidney stones, a urinary alkylating agent, such as allopurinol, is frequently used. As standard practice, the family nurse practitioner should check the patient's serum uric acid level monthly for 3 months to ensure the levels are decreasing to normal ranges, and then annually once serum uric acid levels are normalized. Indomethacin is used for its antiinflammatory properties in the treatment of gout. Urecholine is a cholinergic agent that stimulates the bladder to contract, which improves urine flow. Colchicine is an antigout medication also used for its antiinflammatory properties.

37. Answer: 3

Rationale: Oxybutynin produces anticholinergic effects, and dry mouth is a common side effect. Because this patient is an older adult, the family nurse practitioner should review the patient's list of medications to verify that no other medications will exacerbate dry mouth. If another medication will increase this side effect (e.g., diuretic), then the family nurse practitioner should advise the patient of methods to relieve the dry mouth, such as hard candy or chewing gum. The patient may also be taking other medications with anticholinergic side effects, which could be increased with the addition of oxybutynin to the point the patient could be at risk for falls. Careful review of the patient's medication list is essential before adding a new drug. The other reactions are not consistent with oxybutynin administration.

38. Answer: 1, 3, 5

Rationale: Sedatives and hypnotics (temazepam and diazepam) lead to sedation and muscle relaxation in all groups, but particularly in the older adult population; central nervous system (CNS) changes from aging may lead to increased muscle relaxation, with the addition of a sedative-hypnotic leading to urinary incontinence. Antidepressants (amitriptyline) have anticholinergic effects and lead to sedation. CNS changes and the addition of antidepressants with anticholinergic side effects will increase muscle relaxation in the older adult patient and contribute to urinary incontinence. Antibiotics and laxatives have not been implicated in the development of urinary incontinence in older patients. Opioids (tramadol) increase the tone in the urinary bladder sphincter, leading to urinary retention. Nitrofurantoin (Macrodantin) is on the Beers List and should not be prescribed for an older adult.

39. Answer: 1, 4

Rationale: TMP-SMZ is contraindicated if renal function is impaired, antibacterial concentration in the urine is inadequate, or patient is allergic to sulfa medications. To treat chronic UTI, the family nurse practitioner would consider low-dose TMP-SMZ as treatment. Using this low dose in the adult patient should not cause serum or tissue accumulation of the drug. Liver function studies may be indicated if the patient experiences adverse reactions to the medication. Anticoagulants have not been reported to cause significant drug interactions. The BUN test is not a sensitive indicator of renal creatinine clearance.

40. Answer: 3

Rationale: HCTZ decreases the risk of forming calcium oxalate stones because of decreased renal calcium excretion or hypocalciuria. Hypercalcemia is a possible side effect of this medication. Furosemide, acetazolamide, and triamterene may increase the risk of formation of calcium oxalate stones by causing hypercalciuria. It is important to note that HCTZ may subsequently increase the risk of gout and/or uric acid stone formation caused by hyperuricemia.

41. Answer: 2

Rationale: The severe pain of renal calculi should be addressed before other treatments or diagnostics. Narcotics and nonsteroidal antiinflammatory drugs (NSAIDs) are commonly used for pain relief. In most randomized, blinded studies of NSAIDs versus narcotics, NSAIDs have shown equal or greater efficacy for pain relief and shorter duration of pain relief with equal or fewer side effects. Ketorolac works at the peripheral site of pain production rather than on the central nervous system and, based on clinical findings, has been proven to be as effective as opioid analgesics, with fewer adverse effects. Ketorolac is only indicated for short-term therapy and is contraindicated in patients with renal failure. Because of an increased risk of bleeding, it is not given concurrently with other NSAIDs and should be used with caution in patients aged greater than 65 years.

42. Answer: 1

Rationale: The most important side effects of nitrofurantoin are gastrointestinal upset, which can be decreased if the medication is taken with food or milk, and brown discoloration of the urine. The patient should continue taking nitrofurantoin for at least 3 days after sterile urine is obtained. If applicable to the patient, the drug may interfere with the efficacy of oral contraceptives.

43. Answer: 1

Rationale: The family nurse practitioner should advise the patient that if she experiences yellow discoloration of the sclerae while taking phenazopyridine, she is to return to the office immediately. This may indicate poor renal excretion and requires a renal workup (renal panel, parathyroid and thyroid-stimulating hormone, serum magnesium/calcium, and a 24-hour urine for creatinine clearance) and possible referral to a nephrologist. Phenazopyridine should be administered with food, and no drug interactions occur with aspirin or oral contraceptives.

44. Answer: 3

Rationale: Oxybutynin (Ditropan XL) is contraindicated in patients with narrow-angle glaucoma (angle-closure glaucoma). Patients with open-angle glaucoma may take this medication. Anticholinergics may increase the pressure within the eye, which puts the patient at risk for progression of the glaucoma, which is blindness.

45. Answer: 1

Rationale: This patient most likely has overflow urinary incontinence. Overflow incontinence is caused by an inability to contract the detrusor muscle of the bladder or a bladder outlet obstruction. The patient also likely has decreased sensation or genitourinary autonomic neuropathy bladder caused by uncontrolled diabetes. Other causes of overflow incontinence include anticholinergic medications, neuropathic diseases, and physical obstruction caused by pelvic organ prolapse, strictures, severe constipation, or benign prostatic hyperplasia in men. A postvoid residual urine should be obtained and will likely exceed 100 mL. Treatment options include removing the offending agent and/or self-catheterization, which is typically the best treatment. Medical options include cholinergic agents like bethanechol and alpha blockers such as terazosin and doxazosin. Bethanechol is a cholinergic agent that stimulates the bladder to contract, which improves urine flow. Dicyclomine is an antispasmodic used to treat irritable bowel syndrome. Mirtazapine is an antidepressant. Hyoscyamine (Levsin) is an antispasmodic used to treat bowel or bladder cramping.

46. Answer: 4

Rationale: Although fluoroquinolones are a common and generally effective treatment for urinary tract infections, these drugs received a black box warning in 2016 because of potential side effects, such as tendon ruptures, peripheral neuropathy, and central nervous system effects. Therefore fluoroquinolones should not be used for minor infections as a first-line agent. Fluoroquinolones should not be used in pregnancy.

47. Answer: 1

Rational: Ibuprofen (Motrin) is a nonsteroidal antiinflammatory agent with risk of renal toxicity and should be avoided in patients with preexisting or renal impairment. Levothyroxine is metabolized predominantly in the liver. Metoprolol is a beta blocker and has little effect on the kidneys, unlike the angiotensin-converting enzyme inhibitors. Clopidogrel works on the liver and also has little effect on the kidneys.

48. Answer: 2

Rational: Metformin is contraindicated in patients with heart failure, liver failure, and impaired renal function. It is contraindicated for 2 days before and 2 days after receiving IV radiographic contrast. Metformin combined with IV contrast dye puts the patient at risk for fatal lactic acidosis. Baseline glomerular filtration rate (GFR) should be documented. Captopril is an angiotensin-converting enzyme inhibitor that is renal protective until GFR is noted to be worsening. Glyburide and temazepam minimally effect the renal function, and there is no need to hold these medications before the study.

49. Answer: 3

Rationale: Peripheral neuropathy is most likely to occur in patients with renal impairment and those taking the medication chronically. Symptoms of tingling of the fingers, muscle weakness, and numbness can indicate peripheral neuropathy, which can be an irreversible side effect of nitrofurantoin. The family nurse practitioner would discontinue the medication. The other side effects are not serious and can be reversed by reducing the dosage or after treatment.

50. Answer: 2

Rationale: Methenamine is eliminated by the kidneys and should not be given to patients with renal impairment because crystalluria can occur. The medication is not useful in prevention of catheter-induced UTIs and is indicated for chronic infections of the lower urinary tract. Methenamine should not be combined with sulfonamides because the drug interaction forms an insoluble complex, which poses a risk of urinary tract injury from crystalluria.

51. Answer: 2

Rationale: If a patient continues to have a positive urine culture caused by relapse or reinfection after a 3-day medication regimen of antibiotics, then the drug therapy should be a progressive stepwise approach with a 2-week course of therapy after the short-course 3-day therapy. The next steps would be to begin a 4- to 6-week course of therapy, followed by a 6-month course of therapy if that is unsuccessful. Recommended antibiotics include TMP-SMX, nitrofurantoin, cephalexin, trimethoprim, or a quinolone. If UTIs are thought to be caused by other complicating factors, then an evaluation for structural abnormalities may be warranted by ordering a voiding cystourethrogram. Third-generation cephalosporins (e.g., ceftriaxone) should not be given routinely; instead, they should be given only when conditions demand and the UTI is severe and not responding. Unless the infections are severe or are complicated, IV antibiotics are not indicated.

52. Answer: 2

Rationale: The symptoms of suprapubic discomfort, pyuria, dysuria, and bacteriuria greater than 100,000/mL of urine indicate an uncomplicated cystitis, which is a lower UTI that can be treated with a short course of antibiotics, especially if the symptoms began less than 7 days before starting the treatment. In this case the symptoms occurred during the last 24 hours; short-course therapy is indicated and is more effective than single-dose therapy and is preferred. A complicated lower urinary tract infection would be associated with some predisposing factor, such as renal calculi, an obstruction to the flow of urine, or an indwelling catheter. Upper urinary tract infections often include severe flank pain, fever, and chills and are associated with acute pyelonephritis.

53. Answer: 1

Rationale: Recurrent UTIs are not "normal" for young male patients and need to be evaluated further by a urologist to rule out underlying pathology of urethral stricture, anatomic abnormality, acute prostatitis, or renal stones. UTIs increase in incidence as the male ages. The family nurse practitioner would not start a new medication or discontinue a long-term medication for prophylaxis until the urologist has completed a workup on the patient's condition.

54. Answer: 2

Rationale: Phenazopyridine (Pyridium) is a urinary analgesic. The medication does not treat the urinary infection but does reduce the discomfort of dysuria. Nitrofurantoin and methenamine are urinary antiseptics. Trimethoprim (Primsol) is an antibiotic often used in conjunction with sulfamethoxazole (TMP-SMZ).

55. Answer: 2

Rationale: Nitrofurantoin is not recommended during the last 2 to 4 weeks of pregnancy because of the possibility of hemolytic anemia. Nitrofurantoin is indicated for the treatment of uncomplicated cystitis and should not be used for long-term treatment because of serious side effects of peripheral neuropathy, hepatotoxicity, and pulmonary problems. The medication has only oral preparations and can be administered with food or milk to decrease gastrointestinal upset side effects.

15

Male Reproductive

Physical Exam & Diagnostic Tests

1. Which of the following circumstances is ideal for ordering a prostate-specific antigen (PSA) laboratory test?
   1. A 41-year-old white male with no family history of prostate cancer who "just wants to know if he might have it."
   2. A 60-year-old man with new-onset lower urinary tract symptoms, such as increased urgency and frequency of urination and painful urination.
   3. A 55-year-old male presenting with new symptoms of erectile dysfunction.
   4. A 72-year-old male who recently completed a course of antibiotics for prostatitis.

2. During a sports physical, an adolescent asks the family nurse practitioner if he should be performing testicular self-exams. The nurse practitioner correctly tells him:
   1. Testicular self-exams are necessary if you have a strong family history of testicular cancer.
   2. Testicular self-exams should be done in the shower once a month.
   3. The United States Preventive Services Task Force no long recommends testicular self-exam.
   4. Testicular self-exam has been replaced by regular ultrasound screenings of asymptomatic men.

3. Review of a laboratory report indicating elevated serum gonadotropin would raise suspicion of which disorder?
   1. Seminal vesiculitis.
   2. Vas deferens disease.
   3. Testicular disease.
   4. Benign prostatic hyperplasia (BPH).

4. Which of the following structures can be palpated during an external exam of a male patient?
   1. Epididymis.
   2. Cowper ducts.
   3. Seminal vesicles.
   4. Ejaculatory ducts.

5. What would be most helpful in diagnosing gynecomastia?
   1. History and physical.
   2. Liver function test.
   3. Thyroid function test.
   4. Mammogram.

6. What is the correct position in which to place an adult male patient to examine the rectum and prostate?
   1. Left lateral Sims position with right knee flexed and left leg extended.
   2. Supine position with hips and legs flexed and feet positioned on the examining table.
   3. Modified knee-chest position with patient prone and knees flexed under hips.
   4. Leaning over the exam table with chest and shoulders resting on the table.

7. How is prostate cancer appropriately diagnosed?
   1. An elevated prostatic-specific antigen (PSA).
   2. On palpating a nodule during a digital rectal exam (DRE).
   3. Biopsy via transrectal ultrasonography.
   4. An elevated prostatic acid phosphatase.

8. Which statement is correct about the prostatic-specific antigen (PSA) test?
   1. PSA can be elevated in patients with benign prostatic hyperplasia (BPH).
   2. PSA is not elevated in patients with prostatitis.
   3. Prostatic massage will not elevate PSA levels.
   4. PSA does not increase in recurrence of prostate cancer.

9. The United States Preventive Services Task Force recommends against routine screening for prostate cancer because:
   1. There is a high mortality rate from prostate cancer regardless of screening.
   2. There is harm associated with a high number of false positives.
   3. Digital rectal exam (DRE) is shown to be superior to serologic testing.
   4. Ultrasonography is now the screening of choice.

10. What is the normal finding when examining the scrotum of a man with a dark complexion?
    1. Symmetric scrotal sac with two movable testes.
    2. Smooth, rubbery, saclike surface that is sensitive to gentle compression.
    3. Asymmetric sac with left side lower than right side.
    4. Reddish color that is darker than body skin with sebaceous cysts.

Disorders

11. A 45-year-old male presents with a several-week history of feeling pain in the scrotum that worsens with coughing, lifting, and straining. He states that his scrotum feels "full" at the end of the day. What would the family nurse practitioner be suspicious of?
    1. A spermatocele.
    2. An inguinal hernia.
    3. Epididymitis.
    4. Testicular torsion.

12. A 49-year-old male smoker presents to the clinic with complaints of painless gross hematuria. What is the most serious problem that needs to be considered by the family nurse practitioner?
    1. Bladder cancer.
    2. Benign prostatic hyperplasia.
    3. Erectile dysfunction.
    4. Urinary tract infection.

13. A 65-year-old male presents with a history of well-controlled hypertension and diabetes mellitus. He is a nonsmoker. He has been married for 35 years, is monogamous, and reports that his relationship with wife is good. He complains of new-onset erectile dysfunction (ED). What is the first-line therapy for ED?
    1. Relationship counseling.
    2. Oral phosphodiesterase-5 inhibitors.
    3. Intraurethral injections of alprostadil (Caverject).
    4. Use of a vacuum device.

14. What finding is indicative of testicular torsion?
    1. Scrotal swelling with tenderness that occurs only after age 40.
    2. Sudden onset of pain with a firm, tender mass in the scrotum.
    3. A scrotum that transilluminates.
    4. Cremasteric reflex.

15. A 57-year-old male suffers blunt trauma to the penis. He complains of pain and an inability to urinate. Which of the following should be the family nurse practitioner's priority?
    1. Insertion of an indwelling catheter.
    2. Insertion of an intermittent catheter.
    3. Insertion of a suprapubic catheter.
    4. Order a retrograde urethrogram.

16. On a routine physical exam, a patient expresses concern over the observation that one side of his scrotum is larger than the other side. He states that it has been getting larger for the past few months and that the scrotum is smaller in the morning and enlarges through the day. He has felt a heaviness in the scrotum, denies any acute pain, but does confirm some discomfort in his lower back. He reports no history of trauma to the scrotal area. On exam, the family nurse practitioner confirms the enlargement. Further exam reveals that the scrotum will transilluminate and that manual manipulation of the scrotum does not cause pain. What is the initial diagnosis for the patient?
    1. Hydrocele.
    2. Orchitis.
    3. Epididymitis.
    4. Traumatic injury.

17. A 47-year-old male presents with pain of his right knee and discomfort when grasping objects with his hands lasting 14 days. He reports a low-grade fever of 100.4°F (38°C) for the past 5 days and dysuria 5 days ago. He is sexually active with multiple partners and does not use barrier protection. For which of the following organisms should the family nurse practitioner begin immediate treatment?
    1. *Treponema pallidum.*
    2. *Neisseria gonorrhoeae.*
    3. *Staphylococcus aureus.*
    4. *Chlamydia trachomatis.*

18. Which statement is correct concerning circumcision?
    1. Circumcision is helpful in preventing phimosis.
    2. Circumcision is a cause of paraphimosis.
    3. Balanoposthitis is the direct result of circumcision in older men.
    4. Circumcision increases the incidence of cancer of the penis.

19. A 31-year-old male presents with his fifth diagnosis of gonorrhea in the last 3 years and affirms he completed all treatment regimens as prescribed. Which of the following is an appropriate next step by the family nurse practitioner to evaluate the cause of recurrent infections?
    1. Safe sex education.
    2. Screening for complement deficiency.
    3. Intravenous treatment of the resistant gonococcal infection.
    4. Behavioral therapy for sex addiction.

20. What is acute epididymitis characterized by?
    1. Absence of dysuria.
    2. Nonenlarged scrotum.
    3. Tenderness over epididymis.
    4. Lack of abdominal pain.

21. In a 70-year-old man, which of the following bacteria is likely responsible for epididymitis?
    1. *Escherichia coli.*
    2. *Treponema pallidum.*
    3. *Neisseria gonorrhoeae.*
    4. *Chlamydia trachomatis.*

22. Which of the following is true about hypogonadism?
    1. Usually presents with decreased libido.
    2. May cause an increase in muscle mass.
    3. Causes an increase in body hair.
    4. Does not contribute to infertility.

23. Which of the following is a common cause of erectile dysfunction?
    1. The use of antihypertensives.
    2. Dietary supplements.
    3. Masturbation.
    4. It is a natural part of aging.

24. Which action is true about the prostate?
    1. Secretes fluid that is acidic.
    2. Secretes fluid that is alkaline.
    3. Secretes androgens.
    4. Produces sperm.

25. An older adult man presents to the clinic with complaints of difficulty voiding and hematuria. The digital rectal exam (DRE) reveals a firm prostate about 5 cm in diameter, asymmetric, with firm nodules. The prostatic-specific antigen (PSA) level is 14. What is the next action?
    1. Medicate with finasteride (Proscar) 5 mg PO daily and reevaluate in 3 months.
    2. Advise patient to avoid caffeine, alcohol, and over-the-counter decongestants.
    3. Obtain a urinalysis to determine presence of infection and amount of hematuria.
    4. Refer to urologist for biopsy and diagnostic evaluation for prostatic cancer.

26. A 20-year-old male patient presents with scrotal pain. What is a suspected diagnosis that requires immediate referral?
    1. Testicular torsion.
    2. Hydrocele.
    3. Epididymitis.
    4. Inguinal hernia.

27. The family nurse practitioner has been following an older adult patient who has been treated for benign prostatic hyperplasia with behavioral modifications (limiting fluids before bedtime, avoiding caffeine and alcohol, etc.) and taking an α_1-blocker. Select **two** indications for referral to a urologist.
    1. Urinary tract infection.
    2. Urinary retention.
    3. Prostatic bleeding.
    4. Increased urinary flow rate.
    5. Prostatic-specific antigen level below 4 ng/mL.

28. A 55-year old male presents with a history of burning sensation on urination and difficulty urinating that has been increasing over time. He often feels that he has to void frequently to fully empty his bladder. A digital rectal exam reveals an enlarged prostate. What is the most likely diagnosis considered by the family nurse practitioner?
    1. Bladder cancer.
    2. Testicular torsion.
    3. Benign prostatic hyperplasia (BPH).
    4. Renal failure.

29. A young patient presents with a complaint of a feeling of fullness in the scrotum. Physical exam reveals a round, soft, nontender, nonadherent, bluish testicular mass resembling a "bag of worms." No variation in size occurs with respiration or Valsalva maneuver. The mass transilluminates and is located anterior to the testes. What is the most likely diagnosis?
    1. Varicocele.
    2. Hernia.
    3. Tumor.
    4. Spermatocele.

30. An uncircumcised patient presents with a complaint of not being able to retract the foreskin over the glans penis. What is the most likely diagnosis?
    1. Lateral phimosis.
    2. Phimosis.
    3. Peyronie's disease.
    4. Paraphimosis.

31. An adult, uncircumcised patient presents with tender or pruritic, red pinpoint pustules and papules on the prepuce and glans. What is the most likely diagnosis?
    1. Peyronie's disease.
    2. Balanitis.
    3. Phimosis.
    4. Paraphimosis.

32. A male patient is diagnosed with balanitis. What is the most likely cause?
    1. Candidiasis.
    2. Herpes genitalis.
    3. Lichen planus.
    4. Psoriasis.

33. A male patient presents with a complaint of sexual dysfunction. The family nurse practitioner understands that sexual dysfunction is impairment of:
    1. Erection only.
    2. Emission only.
    3. Ejaculation only.
    4. Erection, emission, or ejaculation.

34. A man presents with a complaint of dysuria, an edematous scrotum, tenderness over the epididymis, and abdominal pain. What is the most likely diagnosis for the patient?
    1. Testicular torsion.
    2. Vas deferens inflammation.
    3. Epididymitis.
    4. Balanitis.

35. The family nurse practitioner knows that erectile dysfunction (ED) is:
    1. Primarily psychologic in origin.
    2. Unusual in older men.
    3. The persistent inability to achieve and maintain an erection adequate for sexual intercourse.
    4. The physiologic dysfunction when smooth muscle contracts, causing a lack of adequate amount of blood in the penis to render a rigid, larger penis.

36. Priapism is classified as which type of sexual dysfunction?
    1. Erection.
    2. Emission.
    3. Ejaculation.
    4. Priapic.

37. Which of the following is correct in response to a patient's question concerning a possible cause of testicular cancer?
    1. Syphilis.
    2. Gonorrhea.
    3. Cryptorchidism.
    4. Balanitis.

38. A male patient complains of erectile dysfunction. Which of the following may be a contributing factor?
    1. Antihypertensive drugs.
    2. Sexual intercourse.
    3. Rheumatoid arthritis.
    4. Frequent masturbation.

39. A 16-year-old boy presents with gynecomastia. The family nurse practitioner knows that it is likely:
    1. A result of hypogonadism.
    2. Caused by medication.
    3. Caused by the hormonal imbalances of adolescence.
    4. An aggressive form of breast cancer.

40. Which is true of prostate cancer?
    1. Rarely diagnosed in men greater than 50 years of age.
    2. Soft, indiscrete, symmetric nodules of the prostate.
    3. Obstructive symptoms rarely present.
    4. Firm prostate, often with hard nodules.

41. Which symptoms would be most concerning about a possible diagnosis of prostate cancer in a male over 50 years of age?
    1. Hesitancy, dribbling, and urgency.
    2. Decreased force of urine stream.

3. Pain and feeling of a full bladder.
4. Urinary symptoms coupled with pain in the hips or back.

42. Which statement is correct concerning testicular cancer?
    1. It is a common problem in men over age 50.
    2. It is directly related to testicular trauma.
    3. It always presents suddenly with pain.
    4. It is primarily found in young men.

43. Which of the following is true about acute bacterial prostatitis?
    1. Characterized by recurrent urinary tract infections.
    2. Involves an ascending infection of the urinary tract.
    3. Always occurs in men under age 30.
    4. Usually treated with 1 month of antibiotics.

44. Which of the following is true of orchitis?
    1. Is rarely viral.
    2. The lesion transilluminates.
    3. Is relatively painless.
    4. Can be associated with a worsening epididymitis.

45. What organism is the most common cause of nongonococcal urethritis (NGU) in men?
    1. *Chlamydia trachomatis.*
    2. *Neisseria gonorrhoeae.*
    3. *Escherichia coli.*
    4. *Streptococcus faecalis.*

46. Which test is a useful tumor marker for testicular cancer?
    1. Alpha-fetoprotein (AFP).
    2. Prostate-specific antigen.
    3. Prostatic acid phosphatase.
    4. Alkaline phosphatase.

47. What is the most common viral causative agent of orchitis?
    1. Arbovirus.
    2. Echovirus.
    3. Mumps.
    4. Rubeola.

48. What are common symptoms of benign prostatic hyperplasia (BPH)?
    1. Dribbling, hesitancy, loss of stream volume and force, and recurrent urinary tract infections.
    2. Dysuria, urgency, frequency, nocturia, and suprapubic heaviness or discomfort.
    3. Obstructive symptoms, such as a weak urine stream, abdominal straining to void, hesitancy, incomplete bladder emptying, and terminal dribbling.
    4. Acute onset of fever, chills, flank pain, headache, malaise, costovertebral angle tenderness, and possibly hematuria.

49. A 25-year-old patient with a history of sickle cell disease complains of a sudden problem with erections that are not sexually oriented. He is currently experiencing a painful erection and he is unable to void. The family nurse practitioner determines the treatment of choice is:
    1. Morphine sulfate and bed rest.
    2. Immediate referral to a urologist.
    3. Increased hydration for sickle cell crisis.
    4. Determination of PSA level.

50. The family nurse practitioner is speaking with a group of male teenagers who are most concerned about symptoms associated with gonorrhea. Which of the following would the family nurse practitioner include in the discussion?
    1. Reddish lesions may appear on the palms of the hands and soles of the feet.
    2. Men may observe a rash over the body of the penis.
    3. Urinary dribbling may result from irritation of the urinary tract.
    4. Painful urination results from inflammation of the urethra.

51. A 65-year-old uncircumcised man presents to the clinic with complaints of a painless "bump" on his penis, difficulty retracting the foreskin, and serosanguineous drainage from beneath the foreskin. The family nurse practitioner must first consider a possible diagnosis of:
    1. Balanitis.
    2. Penile cancer.
    3. Herpes.
    4. Penile trauma.

52. What is considered a major contributing factor in erectile dysfunction?
    1. Diet high in vitamin C.
    2. Diabetes mellitus.
    3. Allergies.
    4. Low-sodium diet.

53. A 30-year-old male presents with a macular-papular rash on his body, including the soles of his feet and his palms. He is also complaining of fatigue, fever, malaise, and swollen lymph nodes. On further questioning, it is revealed that the illness began several weeks ago with several papules on his penis. What does the family nurse practitioner suspect?
    1. Herpes simplex.
    2. Granuloma inguinale.
    3. Gonorrhea.
    4. Syphilis.

54. Which of the following sexually transmitted infections often begins with a prodrome of headaches, fever, malaise, and myalgia?
    1. Genital herpes.
    2. Granuloma inguinale.
    3. Gonorrhea.
    4. Syphilis.

55. Which of the following clinical presentations are commonly associated with genital herpes?
    1. Vesicular lesions on an erythematous base.
    2. Chancres on the penis.
    3. Purulent urethral discharge.
    4. Small, flattened papules and larger verrucous lesions.

56. Which of the following is true of testicular cancer?
    1. It affects hundreds of thousands of adolescent boys each year.
    2. It has a high mortality rate.
    3. Early detection via testicular self-exam improves morbidity and mortality.
    4. Cryptorchidism is a risk factor for testicular cancer.

57. Which one of the following objective findings on a 52-year-old male is consistent with a diagnosis of benign prostatic hyperplasia (BPH)?
    1. Elevated prostatic-specific antigen (PSA).
    2. Gross hematuria.
    3. A nodular firm prostate palpated on digital rectal exam (DRE).
    4. A smooth enlarged prostate palpated on DRE.

58. Which two situations should the family nurse practitioner refer to a urologist?
    1. Patient with a smooth enlarged prostate palpated on digital rectal exam (DRE).
    2. Patient with a nodular firm prostate palpated on DRE.
    3. If initial treatment for benign prostatic hyperplasia (BPH) is not effective.
    4. When the patient with BPH develops a urinary tract infection (UTI).

Pharmacology

59. Which of the following is correct regarding short-acting phosphodiesterase-5 inhibitors, such as sildenafil (Viagra) or vardenafil (Levitra)?
    1. They work best in combination with a large, fatty meal.
    2. They should be taken 30 minutes to 1 hour before intercourse.
    3. They are the only class of medications that is effective for treating erectile dysfunction.
    4. They work in all men.

60. What are the common side effects of phosphodiesterase-5 inhibitors?
    1. Erections lasting longer than 4 hours.
    2. Headaches, flushing, and dyspepsia.
    3. Nausea and vomiting.
    4. Rash, itching, and loss of appetite.

61. What is an important contraindication to phosphodies-terase-5 inhibitors?
    1. Selective serotonin reuptake inhibitors.
    2. Beta blockers.
    3. Nitrates.
    4. Thiazide diuretics.

62. A patient has been taking doxazosin (Cardura) 2 mg PO daily for 3 weeks for treatment of benign prostatic hyperplasia (BPH). He returns to the clinic and is complaining of feeling dizzy when he stands up. Which action would the family nurse practitioner take?
    1. Determine blood pressure with patient lying down, standing, and sitting.
    2. Order urinalysis to determine hematuria and presence of bacteria.
    3. Review with patient his symptoms over the last 3 weeks.
    4. Perform digital rectal exam to determine whether prostate is smaller than previously noted.

63. A 74-year-old male patient has benign prostatic hyperplasia (BPH) and stage 1 hypertension. Which of the following medications would be the most appropriate selection to possibly treat both disorders?
    1. Tamsulosin (Flomax).
    2. Finasteride (Proscar).
    3. Doxazosin (Cardura).
    4. Tadalafil (Cialis).

64. In planning treatment for a patient with balanitis, the family nurse practitioner orders:
    1. Rest, ice, and elevation.
    2. Massage therapy.
    3. Antifungal agents.
    4. Emergency circumcision.

65. A 28-year-old man presents with complaints of fever, low back pain, perineal pain, and intense pain on voiding. Rectal exam reveals a tender, swollen, firm, warm prostate. Based on the patient's symptoms, what is the treatment of choice?
    1. Ceftriaxone (Rocephin) 250 mg IM × 1, followed by doxycycline 100 mg PO bid × 10 days.
    2. Tetracycline (Achromycin) 250 mg PO qid × 10 days.
    3. Amoxicillin (Amoxil) 500 mg PO tid × 14 days.
    4. Erythromycin (Ilosone) 250 mg PO q6h × 24 days.

66. Which of the following side effects is common in a 56-year-old patient taking tamsulosin (Flomax)?
    1. Constipation.
    2. Decreased ejaculate.

3. Anorgasmia.
4. Hypertension.

67. A 70-year-old man complains of scrotal pain with dysuria and frequency that has been increasing over the last 2 weeks. Physical exam reveals extreme scrotal tenderness and swelling, urethral discharge, and testes normal in size and position. Urinalysis reveals pyuria. What is the treatment of choice for the patient?
    1. Nitrofurantoin (Macrodantin) 100 mg PO qid × 14 days.
    2. Levofloxacin (Levaquin) 750 mg PO qd × 10 days.
    3. Doxazosin (Cardura) 1 mg PO qd × 10 days.
    4. Oxybutynin (Ditropan) 5 mg PO tid × 10 days.

68. Finasteride (Proscar) is prescribed for a 50-year-old man who is experiencing a problem with urination secondary to an enlarged prostate. The family nurse practitioner would teach the patient that while he is taking this medication, it is important to:
    1. Increase his fluid intake.
    2. Restrain from sexual activity.
    3. Take special precautions around women of child-bearing age.
    4. Increase intake of folic acid.

69. A 75-year-old patient is diagnosed with chronic bacterial prostatitis, and the family nurse practitioner selects ciprofloxacin (Cipro) as the treatment. How should the ciprofloxacin be prescribed for this patient?
    1. 500 mg PO bid × 10 days.
    2. 500 mg PO tid × 3 days, then 500 mg PO bid × 10 days.
    3. 500 mg PO bid × 21 days.
    4. 500 mg PO bid × 30–45 days.

70. Which of the following would be considered an initial treatment for Peyronie's disease?
    1. Surgery.
    2. Pentoxifylline (Trental).
    3. Circumcision.
    4. Oxybutynin (Ditropan).

71. A patient is diagnosed with benign prostatic hypertrophy. Which medication should be recognized by the family nurse practitioner as likely to aggravate this condition?
    1. Glyburide (DiaBeta).
    2. Oral buspirone (Buspar).
    3. Inhaled ipratropium (Atrovent).
    4. Ophthalmic timolol (Timoptic).

15 Male Reproductive Answers & Rationales

Physical Exam & Diagnostic Tests

1. Answer: 2

Rationale: A PSA is most appropriate to order for a man who presents with lower urinary tract symptoms, which could be indicative of either benign prostatic hyperplasia or prostate cancer. Because of low sensitivity and specificity, the PSA should not be used as a screening test in most men. A man with lower urinary tract symptoms and an elevated PSA should be referred to urology for further evaluation.

2. Answer: 3

Rationale: Neither testicular self-exam nor clinical exam is recommended by the United States Preventive Services Task Force because of a low incidence of disease and the potential harm from anxiety and testing procedures. Similarly, the American Academy of Family Physicians, American Academy of Pediatrics, and the American Cancer Society do not recommend testicular self-exams. Testicular cancer is a low-incidence disease with a high cure rate even in advanced disease.

3. Answer: 3

Rationale: Gonadotropin is often elevated in testicular disease, whereas prostate-specific antigen is elevated in diseases of the prostate, such as BPH, prostate inflammation, and prostate cancer.

4. Answer: 1

Rationale: The epididymis is palpable, whereas the ducts and glands are not. The comma-shaped epididymis is palpated on the posterolateral surface of each testis. The seminal vesicles (pair of glands) lie behind the urinary bladder in front of the rectum. These vesicles join the ampulla of the vas deferens to form the ejaculatory duct.

5. Answer: 1

Rationale: A complete history and physical usually provide the cause of gynecomastia without further testing because it can be caused by medication, starving and refeeding, or lack of androgen production (atrophying testes), which changes the estrogen/androgen ratio. Serologic tests are required only when the history and physical exam suggest other disorders. A serum total testosterone level can be considered in older men to assess for hypogonadism. Gynecomastia is a common finding in adolescents.

6. Answer: 4

Rationale: For patient comfort and ease of exam, the ambulatory adult is asked to lean over the exam table with his chest and upper body resting on the table. Although left lateral Sims position is correct, it is the position used for examining a patient who is confined to bed or requests an alternative to standing.

7. Answer: 3

Rationale: The standard for diagnosing prostate cancer is a biopsy obtained by a urologist via transrectal ultrasonography. An elevated PSA is usually present during prostate cancer, but it can also be present in noncancerous disorders, such as benign prostatic hyperplasia. A nodule palpated on exam is suggestive of prostate cancer but is not diagnostic. The United States Preventive Services Task Force recommends against use of DRE as a screening technique. The prostatic acid phosphatase is an enzyme present in prostate cancer that is an older test for prostate cancer and is present in other diseases and when taking some medications.

8. Answer: 1

Rationale: PSA can be elevated in patients with BPH and those with prostatitis, and after prostate gland massage. PSA does increase with the increasing burden of the tumor, as in recurrent prostate cancer.

9. Answer: 2

Rationale: Prostate cancer has a low mortality regardless of screening, as only 2.5% of men will die of the disease. A large number of prostatic-specific antigen tests are false positives and not attributed to prostate cancer. Biopsies to rule out prostate cancer can cause anxiety, pain, bleeding, and urinary dysfunction. DRE and ultrasonography have not been proven to be effective methods of detecting prostate cancer.

10. Answer: 3

Rationale: The scrotal sac is asymmetric. In men with dark complexions, the scrotal skin is often darker than the body. On all men, the scrotal surface may be coarse with small lumps on the skin, which are sebaceous or epidermoid cysts that may have an oily discharge.

Disorders

11. Answer: 2

Rationale: An inguinal hernia presents with the stated symptoms, along with a bulge in either the groin or scrotum that becomes more obvious when standing. Epididymitis symptoms result from inflammation and lead to scrotal pain and swelling. Testicular torsion is characterized by an acute onset of pain, which is often during a period of inactivity, with nausea and vomiting. A spermatocele is a fluid-filled mass, often painless, and arises from the epididymis and is usually benign.

12. Answer: 1

Rationale: Gross hematuria in a patient over 40 years old should be considered as possible bladder cancer until proven otherwise. Smoking increases the patient's risk of bladder cancer.

13. Answer: 2

Rationale: Oral phosphodiesterase-5 inhibitors are a safe, effective, and reasonable first-line therapy for erectile dysfunction (ED). The class includes commonly known drugs such as sildenafil (Viagra), vardenafil (Levitra), tadalafil (Cialis), and avanafil (Stendra). Patients should be educated on side effects and proper use before first administration. Relationship issues can compound or cause ED and should be investigated as a part of the initial evaluation. Second-line therapies for the treatment of ED include intraurethral suppositories, intracavernous injections, and vacuum pump devices. If the patient has only difficulty in maintaining an erection, a constriction band or a vacuum device is the least invasive and least expensive of the current treatment options for this condition.

14. Answer: 2

Rationale: The sudden pain in testicular torsion is not relieved when the involved testicle is elevated to relieve pressure. Transillumination is associated with cystic masses, such as a hydrocele. The cremasteric reflex is usually absent. Testicular torsion is most common among neonates and adolescents, with the highest incidence during puberty.

15. Answer: 4

Rationale: After stabilization of any life-threatening injuries, patients with suspected urethral trauma should be evaluated with a retrograde urethrogram. Once urethral patency has been established, a urinary catheter can be placed.

16. Answer: 1

Rationale: The lack of pain, increase in size of scrotal contents, and transillumination are characteristic of a hydrocele.

Orchitis and epididymitis are usually characterized by pain; orchitis is most often associated with parotitis or mumps. There is no history of injury, and the scrotum is usually nontender to palpation.

17. Answer: 2

Rationale: A high suspicion of disseminated gonococcal infection (DGI) resulting from an untreated infection by the bacteria *N. gonorrhoeae* should be treated. DGI presents rarely in patients and includes a triad of tenosynovitis, arthritis, and dermatitis. Variable symptoms of DGI include dysuria, penile discharge, and low-grade fever. Treatment includes ceftriaxone and azithromycin or doxycycline and evaluation for other sexually transmitted infections.

18. Answer: 1

Rationale: Circumcision can be helpful in preventing chronic or severe phimosis and paraphimosis because both are a retraction dysfunction of the prepuce. In phimosis, the foreskin is too tight to be retracted backward over the glans penis. In paraphimosis, once the foreskin has been retracted behind the glans penis, it is too constricted to return to a position of covering the glans penis. Balanoposthitis is inflammation of the foreskin in an uncircumcised male.

19. Answer: 2

Rationale: Patients with recurrent or systemic, disseminated *Neisseria* infections should be evaluated for a deficiency of the complement system. Late components of the complement pathway (C5–C9) place patients at high risk of contracting infections by *Neisseria* organisms, especially meningitis. Other reasons for recurrent infections include failure to treat the patient's partner and continued high-risk sexual activity. Safe sex education is indicated in all patients.

20. Answer: 3

Rationale: Acute epididymitis is characterized by an acute scrotal pain, dysuria, and enlarged unilateral scrotum with abdominal pain. Scrotal pain is relieved when the involved testicle is elevated.

21. Answer: 1

Rationale: In men over age 35, the most likely cause of epididymitis is *E. coli*. These men usually have benign prostatic hyperplasia or urinary tract disorders that make them more susceptible to *E. coli*. Sexually active men under age 35 are more likely to have epididymitis because of a sexually transmitted infection, such as *N. gonorrhoeae* or *C. trachomatis*. *T. pallidum* is the causative agent of syphilis.

22. Answer: 1

Rationale: A man with primary hypogonadism will often present with low energy and decreased libido. These same men will often have gynecomastia because of the low or absent production of gonadotropin. Men with hypogonadism often have decreased body hair, which may result in decreased need for shaving. Klinefelter syndrome (chromosomal abnormality with karyotype of 47,XXY–47,XXXXY) is the most common genetic cause of male hypogonadism, with failure of both spermatic function and virilization.

23. Answer: 1

Rationale: Erectile dysfunction can be commonly caused by antihypertensives, particularly thiazide diuretics and beta blockers. Other causes of impotence are diabetes, trauma, vascular disorders, behavioral health disorders, and relationship problems.

24. Answer: 2

Rationale: The prostate secretes an alkaline fluid that helps sperm survive in the acidic environment of the female reproductive tract. Androgens are produced by Leydig cells of the testes. Sperm are produced in the seminiferous tubules of the testes.

25. Answer: 4

Rationale: The DRE findings and elevated levels of PSA in a patient presenting with lower urinary tract symptoms are the primary indicators of prostatic cancer and should be thoroughly evaluated by a urologist. The other options are directed toward the treatment of benign prostatic hyperplasia and should be considered only after prostatic cancer has been ruled out.

26. Answer: 1

Rationale: Testicular torsion can be successfully treated with immediate diagnosis and surgical intervention. Delayed diagnosis may lead to loss of the testicle. Hydrocele, epididymitis, and inguinal hernias also require referral, but they do not require immediate attention.

27. Answer: 2, 3

Rationale: The family nurse practitioner should make a referral to a urologist when symptoms of urinary retention or prostatic bleeding occur. Other indications for referral include the appearance of intractable symptoms related to obstruction, recurrent or persistent urinary tract infection, increase in postvoid residual, very low urinary flow rate, and any significant changes caused by prostatic obstruction or bladder calculi.

28. Answer: 3

Rationale: BPH is often seen in men over age 50. Bladder cancer should be ruled out as a diagnosis in any patient presenting with microscopic or gross hematuria.

29. Answer: 1

Rationale: A varicocele presents as described, whereas a hernia may transilluminate. Hernias vary in size with Valsalva maneuver. Tumors are solid and, therefore, do not transilluminate.

30. Answer: 2

Rationale: Phimosis is a retraction disorder of the penile foreskin or prepuce. It can occur at any age and is often the result of piercings, intercourse, and skin disorders such as eczema or psoriasis. Phimosis is the inability to retract the foreskin back over the glans penis. Paraphimosis is the inability to retract the foreskin from behind the glans penis.

31. Answer: 2

Rationale: Inflammation of the glans penis and prepuce (balanitis) can be associated with poor hygiene and is often found in men with poorly controlled diabetes.

32. Answer: 1

Rationale: Candidiasis is the usual cause of balanitis and is often found in men with poorly controlled diabetes.

33. Answer: 4

Rationale: In sexual dysfunction, erection, emission, or ejaculation may not be functioning because of multifactorial causes, such as medications, vascular disorders, neuropathy, and trauma. Peyronie's disease and priapism are examples of erection dysfunction.

34. Answer: 3

Rationale: Epididymitis presents as described. Testicular torsion does not usually present with dysuria, although if there is any doubt, an ultrasound should be immediately performed.

35. Answer: 3

Rationale: This is the correct definition of ED. The incidence of ED increases significantly in men as they age, particularly at age 60 and over. It involves a dysfunction in the hemodynamic mechanism of smooth muscle relaxation that increases blood flow in the penis and ultimately causes venous trapping (compression of subtunical venules) and rigidity. Patients who present with vascular ED are at a higher risk for cardiovascular events.

36. Answer: 1

Rationale: Priapism is a condition of prolonged penile erection related to venous obstruction and unrelated to sexual arousal. Although rare, men with sickle cell disease are at greatest risk. Men with erections lasting longer than 4 hours are at increased risk for impotence and should be evaluated immediately by a urologist.

37. Answer: 3

Rationale: Patients with undescended testicles are more prone to developing testicular cancer. The other conditions listed are not causes of testicular cancer.

38. Answer: 1

Rationale: Antihypertensive drugs, such as thiazide diuretics and beta blockers can cause impotence. Other common causes include cardiovascular disease, diabetes, smoking, prostate surgeries, antidepressants, relationship problems, and depression.

39. Answer: 3

Rationale: Gynecomastia in adolescent boys is most likely a result of hormonal imbalances experienced during puberty. In older men, it is frequently caused by hypogonadism and medications, such as spironolactone and H_2 blockers. In adolescents, the condition requires reassurance that it rarely persists beyond the age of 17.

40. Answer: 4

Rationale: Prostate cancer is usually found in men over age 65 and causes rapid onset of urinary obstructive symptoms. Palpation reveals a firm, enlarged, hard prostate. Advanced stages may include complaints of bone pain.

41. Answer: 4

Rationale: Urinary symptoms coupled with pain in the hips or back are most concerning for metastatic prostate cancer. It is difficult to differentiate between benign prostatic hyperplasia and prostate cancer based on symptoms alone. Prostate cancer usually has no symptoms in early stages.

42. Answer: 4

Rationale: Although rare, testicular cancer is primarily found in men under age 40 and presents as a scrotal mass with or without pain. It is commonly mistaken for epididymitis. It is second to leukemia as the most common cancer in males aged 15–34. Trauma is not a causal factor. Men with a history of cryptorchidism are at significantly increased risk.

43. Answer: 2

Rationale: Acute bacterial prostatitis is caused by an infection in the urinary tract moving up the urethra into the prostate. The most common organisms in younger men are *Neisseria gonorrhea* and *Chlamydia trachomatis*. In older men they are *Escherichia coli*, Enterobacteriaceae, and *Pseudomonas*. Chronic bacterial prostatitis is characterized by recurrent urinary tract infections. The usual antibiotic course is 2 weeks in acute prostatitis and is 1–3 months for chronic prostatitis.

44. Answer: 4

Rationale: Orchitis can be either bacterial or viral in nature. The viral form is often caused by mumps, and the bacterial form of the disease is often as a result of *Escherichia coli*, spread from a worsening epididymitis. The disorder can range from being uncomfortable to painful, and often presents with constitutional symptoms.

45. Answer: 1

Rationale: *C. trachomatis* is the most common organism in male patients with NGU.

46. Answer: 1

Rationale: AFP, lactate dehydrogenase, and human chorionic gonadotropin are all useful tumor markers for testicular cancer.

47. Answer: 3

Rationale: The mumps virus is responsible for causing orchitis. Arbovirus and echovirus are implicated in meningitis and encephalitis. Rubeola is associated with complications of otitis media, pneumonia, croup, and encephalitis.

48. Answer: 3

Rationale: Obstructive symptoms are common in BPH. Dribbling, hesitancy, loss of normal urine stream, and recurrent urinary tract infections are present in chronic bacterial prostatitis. Dysuria, urgency, frequency, nocturia, and suprapubic heaviness are common symptoms of cystitis. Fever, chills, flank pain, headache, malaise, and costovertebral angle tenderness of acute onset with or without hematuria are indications of pyelonephritis.

49. Answer: 2

Rationale: This is considered a urologic emergency because of the inability to void and because the circulation to the penis may be compromised. The patient should be referred immediately to a urologist.

50. Answer: 4

Rationale: Dysuria is one of the most common complaints of young men with gonorrhea. No lesions, rash, or urinary dribbling accompanies the yellow discharge.

51. Answer: 2

Rationale: The patient's age, presentation, and uncircumcised state put him at risk for the relatively rare condition of penile cancer. Balanitis does not present with a serosanguineous drainage. Human papillomavirus is frequently associated with this type of cancer.

52. Answer: 2

Rationale: Diabetes is a common contributor to erectile dysfunction because of the impaired circulation.

53. Answer: 4

Rationale: This patient has classic symptoms of secondary syphilis. Granuloma inguinale also presents with ulcerative lesions on the penis and lymphadenopathy but lacks the maculopapular rash and the systemic symptoms associated with syphilis. In this stage, syphilis is particularly infectious.

54. Answer: 1

Rationale: Many patients with genital herpes experience a prodrome of constitutional symptoms with their primary infection. In syphilis, systemic symptoms appear weeks to months after the genital lesions. Gonorrhea and granuloma inguinale are not typically associated with constitutional symptoms.

55. Answer: 1

Rationale: Vesicular lesions on an erythematous base are typical of genital herpes. Later in the course of the outbreak, the blisters break and leave a painful sore. Chancres on the penis are associated with syphilis. Purulent urethral discharge is found in those with gonorrhea or chlamydia infection. Small, flattened papules are associated with genital warts.

56. Answer: 4

Rationale: Testicular cancer affects around 8500 men per year in the United States. Treatment is effective, and fewer than 400 will die of the disease. The United States Preventive Services Task Force recommends against screening for testicular cancer because it is unreliable and is of low incidence, and false positives cause anxiety. A major risk factor for testicular cancer is cryptorchidism (undescended testicles).

57. Answer: 4

Rationale: A smooth symmetrically enlarged prostate palpated on DRE is noted on physical exam of a patient with BPH. An elevation in PSA can be found in prostate cancer and BPH but is not diagnostic for either. Gross hematuria may be found in men over the age of 60 with BPH because of the chronicity of the disorder that leads to chronic cystitis. A nodular firm prostate is indicative of prostate cancer.

58. Answers: 2, 3

Rationale: Subsequent testing by a urologist is done if cancer is a concern, which is suspected when the prostate is nodular and firm, or if the patient does not improve with medication management. The subsequent testing may include uroflowmetry to help diagnose obstruction, a cystometrogram that measures bladder compliance for patients with suspected neurologic disease, and a cystoscopy to determine whether surgical intervention is required for obstruction or cancer. Often, one of the symptoms that accompanies initial diagnosis of BPH is a UTI. Unless the patient develops chronic UTIs, the family nurse practitioner can treat UTI with routine antibiotics.

Pharmacology

59. Answer: 2

Rationale: Phosphodiesterase-5 inhibitors should be taken 30–60 minutes before intercourse. Large, fatty meals interfere with absorption and should be avoided. Although this class of medications works best for treating erectile dysfunction, there are other medications that can be prescribed by a urologist should they not prove to be effective.

60. Answer: 2

Rationale: Common side effects of phosphodiesterase-5 inhibitors include headaches and flushing caused by vasodilation. Erectile dysfunction lasting longer than 4 hours is rare but should be promptly evaluated in an emergency room or by a urologist.

61. Answer: 3

Rationale: Patients who are on phosphodiesterase-5 inhibitors cannot concurrently take nitrates because of dangerous effects of synergistic vasodilation. Patients who are on selective serotonin reuptake inhibitors and thiazide diuretics often find that phosphodiesterase-5 inhibitors are effective for treating erectile dysfunction.

62. Answer: 1

Rationale: Doxazosin is also used as an antihypertensive agent; the patient may be experiencing orthostatic hypotension. The other options are directed toward evaluating his BPH, which has already been diagnosed.

63. Answer: 3

Rationale: Doxazosin is indicated as treatment in both BPH and hypertension because of its favorable side effect. Both tamsulosin and doxazosin are α_1-blockers. Tamsulosin has a low potential to cause hypotension and syncope. Finasteride, a 5-α-reductase inhibitor, is indicated for treatment of BPH. Tadalafil is a phosphodiesterase-5 inhibitor indicated for BPH and erectile dysfunction.

64. Answer: 3

Rationale: Topical antifungals, such as clotrimazole, are appropriate for mild-to-moderate disease. Oral agents, such as metronidazole or fluconazole, can also be used to treat this disorder.

65. Answer: 1

Rationale: The patient is presenting with classic symptoms of acute bacterial prostatitis. The treatment of choice is IM ceftriaxone plus oral tetracycline.

66. Answer: 2

Rationale: Tamsulosin (Flomax) is an α_1-blocker indicated for use in benign prostatic hyperplasia. Side effects include syncope caused orthostatic hypotension, dizziness, decreased ejaculate, and loss of libido. Patients should be reassured that the decreased volume of ejaculate is not worrisome.

67. Answer: 2

Rationale: The patient is presenting with classic symptoms of epididymitis. The treatment of choice is a fluoroquinolone, such as levofloxacin or ciprofloxacin. Nitrofurantoin is a urinary antiseptic, doxazosin is given for benign prostatic hyperplasia, and oxybutynin is indicated for incontinence or enuresis.

68. Answer: 3

Rationale: Finasteride has some risk to women of child-bearing age. It is important that women of child-bearing age are not exposed to the sperm of a patient taking finasteride. These women and pregnant women should avoid handling crushed tablets. Exposure can cause fetal abnormalities.

69. Answer: 4

Rationale: The recommended treatment is for at least 30–45 days to prevent recurrence. Patients may require continued suppression therapy for an extended period.

70. Answer: 2

Rationale: Pentoxifylline (Trental) 400 mg PO tid is a reasonable choice in a patient with moderate curvature of the penis. Vitamin E is also commonly used. Oxybutynin (Ditropan) is used to treat symptoms of overactive bladder. Surgical treatment is indicated for patients in the chronic phase when the fibrosis has stabilized and if the deformity significantly limits or interferes with sexual intercourse; otherwise, medical management is more helpful during the initial or acute phase.

71. Answer: 3

Rationale: Benign prostatic hypertrophy is a common cause of urinary retention in older men. Inhaled ipratropium is an atropine-like bronchodilator used to treat chronic bronchitis, and its anticholinergic agent may aggravate urinary retention. Neither glyburide (oral antihyperglycemic) nor buspirone (oral antianxiety agent) has an effect on the urinary system. Timolol is a topical agent used to treat glaucoma and does not have a systemic effect.

16

Female Reproductive

Physical Exam & Diagnostic Tests

1. Which two patients should have a Papanicolaou (Pap) smear test performed by the family nurse practitioner?
   1. An 18-year-old female patient who is not sexually active.
   2. A 45-year-old female patient who denies sexual activity but has two children.
   3. A 21-year-old female patient who denies sexual activity.
   4. A 16-year-old female patient who is not sexually active.

2. A family nurse practitioner has just reviewed the bone mineral density (dual-energy x-ray absorptiometry [DEXA]) report for a 65-year-old postmenopausal woman and noted normal findings. Which interval timeframe should be used for repeated DEXA screening to have more predictive value with regard to fracture risk?
   1. Greater than 2 years.
   2. DEXA should be performed on an annual basis.
   3. In 2 years from the date of the initial screening test.
   4. There is no need for repeated testing.

3. When obtaining a cervical specimen for a conventional Papanicolaou (Pap) smear, what procedure should the family nurse practitioner implement?
   1. Lubricate the speculum with a non–water-soluble lubricant to assist in the insertion of the instrument.
   2. Use a cotton-tipped applicator when obtaining the cervical cells from a prenatal patient.
   3. Use warm water to lubricate the speculum to assist in the insertion of the instrument.
   4. Complete the bimanual portion of the exam first to determine the relative position of the cervix to assist in the comfortable insertion of the speculum.

4. To promote patient comfort before performing a pelvic exam, which action should the family nurse practitioner implement?
   1. Ask the patient to bear down slightly as the speculum is inserted.
   2. Request the patient empty her bladder.
   3. Explain each step of the procedure in a calm manner.
   4. Carefully reassure the patient that the exam will only take a few minutes.

5. What finding is considered a normal surface characteristic of the cervix?
   1. Small, yellow, raised round area on cervix.
   2. Red patches with occasional white spots.
   3. Friable, bleeding tissue at opening of cervical os.
   4. Irregular granular surface with red patches.

6. What is the primary role of a breast ultrasound?
   1. Screen for breast cancer.
   2. Definitively diagnose breast cancer.
   3. Determine whether a breast lesion is cystic or solid.
   4. Locate small lesions before surgery.

7. The screening bone mineral density report ordered for a 60-year-old postmenopausal woman shows a result of −1.5 standard deviations (SDs) at the hip. She gives a past history of myocardial infarction 1 year ago and wrist fracture at age 32. What option would **not** be considered for this patient?
   1. Counsel on smoking cessation and alcohol consumption.
   2. Initiate therapy with continuous conjugated estrogen 0.625 mg and medroxyprogesterone acetate (MPA) 2.5 mg.
   3. Initiate therapy with raloxifene (Evista).
   4. Encourage weight-bearing exercises and increased calcium intake.

8. The use of potassium hydroxide (KOH) when doing a wet mount assists in the diagnosis of:
   1. Bacterial vaginosis and candida vaginitis.
   2. Trichomoniasis and chlamydia cervicitis.
   3. Syphilis and gonorrhea.
   4. Herpes simplex and condyloma.

9. A family nurse practitioner is reviewing a patient's medical history. Which three factors should alert the family nurse practitioner to an increased risk for development of osteoporotic fractures?
   1. Patient is a smoker.
   2. No parental history of hip fractures.
   3. Body mass index (BMI) has been stable for several years at 23.9.
   4. History of rheumatoid arthritis.
   5. Progressive loss of height noted by measurement within the last 2 years.

10. The family nurse practitioner is reviewing the laboratory results of an 18-year-old patient seen recently for a Papanicolaou (Pap) smear. Classification is high-grade squamous intraepithelial lesion, endocervical cells seen, and adequate smear. The family nurse practitioner phones the patient and tells her which of the following?
    1. "Your Pap smear was normal. Follow up in 1 year, or sooner if problems arise."
    2. "Your Pap smear shows invasive cancer. I would like you to see a gynecologic oncologist for treatment."
    3. "Your Pap smear shows abnormal tissue that needs to be evaluated. Please schedule an appointment for a colposcopy."
    4. "Your Pap smear shows a minor abnormality. Sometimes this can signify a disease process just beginning. Please schedule another Pap smear in 4 months for follow-up."

11. A 27-year-old patient reports the desire to become pregnant. She and her husband have had regular, unprotected intercourse for more than 1 year. The family nurse practitioner completes a thorough history and gynecologic exam, which appear normal. What diagnostic test might be ordered early in the workup?
    1. Hysterosalpingogram (HSG).
    2. Tests for antisperm antibodies.
    3. Semen analysis.
    4. Endometrial biopsy.

12. A family nurse practitioner is reviewing the dual-energy x-ray absorptiometry (DEXA) scan screening bone recommendations by the National Osteoporosis Foundation (NOF) for female patients. Which two patients should the nurse identify to undergo a DEXA scan?
    1. A 53-year-old white woman who smokes and has excessive alcohol intake.
    2. A 50-year-old woman having irregular menstrual cycles.
    3. A 51-year-old woman on long-term corticosteroid therapy.
    4. A 54-year-old woman receiving hormone replacement therapy.

5. A 45-year-old woman who plays tennis regularly and recently fractured her ulna while playing.

13. When describing the findings from a normal breast exam, what should the family nurse practitioner document on the patient record?
    1. Left nipple everted, several coarse black hairs arising from areola, enlarged axillary lymph nodes palpated bilaterally, tender nodes in supraclavicular area.
    2. No dimpling or retraction; 1-cm hard, fixed, stellate mass noted next to nipple with scant nipple discharge; no pain or tenderness on palpation.
    3. Right breast slightly larger and denser than left with no nipple discharge, right areola dark pink in color and inverted, left areola dark brown in color and everted, breasts tender to palpation with no axillary nodes noted.
    4. Pendulous breasts with no dimpling, retraction, nipple discharge, or areas of discoloration; numerous small nevi near areola with Montgomery tubercles noted, no supraclavicular or axillary lymph nodes palpated.

14. The family nurse practitioner is reviewing the laboratory results of a 61-year-old patient seen recently for a Papanicolaou (Pap) smear: atrophic changes, scant endocervical cells, and adequate smear. She has been treated for breast cancer with mastectomy and tamoxifen (Nolvadex). She has never received hormone replacement therapy (HRT). What is appropriate for the family nurse practitioner to tell the patient when phoning her with the results?
    1. "Your Pap smear is slightly abnormal. I would recommend the use of some estrogen vaginal cream nightly for 3 weeks, then return to the office to have the Pap smear repeated."
    2. "Your Pap smear is normal but shows a mild thinning of the tissue. This is to be expected in someone who is postmenopausal and not on hormones, and it does not pose a threat to your health. Please return to the office in 1 year for your annual exam, or sooner if needed."
    3. "Your Pap smear shows that you don't have enough endocervical cells. Please make an appointment for endocervical curettage."
    4. "Your Pap smear is abnormal. This could signify a disease state of the cervix. Please schedule a colposcopy at your earliest convenience."

15. Which test is the "gold standard" for the diagnosis of chlamydial infection?
    1. Use of potassium hydroxide wet mount "whiff" test.
    2. Presence of inflammatory cells in Papanicolaou smear.
    3. Direct fluorescent antibody (DFA) test.
    4. Culture with special media and collection technique.

16. Which is the most accurate statement regarding a reactive serologic test for syphilis?
    1. All reactive serologic tests require confirmation with a treponemal test.
    2. Reactive serologic tests are highly suspicious for active syphilis.
    3. A false-positive serologic test, although rare, can be unnecessarily traumatizing to a patient.
    4. A reactive serologic test most likely implies the need for retreatment.

17. In the workup for a patient with secondary amenorrhea, the prolactin serum assay results show a level of 24 ng/mL. What does the appropriate management include?
    1. Administering medroxyprogesterone acetate (Provera) 10 mg PO bid × 5 days.
    2. Referral to a specialist.
    3. Recording the results as within normal limits.
    4. Assessment for nipple discharge.

18. In the evaluation of a young adult with amenorrhea and normal secondary sex characteristics, the purpose of the progesterone challenge is to determine the presence of:
    1. Endogenous estrogen.
    2. Thyroxine.
    3. Prolactin.
    4. Adequate body fat.

19. A patient comes to the office complaining of fatigue, breast tenderness, abdominal bloating, fluid retention, and irritability about a week before onset of her menses. This has been occurring for the last 4 months. What is the most important information for the family nurse practitioner to obtain to assist in determining the diagnosis of premenstrual syndrome (PMS)?
    1. Point in menstrual cycle when symptoms occur.
    2. Severity of symptoms.
    3. Number and frequency of symptoms over last 4 months.
    4. Presence or absence of anxiety or depression.

20. A 65-year-old woman reports to the clinic stating she has been experiencing intermittent vaginal bleeding over the last 2 months. Her last menstrual period was more than 10 years ago. Her last Papanicolaou (Pap) smear at the clinic 9 months ago was within normal limits. She is not taking any hormonal products. She is sexually active with occasional complaints of dyspareunia. What is the most appropriate response of the family nurse practitioner at this time?
    1. Order complete blood count and thyroid-stimulating hormone and repeat Pap smear.
    2. Schedule laparoscopy.
    3. Schedule endometrial biopsy.
    4. Schedule pelvic/transvaginal ultrasonography.

Normal Gynecology

21. What is the best definition of menopause?
    1. Cessation of ability for natural reproduction.
    2. Completion of 12 months of amenorrhea after last menstrual period.
    3. Follicle-stimulating hormone (FSH) level of 30 and estradiol level of 30.
    4. Last menstrual period.

22. An adult patient's last menstrual period (LMP) was 2 months ago. She has had an intrauterine device (IUD) in place for the last 4 months. She is complaining of nausea, fatigue, breast tenderness, and abdominal bloating. Physical exam reveals the following:
    - Abdomen: no abnormalities noted.
    - Pelvic: cervix—positive Chadwick's sign, IUD strings protruding from cervical os.
    - Uterus: enlarged and nontender.
    - Adnexa: nontender, without mass and no cervical motion tenderness.

    What should the family nurse practitioner identify as the most likely diagnosis?
    1. Uterine fibroid.
    2. Ovarian cancer.
    3. Dislodged IUD.
    4. Pregnancy.

23. Which of the following clinical symptoms would occur in response to vaginal changes during menopause?
    1. Increase in acidity causing pelvic discomfort.
    2. Increased vaginal discharge because of increased lubrication.
    3. Hypertrophy of vaginal tissue leading to pelvic discomfort.
    4. Increased likelihood to develop urinary tract infections caused by change in vaginal flora.

24. What function do the Bartholin glands have in reproduction?
    1. Prevent vaginitis by maintaining adequate pH.
    2. Prepare the mucous plug that occurs during early pregnancy.
    3. Produce an alkaline secretion that enhances sperm viability.
    4. Produce small amounts of hormones necessary for ovulation.

25. Which is **not** a risk factor for osteoporosis?
    1. Cigarette smoker.
    2. White race.
    3. Alcohol consumption.
    4. Obesity.

26. A young woman complains to the family nurse practitioner that she is experiencing headaches, irritability, decreased appetite, and fatigue about 1 week before menses. Appropriate management includes which of the following?
    1. Treat premenstrual syndrome (PMS) with increased protein and salt in the diet.
    2. Incorporate daily aerobic exercise and dietary changes into her lifestyle.
    3. Order complete blood count, comprehensive metabolic panel, and urinalysis.
    4. Supplement her diet with an additional 1–2 g of vitamin C.

27. A middle-aged female presents with abnormal uterine bleeding. A hormonal profile reveals increased follicle-stimulating hormone (FSH) and luteinizing hormone (LH) levels. What is the most likely cause for these findings?
    1. Hypothalamic disorder.
    2. Onset of climacteric.
    3. Premature ovarian failure.
    4. Anterior pituitary disorder.

28. Which physical finding would be present in a patient with a clinical diagnosis of uterine fibroids?
    1. Diarrhea.
    2. Shoulder pain.
    3. Increased blood flow during menses.
    4. Amenorrhea.

29. Menopause occurs at a mean age of 51 years. Which of the following factors has been linked to influencing the age at which menopause occurs?
    1. Use of oral contraceptives.
    2. Socioeconomic status.
    3. Age at menarche.
    4. Smoking.

Gynecologic Disorders

30. A female patient presents to the clinic with complaints of pelvic pressure and discomfort. When questioned about her menstrual cycle, the patient relates a history of heavy bleeding recently. Age of menarche was 16. Pelvic exam of the uterus reveals a bicornuate uterus. The family nurse practitioner suspects that the patient may have:
    1. Premenstrual syndrome.
    2. Secondary dysmenorrhea.
    3. Pelvic inflammatory disease.
    4. Dyspareunia.

31. A family nurse practitioner is discussing therapeutic management with a patient who is being actively treated for polycystic ovarian syndrome (PCOS). Which finding would indicate that the disease has progressed?
    1. Positive pregnancy test.
    2. Hemoglobin A1c level is 5.4%.
    3. Blood pressure reading is 150/92 mm Hg.
    4. Menstrual period lasts between 5 and 7 days.

32. During a yearly physical exam, a family nurse practitioner asks a woman if she has any problems or questions about sexual function or activity. Initially the patient hesitates, but with further questioning and discussion, she states that she is unsure if she has ever experienced an orgasm. What does the family nurse practitioner suspect?
    1. Vaginismus.
    2. Primary orgasmic dysfunction.
    3. Secondary orgasmic dysfunction.
    4. Dyspareunia.

33. The family nurse practitioner is talking with a young woman who has been diagnosed with herpes simplex type 2. In discussing her care, it would be important for the family nurse practitioner to include what information?
    1. The initial lesions are usually worse than lesions that occur with outbreaks at a later time.
    2. Her sexual partner will not contract it if she does not have sex when the lesions are present.
    3. This condition can be treated and cured if she takes all of the antibiotics for 2 weeks.
    4. If she becomes pregnant in the future, she will need to have a cesarean delivery.

34. What is the definition of bacterial vaginosis?
    1. A syndrome resulting from homeostatic disruption in the vagina.
    2. Vaginitis caused by a flagellated protozoan.
    3. A bacterial sexually transmitted infection that can be symptomatic or asymptomatic.
    4. A virus characterized by recurrent outbreaks and remissions.

35. A 22-year-old married patient complains of severe dysmenorrhea. Her gynecologic exam is normal. Which management protocol is preferred?
    1. Assess for contraceptive interest and, if interested, suggest use of oral contraceptives (OCs).
    2. Suggest use of a prostaglandin synthetase inhibitor.
    3. Suggest use of over-the-counter ibuprofen.
    4. Assess exercise patterns and use of relaxation techniques.

36. Which is **not** a criterion for the diagnosis of bacterial vaginosis?
    1. Positive amine test (whiff test).
    2. Presence of clue cells.
    3. Vaginal pH greater than 4.5.
    4. Presence of pseudohyphae.

37. A family nurse practitioner is reviewing information about a patient with a history of dilation and curettage (D&C) after a first-trimester spontaneous abortion leading to subsequent amenorrhea. Which working diagnosis should the nurse suspect?
    1. Polycystic ovarian syndrome.
    2. Asherman's syndrome.
    3. Hypogonadism.
    4. Premature ovarian failure.

38. What are common findings in a patient with polycystic ovarian syndrome?
    1. Weight loss, dental caries, and amenorrhea.
    2. Hyperprolactinemia and galactorrhea.
    3. Dysmenorrhea, nodules palpated on bimanual exam, and infertility.
    4. Chronic irregular menses, hirsutism, and increased abdominal girth.

39. A 30-year-old patient presents with scant pubic hair, minimal breast development, absent cervix, and uterus with a 46 XY karyotype. Which diagnosis should the family nurse practitioner suspect?
    1. Turner's syndrome.
    2. Müllerian agenesis.
    3. Testicular feminization.
    4. Gonadal dysgenesis.

40. What is the most common cause of a breast mass in patients ages 15–25?
    1. Fibroadenoma.
    2. Intraductal papilloma.
    3. Infiltrating lobular carcinoma.
    4. Fibrocystic breast syndrome.

41. What is an effective treatment for primary dysmenorrhea?
    1. Nonsteroidal antiinflammatory drugs (NSAIDs).
    2. Tranquilizers.
    3. Progestins.
    4. Steroids.

42. What is a cause of secondary amenorrhea?
    1. Testicular feminization.
    2. Hypogonadotropic hypogonadism.
    3. Congenital absence of uterus.
    4. Extreme exercise.

43. A young woman comes into the clinic for a well-woman checkup. She states that, about 3 weeks ago, she had a sore on her labia that went away. It was not particularly painful, did not itch, and apparently caused no residual problems. How would the family nurse practitioner treat this patient?
    1. Ordering the treponemal-specific test (FTA-ABS).
    2. Swabbing the area of the lesion for a viral culture.
    3. Advising her to notify her sexual contacts to determine whether they have had any symptoms.

4. Ordering nystatin (Mycostatin) cream to be applied to the area three or four times a day.

44. A young woman is complaining of tenderness and burning of her vulva. On exam, the vulva is edematous and excoriated. The family nurse practitioner performs a wet mount preparation of the vaginal secretions. It reveals pseudohyphae and spores. What is the diagnosis for this patient?
    1. Vulvovaginal candidiasis.
    2. Chlamydial infection.
    3. Bacterial vaginosis.
    4. Gonorrhea.

45. What is the leading cause of mortality in women with genital cancer, excluding breast?
    1. Ovarian cancer.
    2. Endometrial cancer.
    3. Cervical cancer.
    4. Vulvar/vaginal cancer.

46. A young woman presents with complaints of an irritation in the vaginal area. This is the first time it has occurred. On vaginal exam, the cervix is inflamed and friable. Flagellated protozoa are seen on the wet mount. What is the most likely diagnosis?
    1. Trichomoniasis.
    2. Cervicitis.
    3. Chlamydial infection.
    4. Bacterial vaginosis.

47. Which is **not** a risk factor for endometrial cancer?
    1. Obesity.
    2. Oral contraceptive (OC) use.
    3. Unopposed estrogen use.
    4. Advancing age, greater than 50 years.

48. Which statement is true regarding the diaphragm?
    1. May be inserted up to 24 hours before intercourse.
    2. May be inserted any time up to 6 hours before intercourse.
    3. Should be removed within 1 hour after intercourse.
    4. Should not be left in place longer than 24 hours.

49. What is a contraceptive method associated with an increase in urinary tract infections (UTIs)?
    1. Intrauterine device.
    2. Diaphragm.
    3. Norplant.
    4. Oral contraception.

50. Which is **not** a risk factor for ovarian cancer?
    1. Family history of ovarian cancer.
    2. Advancing age, greater than 50 years.
    3. Oral contraceptive (OC) use.
    4. Positive *BRCA-2* gene.

51. A 20-year-old college student presents to urgent care with new onset of painful sores in the vulva. These erupted yesterday and are associated with exquisite pain, fever, and flulike symptoms of headache, general body aches, and mild dysuria. She has a new sexual partner. The exam reveals vesicular lesions covering the labia, extreme tenderness of external genitalia to palpation, normal Bartholin glands, and normal vaginal inspection with mild leukorrhea, normal cervical mucosa, and slightly tender, minimally enlarged inguinal lymph nodes bilaterally. What is the most likely diagnosis?
    1. Gonorrhea.
    2. Chlamydial infection.
    3. Herpes simplex virus.
    4. Lymphogranuloma venereum.

52. A 21-year-old patient is seen for her annual gynecologic exam. She is sexually active, rarely uses condoms for sexually transmitted disease (STD) prevention, and has multiple sexual partners. She smokes one pack of cigarettes per day, admits to a sedentary lifestyle, and eats two meals per day, most often at fast-food restaurants. Her exam is negative for any abnormalities. Her family history and personal medical history are negative for major disease. She has no menstrual abnormalities; her last menstrual period was 1 week ago. The family nurse practitioner obtains a Papanicolaou smear. Which action would **not** be appropriate for this patient?
    1. Obtaining cultures for gonorrhea and *Chlamydia*.
    2. Laboratory testing of glucose, cardiac risk profile, and thyroid-stimulating hormone (TSH).
    3. Human immunodeficiency titer and rapid plasma reagin.
    4. Counseling on safe sex practice and contraceptive information.

53. A family nurse practitioner is reviewing development of breast cancer. Which three factors should the nurse identify as leading to increased risk of development of breast cancer?
    1. Early menopause.
    2. High-fat diet.
    3. Advancing age.
    4. Early menarche.
    5. Nonproliferative fibroadenomas.

54. A 32-year-old female patient, G2 T1 P1 A0 L2, is seen in the clinic by the family nurse practitioner for her annual exam and is requesting information on preconception counseling. She has been taking oral contraceptives (OCs) for 3 years without complications. During the past year she has started an exercise program at a health club 5 days a week and is eating three nutritionally sound meals daily. She has lost 33 lb and is now at her ideal body weight. She quit her job as a postal worker and now stays home with her children. As part of her preconception care, what should the family nurse practitioner recommend?
    1. Start prenatal vitamins with folic acid.
    2. Discontinue exercise.
    3. Update measles mumps rubella (MMR) vaccine.
    4. Start genetic counseling because of advanced maternal age.

55. What should the initial workup for abnormal uterine bleeding include?
    1. Referral for diagnostic dilatation and curettage.
    2. Referral for endometrial biopsy to rule out cancer.
    3. Complete blood count, pregnancy test, and endocrine studies.
    4. Coagulation studies and sexually transmitted disease cultures.

56. A 21-year-old female patient presents for her first well-woman exam. She has never been sexually active. Her family history and past medical history are negative for any gynecologic diseases. Her menses occur every 28 days, lasting 5 days, with a relatively moderate flow and no significant abdominal cramps. Her physical exam/visit today should include which tests?
    1. Papanicolaou (Pap) smear.
    2. Cultures for gonorrhea and *Chlamydia*.
    3. Stool hemoccult.
    4. Baseline mammogram.

57. Reactive cellular changes noted on a Papanicolaou smear are most often associated with:
    1. Inflammation.
    2. Use of estrogen vaginal cream.
    3. Drying artifact.
    4. Use of oral contraceptives (OCs).

58. What are the risk factors for cervical cancer?
    1. Pregnancy after age 35.
    2. Viral exposure.
    3. Low parity.
    4. Prolonged contraceptive use.

59. A 48-year-old patient presents to the clinic complaining of hot flashes, no menses for 14 months, insomnia, crying spells, irritability, decreased libido, and fatigue. At the end of her history and physical, she begins to cry and tells the family nurse practitioner that she "thinks she's going crazy." She then begs the family nurse practitioner to tell her what is wrong. Which action is inappropriate for the family nurse practitioner to do at this point?
    1. Obtain laboratory tests, including follicle-stimulating hormone and luteinizing hormone.
    2. Discuss hormone replacement therapy, including risks and benefits and short- and long-term treatment strategies.
    3. Provide antidepressant therapy and a referral for counseling sessions for depression.
    4. Provide written information regarding menopause and options for treatment of symptoms.

60. Care for a patient with chancroid should include:
    1. Screening for HIV and syphilis.
    2. Mandatory notification and treatment of all sexual partners.
    3. Screening for lymphogranuloma venereum.
    4. Culture for gonorrhea.

61. During her annual exam, a 35-year-old patient complains of recent breast changes. She states that her breasts are painful and frequently feel "lumpy." Because of this, she has stopped doing monthly breast self-exam (BSE), believing BSE is a "waste of time." What would be the most appropriate advice for the family nurse practitioner to give to this patient?
    1. Stress the importance of the woman knowing the normal look and feel of her breasts and to report any changes.
    2. Suggest she do BSE at least every 2 months.
    3. Suggest she start having mammograms to establish some baseline data about her breasts.
    4. Determine when her breasts are nontender and least "lumpy," and change her BSE schedule.

62. During a breast exam on a young woman, palpation reveals a painless, 2-cm lobular mass in the right breast that is firm and freely mobile. What should appropriate management include?
    1. Continued observation and rechecking in 3 months.
    2. Referral for a mammogram.
    3. Referral for probable surgical excision.
    4. Detailed family history to determine breast cancer risk.

63. A woman with bilateral breast implants asks if it is really necessary to do monthly breast self-exam (BSE) because she "does not know what to feel for." How should the family nurse practitioner respond?
    1. Suggest she involve her sexual partner in assessing her breasts on a regular basis.
    2. Review the steps in BSE until she feels comfortable with the process.
    3. Acknowledge the difficulty of doing BSE after implant surgery.
    4. Explain the usefulness of regular mammograms for implant patients.

64. An adult patient comes to the clinic complaining of abnormal vaginal discharge (dark watery brown) along with postcoital bleeding. The family nurse practitioner suspects the possibility of cancer of the cervix. During the vaginal exam, suspicious physical exam findings include:
    1. Soft, sill-shaped cervix.
    2. Very firm cervix with an ulcer.
    3. Vague lower abdominal discomfort.
    4. Tender, enlarged lymph nodes.

65. A postmenopausal patient is worried about pain in the upper outer quadrant of her left breast. What action should the family nurse practitioner take?
    1. Do a breast exam and order a mammogram.
    2. Explain that the pain is related to hormone fluctuations, and order laboratory studies.
    3. Reassure the patient that pain is not a presenting symptom of breast cancer, and check for proper fit of the brassiere.
    4. Teach the patient breast self-exam (BSE).

66. A 22-year-old female patient comes to the family nurse practitioner's office with a complaint of 1 day of fever of 102°F (38.9°C), a diffuse macular rash, vomiting, headache, and decreased urine output. Which information obtained in the patient's history would be most significant given the patient's clinical presentation?
    1. Whether the patient's immunizations are up to date.
    2. If the patient is currently menstruating.
    3. If the patient has a history of tuberculosis.
    4. What type of contraception the patient uses.

67. A young female patient presents to the family nurse practitioner's office with a complaint of abdominal pain. Which differential diagnosis should be ruled out given that the patient is of child-bearing age and could lead to increased morbidity and mortality if not treated promptly?
    1. Irritable bowel syndrome.
    2. Cholelithiasis.
    3. Pyelonephritis.
    4. Ectopic pregnancy.

68. A young adult patient presents with a history of vaginal itching and heavy white discharge. The patient gives a history of no sexual activity. On exam, the family nurse practitioner finds a red, edematous vulva and white patches on the vaginal walls. The discharge has no odor. What finding should the family nurse practitioner expect in the patient's history?
    1. Vegetarian diet.
    2. Recent diarrhea.
    3. Early menopause.
    4. Recent antibiotic use.

69. A young patient comes to the office complaining of vaginal bleeding. The patient states that she has used five tampons in the last 3 hours. She admits to sexual activity and takes oral contraceptives (OCs). On further questioning, the patient states that she started her most recent pack of OCs "about 2 weeks late." What priority action should the family nurse practitioner take?
    1. Perform a STAT urine pregnancy test.
    2. Perform a STAT complete blood count (CBC).
    3. Discuss proper use of OCs.
    4. Send the patient for a pelvic sonogram.

70. The family nurse practitioner knows that the majority of breast cancers occur in which area of the breast?
    1. Upper inner quadrant.
    2. Upper outer quadrant.
    3. Beneath the nipple and areola.
    4. Lower outer quadrant.

71. The patient presents with abnormal uterine bleeding and has been found to have endometrial cancer. She returned to the family nurse practitioner because she does not understand how this is possible when the Papanicolaou (Pap) smear 6 months ago was negative. What is the family nurse practitioner's **best** response?
    1. "Uterine cancer develops quickly."
    2. "Pap smears are difficult to read, and mistakes can happen."
    3. "Pap smears are not useful in detecting uterine cancers in most cases."
    4. "The previous Pap smear did not have an adequate sample."

72. A postmenopausal woman is seen in the office with complaints of frequent urination, stress incontinence, vaginal dryness, and dyspareunia. Her last menstrual period was 6 years ago, and she elected not to take hormone replacement therapy. She has increased her intake of soy products. What is the most common cause of her symptoms?
    1. Urinary tract infection.
    2. Cystocele.
    3. Bacterial vaginitis.
    4. Atrophic vaginitis.

73. The family nurse practitioner understands that the following are U.S. Preventive Services Task Force (USPSTF) recommendations about the effectiveness of specific preventive care services for patients without obvious related signs or symptoms of breast cancer.
    1. The USPSTF recommends prescribing risk-reducing medications, such as tamoxifen, raloxifene, or aromatase inhibitors, to women who are at increased risk for breast cancer and at low risk for adverse medication effects.
    2. Women 65 years and older having a history of breast cancer should not take risk-reducing medications.
    3. The USPSTF recommends the routine use of risk-reducing medications, such as tamoxifen, raloxifene, or aromatase inhibitors, in women who are not at increased risk for breast cancer.
    4. Women who have atypical ductal or lobular hyperplasia and lobular carcinoma in situ should not take risk-reducing medication therapy.

Pharmacology

74. A female patient has received treatment for *Trichomonas vaginalis* and completed the course of therapy, but the patient remains symptomatic. Which two findings might prompt the family nurse practitioner that the patient has not been compliant with treatment?
    1. States that she had a few alcohol drinks during the course of therapy.
    2. Uses cotton underwear as an undergarment.
    3. Did not douche during the course of therapy.
    4. Took 2-g dose of metronidazole (Flagyl) as a single dose as opposed to 500 mg twice a day dosage for 7 days.
    5. Reports that she has not abstained from sexual intercourse.

75. The results of the Women's Health Initiative (WHI) provided evidence-based data that have led to new guidelines in assessing the risk/benefit ratio for initiation of hormone replacement therapy (HRT) in postmenopausal women. Which statement is **not** correct?
    1. HRT is indicated for the treatment of menopausal symptoms, such as vasomotor and urogenital symptoms.
    2. HRT should be continued for primary prevention of coronary heart disease.
    3. HRT can be continued for the prevention of postmenopausal fractures caused by osteoporosis.
    4. HRT should be limited to the shortest duration consistent with treatment goals and benefits in consideration with risks in the individual woman.

76. A 46-year-old female patient is being seen in the clinic by the family nurse practitioner. She was last seen 2 weeks ago for an upper respiratory tract infection and was treated with amoxicillin (Amoxil) 250 mg PO tid × 10 days. She completed her medication last week, but now is aware of vaginal itching and has cottage cheese–like vaginal discharge. She states that she has never experienced such intense itching. She is in a mutually monogamous relationship. Her last menstrual period was 2 weeks ago. Her partner had a vasectomy 2 years ago. Wet mount with potassium hydroxide shows negative whiff test, rare clue cells, positive lactobacilli, positive hyphae and spores, few white blood cells, and no trichomonads. She is leaving tomorrow for a week-long cruise. She is not taking any medications and has no known drug allergies. The family nurse practitioner knows that the best treatment for this problem is:
    1. Metronidazole (Flagyl) 500 mg PO bid × 7 days.
    2. Clindamycin (Cleocin) vaginal cream one applicator full vaginally hs × 7 days.
    3. Fluconazole (Diflucan) 150 mg 1 tab PO one time.
    4. Hydrocortisone (Cortaid) 1% cream sparingly bid × 7 days.

77. A 25-year-old patient presents with complaints of a malodorous vaginal discharge, which is described as white and watery. She douches with vinegar and water every 2 weeks. She uses a diaphragm for contraception. She and her boyfriend have been sexually active for 2 years, using condoms for sexually transmitted disease (STD) prevention with every act of coitus. She denies any dyspareunia. Her last menstrual period (LMP) was 1 week ago, and there are no noted changes in her normal menstrual pattern. Her wet mount with potassium hydroxide results show a positive whiff test, clue cells too numerous to count/high-power field, no lactobacilli, no hyphae or spores, no trichomonads, and few white blood cells. What is the diagnosis and treatment for this patient?
    1. *Chlamydia;* doxycycline (Vibra-Tabs) 100 mg PO bid × 10 days.
    2. *Candida albicans;* terconazole (Terazol 7) vaginal cream 1 applicator hs × 7 days.
    3. Herpes simplex type 2; acyclovir (Zovirax) 200 mg PO q4h × 5 days.
    4. Bacterial vaginosis; metronidazole (Metrogel) vaginal gel 1 applicator hs × 5 days.

78. A 55-year-old patient, G2 T2 P0 A0 L2, is being seen in the clinic for her annual exam. She went through a natural menopause 5 years ago and has never been interested in hormone replacement therapy (HRT). She smokes one pack per day and does no formal exercise. Her family history is positive for osteoporosis in her mother, positive for myocardial infarction in her father, and negative for cancer. She has a normal physical exam today and had a negative mammogram yesterday. She is now interested in HRT but wants to know her alternatives. Which choice has **not** been clinically proven for prevention of osteoporosis?
    1. Estradiol (Estrace) 0.5 mg 1 tab PO qd and micronized progesterone (Prometrium) 100 mg 1 tablet PO qd.
    2. Weight-bearing exercise three times weekly.
    3. Discontinue cigarette smoking.
    4. Wild Mexican yam cream applied to skin tid.

79. A young woman is seen in the sexually transmitted disease (STD) clinic. She noticed some itchy bumps in the vulvar area and is concerned that they could be cancer. On careful inspection, the family nurse practitioner notes five cauliflower-like, warty, pinkish lesions in the lower introitus. Two smaller lesions nestled anterior to the hymeneal ring of the vagina and cervix fail to reveal any abnormalities. Wet mount with potassium hydroxide is negative. Culture for gonorrhea and *Chlamydia* was obtained, Papanicolaou smear done, and HIV titer and rapid plasma reagin drawn. Which is **not** an appropriate treatment for this patient?
    1. Podophyllin (Podoben) application; wash off in 6 hours with soap and water.
    2. Trichloroacetic acid application; do not wash off.
    3. Cryotherapy with liquid nitrogen to lesions.
    4. Benzathine penicillin 2.4 million units IM weekly × 3 weeks.

80. A young adult complaining of vaginal itching, thick yellow mucous discharge, and urinary discomfort is seen in the urgent care unit by the family nurse practitioner. She is sexually active and uses condoms with only one of her two partners. On physical exam, the abdomen is negative; pelvic exam reveals the Bartholin glands within normal limits, cervix with mucopurulent discharge from the os, and mucosa friable to palpation; bimanual exam is negative. Cultures were taken but are not yet available. Wet mount with potassium hydroxide reveals a negative whiff test, few clue cells, white blood cells too numerous to count/high-power field, no yeast, and no trichomonads. What is the most likely diagnosis and appropriate treatment?
    1. *Chlamydia;* azithromycin (Zithromax) 1 g PO single dose.
    2. *Chlamydia;* ceftriaxone (Rocephin) 125 mg IM.
    3. Herpes simplex virus; acyclovir (Zovirax) 200 mg 1 cap PO q4h × 5 days.
    4. Trichomoniasis; metronidazole (Flagyl) 2 g PO single dose.

81. A 52-year-old woman presents for her annual gynecologic exam from her primary care provider. She received a hysterectomy with ovarian conservation at age 40 for uterine fibroids and dysfunctional uterine bleeding. She has been taking oral estrogen (conjugated equine estrogen 0.625 mg) hormone replacement therapy (HRT) for 1 year. Although HRT has definitely reduced the discomfort of hot flashes, vaginal dryness, and mood swings from insomnia, she still experiences flashes and some night sweats. Her diagnostic lipid panel shows total cholesterol 180 mg/dL, LDL low-density lipoprotein (LDL) 112 mg/dL, high-density lipoprotein (HDL) 52 mg/dL, and triglycerides 325 mg/dL. What, if any, change should the family nurse practitioner consider in her medication regimen?
    1. No change should be considered at this time.
    2. Decrease estrogen dosage to 0.3 mg daily.
    3. Recommend stopping estrogen therapy.
    4. Suggest changing route of administration to transdermal.

82. An adult female patient is seen in the family planning clinic for a consultation on contraception with the family nurse practitioner. She is using oral contraceptives but forgets to take them because her work schedule changes every week; she is looking for an effective method that will be easy to remember. She has been married for 14 years, is G2 T2 P0 A0 L2, and is a nonsmoker. She has a negative past history for major diseases and a negative gynecologic history for abnormalities. She has never been treated for a sexually transmitted infection and is in a mutually monogamous relationship. She is needle phobic and faints when she has to have blood drawn. What contraceptive method would be the best choice for the patient?
    1. Depo-Provera injection every 3 months.
    2. Implantation system for 5 years.
    3. Intrauterine device (IUD).
    4. Diaphragm.

83. A young woman is seen at the family planning clinic by the family nurse practitioner. The patient wants birth control pills but has heard that oral contraceptives (OCs) are "dangerous to one's health." When asked for clarification, she lists weight gain, ovarian cancer, heavy or irregular periods, and infertility. After saying, "I can see that you are concerned about your health," what would be the most appropriate for the family nurse practitioner to tell the patient?
    1. "There are a lot of fallacies about birth control pills. They actually are thought to reduce the risk of ovarian cancers and to help regulate the bleeding, and they are not associated with causing infertility. There can be a minor increase in body weight of 3–5 pounds."
    2. "Perhaps you would be better off trying the implantation system or Depo-Provera."
    3. "What you have heard is true. They can be dangerous to your health, and many women experience these problems."
    4. "There are a lot of fallacies about birth control pills. Ovarian cancer and infertility are risks when taking the pills, but they do not cause weight gain or bleeding changes during periods. Papanicolaou (Pap) smears done every year will detect such problems as ovarian cancer."

84. An adult female patient is taking oral contraceptives (OCs). She calls into the clinic with complaints of bleeding through the first 2 weeks of every package of pills. She has been taking this pill for 4 months at the same time every day. Her present OC is a low-dose monophasic pill.

She is not taking any other medications and denies any adverse effects from the OCs. She would prefer to keep taking the OCs if possible. What should the family nurse practitioner's advice include?
    1. Discontinue the pills and do not restart them. Use an alternative contraceptive method.
    2. Change to a higher dosage, and higher progestational agent.
    3. Try taking the pills early in the morning on an empty stomach to improve their metabolism.
    4. There is no cause for concern; breakthrough bleeding is a normal side effect of OCs.

85. An adult female patient is seen by the family nurse practitioner at the family planning clinic. The patient notes heavy, irregular menses and an increase in facial acne and facial/abdominal hair growth over the past few years. She is G1 T1 P0 A0 L1 and is not planning future pregnancies. After a normal pelvic exam, she decides she wants oral contraceptives (OCs). What is the best medication choice for this patient?
    1. Loestrin 1/20.
    2. Triphasil.
    3. Demulen 1/35.
    4. OCs are inappropriate for this patient.

86. A 41-year-old patient is seen for her 6-week postpartum exam by the family nurse practitioner. She is breast-feeding without difficulty and plans to continue for a year. She wants to begin using a contraceptive and plans no further pregnancies. Which of the following is an inappropriate choice for this patient?
    1. Depo-Provera 150 mg IM every 3 months.
    2. Intrauterine device (IUD).
    3. Progestin-only oral contraceptive (OC).
    4. Combination OC.

87. A 38-year-old patient is seen for her 6-week postpartum exam by the family nurse practitioner. The patient was breast-feeding for a short time but discontinued 4 weeks ago. Her menses have resumed. She is contemplating another pregnancy in about a year, but if she became pregnant before then, she "wouldn't mind." She is seeking contraception. She smokes one pack per day. Her exam is normal, with the uterus well involuted. Which of the following is contraindicated in this patient?
    1. Progestasert intrauterine device (IUD).
    2. Oral contraception.
    3. Depo-Provera injection.
    4. Condoms and spermicide.

88. A 22-year-old female patient presents to the urgent care department and is seen by the family nurse practitioner. She is complaining of abdominal pain, low-grade fever, and mucopurulent vaginal discharge. Her symptoms began 3 days ago and are worsening. She has a new sexual partner and has not yet used condoms with him. Her menses just ended; she is taking oral contraceptives. She denies nausea, vomiting, or anorexia. Her exam reveals findings consistent with pelvic inflammatory disease (PID). Cultures are taken for gonorrhea and *Chlamydia*. Which of the following represents an inappropriate treatment plan for the family nurse practitioner to follow?
    1. Ceftriaxone (Rocephin) 250 mg IM.
    2. Doxycycline (Vibra-Tabs) 100 mg PO bid × 10 days.
    3. Complete blood count (CBC), erythrocyte sedimentation rate (ESR).
    4. Hospitalization.

89. What is the primary role of progestins in prescribing postmenopausal hormone replacement therapy (HRT)?
    1. Reduce side effects of estrogen-related breast tenderness.
    2. Provide endometrial protection against hyperplasia.
    3. Stabilize mood swings and reduce hot flashes.
    4. Reduce occurrence of breakthrough bleeding.

90. An older female patient is seen by the family nurse practitioner for her annual exam. She has been on hormone replacement therapy (HRT) for 6 months, having started herself on the pills left over by her deceased mother. She brings the pills, which she wants to keep taking, and requests a prescription for Estrace 1 mg daily. She has an intact uterus, is in excellent health, and denies any complaints. She does not have any contraindications to the use of HRT. Her exam is normal. Which represents an incorrect and potentially dangerous plan for the family nurse practitioner to follow?
    1. Endometrial biopsy.
    2. Prescription for Estrace 1 mg daily plus medroxyprogesterone acetate (Provera) 2.5 mg daily.
    3. Prescription for Estrace 1 mg daily.
    4. Instruct patient on the risks and benefits of HRT.

91. An older adult patient is seen for follow-up to discuss her hormone replacement therapy (HRT) that she began 3 months ago. She needs a refill on her HRT but is not sure "if it is working right." She continues to feel hot flashes, moodiness, and decreased libido, and she has many sleep disturbances. She is taking Premarin 0.625 mg daily and Provera 2.5 mg daily. She denies any vaginal bleeding. Which is **not** an acceptable choice for the patient?
    1. Premarin 0.9 mg 1 tab PO qd and Provera 5 mg 1 tab PO qd days 1–12.
    2. Premarin 0.9 mg 1 tab PO qd and Provera 5 mg 1 tab PO qd days 16–25.
    3. Premarin 0.3 mg 1 tab PO qd and Provera 2.5 mg 1 tab PO qd.

    4. Premarin 1.25 mg 1 tab PO qd and Provera 10 mg 1 tab PO qd days 1–12.

92. A young adult patient presents to the clinic with complaints of a malodorous, yellowish vaginal discharge and vulvovaginal itching. She has never had a gynecologic exam and is extremely apprehensive. She is sexually active and has had a new sexual partner for 2 months. She states that they use condoms "most of the time" and are not interested in alternate forms of contraception at this time. Her last menstrual period (LMP) was 1 week ago. Her wet mount with potassium hydroxide shows few clue cells, moderate lactobacilli, few white blood cells, no yeast, and mobile trichomonads too numerous to count. What would the appropriate treatment for this patient include?
    1. Metronidazole (Flagyl) 2 g PO single dose.
    2. Metronidazole (Metrogel) vaginal cream 1 applicator hs × 5 days.
    3. Fluconazole (Diflucan) 150 mg PO single dose.
    4. Terconazole (Terazol) vaginal cream 1 applicator hs × 7 days.

93. Which dose of conjugated equine estrogen (Premarin) is the minimal effective dose to prevent osteoporosis?
    1. 0.3 mg.
    2. 0.625 mg.
    3. 0.9 mg.
    4. Premarin is inappropriate.

94. A single woman presents for contraceptive counseling, expressing preference for a diaphragm. Which factor in her history would make a diaphragm a poor choice?
    1. Three urinary tract infections (UTIs) in the past year.
    2. Strong desire to avoid pregnancy.
    3. Last two Papanicolaou smears showing atypical cells.
    4. Nulliparous cervix.

95. Combination oral contraceptives (OCs) prevent pregnancy primarily by:
    1. Decreasing fallopian tube motility.
    2. Thinning of cervical mucus.
    3. Suppressing ovulation.
    4. Causing inflammation of the endometrium.

96. A young adult patient is hesitant to be fitted for an intrauterine device (IUD) because of strong antiabortion views and asks for the family nurse practitioner's opinion. Which explanation **least** accurately describes an IUD's probable action?
    1. Slows transport of ovum through the fallopian tube, causing it to age and die in transit.
    2. Prevents effective implantation of a fertilized ovum.
    3. Action is no different than that of a spermicide.
    4. Slows transport of sperm.

97. What is a unique advantage of a Progesterone T intrauterine device (IUD)?
    1. Lowest failure rate of IUDs.
    2. May be left in place for up to 10 years.
    3. Decreases menstrual blood loss and dysmenorrhea.
    4. Must be replaced annually.

98. An older female patient is seen by the family nurse practitioner for her annual exam and needs a refill on her hormone replacement therapy (HRT). She is feeling well and has not voiced concerns. The patient had a total abdominal hysterectomy and bilateral salpingo-oophorectomy 2 years ago for benign fibroids. Her exam is normal. She takes conjugated estrogen (Premarin) 0.625 mg days 1–25 and medroxyprogesterone acetate (Provera) 10 mg from days 16–25. What changes would be appropriate for the family nurse practitioner to make in the HRT regimen?
    1. No changes needed; the patient is doing well on the present regimen.
    2. Premarin 0.625 mg daily and discontinue the Provera.
    3. Premarin 0.625 mg daily and Provera 2.5 mg daily.
    4. Premarin 0.625 mg days 1–25 and Provera 5 mg days 16–25.

99. Which statement about progestin-only pills is true?
    1. Women who are breast-feeding should not use progestin-only pills.
    2. Ovulation suppression is as effective with progestin-only pills as with combination oral contraceptives (OCs).
    3. There is an increased incidence of functional ovarian cysts.
    4. The risk of ectopic pregnancy is lower for women using progestin-only pills.

100. Before prescribing hormone replacement therapy (HRT), which clinical approach should have the highest priority?
    1. The decision about use should rest primarily with the patient after providing appropriate education and counseling.
    2. For most women the benefits of HRT far outweigh any possible side effects, so HRT should be actively encouraged.
    3. Involving the sexual partner in the counseling session is likely to lead to a higher compliance rate for HRT.
    4. Education regarding HRT should include a thorough review of risk factors and possible side effects to avoid liability issues.

101. What is the most common side effect associated with depo-medroxyprogesterone (Depo-Provera)?
    1. Nausea.
    2. Acne.
    3. Menstrual cycle changes.
    4. Increased menstrual cramps.

102. What information should the family nurse practitioner include when teaching a patient about taking alendronate (Fosamax)?
    1. Take it midmorning.
    2. Take with food.
    3. Take with a full glass of orange juice.
    4. Remain upright after taking medication.

103. The addition of a progesterone to an estrogen regimen in a postmenopausal woman with a uterus reduces the risk of:
    1. Endometrial cancer.
    2. Cervical cancer.
    3. Gallbladder disease.
    4. Breast cancer.

104. What is the single-dose treatment of choice for trichomoniasis?
    1. Azithromycin (Zithromax) 1 g PO.
    2. Ofloxacin (Floxin) 500 mg PO.
    3. Metronidazole (Flagyl) 2 g PO.
    4. Clindamycin (Cleocin) 300 mg PO.

105. A young woman who is taking a low-dose oral contraceptive (OC) calls the clinic in a panic, stating that she forgot her pill 2 days ago. She is taking phenytoin (Dilantin) for seizure activity and has been seizure free for over a year. She asks, "What should I do about my pills?" What would be the family nurse practitioner's most appropriate response?
    1. "Take the forgotten dose today along with the regular dose."
    2. "See your physician for advice about the Dilantin."
    3. "Continue the pills but use another contraceptive through the rest of this cycle."
    4. "Come to the clinic for a 'morning-after' pill."

106. A vaginal culture has confirmed the presence of a chancroid in a homeless woman who presented with a painful genital ulcer. What should be the treatment regimen of choice?
    1. Ceftriaxone (Rocephin) 250 mg IM single dose.
    2. Erythromycin (E-Mycin) 500 mg PO qid × 7 days.
    3. Metronidazole (Flagyl) 2 mg PO single dose.
    4. Clindamycin (Cleocin) 2% vaginal cream 1 applicator × 5 days.

107. You are counseling a 49-year-old woman who had her last menstrual period (LMP) 10 months ago. She is experiencing some hot flashes and night sweats and is not sleeping well. These symptoms are affecting her ability to work effectively because she finds herself tired and "cranky." She does not want hormone replacement therapy (HRT). Which of the following evidence-based alternative measures is most accurately described?
    1. Venlafaxine (Effexor SR) has been effective in reducing hot flashes in randomized controlled trials.
    2. Raloxifene (Evista) has demonstrated a significant reduction in hot flashes compared with placebo in clinical trials.
    3. Black cohosh (*Cimicifuga racemosa*) has been reported as efficacious in treating menopausal symptoms in many large, controlled trials.
    4. Isoflavones, specifically soy, have been shown in studies to be significantly more effective than placebo in reducing hot flashes.

108. A 65-year-old postmenopausal female has been treated with alendronate (Fosamax) for 6 years. Current screening indicates no increase in risk factors. Based on clinical guidelines, which treatment option would the family nurse practitioner suggest to the patient?
    1. Discontinue medication at this time.
    2. Switch medication from oral to intravenous route to maintain adequate coverage.
    3. Add vitamin D 500 IU daily to treatment regimen.
    4. Increase calcium supplementation to 1500 mg per day.

109. A young woman presents to the office for evaluation of abdominal pain. The patient admits to recent sexual activity and states that she does not have her partner use condoms. On exam, the family nurse practitioner finds vaginal discharge and cervical motion tenderness. Along with sending cultures to the laboratory, the family nurse practitioner's treatment plan for the patient would also include which two medications?
    1. Penicillin G 2.4 million units IM.
    2. Metronidazole (Flagyl) 500 mg PO bid × 7 days.
    3. Ceftriaxone (Rocephin) 125 mg IM.
    4. Azithromycin (Zithromax) 1 g PO.
    5. Acyclovir (Zovirax) 400 mg PO bid × 7 days.

110. Which information about hormone replacement therapy (HRT) should the family nurse practitioner understand when discussing HRT with patients?
    1. Estrogen replacement delays the onset of menopause.
    2. Estrogen and progesterone cause vasomotor symptoms.
    3. Estrogen decreases the risk of osteoporosis.
    4. Estrogen replacement with progesterone increases risk of ovarian cancer.

16 Female Reproductive Answers & Rationales

Physical Exam & Diagnostic Tests

1. Answer: 2, 3

Rationale: Based on current cervical screening guidelines by the U.S. Preventive Services Task Force (USPSTF), Pap smear tests should be performed on female patients aged 21 and older.

2. Answer: 1

Rationale: Recommendations made by the U.S. Preventive Services Task Force (USPSTF) with regard to screening intervals to establish better risk fracture prediction suggest intervals longer than the minimum of 2 years.

3. Answer: 3

Rationale: Lubricants, other than water, should not be used if a cervical specimen is being obtained for conventional Pap smear analysis; some lubricants can alter the appearance of the cells and affect cytologic accuracy. For a liquid-based Pap test, in addition to the use of water, the posterior blade of the speculum also may be lubricated with a small amount of water-based lubricant before insertion. The endocervical cell retrieval is diminished with use of a cotton-tipped applicator and is not recommended in any female patient regardless of pregnancy status. The bimanual exam is performed after the internal vaginal exam.

4. Answer: 2

Rationale: To aid in the exam, an empty bladder provides comfort for the patient and assists the family nurse practitioner in making a more accurate assessment during the bimanual portion of the exam. Asking the patient to bear down slightly while the speculum is inserted and explaining each step of the procedure help reduce the patient's anxiety, which ultimately may help achieve comfort.

5. Answer: 1

Rationale: A nabothian cyst (Naboth follicle) is a small, white or yellow, raised, round area on the cervix and is considered to be a normal variant. The surface of the cervix should be smooth and may have a symmetric, reddened circle around the os (squamocolumnar epithelium, or ectropion). The other options are all unexpected, abnormal findings.

6. Answer: 3

Rationale: A breast ultrasound is used to determine whether a lesion is solid or cystic. Ultrasound misses 50% of lesions less than 2 cm. The test is not sensitive enough to be used for routine screening and cannot replace mammography. The definitive diagnosis of breast cancer is the breast biopsy.

7. Answer: 2

Rationale: The World Health Organization defines osteoporosis as a bone mineral density T-score below −2.5 SD and osteopenia as a T-score between −1 and −2.5. The woman has early signs of osteopenia. She is not a candidate for hormone replacement therapy (HRT; estrogen + MPA) because of her past cardiovascular history. Raloxifene has been shown to prevent the progression of osteoporosis and, as a selective estrogen-receptor modulator (SERM), may be a good alternative to HRT. The other two lifestyle modifications are important counseling issues to reduce the risk of developing osteoporosis.

8. Answer: 1

Rationale: KOH lyses epithelial and white blood cells, making it easier to visualize *Candida albicans* (yeast). *Candida* cells are resistant and remain intact. KOH also assists with diagnosing bacterial vaginosis by alkalinizing vaginal discharge, causing a distinct fishy odor. This is a positive amine or whiff test.

9. Answer: 1, 4, 5

Rationale: Smoking, history of rheumatoid arthritis, and progressive loss of height in an individual indicate an increased risk for the development of osteoporotic fracture. No parental history of hip fractures and a stable BMI within normal range do not support evidence of increased risk of osteoporotic fracture.

10. Answer: 3

Rationale: The Pap smear is a screening test for cervical cancer and precancerous states. The diagnostic test needed to confirm the diagnosis of a high-grade lesion is the colposcopy with guided biopsies. The results of this test are clearly abnormal and must be addressed. Waiting a year could be deleterious to the patient's health. This is not a Pap smear report that one would choose to redo in 4 months; the patient needs a diagnostic test, not another screening test. Because there is no diagnosis of cervical cancer on this Pap smear, referral to a gynecologic oncologist is premature at this time.

11. Answer: 3

Rationale: All the tests listed may be included in the workup for infertility. Because male factors account for 35%–40% of infertility, a semen analysis should be done early in the workup. HSG and endometrial biopsy require scheduling at specific times of the menstrual cycle. Tests for antisperm antibodies would be done if the postcoital test revealed abnormalities.

12. Answer: 1, 3

Rationale: The NOF has conducted cost analyses on the value of screening bone DEXAs for evaluation of bone mineral density (BMD). NOF reports that BMD testing is cost-effective for postmenopausal women ages 50–60 who have other risk factors for development of osteoporosis, including lifestyle factors of minimal exercise, smoking, excessive alcohol intake, and low calcium intake. Other risk factors include genetic history of disease, slender physical frame, premature menopause, hyperthyroidism, multiple myeloma, rheumatoid arthritis, chronic renal disease, corticosteroid use, and long-term anticonvulsant therapy. The woman with the history of long-term corticosteroid therapy would meet the NOF criteria.

13. Answer: 4

Rationale: Long-standing nevi and Montgomery tubercles are normal findings; pendulous breast is a description of size, which is important to note. Enlarged lymph nodes and tender supraclavicular nodes are potential causes for concern. A fixed stellate mass with nipple discharge is not normal, and although asymmetry might be normal, the different colors of the areolae and unilateral nipple inversion could represent a problem.

14. Answer: 2

Rationale: Atrophic changes on the cervix of a postmenopausal woman are to be expected, as is the paucity of endocervical cells. Because of her past medical history of breast cancer, she is not a candidate for the use of estrogen vaginal cream, and the Pap smear interpretation is not abnormal. Endocervical curettage is used as a biopsy technique for sampling tissue from the endocervical canal; however, it is not appropriate to recommend this invasive procedure for someone with scant endocervical cells. It is appropriate for someone with abnormal endocervical cells. Because this Pap smear report is not really classified as abnormal, there is no need to recommend a diagnostic procedure for the patient.

15. Answer: 4

Rationale: Culture is a definitive method of diagnosis. It is a collected cervical specimen, and the results take about 2–6 days to obtain. Blood titers and a urine screen can also be used to diagnose a chlamydial infection. The DFA is fast and has good sensitivity and specificity.

16. Answer: 1

Rationale: Serologic tests are used as screening tests, but positive results require follow-up with a treponemal test to detect specific antibodies.

17. Answer: 2

Rationale: Serum prolactin assay levels greater than 20 ng/mL indicate the need for medical referral, usually to an endocrinologist. The most common cause of hyperprolactinemia and galactorrhea is a pituitary tumor or lesion of the hypothalamus. Other causes include hypothyroidism, medications (narcotics, tranquilizers, and antihypertensives), and oral contraceptives.

18. Answer: 1

Rationale: A positive withdrawal bleed after a progesterone challenge indicates adequate levels of endogenous estrogen. A serum prolactin level should be obtained as part of the amenorrhea workup in addition to a serum pregnancy test. A diagnosis of anovulation can be made on the basis of the successful withdrawal bleed and normal prolactin levels. Low body fat and abnormal thyroxine levels also can lead to amenorrhea, but they do not affect the progesterone challenge test.

19. Answer: 1

Rationale: The occurrence of the symptoms during the luteal phase of the cycle (after ovulation) will assist the family nurse practitioner in making the diagnosis of PMS. Having the patient keep a calendar to track her symptoms for three cycles is helpful in making the diagnosis and measuring successful treatment. Severity of symptoms, although important, is not the most important information.

20. Answer: 3

Rationale: If bleeding resumes after 1 year of amenorrhea in a postmenopausal woman or persists longer than 6 months after hormone replacement therapy initiation, further evaluation is necessary. The most common cause of this abnormal finding is endometrial atrophy, but more serious pathology must be definitively ruled out. An endometrial biopsy should be scheduled to further evaluate the cause of bleeding.

Normal Gynecology

21. Answer: 2

Rationale: Menopause is one point in time and is defined after 12 months of amenorrhea, after the final menstrual period. In postmenopause, FSH levels rise 10- to 15-fold with marked reductions in estradiol, but other menstrual irregularities can create a variation in these levels. Therefore these levels are not considered the best definition for menopause.

22. Answer: 4

Rationale: Pregnancy is the most likely diagnosis in this patient, given the list of symptoms and physical findings. She could have a uterine fibroid, but it is not contributing to the symptoms listed. Ovarian cancer could present with nausea, fatigue, and abdominal bloating, but it would not cause the enlarged uterus or the positive Chadwick's sign. A dislodged IUD will usually change the position of the IUD, decreasing visibility of the strings or causing the IUD itself to be expelled into the vagina or endocervical canal.

23. Answer: 4

Rationale: During menopause, vaginal flora changes leading to an increased likelihood for pathogenic growth and urinary symptoms. Vaginal tissue becomes more alkaline, drier (decreased lubrication), and thinner.

24. Answer: 3

Rationale: Maintaining an alkaline pH is important to promote viability of sperm that are deposited into the vaginal vault.

25. Answer: 4

Rationale: Obesity is not a risk factor for osteoporosis. Cigarette use, white race, and alcohol consumption, among others, are considered risk factors for osteoporosis.

26. Answer: 2

Rationale: Conservative management for PMS, including daily exercise, stress reduction, dietary changes, and reassurance that her symptoms are valid, should help the patient gain more control. A low-salt diet is encouraged; when necessary, a diuretic may be used for fluid retention. The use of vitamins B_6, A, and E may be helpful as well. Laboratory studies are not indicated here but might be helpful if the symptoms were sustained throughout the menstrual cycle.

27. Answer: 2

Rationale: As the function of the ovaries declines and the amount of circulating estrogen begins to fall, the middle-aged woman may begin to experience the symptoms typically associated with menopause. The body's feedback system will attempt to stimulate the ovaries and increase estrogen level. FSH and LH levels rise in response to these efforts.

28. Answer: 3

Rationale: Uterine fibroids are associated with heavy menstrual blood flow, which can be prolonged. Constipation and pelvic, leg, and back pain are also associated with uterine fibroids.

29. Answer: 4

Rationale: The age of menopause has fluctuated little over the past several centuries, even though life expectancy has increased. Of the options, only smoking has been found to cause an earlier menopause. Research shows a direct correlation among number of cigarettes smoked, number of years of smoking, and age at menopause. Nulliparity and epilepsy have also been associated with an earlier age at menopause.

Gynecologic Disorders

30. Answer: 2

Rationale: Secondary dysmenorrhea is associated with clinical symptoms that are caused by anatomic abnormalities in the pelvis. Premenstrual syndrome presents with both physical and psychologic clinical symptoms that typically occur before menses. Pelvic inflammatory disease is an infectious process that affects uterine and pelvic structures that can affect fertility. Dyspareunia is pain experienced during intercourse.

31. Answer: 3

Rationale: Complications associated with polycystic ovarian syndrome (PCOS) include hypertension, increased glucose levels, and infertility. Hemoglobin A1c level between 4% and 5.6% is within normal range, as is a menstrual period lasting between 5 and 7 days.

32. Answer: 2

Rationale: Dyspareunia is painful intercourse, and vaginismus is painful vaginal spasms on penetration. Primary orgasmic disorder is when an individual has never achieved orgasm, usually a lifelong problem. Secondary orgasmic dysfunction refers to an acquired problem of loss of orgasmic function after an individual has experienced orgasm.

33. Answer: 1

Rationale: The initial outbreak is usually the worst. It can be transmitted even when there is no lesion present, and it cannot be cured. Vaginal delivery is allowed if there are no genital lesions at the time of labor.

34. Answer: 1

Rationale: Bacterial vaginosis results when the normal environment in the vagina is disrupted. The normal vaginal lactobacilli are decreased or absent, and there is an overgrowth of many different types of anaerobic bacteria. Trichomoniasis is caused by a flagellated protozoan, and gonorrhea is caused by a bacterium and may be asymptomatic. The virus that causes recurrent outbreaks of genital lesions is herpes simplex type 2.

35. Answer: 1

Rationale: OCs will reduce prostaglandin production, which is thought to be the primary cause of dysmenorrhea.

36. Answer: 4

Rationale: The criteria for the diagnosis of bacterial vaginosis are characteristic milky homogeneous discharge, pH greater than 4.5, amine odor (positive whiff test) with addition of potassium hydroxide, and presence of epithelial cells studded with coccobacilli that obscure the borders (clue cells). Pseudohyphae are present in candidiasis.

37. Answer: 2

Rationale: In Asherman's syndrome, a normally functioning uterus has been damaged and scarred secondary to surgical intervention with resultant trauma, primarily following a D&C. Ovulation may be occurring normally, but no endometrium is built up; therefore no endometrium is shed (menstruation does not occur). Pregnancy, and the other diseases listed, should be ruled out in this patient.

38. Answer: 4

Rationale: The criteria for the diagnosis of polycystic ovarian syndrome include menstrual irregularity, increased body weight, hirsutism, and androgen excess evidenced by laboratory studies and physical findings, chronic anovulation, and multiple bilateral ovarian cysts. Weight loss, dental caries, and amenorrhea would be more common in anorexia nervosa/bulimia. Hyperprolactinemia and galactorrhea are found with a prolactin-secreting pituitary tumor. Dysmenorrhea, nodules palpated on bimanual exam, and infertility are associated with endometriosis.

39. Answer: 3

Rationale: A female-appearing person with a 46 XY karyotype has androgen insensitivity syndrome, or testicular feminization. This maternal X-linked recessive disorder accounts for approximately 10% of all cases of amenorrhea, and these persons appear normal until puberty. These patients present with amenorrhea, scant or absent pubic hair, and abnormal or no breast development. Persons with Müllerian abnormalities have a normal XX karyotype with abnormalities of fallopian tubes, uterus, and upper vagina occurring in fetal development. In Turner's syndrome, congenital absence of ovaries results from loss of one X chromosome.

40. Answer: 1

Rationale: The most common breast mass in young women less than 30 years old is the fibroadenoma. This benign breast mass is the third most common breast mass after fibrocystic changes and carcinoma. Fibrocystic breast changes are seen most commonly in women 30–50 years old. Intraductal papilloma is a wartlike growth located in the mammary duct and occurs in women 40–50 years old. Malignant breast neoplasms occur most frequently in women over 40 and are rarely seen in women 15–25 years old.

41. Answer: 1

Rationale: NSAIDs inhibit prostaglandin synthesis and are effective agents in primary dysmenorrhea. The other agents listed have not demonstrated effectiveness in primary dysmenorrhea. Other measures to decrease discomfort are exercise, relaxation techniques, heat application, and low-dose oral contraceptives.

42. Answer: 4

Rationale: Secondary amenorrhea is defined as no menses for three cycle lengths or 6 months in a woman with previously established menses. Exercise can cause an increase in estrogen and endorphin levels, which influences the release of gonadotropin-releasing hormone (GnRH). Without appropriate GnRH release, follicle-stimulating hormone and luteinizing hormone are not released adequately, resulting in anovulation, which may lead to amenorrhea. The other conditions listed are causes of primary amenorrhea.

43. Answer: 1

Rationale: This has the characteristics of a syphilitic lesion and needs to be evaluated. Only after determining the presence or type of sexually transmitted infection can it be treated effectively. The herpes viral culture should be done while the lesion is present and the fluid from the vesicles can be obtained.

44. Answer: 1

Rationale: The pseudohyphae and spores on the wet mount with potassium hydroxide are diagnostic for candida infection. *Chlamydia trachomatis* is diagnosed by direct immunofluorescent assay or by chlamydial culture. Gonorrhea is diagnosed by cervical culture, and bacterial vaginosis has microscopic findings of clue cells and positive amine odor.

45. Answer: 1

Rationale: Cancer of the ovary is the leading cause of death from female genital cancer, excluding the breast, in the United States.

46. Answer: 1

Rationale: Flagellated protozoan confirms the diagnosis of trichomoniasis. Chlamydial infection is best diagnosed by direct immunofluorescent assay or culture. Bacterial vaginosis is diagnosed by wet mount revealing clue cells and positive amine test. Inflammatory cervicitis is generally asymptomatic and will not cause vaginal irritation.

47. Answer: 2

Rationale: OCs have been shown to reduce the risk of endometrial cancer. Obesity, unopposed estrogen use, and advanced age, in addition to others not listed here, are considered to be risk factors for developing endometrial cancer.

48. Answer: 4

Rationale: The diaphragm may be inserted up to 2 hours before intercourse and should be removed no sooner than 6 hours after intercourse has ended. It should not be left in place longer than 24 hours.

49. Answer: 2

Rationale: Urethral discomfort and recurrent UTIs are associated with diaphragm use and are the most common reasons for discontinuing use and changing birth control methods.

50. Answer: 3

Rationale: OC use has been shown to reduce the risk of ovarian cancer. Family history of ovarian cancer, advancing age, and positive *BRCA-2* gene are considered risk factors for developing ovarian cancer.

51. Answer: 3

Rationale: Herpes simplex virus type 2 typically presents dramatically in the newly infected primary outbreak. Gonorrhea generally is associated with a mucopurulent vaginal discharge and is not accompanied by vesicular lesions. Chlamydial infection may be associated with dysuria and, unless accompanied by pelvic inflammatory disease, it is not generally accompanied by fever or body aches and is not associated with vesicular lesions. Lymphogranuloma venereum is a rare disease classically accompanied by pustular enlargement of the lymph nodes, particularly the inguinal nodes. It is associated not with vesicles, but buboes.

52. Answer: 2

Rationale: Screening blood studies for glucose, cardiac risk profile, and TSH in this age group without any stated risk factors is not cost-effective and is of little value. The patient can be better served with a discussion regarding diet and exercise. Because this patient is at risk for STDs, counseling and testing for these is a reasonable approach. Contraceptive information educates the patient and allows her to make wiser choices in her family planning.

53. Answer: 2, 3, 4

Rationale: High-fat diet, advancing age, and early menarche have been identified as risk factors in the development of breast cancer. Early menopause and nonproliferative fibroadenomas have not been associated with the development of breast cancer.

54. Answer: 1

Rationale: The use of prenatal vitamins with folic acid before conception has been found to reduce the risk of neural tube defects in the fetus. It is important for the patient to continue her exercise program, although some discussion about the type of exercise and any limitations are important once pregnancy is achieved. Because the patient has had two previous pregnancies, it is likely that her rubella immune status has been determined; if she is found to not be immune to rubella, an MMR vaccination should be recommended. This patient is not of advanced maternal age so she does not require genetic counseling for this reason.

55. Answer: 3

Rationale: Baseline laboratory work should be obtained to determine the presence of anemia, possible pregnancy, and endocrine dysfunction.

56. Answer: 1

Rationale: The recommended age for a female to begin screening Pap smears is at the onset of sexual activity or at 21 years of age. Because this patient is 21 years old and has not yet had her first Pap smear, this would be the most appropriate test to perform. It is not necessary to perform sexually transmitted disease screening on patients who have not been sexually active. Stool guaiac (hemoccult) testing and mammography are not recommended as screening procedures in the young adult.

57. Answer: 1

Rationale: Reactive cellular changes are most often associated with inflammation, including typical repair. Other causes include atrophy with inflammation (atrophic vaginitis), intrauterine device use, radiation, and diethylstilbestrol exposure in utero. OCs do not cause reactive changes, and estrogen vaginal cream may be used to improve atrophy.

58. Answer: 2

Rationale: Cervical cancer has been directly linked with high-risk types of human papillomavirus. Pregnancy after age 35, low parity, and prolonged contraceptive use are not risk factors for cervical cancer.

59. Answer: 3

Rationale: These symptoms are classic for menopausal syndrome, although some depressive symptoms are listed. Antidepressant therapy and counseling for depression at this stage of treatment is not appropriate. Testing, teaching, and treatment in this case should be aimed at the menopause. The depressive symptoms will undoubtedly improve with greater understanding and treatment of the menopausal symptoms.

60. Answer: 1

Rationale: Chancroid is well established as a cofactor for HIV transmission. Chancroid is a sexually transmitted infection of the genitals that is caused by the bacteria *Haemophilus ducreyi*. It is characterized by an open sore or ulcer and can be transmitted from skin-to-skin contact with an infected person. It should be noted that it is rarely seen in the United States but occurs more in third-world countries.

61. Answer: 1

Rationale: According to the American Cancer Society, women should be advised of the benefits and limitations of monthly BSE and should be aware of how their breasts normally look and feel and to report any new breast changes.

62. Answer: 2

Rationale: Symptoms are most likely indicative of benign fibroadenoma. Mammography is indicated. Surgical excision is unlikely for a young woman.

63. Answer: 2

Rationale: This patient needs to become more knowledgeable about the normal feel of implants and her own breast tissue. Mammography is not a substitute for BSE.

64. Answer: 2

Rationale: A very firm cervix along with a cervical lesion/ulcer is suspicious for cancer of the cervix, which can be confirmed with a Papanicolaou smear.

65. Answer: 1

Rationale: This complaint is an indication for clinical breast exam and mammography. Although uncommon, breast pain can be a presenting symptom for breast cancer. Teaching BSE is important, but not the most important action at this point. Hormonal fluctuations can explain breast pain, as can excessive caffeine intake, but should be a diagnosis of exclusion after ruling out malignancy.

66. Answer: 2

Rationale: Toxic shock syndrome occurs primarily in menstruating women ages 12–24 who use tampons. The diagnosis is made with the presence of fever over 102°F (38.9°C), macular rash, hypotension, and involvement of three or more organ systems.

67. Answer: 4

Rationale: Ectopic pregnancies, if not diagnosed and treated promptly, can lead to increased morbidity and mortality accounting for up to 4% of all pregnancy-related deaths. This is especially evident if the death occurred during the first trimester.

68. Answer: 4

Rationale: Almost half of all vaginal infections are caused by candidiasis. The majority of women who develop the infection have recently taken antibiotics. It is not a sexually transmitted infection.

69. Answer: 1

Rationale: It is important to evaluate the patient for threatened abortion as soon as possible. It is most likely too soon for the CBC to reflect blood loss. A pelvic sonogram takes longer than a urine pregnancy test, and the patient must be immediately referred for a dilatation and curettage if her pregnancy test is positive.

70. Answer: 2

Rationale: The most common site for breast cancer occurrence is the upper outer quadrant (Tail of Spence), followed by the area beneath the nipple.

71. Answer: 3

Rationale: Pap smears are crucial for the detection of cervical cancer but do not diagnose uterine cancer. In the early stages, uterine cancer can be asymptomatic and would not be detectable even on bimanual exam.

72. Answer: 4

Rationale: Vulvovaginal changes, such as atrophic vaginitis, often become apparent and bothersome several years after the last menstrual period in women not receiving estrogen therapy. Insufficient data are available to demonstrate that isoflavones have a positive effect on vaginal symptoms. Vaginal lubricants are therapeutic in relieving symptoms of vaginal dryness. If nonprescription remedies do not provide relief and no contraindications exist, estrogen (often topical) is the treatment of choice.

73. Answer: 1

Rationale: The USPSTF recommends that clinicians offer to prescribe risk-reducing medications, such as tamoxifen, raloxifene, or aromatase inhibitors, to women who are at increased risk for breast cancer and at low risk for adverse medication effects. This recommendation applies to asymptomatic women 35 years and older, including women with previous benign breast lesions on biopsy (such as atypical ductal or lobular hyperplasia and lobular carcinoma in situ). The USPSTF recommends against the routine use of risk-reducing medications, such as tamoxifen, raloxifene, or aromatase inhibitors, in women who are not at increased risk for breast cancer.

Pharmacology

74. Answer: 1, 5

Rationale: Recommended treatment for *T. vaginalis* is metronidazole (Flagyl), which can be delivered as a single dose (2 g) or as 500 g dose, twice a day for 7 days. During the course of therapy, both alcohol and sexual activity avoidance are recommended. As the patient relates drinking and sexual activity, this is indicative of noncompliance with treatment therapy. Using cotton underwear and avoiding douching are part of the treatment plan.

75. Answer: 2

Rationale: The WHI study was stopped early because after 5.2 years, in the opinion of the Safety/Data Monitoring Board, the health risks for the women on the study (mean age 63) taking estrogen plus progestin exceeded the benefits. Women taking estrogen/progestin were at higher risk for developing myocardial infarctions, strokes, and thromboemboli and developing breast cancer than women taking placebo. However, women taking HRT were less likely to have a fracture caused by osteoporosis and less likely to develop colorectal cancer. The study did not address the shorter term use of HRT for treatment of menopausal symptoms, the primary indication for initiating the therapy. This landmark study stresses the need for providers to discuss the risks/benefits of initiating or continuing HRT with postmenopausal women.

76. Answer: 3

Rationale: Fluconazole is now approved for a single-dose oral treatment of uncomplicated vulvovaginal candidiasis. It is the most convenient approach for this patient, who is unlikely to be compliant with vaginal creams, given the upcoming travel. She does not have contraindications to its use. Metronidazole and clindamycin are for bacterial vaginosis, not *Candida* infections. Hydrocortisone is a topical steroid used for inflammatory dermatologic conditions, and although it may help the itching, it would not treat the candidiasis.

77. Answer: 4

Rationale: Metronidazole vaginal gel is the treatment of choice for bacterial vaginosis in the nonpregnant female. The presence of clue cells, and the associated malodorous discharge and absence of lactobacilli, are markers for the diagnosis of bacterial vaginosis.

78. Answer: 4

Rationale: Although some authors may recommend herbal treatments for menopausal symptoms, more controlled studies need to be done to provide recommendations that it is effective toward disease prevention. Traditional allopathic Western medicine supports the use of HRT for the prevention of osteoporosis. Weight-bearing exercise and increased calcium intake have been shown to help maintain bone health. Cigarette smoking increases the risk for bone loss. This patient can reduce her risk by quitting smoking.

89. Answer: 4

Rationale: Benzathine penicillin 2.4 million units IM is the treatment of choice for syphilis, but this patient has condyloma acuminatum, not condyloma latum. Topical use of podophyllin, trichloroacetic acid, and cryotherapy are all accepted treatment modalities for condyloma acuminatum.

80. Answer: 1

Rationale: *Chlamydia* often presents this way (dysuria, mucopurulent discharge, and cervical friability). The treatment of choice in ambulatory care settings is single-dose azithromycin 1 g PO. Another treatment dose regimen would be 250 mg IM of ceftriaxone for a chlamydial infection, not 125 mg, plus doxycycline 100 mg PO for 14 days with or without metronidazole 500 mg PO bid for 14 days. Herpes simplex virus will present with painful vesicles in the vulvovaginal region and is treated with acyclovir 200 mg 1 cap PO q4h × 5 days for recurrences. Trichomoniasis can present this way, but trichomonads on the wet mount are absent. Therapy for trichomoniasis is single-dose metronidazole 2 g PO.

81. Answer: 4

Rationale: A hepatic effect caused by the first-pass metabolism in the liver occurs with oral estrogen products. A 25% increase in triglycerides has been associated with this route of administration. Because transdermal estrogen is not dependent on gastrointestinal absorption or affected by the first-pass metabolic effect, this option should be considered. A discussion regarding risks/benefits of continuing HRT is appropriate from the primary provider. Because the patient is only 52 years old and is still experiencing menopausal symptoms, reducing the most common dosage or stopping the medication, unless significant risks are apparent, is probably not the most therapeutic option.

82. Answer: 3

Rationale: The IUD would be a good choice for this patient because it is extremely effective (greater than 99%). Maintenance is minimal, and no injections are involved for insertion or removal. The Depo-Provera injections, although extremely effective as well (greater than 99%), require an injection every 3 months, which could lead to decreased patient compliance. The system of implants is also very effective (greater than 99%) but also requires injections for insertion and removal, which this patient is trying to avoid. The diaphragm is a noninvasive contraceptive that is effective (88%) but requires her to be more active in its use. None of these methods is contraindicated for this patient, but an attempt should be made to help her choose one with which she is likely to be comfortable.

83. Answer: 1

Rationale: The family nurse practitioner should try to determine what the patient has heard and dispel the fallacies if possible. Recent research supports the protective benefit of OCs against ovarian cancer and endometrial cancer. Amount of menstrual bleeding usually is decreased and the cycle regulated. Minimal weight fluctuations are reported. Infertility is not associated with OC use. To suggest either implantation system or Depo-Provera injections to someone who voices concerns about irregular menses or weight gain is sure to lead to an unhappy patient because these are common side effects of both methods. Pap smears do not screen for ovarian cancer.

84. Answer: 2

Rationale: Changing to a pill with a stronger progestational agent or changing to a different progestational agent often will resolve the problem of bleeding irregularities with OCs. Many choices are available regarding the dose or strength of an OC, and her problem likely can be resolved with a different pill. Taking the pills at a different time of day or on an empty stomach will do nothing to resolve the stated problem, which is not breakthrough bleeding, but rather prolonged bleeding, probably secondary to poor endometrial support. If a change is not made in the pills, the patient will continue to bleed and may eventually develop anemia.

85. Answer: 3

Rationale: An OC such as Demulen 1/35 is a good choice for women with more androgenic characteristics because of its strong estrogenic effect with moderate progestational effect. Loestrin 1/20 is a poor choice; the weaker dose of estrogen and progestin may not adequately support her endometrium and will not have a positive effect on this patient's androgenic characteristics. Triphasil is a triphasic pill and does have a positive progestational effect that should support the endometrium, but the progestin in this OC tends to be slightly more androgenic, which is undesirable in this patient.

86. Answer: 4

Rationale: Combination OCs are not recommended for breast-feeding mothers because of the potential effect on decreasing milk quantity and quality. Progestin-only OCs are approved for nursing mothers because no deleterious effect on milk quantity or quality have been shown. Depo-Provera and the IUD are also accepted contraceptive methods for lactating females.

87. Answer: 2

Rationale: Oral contraceptives are contraindicated in a cigarette smoker age 35 years or older. No contraindication exists to the use of Depo-Provera injection in the cigarette smoker. The Progestasert IUD would probably be a good IUD choice

for this patient because it is approved for only 1 year's use and is safe in a cigarette smoker. The only contraindication to condoms and spermicide is allergy to either substance.

88. Answer: 4

Rationale: It is not necessary to hospitalize the patient with acute PID who is not vomiting or pregnant. If she does not respond well to outpatient treatment, hospitalization may be recommended. The medications listed are the accepted treatment of choice for outpatient management of PID and should be started before laboratory results are available, based on the patient's clinical presentation. The CBC and ESR are helpful to track the white blood cell count and inflammatory response of the body.

89. Answer: 2

Rationale: Unopposed estrogen in a woman with an intact uterus increases her risk of endometrial hyperplasia and progression to endometrial cancer. Women who have taken unopposed estrogen for more than 3 years have a fivefold increased risk of endometrial cancer compared with women not on this regimen. The addition of progesterone to the regimen provides uterine protection. However, the progestin component of HRT is responsible for the breakthrough bleeding, a chief complaint at the initiation of therapy that may lead to discontinuance of the drug. Some women also are intolerant of progestins, which have been linked to irritability.

90. Answer: 3

Rationale: The use of unopposed estrogen in the patient with an intact uterus could put her at risk for endometrial hyperplasia or cancer. The addition of a progestin protects the endometrium adequately. The patient is an excellent candidate for endometrial biopsy to document the status of the endometrium. This patient also needs to be educated on the risks and benefits of HRT.

91. Answer: 3

Rationale: Lowering the dose of the estrogen would not help this patient's symptoms. The other dosage regimens listed are all acceptable choices for this patient, proving that there are many effective ways to use HRT, allowing for individualization of the regimen to the patient.

92. Answer: 1

Rationale: Metronidazole 2 g PO in a single dose is the treatment of choice for trichomoniasis. Metronidazole vaginal cream does not effectively treat vaginal trichomoniasis. Fluconazole and terconazole are treatments for vaginal candidiasis.

93. Answer: 1

Rationale: A dose of 0.3 mg of conjugated equine estrogen (Premarin) is the minimal effective dose to prevent osteoporosis. Hormone replacement therapy (HRT) helps maintain bones, but this effect lasts only as long as HRT is taken. Because of the risks for cardiovascular disease from using HRT, it is no longer recommended for osteoporosis prevention. Other methods of osteoporosis prevention include regular exercise, smoking cessation, and sufficient calcium (1200–1500 mg of elemental calcium) and vitamin D (400–800 IU) daily.

94. Answer: 1

Rationale: The diaphragm predisposes many women to UTIs. Some women are sensitive to the contraceptive cream or jelly. The diaphragm has been associated with toxic shock syndrome, so its use should be avoided during menses, and it should not be left in place longer than 24 hours.

95. Answer: 3

Rationale: The primary mechanism of action of OCs is suppression of ovulation. Ovulation is suppressed in 95%–98% of patients. Should ovulation occur, the other mechanisms of action likely to prevent conception are thickening of cervical mucus, causing the endometrium to become atrophic and making the uterine environment unfavorable for implantation.

96. Answer: 3

Rationale: Although still unproven conclusively, mechanisms of action for IUDs include prevention of blastocyst implantation by inducing low-grade endometritis, the copper's effects on enzymes, progesterone's actions on the endometrium, and inhibition of sperm/ovum migration.

97. Answer: 3

Rationale: A progesterone-releasing IUD acts to decrease blood loss and cramping. Progesterone-releasing IUDs thicken the cervical mucus, thicken the endometrium, and inhibit ovulation. Copper-containing IUDs can increase bleeding and dysmenorrhea. There are two hormonal IUDs available; one works for 3 years and the other for 5 years. The copper IUD can stay in place for up to 10 years.

98. Answer: 2

Rationale: The patient no longer requires Provera to protect the endometrium from the potential effects of estrogen; therefore the progestin can be discontinued, and the patient given continuous estrogen therapy without concern. The other dosage regimens listed are appropriate for an HRT patient with an intact uterus.

99. Answer: 3

Rationale: The progestin-only pill does not consistently suppress ovulation. This suppression occurs in only 40%–60% of cycles, which makes the progestin-only pill less effective than combination OCs. Mechanisms of action that contribute to the progestin-only pill's effectiveness include creating an atrophic endometrium and possibly altering tubal physiology by decreasing ovum transport. Progestin-only pills contain no estrogen and are a good choice for the breast-feeding woman. There is an increased incidence of functional ovarian cyst.

100. Answer: 1

Rationale: Informed consent is essential. The pros and cons of HRT should be explained, but the choice is up to the patient.

101. Answer: 3

Rationale: Depo-Provera is frequently associated with menstrual cycle changes. In fact, this irregular bleeding is the most frequently cited reason for discontinuation. These menstrual changes range from heavy, irregular bleeding to spotting and even amenorrhea. Nausea and acne are usually effects of estrogen and are not seen with Depo-Provera.

102. Answer: 4

Rationale: Patients taking alendronate are instructed to take the medication on awakening, 30 minutes before eating, and with a full glass of water. Patients should be instructed to remain upright to prevent esophageal irritation. Taking medication with food (reduces bioavailability by 40%), coffee, orange juice (decreases bioavailability by 60%), or after eating significantly reduces absorption.

103. Answer: 1

Rationale: Women with a uterus taking unopposed exogenous estrogen have an increased risk of endometrial cancer. The addition of progesterone decreases this risk. The addition of progesterone may prompt bleeding, which many women view unfavorably. Progesterone does not affect cervical cancer, breast cancer, or gallbladder disease.

104. Answer: 3

Rationale: Metronidazole in a single 2-g dose is the treatment of choice for trichomoniasis. An alternative is giving the 2 g in divided doses the same day to reduce nausea and improve compliance.

105. Answer: 3

Rationale: This patient requires added protection through this cycle because of the low-dose OC. Phenytoin may also decrease the effectiveness of OCs, especially low-dose forms.

106. Answer: 1

Rationale: Because of the patient's homeless status, the family nurse practitioner needs to use a single-dose treatment. Erythromycin, although a correct medication, is a poor dosing choice for this patient.

107. Answer: 1

Rationale: The most accurate answer is venlafaxine. This combination serotonin and norepinephrine reuptake inhibitor has been found to reduce hot flashes at doses of 25–150 mg/day in several clinical trials. Although many individuals consider the "natural" over-the-counter products to be safer than prescription drugs, these products can have pharmacologic effects and side effects. Use of these drugs by patients should be questioned at the time of the exam. Critics argue that the trials studying black cohosh (*C. racemosa*) have been too small, uncontrolled, and not randomized to provide evidence-based information on the herb's efficacy and safety. Soy has been found to be moderately effective in reducing hot flashes, but comparable results have been seen in the placebo groups as well. A side effect of raloxifene, used to prevent postmenopausal osteoporosis, is hot flashes.

108. Answer: 1

Rationale: Patients who have low fracture risk after being treated with alendronate (Fosamax) for at least 5 years qualify for a drug holiday because the effects of the medication are still present. There is no need to switch the route of medication. Vitamin D supplementation should be within 800–1000 IU per day. Calcium supplementation greater than 1200 mg per day maybe associated with increased risk of complications ranging from kidney stones to cardiac events.

109. Answer: 3, 4

Rationale: The most common cause of pelvic inflammatory disease in sexually active women is gonococcal infections. These infections are often accompanied by *Chlamydia,* and usually both are treated.

110. Answer: 3

Rationale: HRT may be considered for short-term use (3–4 years) to alleviate menopausal symptoms and the risk of osteoporosis in high-risk patients. The ovarian cancer risk may increase for women using estrogen alone for 10 years or longer. Current data are insufficient to know if combination HRT has the same risk. HRT reduces colorectal cancer risk.

17

Maternity

Physiology of Pregnancy

1. What are the normal cardiovascular physiologic responses to pregnancy?
   1. Increased heart rate, increased cardiac output, decreased blood volume, and systolic murmur.
   2. Increased heart rate, decreased cardiac output, increased blood volume, and systolic murmur.
   3. Increased heart rate, increased cardiac output, increased blood volume, and systolic murmur.
   4. Decreased heart rate, increased cardiac output, increased blood volume, and diastolic murmur.

2. How does progesterone affect the gastrointestinal (GI) system during pregnancy?
   1. Causes nausea and vomiting early in pregnancy.
   2. Causes hypertrophy and bleeding of gums.
   3. Delays gastric emptying time and decreases intestinal peristalsis.
   4. Causes diarrhea caused by increased intestinal peristalsis.

3. A pregnant patient has a hemoglobin value of 11.7 g/dL. What is the most likely explanation for this finding?
   1. Presence of iron-deficiency anemia.
   2. Nausea and vomiting.
   3. Physiologic anemia of pregnancy.
   4. Anemia of chronic disease.

4. Several physiologic changes in pregnancy may mimic heart disease. Which of the following is an abnormal finding in pregnancy?
   1. Third heart sound.
   2. Leg edema.
   3. Systolic murmur.
   4. Diastolic murmur.

5. What are three common urinary system findings that the nurse should expect to find in the pregnant patient?
   1. Physiologic hydronephrosis.
   2. Increased glomerular filtration rate.
   3. Increased urinary frequency.
   4. Proteinuria.
   5. Decreased renal plasma blood flow.

6. Which laboratory finding remains unchanged during pregnancy?
   1. White blood cell (WBC) count.
   2. Red blood cell (RBC) volume.
   3. Fibrinogen level.
   4. Prothrombin level.

7. During pregnancy, what is estrogen is responsible for?
   1. Hyperpigmentation.
   2. Facilitating implantation.
   3. Reducing smooth muscle tone.
   4. Decreased uterine contractility.

8. Which is **not** a placental hormone?
   1. Human chorionic gonadotropin (hCG).
   2. Estrogen.
   3. Relaxin.
   4. Cortisol.

9. What is the function of the placental hormone relaxin?
   1. Causes changes in endometrium and relaxes smooth muscle.
   2. Stimulates development of the ductal system of the breasts and causes hypertrophy and hyperplasia of the uterus.
   3. Aids in softening smooth muscle and connective tissue.
   4. Involved with metabolizing certain nutrients and aids in the growth of breasts and other maternal tissues.

10. The family nurse practitioner understands that at 12 weeks of fetal development, which finding is seen?
    1. Quickening is felt.
    2. Fetal heart tones should be heard with Doppler ultrasound.
    3. Fetal heart tones are heard with the stethoscope.
    4. Respiratory movements occur.

11. What is a positive sign of pregnancy?
    1. Softening of the cervix.
    2. Fetal heartbeat.
    3. Enlargement of uterus and abdomen.
    4. Mother's perception of fetal movement.

12. What is the bluish discoloration of the cervix and vagina called?
    1. Goodell's sign.
    2. Chadwick's sign.
    3. Hegar's sign.
    4. Braxton Hicks sign.

13. What is MacDonald's method of abdominal measurement in the pregnant woman?
    1. With the woman on her back and knees slightly flexed, top of fundus is palpated, and measuring tape is stretched from top of symphysis pubis over the abdomen to top of fundus.
    2. Midline of abdomen is determined, and measuring tape is placed around abdomen and measured at the point where fundus is determined to be at midline.
    3. Distance from xiphoid process to symphysis pubis is measured, and dimensions of abdominal curve or fundus is calculated.
    4. With the woman on her back and knees flexed, bony pelvis is determined, ischial tuberosities are identified, and distance from tuberosities to top of fundus is measured.

14. During the regular prenatal visits, what assessment data other than vital signs and weight are determined with each visit?
    1. Fundal height, fetal heart rate, urine dip for protein and glucose, and presence of edema.
    2. Urinalysis, glucose screen, fundal height, and fetal heart rate.
    3. Presence of/changes in Chadwick's sign, complete blood count, and blood glucose screening.
    4. Pelvic measurements, fundal height, urinalysis, and complete blood count.

Perinatal Care & Newborn

15. A patient is pregnant for the fifth time and is in her 7th month. She had two spontaneous abortions in the first trimester. She has a son and daughter, both full-term pregnancies. How should the family nurse practitioner designate the patient's gravida and para status using the TPAL acronym?
    1. Gravida 2, para 5, T1, P1, A2, L4.
    2. Gravida 5, para 2, T2, P0, A2, L2.
    3. Gravida 2, para 4, T0, P2, A0, L2.
    4. Gravida 5, para 2, T0, P2, A2, L2.

16. A patient comes in for her first prenatal visit. Her last menstrual period was on June 15, 2020. Using Nagele's rule, the family nurse practitioner computes the estimated date of delivery as:
    1. March 22, 2021.
    2. April 20, 2021.
    3. February 15, 2021.
    4. April 3, 2021.

17. Dietary changes to reduce nausea and vomiting in pregnancy include:
    1. Consuming small, frequent, low-fat meals and avoiding spicy foods.
    2. Avoiding carbonated beverages.
    3. Avoiding eating when awakening in the morning.
    4. Increasing iron and prenatal vitamins to twice daily.

18. The pregnant woman requires an average of how many extra calories per day?
    1. 100.
    2. 300.
    3. 500.
    4. 800.

19. A pregnant patient at 22 weeks' gestation is planning a prolonged car trip. The family nurse practitioner's recommendations would **not** include:
    1. Support stockings.
    2. Frequent (every 1–2 hours) walking.
    3. Wearing a seat belt.
    4. Knee-high stockings.

20. The recommended office visit interval for a low-risk patient at 28 weeks of pregnancy is every:
    1. 4 weeks.
    2. Week.
    3. 2 weeks.
    4. 6 weeks.

21. At 20 weeks' gestation, where would the family nurse practitioner expect to palpate the fundus?
    1. The symphysis pubis.
    2. The umbilicus.
    3. Halfway between symphysis pubis and umbilicus.
    4. The xiphoid.

22. At an initial prenatal visit occurring in the first trimester, which blood test is **not** recommended?
    1. Antibody screen.
    2. Rubella.
    3. Maternal serum alpha-fetoprotein (MSAFP).
    4. Hepatitis B surface antigen.

23. What is the most common indication for genetic counseling?
    1. Maternal age.
    2. Drug exposure during the first trimester.
    3. Increased maternal alpha-fetoprotein.
    4. History of previous stillbirth.

24. What patients are at highest risk for having a child with Tay-Sachs disease?
    1. Black.
    2. Jewish.
    3. Asian.
    4. 35 years or older at conception.

25. The family nurse practitioner teaches a prenatal patient that a significant source of toxoplasmosis is:
    1. Rare hamburger.
    2. Fresh fruits.
    3. Raw oysters.
    4. Raw vegetables.

26. Which finding would the family nurse practitioner assess in a patient with a ruptured tubal pregnancy?
    1. Sharp, stabbing pain localized to left lower quadrant with a blood pressure (BP) of 90/58 mm Hg.
    2. Boardlike rigidity of the uterus with abdominal distention.
    3. Dilatation of the cervix and rapidly falling BP and pulse.
    4. Serosanguineous vaginal fluid with grapelike vesicles.

27. A pregnant patient at 20 weeks' gestation comes into the clinic with complaints of vaginal bleeding for the last 6 hours and abdominal cramping before the bleeding started. Vaginal exam reveals a decrease in the uterine size, loss of pregnancy symptoms, and a closed, firm cervix. What is the most likely diagnosis for this patient?
    1. Threatened abortion.
    2. Braxton Hicks contractions.
    3. Placenta previa.
    4. Missed abortion.

28. The family nurse practitioner schedules a 38-year-old primigravida for an amniocentesis at 16 weeks' gestation. The family nurse practitioner would explain that the purpose of this procedure is to:
    1. Assess for the possibility of twins.
    2. Determine the bilirubin level.
    3. Perform genetic studies.
    4. Assess lecithin/sphingomyelin (L/S) ratio.

29. Management of a patient after an amniocentesis includes assessing for:
    1. Increased fetal activity.
    2. Elevated temperature.
    3. Spontaneous rupture of the membranes.
    4. Abnormal lung sounds.

30. What would be appropriate management for a primigravida at term who experiences rupture of the membranes?
    1. Begin timing contractions.
    2. Begin pushing.
    3. Take a warm bath.
    4. Immediately go to the emergency department (ED).

31. The family nurse practitioner would note which finding as a possible sign of preeclampsia?
    1. Urgency to urinate at night.
    2. Edema in extremities and puffy face.
    3. Stomach cramps.
    4. Clear fluid discharge from nipple.

32. The family nurse practitioner is discussing the monitoring of the growth of twins during the pregnancy with a patient in the first trimester. Which test should the family nurse practitioner explain to the patient at this time?
    1. Nonstress test (NST).
    2. Sonogram.
    3. Lecithin/sphingomyelin (L/S) ratio.
    4. Amniocentesis.

33. A woman who has missed her period for 5 weeks states that she has been having nausea with some vomiting in the morning hours. The woman also states that she may have a urinary tract infection because of frequency and fatigue. What would the family nurse practitioner recognize these symptoms to be?
    1. A possible systemic infection.
    2. Positive signs of pregnancy.
    3. Presumptive signs of pregnancy.
    4. Probable signs of pregnancy.

34. The family nurse practitioner managing a pregnant patient with sickle cell trait would include which information in the plan?
    1. Complete blood count each trimester.
    2. Weekly nonstress test.
    3. Urine cultures each trimester.
    4. Frequent ultrasounds for growth.

35. Screening based on American Diabetic Association (ADA) guidelines for gestational diabetes mellitus (GDM) during pregnancy includes:
    1. 1-hour postprandial 100-g glucose screen for all women at 24–28 weeks' gestation.
    2. 3-hour, 150-g glucose tolerance test at initial visit for all women with GDM history.
    3. 1-hour postprandial 50-g glucose screen at initial visit for women at risk.
    4. Glycosylated hemoglobin A1c for all women at 24–28 weeks' gestation.

36. A 23-year-old (G3, P0) has a 75-g glucose load with a 1-hour postprandial glucose screen result of 210 mg/dL. What is the next appropriate step for the family nurse practitioner to take?
    1. Order 3-hour 100-g glucose tolerance test (GTT).
    2. Order fasting blood sugar (FBS).
    3. Order A1c.
    4. Refer immediately for diabetic treatment.

37. A teenager returns to the clinic for contraceptive follow-up after being on a low-dose oral contraceptive (OC) for 3 months. She complains of amenorrhea for 2 months, urinary frequency, and leukorrhea. Vaginal exam reveals the uterus to be about 6 cm and the presence of Chadwick's sign. The first diagnostic test indicated should be:
    1. Pregnancy test.
    2. Complete blood count.
    3. Microscopic urinalysis.
    4. Culture for gonorrhea and *Chlamydia.*

38. An adult patient presents with her spouse for a prenatal visit. During the exam, the family nurse practitioner notices bruises on her abdomen and back. The spouse does most of talking during the history. What is the best approach for the family nurse practitioner to take in this situation?
    1. Ask the spouse to leave the room so the nurse can do a pelvic exam.
    2. Ask the woman to accompany the nurse to the laboratory for blood work and ask about bruises.
    3. Ask the woman about the bruises during the exam.
    4. Do nothing; domestic violence is beyond the scope of the nurse's practice.

39. A pregnant employee who works at a day care center is concerned about a recent outbreak of "fifth disease." The family nurse practitioner understands that:
    1. Most parvovirus B19 infections in utero are associated with an increased number of congenital anomalies.
    2. There are no isoimmunization-associated problems for the mother exposed to a young child with fifth disease.
    3. Parvovirus B19 has caused hydrops fetalis and death in some fetuses infected in utero.
    4. Mortality risk for a fetus is extremely high, especially if the mother has never had fifth disease.

40. Which is an abnormal complaint in the second trimester of pregnancy?
    1. Frequent uterine contractions.
    2. Frequent fetal movement.
    3. Calf cramps.
    4. Heartburn.

41. Which statement is true about smoking during pregnancy?
    1. The rate of spontaneous abortion among smokers is the same as in nonsmokers.
    2. Risks of complications increase with the number of cigarettes smoked.
    3. Discontinuation of smoking during pregnancy has no effect on pregnancy outcome.
    4. No relationship exists between smoking and sudden infant death syndrome.

42. Chlamydial infections during pregnancy may be associated with:
    1. Transplacental transmission to fetus.
    2. Congenital anomalies of the eyes.
    3. Premature rupture of membranes.
    4. Fetal hydrops.

43. Cocaine use during pregnancy is associated with:
    1. Abruptio placentae.
    2. Postdate pregnancy.
    3. Macrosomatia infant.
    4. Maternal hypotension.

44. During pregnancy, sexual relations are contraindicated:
    1. During the first trimester when patient has a history of spontaneous abortion.
    2. After 36 weeks' gestation.
    3. With the diagnosis of placenta previa.
    4. With excessive maternal weight gain.

45. Which is an abnormal complaint in the first trimester of pregnancy?
    1. Nausea and vomiting.
    2. Fatigue.
    3. Vaginal bleeding.
    4. Low backache.

46. What is a recommended screening test for gestational diabetes mellitus?
    1. 3-hour glucose tolerance test (GTT).
    2. 1-hour postprandial 50-g glucose screen.
    3. 2-hour postprandial blood sugar measurement.
    4. Random blood sugar measurement.

47. Which is an abnormal complaint of the third trimester of pregnancy?
    1. Leukorrhea.
    2. Headache with blurred vision.
    3. Urinary frequency.
    4. Uterine contractions.

48. Which would be incorrect for the treatment of preeclampsia without severe features?
    1. Modified bed rest.
    2. Monitor blood pressure (BP), weight, and urinary protein.
    3. Methyldopa (Aldomet) 250 mg PO tid.
    4. Daily urine dipstick for protein.

49. A pregnant patient requests further information regarding exercise guidelines from the family nurse practitioner. She runs on the treadmill 4 mph for 30 minutes daily, and then does 30 additional minutes of free weight and lower leg exercises at the gym. Which general guideline should not be included?
    1. Keep the heart rate less than 140 beats/min.
    2. Limit free weight for upper body to less than 10 lb each.
    3. Limit exercise time to 30 minutes total.
    4. Avoid breathlessness and excessive heat.

50. Testing for gestational diabetes mellitus (GDM) should be done in which of the following patients?
    1. Patient with previous macrosomatia infant.
    2. Obese patients.
    3. All pregnant patients.
    4. Patient with glycosuria.

51. For a pregnant patient at 32 weeks' gestation with a blood pressure (BP) of 140/92 mm Hg, weight gain the last 2 weeks of 4 lb, trace protein on urine dip, 1+ pitting edema in the feet, and 2+ reflexes, which clinical diagnosis should the family nurse practitioner suspect as being most likely?
    1. Preeclampsia without severe features.
    2. Preeclampsia with severe features.
    3. Eclampsia.
    4. Hemolysis, elevated liver enzymes, low platelets (HELLP) syndrome.

52. The family nurse practitioner is assessing a patient who has a positive pregnancy test. Laboratory data indicate that the mother's blood group is O positive and the father's blood group is AB negative. What risk is associated with this pregnancy?
    1. The mother may build up antibodies to the infant's blood if the infant is type B positive, which will be significant in future pregnancies.
    2. The mother is Rh positive; if the infant is Rh negative, there is an increased incidence of the infant building up Rh antibodies.
    3. Because the mother is O and the father is AB, there is an increased risk for the development of an ABO incompatibility.
    4. Type O blood is the dominant characteristic; the infant's blood will be in the O group, with no complications.

53. A young adult patient, G2 P1 A0 L1, 10 weeks' gestation with intrauterine pregnancy (IUP), is seen for her first obstetric intake history and physical. She knows when she conceived and denies any vaginal bleeding or abdominal pain. The patient has a soft, nontender fundus that measures 14 cm; adnexal exam negative for mass or tenderness; no fetal heart rate (FHR) audible with Doppler. What is the most likely diagnosis seen on ultrasound?
    1. Multiple gestations.
    2. Fibroid uterus.
    3. Ectopic pregnancy.
    4. 14-week viable IUP.

54. A healthy patient is at 36 weeks' gestation. On her regular clinical visit, the fundus is measured at the level of the xiphoid process. At the 40-week gestational visit, the fundus is measured at just below the xiphoid process. What is the **most** likely interpretation of this observation?
    1. Fetus has stopped growing.
    2. Fetal head has descended into pelvic cavity.
    3. Labor will probably begin within 24 hours.
    4. Amount of amniotic fluid is decreased.

55. On her first prenatal visit, a patient's blood work indicates that she is Rh negative. This is her first pregnancy, and she has no history of abortions. What will the family nurse practitioner explain to the patient regarding this information?
    1. To prevent complications of future pregnancies, the patient will receive an injection of $Rh_o(D)$ immune globulin (RhoGAM) at about 28 weeks' gestation and after the birth of an Rh-positive infant.
    2. Her husband needs to be tested to determine whether his blood type is Rh positive and if there is a problem.
    3. The patient needs to receive RhoGAM at about 20 weeks' gestation and after the birth of the first child to prevent hemolytic disease.
    4. There could be a problem with the mother's blood sensitizing the infant's blood to the Rh factor; the mother will receive RhoGAM after the birth of each child.

56. A 28-year-old female patient is seen by the family nurse practitioner for an office visit. Her last menstrual period was 8 weeks ago; she is complaining of left lower quadrant abdominal pain, spotting, and fatigue. Her pelvic exam reveals cervical os closed, minimal blood in vaginal vault, uterus minimally enlarged, mild cervical motion tenderness, left adnexal fullness and tenderness, and right adnexa within normal limits. Vital signs are stable. The serum pregnancy test is positive. What is the most cost-effective and useful test for the family nurse practitioner to order?
    1. Abdominopelvic computed tomography (CT) scan.
    2. Barium enema.
    3. Pelvic ultrasound.
    4. Flat plate of abdomen.

57. Ten days after delivery, a patient is diagnosed with mastitis. Which of the following should the family nurse practitioner expect to find on physical exam?
    1. Tender, hard, hot, and reddened area on breast.
    2. Dimpled skin on breasts and firm nodules around areola.
    3. Decreased milk production, inverted nipple, and firm, inflamed breast tissue.
    4. Soft, tender palpable masses with cracked, bleeding nipples.

58. In discussing the timing of contractions with a patient, the family nurse practitioner explains "frequency" as the interval from the:
    1. Beginning of one contraction to the beginning of the next.
    2. Beginning of one contraction to the end of that contraction.
    3. End of one contraction to the start of the next.
    4. End of one contraction to the end of the next.

59. The biophysical profile includes which of the following parameters?
    1. Fetal breathing movements, fetal muscle tone, and amniotic fluid volume.
    2. Ultrasonography, alpha-fetoprotein screening, and fetal heart reactivity.
    3. Amniocentesis, amniotic fluid volume, and nonstress test.
    4. Contraction stress test, nonstress test, and gross fetal movement.

60. What is the most common reason for a nonreactive nonstress test (NST)?
    1. Fetal hypoxia.
    2. Maternal drug use.
    3. Fetal inactivity or sleep.
    4. Congenital heart defect.

61. Which is least likely to be found in a patient presenting with an ectopic pregnancy?
    1. Pain.
    2. Missed menses.
    3. Vaginal bleeding.
    4. Abdominal mass.

62. A patient presents to the clinic with a diagnosis of threatened abortion. The family nurse practitioner describes this as:
    1. Vaginal bleeding with or without cramping and no cervical change.
    2. Vaginal bleeding with cramping and cervical change.
    3. Loss of pregnancy symptoms, decrease in uterine size, and cervix closed and firm.
    4. Cramping, bleeding, and incomplete expulsion of products of conception.

63. What is a predisposing factor in preterm labor?
    1. Obesity.
    2. Previous spontaneous abortions.
    3. Prior preterm delivery.
    4. Caucasian race.

64. The ability of amniotic fluid to produce a ferning pattern when dried may be altered by:
    1. Meconium.
    2. Changes in vaginal pH.
    3. Presence of cervical mucus.
    4. Heavy contamination with blood.

65. Ten weeks into her pregnancy, a patient begins to experience light vaginal bleeding. Her human chorionic gonadotropin levels remain elevated. The family nurse practitioner would instruct the patient to report which of the following symptoms?
    1. Nausea and vomiting.
    2. Abdominal pain or severe cramping.
    3. Urinary frequency.
    4. Fatigue.

66. Which statement is true regarding the course of pruritic urticarial papules and plaques of pregnancy (PUPPP)?
    1. Perinatal mortality is increased.
    2. Pruritus is increased postpartum.
    3. Lesions first appear on abdomen.
    4. Onset is usually in the first trimester.

67. Why does an infant have increased loss of scalp hair 2–4 months after delivery?
    1. Increased number of hairs in telogen.
    2. Hyperthyroidism.
    3. Fatigue.
    4. Sudden postpartum cardiovascular changes.

68. In a breast-feeding patient having difficulty with milk production, the family nurse practitioner understands that milk production will be increased by:
    1. More frequent suckling of infant.
    2. Longer duration of suckling.
    3. Cessation of suckling for 24 hours.
    4. Cold compresses to the breast.

69. A new first-time mother is being evaluated for a complaint of breast pain. Her infant is 3 weeks old, and she is breast-feeding. The infant is gaining weight and seems satisfied after feeding. On exam, the family nurse practitioner finds red, irritated nipples on both breasts, but no masses and tenderness to the breasts themselves. What is the most important part of the family nurse practitioner's evaluation?
    1. Mammogram of the breast.
    2. Exam of the infant's mouth.
    3. STAT complete blood count.
    4. Analysis of the milk.

70. A patient delivers a healthy newborn with a cleft lip and cleft palate. Which action by the family nurse practitioner would promote maternal–infant bonding?
    1. Point out the newborn's normal characteristics.
    2. Explain to the mother how the problem is not significant.
    3. Have the mother begin taking care of the newborn immediately after delivery.
    4. Explain to the mother that orofacial surgery will completely correct the defect.

71. When do most nonnursing mothers resume menstruation after childbirth?
    1. 30 days.
    2. 7–9 weeks.
    3. 45 days.
    4. 2–4 weeks.

72. A 57-year-old female complains of fecal leakage intermittently and one episode of incontinence over the last 2 months. The family nurse practitioner elicits the following history: 3 vaginal childbirths, 8-lb babies, 1 forceps delivery, 1985–1990. Why was this history important?
    1. It is a routine aspect of past medical history that is elicited at each female patient visit.
    2. It may provide a clue to possible etiology of fecal leakage and incontinence.
    3. It indicates that the patient now has adult children and may be dealing with stress of the "empty nest."
    4. Vaginal deliveries with large babies can cause a rectocele which would contribute to her incontinence.

73. The family nurse practitioner is assessing a postpartum patient about 12 hours after delivery. On assessment of the uterus, at what position would the family nurse practitioner expect to palpate it?
    1. At the level of the umbilicus.
    2. Two fingerbreadths below the umbilicus.
    3. About 2 cm above the umbilicus.
    4. Three fingerbreadths above the symphysis pubis.

Pharmacology

74. Which immunization is contraindicated in pregnancy?
    1. Polio vaccine.
    2. Hepatitis B vaccine.
    3. Measles mumps rubella (MMR).
    4. Tetanus.

75. If studies in animals or pregnant women demonstrate evidence of fetal abnormality or risk, or if the potential for fetal risk clearly outweighs the possible benefit of a drug, the U.S. Food and Drug Administration (FDA) category for this drug is:
    1. B.
    2. C.
    3. D.
    4. X.

76. The family nurse practitioner is aware that fetal exposure to tetracycline (Tetracap) causes:
    1. Blindness.
    2. Hearing loss.
    3. Tooth discoloration.
    4. Limb deformities.

77. Which of the following may reduce the risk of neural tube defects when taken before conception?
    1. Vitamin A.
    2. Pyridoxine.
    3. Folic acid.
    4. Vitamin C.

78. The current recommendation for antepartum treatment of Rh-negative pregnant women with $Rh_o(D)$ immune globulin (RhoGAM) includes:
    1. Administration of 300 mcg at 28 and 36 weeks' gestation.
    2. Administration of 300 mcg at 28 weeks' gestation.
    3. Administration of 300 mcg in each trimester.
    4. No administration is needed until postpartum.

79. The patient comes in for her first prenatal visit. She is healthy and has no history that would contribute to complications during the pregnancy. She asks the family nurse practitioner what she can take for her occasional headaches caused by eyestrain and allergies. Which of the following would the family nurse practitioner recommend for the patient?
    1. Ibuprofen (Advil) 200 mg q4–6h, not to exceed 600 mg over 24 hours.
    2. Naproxen (Aleve) 220 mg q8–12h.
    3. Aspirin (ASA) 60 mg q6h, not to exceed 300 mg over 24 hours.
    4. Acetaminophen (Tylenol) 650 mg q4–6h, not to exceed 650 mg over 24 hours.

80. Which medication would be considered safe to use in all trimesters of pregnancy?
    1. Metronidazole (Flagyl).
    2. Tetracycline (Achromycin).
    3. Isotretinoin (Accutane).
    4. Angiotensin-converting enzyme (ACE) inhibitors.

81. For the patient who wants to breast-feed and take oral contraceptives (OCs), what is the pill of choice?
    1. 1/35 preparation.
    2. Triphasic preparation.
    3. Progestin-only preparation.
    4. 1/50 preparation.

82. A pregnant patient in the last trimester complains of a constant backache aggravated by walking, moving, and bending. The pain does not radiate to either leg. In addition to rest, massage, and physiotherapy, which of the following medications is appropriate?
    1. Acetaminophen.
    2. Codeine.
    3. Naproxen.
    4. Aspirin.

83. The family nurse practitioner has diagnosed mastitis in a 6-week postpartum patient. The patient has no known drug allergies. Which medication is appropriate for treatment?
    1. Doxycycline (Vibramycin) 100 mg PO bid × 10 days.
    2. Dicloxacillin (Dynapen) 250 mg PO qid × 10 days.
    3. Metronidazole (Flagyl) 500 mg PO bid × 10 days.
    4. Ciprofloxacin (Cipro) 500 mg PO bid × 7 days.

84. The family nurse practitioner is choosing an antidepressant for a prenatal patient who has a history of depression. Which antidepressant would be an acceptable choice to prescribe?
    1. Risperidone (Risperdal).
    2. Alprazolam (Xanax).
    3. Imipramine (Tofranil).
    4. Sertraline (Zoloft).

17 Maternity Answers & Rationales

Physiology of Pregnancy

1. Answer: 3

Rationale: During pregnancy, a hyperdynamic state is caused by an increase in blood volume, which results in a slightly increased heart rate and increased cardiac output. Systolic ejection murmurs are common and caused by increased flow across the pulmonic and aortic valves. Diastolic murmurs are abnormal and require referral.

2. Answer: 3

Rationale: Progesterone affects the GI system by decreasing smooth muscle tone, delaying gastric emptying, and decreasing intestinal peristalsis. Human chorionic gonadotropin is associated with nausea and vomiting early in pregnancy. Estrogen causes the gums to become hyperemic, soft, and swollen with a tendency to bleed.

3. Answer: 3

Rationale: The increase in plasma volume combined with a slower rise in red blood cell production produces a dilutional anemia. Hemoglobin and hematocrit decrease in relation to plasma volume, reaching the lowest levels during the second trimester. True anemia occurs with hemoglobin less than 11 g/dL and hematocrit less than 35%, although some providers will allow the hemoglobin to drop to 10 g/dL and hematocrit to drop to 33% before treating. Nausea and vomiting will increase hemoglobin and hematocrit.

4. Answer: 4

Rationale: Leg edema is caused by increased venous pressure in the legs. Both components of the first heart sound become louder, with exaggerated splitting, and a third heart sound gallop is common after midpregnancy. Systolic ejection murmurs are common and result from the increased flow across the aortic and pulmonic valves. Diastolic murmurs are an abnormal finding and should always be referred.

5. Answer: 1, 2, 3

Rationale: Changes in renal structure are influenced by estrogen, progesterone, increased blood volume, and uterine pressure. Changes in the collection system, such as dilation of the renal pelvis and ureters, cause a physiologic hydronephrosis. The glomerular filtration rate does increase during pregnancy, along with renal plasma flow. Increased urinary frequency is related to increasing size of uterus and its pressure on the bladder. Proteinuria is abnormal when the amount exceeds 300 mg/24 hours or albuminuria is greater than 30 mg/24 hours, except in very concentrated urine or in the first voided specimen on arising. Proteinuria is a warning of impaired kidney function or preeclampsia.

6. Answer: 4

Rationale: RBC volume increases approximately 30%, and WBCs increase 5000–12,000/mm^3. Fibrin, fibrinogen, and plasma levels of factors VII, IX, and X are also increased. Prothrombin levels remain unchanged.

7. Answer: 1

Rationale: During pregnancy, estrogen is responsible for stimulation of melanin-stimulating hormone, resulting in hyperpigmentation. Progesterone from the corpus luteum and later the placenta is responsible for facilitating implantation, decreasing uterine contractility, and reducing smooth muscle tone.

8. Answer: 4

Rationale: There are five placental hormones: hCG, estrogen, progesterone, human placental lactogen, and relaxin. Cortisol is produced in the adrenal glands.

9. Answer: 3

Rationale: Relaxin helps soften smooth muscle and connective tissue in preparation for labor and delivery. Progesterone relaxes smooth muscle and causes changes in the endometrium. Estrogen stimulates the development of the ductal system of the breasts and causes hypertrophy and hyperplasia of the uterus. Human placental lactogen is involved with metabolism of glucose, fatty acids, and amino acids. It also aids in the growth of the breasts and other maternal tissues.

10. Answer: 2

Rationale: Fetal heart rate should be heard by 12 weeks' gestation and may be heard as early as 10 weeks, depending on the maternal adipose tissue and amniotic fluid. Quickening is felt at 16–22 weeks. Fetal heart rate can be heard by stethoscope at 20 weeks. Respiratory movements occur later in fetal development, at about 24 weeks.

11. Answer: 2

Rationale: Positive evidence of pregnancy includes fetal heartbeat, palpation of fetal movement by examiner, and visualization of fetus by ultrasonography. Amenorrhea, nausea, emesis, urinary frequency, fatigue, skin changes, and mother's perception of fetal movement are presumptive evidence of pregnancy. Probable evidence of pregnancy includes softening of cervix, softening of lower uterine segment, cyanosis of cervix and vagina, Braxton Hicks contractions, ballottement, palpation of fetal outline by examiner, and pregnancy tests.

12. Answer: 2

Rationale: Chadwick's sign occurs at 6–8 weeks' gestation and is the bluish discoloration of the cervix and vagina. Goodell's sign is the softening of the cervix that is seen as early as 4 weeks' gestation. Hegar's sign is the softening of the lower uterine segment. Braxton Hicks sign consists of contractions of the uterus that can occur as early as 16 weeks' gestation.

13. Answer: 1

Rationale: MacDonald's measurement is taken at each prenatal visit to estimate uterine size. Fundal height is measured with a measuring tape that is stretched from the top of the fundus to the symphysis pubis. If the fundal height is less or more than expected based on the gestational age, the estimated date of delivery should be reevaluated and confirmed. Further fetal assessment may be necessary.

14. Answer: 1

Rationale: Fundal height, fetal heart rate, urine dip for protein and glucose, and assessment for edema are determined with each prenatal visit. Urinalysis and complete blood count are done as part of initial exam and are repeated as necessary. Chadwick's sign is an early indication of pregnancy, and pelvic measurements are done to determine adequacy of the pelvic outlet for delivery.

Perinatal Care & Newborn

15. Answer: 2

Rationale: Gravida is the number of pregnancies, including the present pregnancy, gravida 5 for this patient. Para is the number of pregnancies that have progressed past 20 weeks, para 2. T is the number of pregnancies that have progressed to term, T2. P is the number of pregnancies with delivery preterm, P0. A is abortions, A2. L is living children, L2.

16. Answer: 1

Rationale: The family nurse practitioner counts back 3 months to March 15 and adds 7 days. This brings the date to March 22 of the next year.

17. Answer: 1

Rationale: Patients should eat frequent small meals to keep some food in the stomach at all times and to avoid stomach distention. Sipping on carbonated beverages may be helpful. Having crackers at the bedside to take before rising in the morning may be a successful preventive measure.

18. Answer: 2

Rationale: The pregnant woman requires about 15% more calories per day than the nonpregnant woman. This is approximately 300 calories per day and depends on the patient's weight and activity level.

19. Answer: 4

Rationale: Venous stasis occurs with prolonged sitting and may be a risk factor for thrombophlebitis. Support stockings and frequent walking should be encouraged. Knee-high stockings have elastic around the calf that may act as a tourniquet. They should be avoided during pregnancy. Seat belts are recommended.

20. Answer: 3

Rationale: The American College of Obstetricians and Gynecologists recommends visits every 2 weeks starting at 28 weeks until 36 weeks of pregnancy. At 36 weeks of pregnancy, visits are weekly until delivery.

21. Answer: 2

Rationale: The expected fundal height at 20 weeks' gestation is at the umbilicus. At 12 weeks' gestation, the fundus can be palpated just above the symphysis pubis, and at 16 weeks' gestation it is palpated between the symphysis and umbilicus. The fundus is palpated at the xiphoid process at approximately 36 weeks' gestation.

22. Answer: 3

Rationale: Routine prenatal laboratory studies include complete blood count, blood type and Rh, antibody screen, hepatitis B surface antigen, syphilis screen, and rubella immune status. The MSAFP is done between 15 and 20 weeks. Before this time the fetus produces little alpha-fetoprotein, and results would be inaccurate.

23. Answer: 1

Rationale: The largest group of women who potentially benefit from genetic counseling are those age 35 and older. The number of births to women between age 35 and 40 years old increased by approximately 35% in the 1990s. The primary cause of congenital abnormalities in women older than age 35 years is chromosomal abnormalities. The other answers are all reasons for genetic counseling but to a much lesser degree.

24. Answer: 2

Rationale: The incidence of the Tay-Sachs gene in the Jewish population is 1 in 30, compared with 1 in 300 for the non-Jewish population.

25. Answer: 1

Rationale: Undercooked red meat is a major source of toxoplasmosis. Pregnant women should be cautioned against eating undercooked meats. Cats are also shown to be hosts. Toxoplasmosis is spread through cat feces. Pregnant women should be warned about cleaning the litter box and about contaminated soil.

26. Answer: 1

Rationale: The ruptured fallopian tube causes a sharp, sudden, stabbing pain. Symptoms of shock (decreased BP, increased pulse, and increased respiration) occur, and the situation quickly becomes a surgical emergency. The cervix does not dilate. Boardlike abdominal rigidity is often noted with abruptio placentae. Grapelike vesicles are associated with hydatidiform mole, a gestational trophoblastic disease.

27. Answer: 4

Rationale: A missed abortion is characterized by a loss of pregnancy symptoms, vaginal bleeding, and a closed cervix. A threatened abortion has vaginal bleeding and cramping, but the symptoms of pregnancy are still present. Placenta previa is bleeding without pain, and symptoms of pregnancy are present. Braxton Hicks contractions can occur as early as the second trimester but are more commonly experienced in the third trimester. The uterine muscles tighten for 30–60 seconds and then relax.

28. Answer: 3

Rationale: The woman's age places her at risk for a Down's syndrome baby. Amniocentesis for L/S ratio is performed in the third trimester for fetal lung maturity, and amniocentesis for bilirubin level (delta optical density) is performed for a pregnancy complicated by isoimmunization.

29. Answer: 3

Rationale: Damage to the membranes is a possibility and a high-priority situation. Fever would not be an immediate problem. Fetal heart rate is monitored, not activity.

30. Answer: 1

Rationale: The patient should begin to count the contractions to determine the progress of beginning labor. Because she is a primigravida, delivery probably is not imminent, so going to the ED is not appropriate. She should not try to "push" this early in labor. Without the protective barrier of the amniotic membrane, the mother and fetus are susceptible to infection. Bathing would be a hazard because of the possibility of contracting an infection from the bath water. The patient should count the contractions and call the physician.

31. Answer: 2

Rationale: Classic signs of preeclampsia are hypertension and proteinuria. Generalized edema of the extremities and around the face occurs because of increased permeability and capillary leakage. Stomach cramps could be an indication of early labor or gastrointestinal upset. Clear nipple fluid would be an early sign of colostrum.

32. Answer: 2

Rationale: The ultrasound (sonogram) test is used to assess growth of the fetus and position of the placenta and fetus. The NST is used to observe the response of the fetal heart rate to activity. The L/S ratio determines whether there is sufficient surfactant. An amniocentesis is performed to obtain amniotic fluid for analysis later in the pregnancy, if indicated.

33. Answer: 3

Rationale: Missed menstrual periods, nausea, vomiting, frequency, and fatigue are presumptive signs (subjective) of pregnancy. Probable signs of pregnancy are objective, such as Chadwick's sign, ballottement, and a positive pregnancy test. Positive signs of pregnancy are fetal heart rate, fetal movement felt by a health care provider, and sonographic evidence.

34. Answer: 3

Rationale: Sickle cell trait occurs in 8% of African Americans. These women are asymptomatic, not anemic, and usually have no problems except under conditions of hypoxia. There is no difference in perinatal outcome, and these women do not require frequent ultrasounds or nonstress testing. They are at increased risk for asymptomatic bacteriuria and require a urine culture each trimester.

35. Answer: 3

Rationale: This is standard screening for women at risk of GDM. The American College of Obstetricians and Gynecologists (ACOG) recommends a two-step screening method that has been used for many years. The first step is a screen consisting of a 50-g oral glucose load, followed by a plasma glucose measurement 1 hour later. An initial positive screening result is followed by step 2, a 3-hour (100-g) oral glucose tolerance test (OGTT) on another day. ACOG recommends use of the two-step screening procedure because there is no evidence that the one-step method leads to clinically significant improvement in maternal or newborn outcomes. This glucose screen should also be done for all other pregnant women between 24 and 28 weeks of gestation.

36. Answer: 4

Rationale: An elevated result, greater than 200 mg/dL, on the glucose challenge is considered diagnostic, alleviating the need for an oral GTT or FBS.

37. Answer: 1

Rationale: This clinical picture is highly indicative of pregnancy, especially the presence of Chadwick's sign.

38. Answer: 2

Rationale: Although asking the spouse to leave the room during a pelvic exam may work, it may also arouse the spouse's suspicion. Asking the woman to accompany the nurse to the laboratory and asking about the bruising is best because it gives a legitimate reason to move the woman quickly from the room, offers privacy to inquire about the bruises, and provides an opportunity to move the woman to a safe place, if needed, without creating confrontation.

39. Answer: 3

Rationale: Most fetuses are not affected; however, some undergo isoimmunization, which leads to hydrops fetalis and death. The mortality risk is actually low, and there are usually no associated congenital anomalies.

40. Answer: 1

Rationale: Contractions could represent early premature labor and should be monitored to rule out early cervical change. Not all contractions are "Braxton Hicks," and contractions require serious consideration. The other symptoms listed are important to discuss and to rule out other associated symptomatology.

41. Answer: 2

Rationale: The risk of complications and perinatal loss increases with the number of cigarettes smoked. Discontinuation of or decrease in the amount of cigarettes smoked during pregnancy can reduce the risk of complications, especially for high-risk women.

42. Answer: 3

Rationale: Premature rupture of membranes may be associated with chlamydial infections. Intrauterine transmission of *Chlamydia trachomatis* to the fetus has not been demonstrated. There is no evidence of fetal eye anomalies; without prophylaxis, however, conjunctivitis will develop in 30%–50% of infants 7 days after birth.

43. Answer: 1

Rationale: Use of cocaine during pregnancy is associated with placental abruption, spontaneous abortion, and preterm labor. Maternal blood pressure and heart rate are increased. The fetus is at risk for intrauterine growth retardation, fetal distress, seizures, and death.

44. Answer: 3

Rationale: In placenta previa, the placenta is improperly positioned in the lower uterine segment, covering all or part of the cervical os. There is an increased risk of bleeding. Management includes bed rest, no intercourse, no vaginal exams, instruction on managing bleeding, and close fetal surveillance.

45. Answer: 3

Rationale: Vaginal bleeding could represent a potential problem in the pregnancy during the first trimester. The other symptoms listed are important as well and warrant further discussion to rule out a problem.

46. Answer: 2

Rationale: The recommended screening test for gestational diabetes is a blood sugar measurement 1 hour after 50 g of glucose at 24–28 weeks' gestation. If the result of this test is 140 or above, a 3-hour GTT is done.

47. Answer: 2

Rationale: Headache associated with blurred vision could represent early symptoms of preeclampsia and warrants further workup to rule out a problem. The other symptoms are not of concern if not associated with other symptoms.

48. Answer: 3

Rationale: The use of medication is no longer thought to be useful in the treatment of preeclampsia without severe features and could be hazardous. The patient is best treated conservatively with modified bed rest on the left side and dietary counseling, along with close monitoring of BP, weight, and urinary protein. Close follow-up with exam for edema or symptomatic change and monitoring of the fetus are also performed.

49. Answer: 3

Rationale: No reason exists to limit the amount of time for exercise, provided the patient is feeling well. Keeping the heart rate below 140 beats/min reduces the risk of internal overheating and exhaustion. The American College of Obstetricians and Gynecologists suggests limiting free weights to less than 10 lb to avoid undue stress and strain on muscles and ligaments. Avoidance of breathlessness and excessive heat allows for better circulation to the fetus.

50. Answer: 3

Rationale: More than one half of pregnant women who exhibit GDM lack the classic risk factors of family history of diabetes, unexpected stillbirth, prior macrosomatia infant, obesity, and advanced maternal age. Glycosuria in pregnancy is not necessarily an indication of diabetes. The best answer is that all women should be screened for gestational diabetes.

51. Answer: 1

Rationale: Preeclampsia without severe features is consistent with systolic BP greater than 140 mm Hg or systolic rise greater than 30 mm Hg, diastolic greater than 90 or diastolic rise greater than 15 mm Hg, weight gain greater than 2 lb/week, and nondependent edema greater than 1+ with normal reflexes. Severe features of preeclampsia include BP greater than 160/110 mm Hg, proteinuria greater than 2 g/24 hours, serum creatinine greater than 1.2 mg/dL, platelets less than 100,000, ↑ lactic dehydrogenase, ↑ alanine aminotransferase, persistent headache or cerebral/visual disturbances, and persistent epigastric pain. Eclampsia includes the above plus seizures. HELLP syndrome includes signs and symptoms of severe preeclampsia, an enlarged and firm liver, and epigastric or right upper quadrant pain.

52. Answer: 3

Rationale: There is an increased incidence of ABO incompatibility if the mother is blood group O and the infant is either blood group A or B. Rh incompatibility occurs only when the mother is Rh negative and is carrying an Rh-positive infant. In the most common cases of ABO incompatibility, there is production of maternal antibodies against the A or B cells.

53. Answer: 1

Rationale: Multiple gestations will cause the uterus to enlarge faster than normal. FHR may be inaudible with the doptone at 10 weeks' gestation. A fibroid could cause the uterus to enlarge, but it is generally accompanied by firmness to palpation of the uterus. Ectopic pregnancy could be the cause of an inaudible FHR, but it is usually accompanied by adnexal tenderness, a mass, or vaginal bleeding. A 14-week viable IUP should have an audible FHR with the Doppler.

54. Answer: 2

Rationale: "Lightening" often occurs at about 40 weeks' gestation when the infant's head descends into the pelvic cavity and becomes "engaged." At any other time during pregnancy, a decrease in fundal height would cause concern for the infant's growth. There has been no decrease in amniotic fluid, and it does not indicate that labor is imminent.

55. Answer: 1

Rationale: The unsensitized Rh-negative pregnant woman is given RhoGAM at 28 weeks' gestation as a preventive measure. It effectively prevents the formation of active antibodies if there is accidental transport of fetal Rh-positive blood cells into the circulation during the remainder of the pregnancy. At delivery, the infant's blood type is determined. If the infant is Rh positive, the mother will receive another dose of RhoGAM within 72 hours of delivery. If the infant is Rh negative, there is no antibody formation and RhoGAM is unnecessary.

56. Answer: 3

Rationale: This easy, inexpensive, and relatively noninvasive test assists the family nurse practitioner with confirming the diagnosis of ectopic pregnancy. It can be obtained quickly and is often available rapidly. Abdominopelvic CT will also show an ectopic pregnancy but is neither cost-effective nor noninvasive. Barium enema and flat plate of the abdomen are not useful in this patient.

57. Answer: 1

Rationale: A tender, hard, hot, and reddened area on the breast over the affected area is typically found with mastitis. The patient with mastitis will also typically be febrile. Dimpled skin (peau d'orange or orange-peel appearance) is a potential sign of breast cancer. Decreased milk production, inverted nipple, and firm breast tissue may be complications of engorgement. Cracked nipples may result from improper positioning or oversuckling. Soft, tender breast masses may be engorged milk ducts.

58. Answer: 1

Rationale: Frequency of contractions should be timed from the beginning of one contraction to the beginning of the next contraction.

59. Answer: 1

Rationale: The biophysical profile includes observation of fetal respiratory movement, fetal tone, gross fetal movement, measurement of amniotic fluid volume, and fetal heart reactivity. Each parameter is given a score of 0 or 2. The scores from all parameters are then added together, and the normal score is 8–10. Ultrasonography, alpha-fetoprotein screening, nonstress testing, and stress test are not part of this profile.

60. Answer: 3

Rationale: The most common reason for a nonreactive NST is fetal sleep or inactivity. The fetal sleep-wake cycle ranges from 20–40 minutes. If reactivity is not demonstrated in 20 minutes, continuing to 40 minutes usually accommodates the sleep-wake cycles. Fetal hypoxia and maternal smoking and drug use certainly affect fetal heart rate but are not the most common causes. Infants with a congenital heart defect do not exhibit a significant incidence of nonreactive NSTs.

61. Answer: 4

Rationale: Greater than 90% of patients presenting with ectopic pregnancies will complain of pain and report a missed period. Approximately 80% will describe vaginal bleeding. Only 50% will have a palpable abdominal mass.

62. Answer: 1

Rationale: A threatened abortion progresses to complete spontaneous abortion in 50% of cases. Clinical findings are vaginal bleeding with or without cramping and no cervical change. Vaginal bleeding with cramping and cervical change is an inevitable abortion. An incomplete abortion is demonstrated by vaginal bleeding, cramping, and incomplete expulsion of the products of conception. A missed abortion is diagnosed when products of conception are retained after fetal death. There is a decrease in uterine size, loss of pregnancy symptoms, and often a closed and firm cervix.

63. Answer: 3

Rationale: History of preterm birth is associated with a 20%–40% recurrence risk. Low prepregnancy weight and inadequate weight gain, not obesity, are associated with preterm labor. Maternal smoking, drug use (especially cocaine), low socioeconomic status, maternal age less than 17 and greater than 35 years, and non-Caucasian race are all predisposing factors for preterm labor. Previous spontaneous and elective abortions are not risk factors.

64. Answer: 4

Rationale: Ferning is caused by high levels of estrogen; when air-dried, amniotic fluid produces a fern pattern. This microscopic arborization is accurate in confirming rupture of membranes in 90%–95% of cases. Samples heavily contaminated with blood may not fern.

65. Answer: 2

Rationale: Contractions, cramping, or abdominal pain along with continued bleeding could signify a spontaneous abortion. The other symptoms are common during the first trimester.

66. Answer: 3

Rationale: PUPPP skin rash typically starts on the abdomen and spreads to the thighs and possibly the buttocks. Onset of lesions is usually in the third trimester and usually resolves postpartum. It is thought to be related to the stretching of the skin. There is no associated adverse perinatal outcome.

67. Answer: 1

Rationale: Normally, 15%–20% of hairs are in telogen (resting phase of hair cycle). In late pregnancy, this is reduced to less than 10%. After delivery the percentage increases, and by 2 months postpartum, 20% of hairs are in telogen. Therefore, a marked increase occurs in hair loss at 2–4 months after delivery.

68. Answer: 1

Rationale: More frequent suckling will increase production of milk more effectively than increasing the duration of suckling. Stopping or decreasing breast-feeding or applying cold compresses to the breasts will decrease milk production.

69. Answer: 2

Rationale: Breast irritation in nursing mothers is often caused by *Candida albicans*. The source of infection is most likely the infant's mouth (thrush).

70. Answer: 1

Rationale: Initially after delivery, the mother needs an opportunity to accept that her newborn has a congenital defect. Pointing out normal characteristics of the newborn will allow her to put the problem in perspective. Often the mother will focus on the defect. Orofacial surgery will provide closure of the defect but will not completely correct it because scarring will undoubtedly occur.

71. Answer: 2

Rationale: Most nonnursing mothers will resume menstruation 7–9 weeks after birth. About one-half of them will ovulate during the first cycle. Most lactating women will resume menstruation in 12 weeks, although some do not menstruate during the entire lactation period.

72. Answer: 2

Rationale: A history of vaginal delivery of large babies and possible complications such as use of forceps can indicate she has weakened pelvic floor muscles and has lost the ability to maintain a closed external anal sphincter to control leakage. Typically, the development of incontinence can occur 20–30 years after the delivery. Diagnostic testing would include anorectal manometry, and treatment with physical therapy and biofeedback may be helpful. Although the past medical history should include the childbirth history, it is not necessarily obtained in detail and may not be relevant depending on the reason for the office visit. Stress can play a role in worsening many symptoms, but it is less likely to be affecting her bowel control. A rectocele is a rectal prolapse into the vagina that can occur after delivery when the ligaments and muscles weaken. However, the main complaint with a rectocele is constipation, not stool leakage.

73. Answer: 1

Rationale: Within a few hours after birth, the fundus rises to the level of the umbilicus and remains there for about 24 hours. After 24 hours, the fundus begins to descend by about 1 cm or one fingerbreadth per day. It often is not palpable by day 10.

Pharmacology

74. Answer: 3

Rationale: The MMR is a live virus vaccination and is contraindicated in pregnancy. Polio, tetanus, and hepatitis B vaccine are inactivated bacterial or DNA-based vaccines and are safe when indicated.

75. Answer: 4

Rationale: The FDA has five pregnancy risk categories for drugs. Category X indicates that fetal risk outweighs any benefit and use in pregnancy is contraindicated. Category B drugs show no evidence of fetal abnormalities, and risk to the fetus is relatively unlikely. Category C drugs have the potential for animal fetal abnormalities and/or no adequate well-controlled studies in pregnant women but benefits of drugs are thought to justify risks to the fetus. Drugs classified as Category D demonstrate positive evidence of human fetal risk and should be used only in serious disease or life-threatening situations when safer drugs are ineffective.

76. Answer: 3

Rationale: Tetracycline binds with developing enamel and discolors the deciduous teeth between 26 weeks' gestation and 6 months of infancy.

77. Answer: 3

Rationale: Recent studies have confirmed that folic acid taken before conception can reduce the risk of neural tube defect.

78. Answer: 2

Rationale: The current recommendation for RhoGAM is administration of 300 mcg to all Rh-negative women at 28 weeks' pregnancy. This is considered protective for the remainder of the pregnancy.

79. Answer: 4

Rationale: Acetaminophen is a risk category B drug, but problems have not been documented; it should be used with caution. Aspirin is risk category D and may cause bleeding disorders. Nonsteroidal antiinflammatory drugs (ibuprofen; naproxen) are risk category B but have been associated with prolonging pregnancy and prematurely closing the fetal ductus arteriosus because of antiprostaglandin effects.

80. Answer: 1

Rationale: Metronidazole is safe to use in all trimesters of pregnancy. The other medications are known teratogens and contraindicated in pregnancy.

81. Answer: 3

Rationale: Estrogen inhibits milk production. Progestin-only preparations are ideal for the breast-feeding patient because they do not contain estrogen and, therefore, do not inhibit milk production. The other OCs listed contain estrogen in varying amounts.

82. Answer: 1

Rationale: Acetaminophen can be safely prescribed to the pregnant patient. Aspirin and nonsteroidal antiinflammatory drugs are contraindicated in the third trimester. The use of narcotics for the patient is inappropriate.

83. Answer: 2

Rationale: Dicloxacillin will treat *Staphylococcus aureus,* which is the most common organism associated with mastitis. None of the other medications is appropriate for treatment of mastitis, and both doxycycline and ciprofloxacin are contraindicated when breast-feeding.

84. Answer: 4

Rationale: Sertraline, a selective serotonin reuptake inhibitor (SSRI), is not associated with any reported birth defects. Certain SSRI antidepressants, such as fluoxetine (Prozac) and paroxetine (Paxil), have been associated with cardiac defects, anencephaly, craniosynostosis, and abdominal wall defects and should not be prescribed. Risperidone (Risperdal) is an atypical antipsychotic medication (pregnancy category C) and is contraindicated in pregnancy. Alprazolam (Xanax) is an antianxiety medication (pregnancy category D) and causes fetal defects. Imipramine (Tofranil) is a tricyclic antidepressant (pregnancy category D) and causes fetal defects.

Pediatrics

18

Endocrine

1. An infant with congenital hypothyroidism is being discharged home. What would the family nurse practitioner instruct the parents to do?
   1. Watch for constipation and slow pulse as signs of toxicity.
   2. Reduce the medication as symptoms decrease.
   3. Give the medication as a single dose in the early morning on an empty stomach.
   4. Expect weight loss until the child adjusts to the dose of medication.

2. A mother presents her school-age child to the family nurse practitioner and expresses her concern that her son is the shortest child in his class and asks if something is wrong with him. What would the initial differential of short stature in this patient by the family nurse practitioner include?
   1. History with familial height patterns, physical exam with Tanner stage, and radiography to assess skeletal maturation, if indicated.
   2. History with familial height patterns, physical exam, and trial treatment with growth hormone.
   3. Immediate referral to an endocrinologist.
   4. Physical exam and complete blood count, thyroid function panel, urinalysis, karyotyping, chemistry profile, and insulin sensitivity tests.

3. Which of the following findings would the family nurse practitioner expect to find in a child with pubertal gynecomastia?
   1. Tanner stage II with testes less than or equal to 4 cm in length.
   2. Breasts and nipples nontender and equal in size.
   3. Breast tissue enlargement mainly glandular, movable, and nonadherent to skin or underlying tissue.
   4. Lymphadenopathy, goiter, asymmetric testes, and repaired hypospadias.

4. Which of the following is true regarding hyperthyroidism in children?
   1. Boys have a higher incidence of Graves' disease.
   2. Autoimmune response is most often triggered by the body's reaction to a bacterial or viral infection.

3. Decreased production and secretion of thyroid hormone and presence of goiter.
4. Common, endemic congenital disorder caused by iodine deficiency.

5. On physical exam of a 14-year-old girl complaining of amenorrhea, the family nurse practitioner notes blood pressure 138/90 mm Hg; pulse of 98 beats/min; broad chest with widely spaced nipples; Tanner stage I; webbing of neck; low hairline; and prominent, anomalous ears. What does the family nurse practitioner suspect?
   1. Klinefelter's syndrome.
   2. Marfan's syndrome.
   3. Fragile X syndrome.
   4. Turner's syndrome.

6. The family nurse practitioner understands that growth retardation that appears after age 12 in boys is usually caused by:
   1. Chromosomal abnormalities.
   2. Hyperthyroidism.
   3. Hyperpituitarism.
   4. Hypogonadism.

7. The family nurse practitioner understands that the blood glucose level in diabetic children 7–12 years of age who can recognize the symptoms of hypoglycemia should target which range before meals?
   1. 60–75 mg/dL.
   2. 100–175 mg/dL.
   3. 90–130 mg/dL.
   4. Greater than 180 mg/dL.

8. An adolescent male patient presenting with recent-onset nocturia, polydipsia, polyphagia, weight loss, and blurred vision is most likely experiencing the symptoms of:
   1. Type 1 diabetes.
   2. Type 2 diabetes.
   3. Urinary tract infection.
   4. Mononucleosis.

9. In which of the following groups of patients is tight glycemic control contraindicated?
   1. Adolescent males.
   2. Middle-aged females.
   3. Middle-aged males.
   4. Children under age 6.

10. An infant with an abnormally pitched cry may demonstrate a genetic disorder or other problems, such as:
    1. Hypothyroidism.
    2. Hypertelorism.
    3. Cleft palate.
    4. Pyloric stenosis.

11. A 6-year-old child with hypothyroidism diagnosed shortly after birth is seen by the family nurse practitioner for a routine physical exam. Temperature is 96.8°F (36°C) and pulse is 68 beats/min. The mother states that the child has been constipated and seems to be more tired than usual. Based on this history, what should the family nurse practitioner suspect?
    1. The child has been taking too much levothyroxine (Synthroid) and is exhibiting symptoms of toxicity.
    2. The child needs to add more fluids to his diet to correct the constipation.
    3. The child needs to have the dose of levothyroxine (Synthroid) increased because he is exhibiting signs of hypothyroidism.
    4. The child has "outgrown" the hypothyroidism and no longer needs levothyroxine.

12. A mother brings her school-age child to the clinic and reports a recent history of easy fatigability ("he can't keep up with his brother anymore"), unexplained bruising, and multiple courses of antibiotics for symptoms of upper respiratory infection (URI) during the last 6 months. Physical exam reveals scattered bruising in no apparent pattern, pallor, and cervical lymphadenopathy. What should be the first step of the diagnostic workup for this child?
    1. Chest x-ray and electrocardiogram.
    2. Liver function tests and abdominal ultrasound.
    3. Prothrombin/partial thromboplastin time.
    4. Complete blood count (CBC) with differential and platelet count.

13. In evaluating the laboratory findings for a child with iron-deficiency anemia, what should the family nurse practitioner expect?
    1. Low mean corpuscular volume (MCV) and low reticulocyte count.
    2. High MCV and hemoglobin 12 g/dL.
    3. Normal MCV and hematocrit 34%.
    4. High MCV and normal reticulocyte count.

14. The family nurse practitioner explains a bone marrow aspiration procedure to a 4-year-old child. Which behavior of the child would reflect effective teaching?
    1. Appears calm as the nurse takes her for the procedure.
    2. Asks if she can have ice cream after the procedure.
    3. States that her blood is bad and "the doctor will make it better."
    4. Points at her doll and says, "They have to put a needle here to look at my blood."

15. Which of the following signs and symptoms are associated with a diagnosis of childhood acute lymphocytic leukemia (ALL)?
    1. Splenomegaly, facial rash, and cough.
    2. Expiratory wheezing, bleeding, and hepatomegaly.
    3. Bleeding, fever, and pain.
    4. Bone pain, fever, and night sweats.

16. The family nurse practitioner is concerned about the development of which complication in a young child with a diagnosis of iron-deficiency anemia?
    1. Crohn's disease.
    2. Pernicious anemia.
    3. Impaired cognitive development.
    4. Hepatic and spleen dysfunction.

17. The family nurse practitioner is counseling a parent who has a child with sickle cell disease. The parent asks, "If my child has sickle cell disease, does that mean that I'm at an increased risk for developing the same problems?" The family nurse practitioner's response would be based on which principle of sickle cell disease?
    1. The mother is at an increased risk because the condition is inherited and she probably has the condition and has not had an active episode.
    2. The mother is not at risk for developing the condition because males are carriers of the trait.
    3. The mother has a 25% chance of being affected by the disease, especially during times of stress.
    4. Both parents are either carriers of the trait or have disease, and each child has a 25% chance of having the condition.

18. During a clinic visit, the family nurse practitioner notes that an 11-month-old infant is pale. The physical exam reveals a pulse of 170 beats/min, height at the 25th percentile, and weight at the 95th percentile. The nurse questions the mother about the infant's diet. The mother states that the infant eats mostly puréed fruits and whole milk. Which diagnostic finding does the family nurse practitioner expect?
    1. Normal hemoglobin.
    2. Elevated mean corpuscular volume (MCV).
    3. Low serum ferritin level.
    4. Macrocytic, hyperchromic anemia.

19. The family nurse practitioner knows that an infant who is exclusively breast-fed is at risk for developing iron-deficiency anemia after what age?
    1. 1 month.
    2. 2 months.
    3. 4 months.
    4. 6 months.

20. In children, hypertension and history of a sore throat may indicate which disorder?
    1. Heart failure.
    2. Glomerulonephritis.
    3. Vasculitis.
    4. Cushing's syndrome.

21. When assessing a child with glomerulonephritis, what symptoms would the family nurse practitioner expect to be present?
    1. Fever greater than 102°F (38.9°C) and bilateral flank pain.
    2. Periorbital edema and increased blood pressure (BP).
    3. Anorexia and complaints of dysuria.
    4. Oliguria with strong concentrated urine.

22. When instructing the parents regarding the course of poststreptococcal glomerulonephritis in their child, the family nurse practitioner would tell them to expect bloody urine for how long after onset of diuresis?
    1. 1 week.
    2. 1–2 weeks.
    3. 2–3 weeks.
    4. 4–7 days.

23. A mother brings her 3-year-old daughter to the clinic, stating that she noticed a swelling in the child's abdominal area just below the rib cage on the left side. The family nurse practitioner observes a bulging of the area, and the child does not want to be touched because of abdominal tenderness. What is the best action for the family nurse practitioner at this visit?
    1. Immediately contact a surgeon, radiologist, or pediatrician for discussion of further radiologic workup.
    2. Schedule a referral with a pediatrician in the near future.
    3. Perform a urinalysis (UA) and draw blood for creatinine and potassium.
    4. Explain to the child that it is necessary to examine the abdomen.

24. A mother brings her 6-year-old daughter to the clinic. The child is complaining of burning on urination, and the urine is cloudy. A dipstick test of the urine is positive for leukocyte esterase. The mother states the child had a fever with nausea and vomiting the last time she took sulfisoxazole (Gantrisin). What would be an appropriate medication for this child?
    1. Nitrofurantoin (Macrodantin) 50 mg PO qid × 7 days.
    2. Trimethoprim-sulfamethoxazole (Septra DS) 1 tab PO bid × 10 days.
    3. Ciprofloxacin (Cipro) 200 mg PO bid × 10 days.
    4. Clarithromycin (Biaxin) 250 mg PO bid × 10 days.

Cardiac

25. On exam of a child, the family nurse practitioner notes weak femoral pulses. This finding is associated with what condition?
    1. Patent ductus arteriosus.
    2. Coarctation of the aorta.
    3. Tetralogy of Fallot.
    4. Pulmonary stenosis.

26. In doing a cardiac assessment of a 4-month-old infant, the family nurse practitioner notes a continuous murmur. This finding is consistent with a diagnosis of:
    1. Coarctation of the aorta.
    2. Patent ductus arteriosus (PDA).
    3. Ventricular septal defect.
    4. Aortic stenosis.

27. Heart failure (HF) is a common clinical presentation occurring in a child with congenital heart disease (CHD). What is another common clinical presentation with CHD?
    1. Hypoglycemia.
    2. Hypertension.
    3. Peripheral edema.
    4. Cyanosis.

28. What are the clinical manifestations of heart failure (HF) in an infant?
    1. Easily fatigued, central cyanosis, tachycardia, tachypnea, hepatomegaly.
    2. Coughing, diaphoresis, peripheral edema, hepatomegaly.
    3. Tachycardia, tachypnea, easily fatigued, pallor, hepatomegaly.
    4. Peripheral edema, coughing, splenomegaly, hepatomegaly, tachycardia.

29. A young child is scheduled for surgical repair of tetralogy of Fallot. The family nurse practitioner is doing the preoperative physical exam. What does the family nurse practitioner expect the child's hemoglobin (Hgb) values to show, and what kind of lesion does the child have?
    1. Hgb 18 g/dL, decreased pulmonary blood flow lesion.
    2. Hgb 3 g/dL, decreased pulmonary blood flow lesion.
    3. Hgb 10 g/dL, mixed blood flow lesion.
    4. Hgb 18 g/dL, obstructive lesion.

30. The family nurse practitioner understands that the most likely cause of hypertension in a young child is:
    1. Glomerulonephritis.
    2. Pheochromocytoma.
    3. Rheumatic fever.
    4. Hyperthyroidism.

31. Which of the following would be pertinent in the past medical history of a child who is being evaluated for cardiovascular disease?
    1. Kawasaki disease.
    2. Hypothyroidism.
    3. Osteogenic sarcoma.
    4. Tourette's syndrome.

32. Infective endocarditis prophylaxis may be required for children with congenital heart defects in which of the following procedures?
    1. Dental procedures such as simple adjustment of orthodontic appliances.
    2. Cardiac catheterization.
    3. Tonsillectomy and/or adenoidectomy.
    4. Insertion of tympanostomy tubes.

33. For the child with congenital heart disease (CHD) and a permanent pacemaker, electrical safety precautions include avoidance of:
    1. Cellular phones.
    2. Microwave ovens.
    3. Household electrical appliances.
    4. Metal detectors.

34. A child is having a workup for rheumatic fever. His physical findings are temperature of 103.6°F (39.8°C), migratory joint pain, and increased erythrocyte sedimentation rate (ESR). According to the Jones Criteria, what is essential for the diagnosis of rheumatic fever?
    1. History of group A β-hemolytic streptococcal throat infection.
    2. Carditis.
    3. Sydenham's chorea.
    4. History of erythema marginatum for the last 3 days.

35. A toddler has ingested some of his grandfather's pills. The toddler is vomiting, feels weak, and has a first-degree atrioventricular (AV) block pattern on the electrocardiogram. The grandfather brings in four medication bottles. Which medication did the toddler most likely ingest?
    1. Amitriptyline (Elavil).
    2. Digoxin (Lanoxin).
    3. Furosemide (Lasix).
    4. Aspirin.

Respiratory

36. Cystic fibrosis (CF) is the preliminary diagnosis for a young girl who was brought to the clinic for evaluation. What is the test used to rule out CF?
    1. Hemoccult test.
    2. Sweat chloride test.
    3. Sputum culture and sensitivity.
    4. Glucose tolerance test.

37. An 18-month-old infant brought to the emergency department is awake, lethargic, and in severe respiratory distress. His mother states that he has not been sick and was playing on the floor when he suddenly began coughing, choking, and gagging. He has expiratory wheezes, with decreased breath sounds over right lower lobes; respirations of 36 breaths/min, pulse of 130 beats/min, and normal temperature. Portable chest x-ray shows hyperinflation on expiratory views. What is the best treatment for the infant?
    1. Bronchoscopy as soon as possible.
    2. Cool-mist therapy with racemic epinephrine.
    3. Antibiotics with chest physiotherapy.
    4. Immediate endotracheal intubation and ventilation.

38. A 4-month-old patient presents to the office with a history of several days of rhinorrhea, cough, low-grade fever, increased respiratory rate, mild subcostal retractions, wheezes, and crackles. What is the most likely diagnosis?
    1. Croup.
    2. Epiglottitis.
    3. Tracheitis.
    4. Bronchiolitis.

39. During a physical exam of a 2-year-old diagnosed with possible cystic fibrosis (CF), the child passes a stool. The family nurse practitioner would expect the stool's appearance to be:
    1. Yellow and loose.
    2. Small and constipated.
    3. Green and odorous.
    4. Large and bulky.

40. A 6-year-old patient with a history of asthma has never used a peak flowmeter. What quick tool can be used to assess the severity of the child's distress?
    1. Arterial blood gases (ABGs).
    2. Child's inability to complete a sentence.
    3. Chest x-ray.
    4. Presence of runny nose.

41. During a visit to the clinic for routine care, the mother reports that her infant was diagnosed with bronchopulmonary dysplasia (BPD). In addition, the infant has been vomiting after each gastrostomy feeding. The family nurse practitioner notes that the infant's weight gain is adequate and would recommend:
    1. Referral to the pediatrician for follow-up.
    2. Reduction in amount of formula for the gastrostomy feeding.
    3. Addition of 3 oz of Pedialyte for the next two feedings.
    4. Positioning of the infant after feedings with head and trunk elevated.

42. A 3-year-old child with up-to-date immunizations is brought to the office by his mother with a fairly rapid onset of stridor and a high-pitched wheeze. In view of this information, what would be the least important condition to consider for the differential diagnosis?
    1. Croup.
    2. Foreign body aspiration.
    3. Epiglottitis.
    4. Bacterial tracheitis.

43. A 15-year-old girl comes to the emergency department (ED) with complaints of extreme shortness of breath. She is confused, and her past medical history is not available. Her vital signs are pulse of 124 beats/min, respirations of 32 breaths/min, blood pressure of 124/80 mm Hg, and normal temperature. Physical exam reveals diffuse expiratory wheezes, hyperresonance on percussion, and prolonged expiratory phase. What should the best treatment for this patient include?
    1. Aminophylline by mouth.
    2. Beclomethasone (Beclovent) inhaler.
    3. Epinephrine by injection.
    4. Albuterol (Proventil) by metered-dose inhaler (MDI).

44. An appropriate medication regimen for a child with drug-susceptible pulmonary tuberculosis (TB) is:
    1. Montelukast (Singulair) therapy with rifampin (Rifadin).
    2. Streptomycin, pyrazinamide, and rimantadine (Flumadine).
    3. Isoniazid, pyrazinamide, and rifampin.
    4. Montelukast therapy with pyrimethamine (Fansidar).

45. During a routine well-child exam of a 4 year old, the family nurse practitioner learns that the paternal grandmother has just been diagnosed with active tuberculosis (TB). The mother states that the grandmother had stayed in their home for a week during the summer. The child has no signs of TB and has a negative purified protein derivative (PPD). What action should the family nurse practitioner take?
    1. Prescribe no medications but schedule a repeat PPD in 2 months.
    2. Administer 1 mL gamma globulin IM.
    3. Start combination therapy with isoniazid (INH) and rifampin (Rifadin) for 15 months.
    4. Start INH therapy for 4 months and then reevaluate.

46. Indications for antibiotic use in a child with bronchiolitis would include:
    1. History of two episodes of bronchiolitis in 4 months.
    2. Rhinitis and a productive cough for 3 days.
    3. High fever and increased crackles after patient had been improving for several days.
    4. Low-grade fever, increased nasal secretions, and retractions while febrile.

47. A 10-year-old taking isoniazid (INH) prophylactically for exposure to TB complains of headache, palpitations, rash, and diarrhea. What would the management be based on?
    1. Avoidance of foods containing tyramine and histamine.
    2. Addition of pyridoxine to the diet.
    3. Change in therapy from INH to rifampin.
    4. Evaluation for hepatic impairment.

48. What is the initial treatment of choice for children diagnosed with bronchiolitis?
    1. Increase fluids; antipyretics as needed.
    2. Prednisolone (Pediapred) immediately and continue over 3–5 days.
    3. Albuterol 2 puffs q4 hours prn wheezing.
    4. Amoxicillin over 10–14 days; aerosol humidification.

49. A 10-year-old boy is experiencing problems with wheezing, coughing, and shortness of breath for about 4 hours after basketball practice. He has normal respirations and experiences the problems only after exercise. He is experiencing no other respiratory problems, and the physical findings are within normal limits. What is the treatment of choice for this child?
    1. Albuterol (Ventolin) 2 puffs metered-dose inhaler 20–30 minutes before exercise.
    2. Cromolyn sodium (Intal) 2 puffs each morning.
    3. Theophylline (Theo-24; methylxanthine) 100 mg PO bid.
    4. Beclomethasone (Beclovent) 2 puffs 3–4 times daily.

50. What test is ordered for all newborns to screen for cystic fibrosis (CF)?
    1. Serum amylase.
    2. Immunoreactive trypsinogen (IRT).
    3. Sweat chloride test.
    4. DNA analysis.

Immune and Allergy

51. A tuberculosis (TB) skin test on an immunocompetent 6-year-old child who has no risk factors for TB is considered positive for this patient when it measures:
    1. 5 mm.
    2. 10 mm.
    3. 15 mm.
    4. 20 mm.

52. Children who have chronic allergic rhinitis often present with clinical symptoms that include:
    1. Mouth breathing and nasal polyps.
    2. Allergic "shiners" and Dennie-Morgan lines.
    3. Thick nasal discharge and sneezing.
    4. Flushed face and fever.

53. What are common sites for adolescent atopic dermatitis?
    1. Cheeks, forehead, and scalp.
    2. Wrists, ankles, and antecubital fossae.
    3. Antecubital fossae, face, neck, and back.
    4. Palmar creases and extensor surface of legs.

54. The clinic is notified that a 2-year-old child is being brought in with a bee sting and that the child is having difficulty breathing. Which medication should the family nurse practitioner have available for the child's initial care?
    1. Epinephrine 0.3 mg, IM.
    2. Epinephrine 0.15 mg, IM.
    3. Prednisone 10 mg, PO, q12 hours × 3 doses.
    4. Diphenhydramine (Benadryl) elixir 12.5 mg, PO × 1.

55. What is an appropriate antihistamine to recommend for a child with allergic rhinitis?
    1. Diphenhydramine (Benadryl).
    2. Chlorpheniramine (Chlor-Trimeton).
    3. Brompheniramine (Dimetane).
    4. Loratadine (Claritin).

56. A child who weighs 30 lb (13.6 kg) arrives in the office. The mother is concerned that the child is having an allergic reaction to peanuts. The child has hives on most of her body and is beginning to wheeze; she is in acute distress. What does the family nurse practitioner administer?
    1. Diphenhydramine (Benadryl) 50 mg PO.
    2. Diphenhydramine (Benadryl) 25 mg PO.
    3. Epinephrine (Adrenalin) 0.15 mL of a 1:1000 solution.
    4. Epinephrine (Adrenalin) 0.3 mL of a 1:1000 solution.

57. A 2-year-old presents with symptoms of atopic dermatitis, rhinorrhea, and recurrent otitis media with effusion. The house is nonsmoking and there are no pets in the home. The family nurse practitioner recognizes that the most likely cause of these symptoms in this age group would be from:
    1. Dust mite exposure.
    2. Internal mold exposure.
    3. Milk ingestion.
    4. Wheat ingestion.

58. A mother of a 5-year-old patient is concerned that the child has a significant reaction to poison ivy every spring with a rash that appears on the ventral surfaces of the arms in the antecubital fossa. The rash is flat and erythematous and comes on suddenly with exposure to grass. Which statement would best describe the trigger of this dermatologic symptom?
    1. Poison ivy is very common in the spring and exposure results in immediate onset of symptoms.

2. Plants that flower in the spring are laden with pollen that most likely will cause this type of symptom.
3. Type IV hypersensitivity reactions are common in the spring with direct exposure to the allergen.
4. Type I hypersensitivity reactions result in immediate symptoms on exposure to the allergen.

Head, Eyes, Ears, Nose, & Throat (HEENT)

59. In examining the mouth of a school-age child, the family nurse practitioner notes that the central and lateral permanent incisors have surface pitting and are stained brown. What is this condition most suggestive of?
    1. The mother taking tetracycline during pregnancy.
    2. Poor dental hygiene.
    3. Dental fluorosis.
    4. Going to bed with a bottle during infancy.

60. During a preschool screening for visual acuity, what else would the family nurse practitioner assess for?
    1. Pupils that are equal and reactive.
    2. Intraocular pressure by tonometry.
    3. Diplopia.
    4. Strabismus.

61. A 4-year-old child's pure-tone audiometry reveals 25 decibels (dB) in the left ear and 43 dB in the right ear. The family nurse practitioner would interpret these findings as:
    1. Inconclusive; pure-tone audiometry is not accurate in children less than 5 years of age.
    2. Within normal limits for age.
    3. Normal hearing in the left ear and moderate hearing loss in the right ear.
    4. Mild hearing loss in the left ear and normal hearing in the right ear.

62. An infant with low or obliquely set ears also has an increased incidence of:
    1. Cataracts.
    2. Hyaline membrane disease.
    3. Genitourinary defects.
    4. Cardiovascular anomalies.

63. Which of the following statements is true regarding tonsils?
    1. Children with large tonsils are more prone to tonsillitis than those with small tonsils.
    2. Tonsils enlarge as the child grows older.
    3. Hypertrophied tonsils in children usually represent a normal finding.
    4. Most cases of tonsillitis are caused by a β-hemolytic streptococcal infection.

64. An adolescent arrives at the clinic with a complaint of low-grade fever, sore throat, slight headache, and fatigue for the past week. On physical exam, the family nurse practitioner finds exudative tonsils bilaterally, red pharynx with white patches, and enlarged posterior cervical neck nodes. The family nurse practitioner would expect which laboratory test result?
    1. Positive rapid strep test.
    2. Positive monospot test.
    3. Increased white blood cell (WBC) count.
    4. Positive viral throat cultures.

65. The family nurse practitioner taking a preschooler's history learns that the family does not have fluoridated drinking water. With consideration of the concerns about fluorosis, what is the most appropriate nursing intervention?
    1. Prescribe 5 mL of 0.02% fluoride solution (Fluorinse) once daily.
    2. Instruct parents to use a pea-size fluoridated dentifrice and to supervise toothbrushing.
    3. Instruct parents to use bottled drinking water.
    4. Refer to dentist for topical application of fluoride.

66. A mother reports that her toddler awoke this morning with eyelid redness and swelling. The child is afebrile and the eyelid is nontender and uniformly swollen. What is the most likely diagnosis?
    1. Blepharitis.
    2. Hordeolum.
    3. Insect bite.
    4. Dacryocystitis.

67. On exam, the family nurse practitioner notes that a 2-week-old infant's left eye is watering and crusted material is on the eyelids. No edema or erythema is noted. What is the diagnosis the family nurse practitioner would make?
    1. Nasolacrimal duct obstruction.
    2. Conjunctivitis.
    3. Congenital dacryocystocele.
    4. Corneal abrasion.

68. A mother brings her 6-week-old infant to the clinic because she is concerned that the child's eyes are crossed. What is the family nurse practitioner's most appropriate response?
    1. Explain to the mother that this is normal; reevaluate the child at 3 months of age.
    2. Refer the infant to an ophthalmologist.
    3. Provide the mother with normal saline eye drops for the infant.
    4. Have the mother alternate patching one eye and then the other every 6 hours.

69. In assessing a child with bacterial conjunctivitis, the family nurse practitioner finds:
    1. Minimal tearing, moderate itching, and profuse exudate.
    2. Severe itching, moderate tearing, and minimal discharge.

    3. Minimal itching, moderate tearing, and mucoid exudate.
    4. Minimal itching, moderate tearing, and profuse exudate.

70. The family nurse practitioner makes the diagnosis of nasolacrimal obstruction in a 1-week-old infant who presents with "leaking" of the right eye and a yellow discharge in the inner canthus of both eyes. Which of the following interventions would be contraindicated?
    1. Neosporin ophthalmic drops.
    2. Massaging the lacrimal duct for 1 minute four times daily.
    3. Cleansing the eye with warm water four times daily.
    4. Dexamethasone (Decadron) ophthalmic drops.

71. A child is diagnosed by the family nurse practitioner with acute otitis media (AOM). During a pneumatic otoscopy, the family nurse practitioner expects the tympanic membrane (TM) to be:
    1. Immobile, painful, with absent or decreased landmarks.
    2. Mobile, painful, with absent or decreased landmarks.
    3. Immobile, not painful, with landmarks visualized.
    4. Mobile, not painful, full and bulging.

72. A 6-year-old child is seen by the family nurse practitioner for ear pain. The child is afebrile. The left ear canal is extremely edematous and moderately inflamed, with thick yellowish drainage at the external meatus. The child denies putting anything in the ear canal, but the family nurse practitioner finds that the child swims frequently. What is the most likely diagnosis?
    1. Acute otitis media.
    2. Serous otitis media.
    3. Sinusitis.
    4. Otitis externa.

73. What risk factors are included for acute otitis media (AOM)?
    1. Second-hand smoke, attending day care, American Indians and Eskimos.
    2. Chinese race, previous otitis media, many siblings.
    3. Higher socioeconomic level, full-time day care, allergies.
    4. Summer season, full-time day care, premature at birth.

74. A 6-year-old child is examined by the family nurse practitioner because of fluctuating hearing problems. The child is afebrile and denies otalgia. The mobility of the tympanic membrane (TM) is decreased when the family nurse practitioner performs pneumatic otoscopy. The TM is opaque with no visible landmarks. The child denies putting anything in the ear, and the mother states the child does not swim frequently. What is the most likely diagnosis?
    1. Acute otitis media (AOM).
    2. A foreign body.
    3. Otitis media with effusion (OME).
    4. Otitis externa.

75. The family nurse practitioner teaches the mother of a school-age child the following as the most effective preventive measure against the common cold:
    1. Judicious use of vitamin C during cold season.
    2. Ensuring adequate sleep and fluids.
    3. Meticulous handwashing, preferably with an antibacterial soap and warm water.
    4. Avoiding contact with children and adults who have a runny nose, cough, and sore throat.

76. Which antibiotic would be appropriate for the family nurse practitioner to prescribe for β-lactamase production by strains of *Haemophilus influenzae* and *Moraxella catarrhalis* in a child with acute otitis media?
    1. Amoxicillin (Amoxil).
    2. Erythromycin-sulfisoxazole (Pediazole).
    3. Penicillin V potassium (Pen-Vee K).
    4. Amoxicillin with clavulanic acid (Augmentin).

77. A 4-year-old boy (weight 18 kg) is diagnosed with bilateral otitis media. His last ear infection was 6 months ago, and he has no known drug allergies. What would be an appropriate medication to prescribe?
    1. Ampicillin 40–50 mg/kg/day tid × 7 days.
    2. Corticosteroid otic solution 3 gtt both ears × 10 days.
    3. Amoxicillin 75–90 mg/kg/day bid × 10 days.
    4. Doxycycline 250 mg 1 tsp PO tid × 10 days.

78. An adolescent patient has had yellowish-green nasal discharge and a frontal headache for a week. The adolescent's temperature has gone up to 101.2°F (38.4°C) on most afternoons, and she has a cough that worsens when she lies down. The physical exam is within normal limits except for the drainage and a slightly erythematous pharynx. She does not have any drug allergies and has not been taking any medications in the last few months. Which medication would be best to prescribe for her?
    1. Diphenhydramine (Benadryl).
    2. Erythromycin (E-Mycin).
    3. Pseudoephedrine (Sudafed).
    4. Amoxicillin/clavulanate (Augmentin).

Integumentary

79. The nurse is examining a 6-week-old infant of Latin American descent. There are irregular areas of deep-blue pigmentation across the infant's buttocks. The nurse would identify this as characteristic of:
    1. Child abuse.
    2. Telangiectatic nevi.
    3. Cutis marmorata.
    4. Mongolian spots.

80. A mother brings her school-age child in for an exam. She reports that the child frequently scratches and that the itching seems to be worse at night. On exam, the family nurse practitioner notes lesions on the sides of the fingers and inner aspect of the elbows. These lesions are short, irregular "runs" that are approximately 2–3 mm long and the width of a hair. The family nurse practitioner tells the mother she suspects:
    1. Scabies.
    2. Hives.
    3. Fleas.
    4. Ticks.

81. When treating atopic dermatitis in children, which of the following instructions are applicable?
    1. Eliminate common foods thought to induce flares, one food at a time.
    2. Encourage moisturizing bubble baths.
    3. Keep well dressed during winter.
    4. Encourage bathing two or three times a day.

82. A family nurse practitioner is teaching the mother of a child how to use permethrin 1% cream rinse (Nix) for treatment of pediculosis capitis. What is the most important information the family nurse practitioner should give to the mother?
    1. Shampoo the child's hair daily for 1 week, followed by permethrin rinse.
    2. Shampoo and towel-dry hair, apply permethrin to scalp and hair, and wait 10 minutes before rinsing.
    3. The shampoo should not be used again because it is toxic and may absorb systemically.
    4. It is not necessary to launder bedding or clothing.

83. The family nurse practitioner understands that nonintentional scalding in young children usually occurs:
    1. On the back of the body.
    2. On the front of the body.
    3. In a circular or glove pattern.
    4. With no specific pattern.

84. An infant has pruritus caused by eczema. The family nurse practitioner teaches the mother the following regarding the infant's care:
    1. Dress the infant in cotton shorts and short-sleeved shirts.
    2. Dress the infant in wool-blend, long-sleeved jump suits.
    3. Give the infant cornstarch or Aveeno baths.
    4. Give the infant salt baths three times a day.

85. A new mother is concerned about the hemangioma on her infant's neck. What is the treatment of choice for the majority of infants with hemangioma?
    1. Cryosurgery.
    2. Intralesional injection of steroids.
    3. Observation.
    4. Injection of a sclerosing agent.

86. The family nurse practitioner is examining an infant with atopic dermatitis. What would the physical exam reveal?
    1. Dry, scaly rash with pruritus.
    2. Distribution of rash on face and extensor surfaces.
    3. Erythematous raised areas on flexor surfaces.
    4. Moist, crusting rash with no pruritus.

87. The family nurse practitioner is examining a 6-year-old child and identifies 8–10 patches of coffee-colored areas on the trunk. The areas are nontender, the border is irregular, and most of the areas are larger than 1.5 cm and nonpalpable. What is the best recommendation to the child's parents?
    1. The child should be referred to a neurologist.
    2. These areas are normal pigmentation and will disappear.
    3. A dermatologist should be consulted for removal of lesions.
    4. Emollients should be applied to keep skin moist, and sunlight on the areas should be avoided.

88. An infant is noted at his well-child visit to have a yellowish, greasy scaly rash on his scalp, forehead, and ears. What is the most likely diagnosis?
    1. Seborrheic dermatitis.
    2. Atopic dermatitis.
    3. Erythema toxicum.
    4. Eczema.

89. A 1-month-old infant is being seen by the family nurse practitioner for a diaper rash. On exam, the family nurse practitioner notes moderate erythema and poorly marginated, dry patches of skin localized to the buttocks. The deep folds are not affected. There are no satellite lesions. What is the most likely diagnosis?
    1. Infantile seborrheic dermatitis.
    2. Allergy to disposable diapers.
    3. Contact dermatitis.
    4. *Candida* diaper rash.

90. A mother brings her preschool child to see the family nurse practitioner because of sores on his arms and legs. On exam, the family nurse practitioner notes several honey-colored crusted lesions with an erythematous base on the arms and legs. There is a history of exposure to mosquitoes. The rest of the exam is essentially negative. What is the most likely diagnosis?
    1. Scabies.
    2. Impetigo.
    3. Pityriasis rosea.
    4. Varicella.

91. A mother returns to the clinic with her 6-month-old infant to have his ears rechecked after a 10-day course of antibiotics for an ear infection. During the visit, the mother states that the child is now eating better and appears to be recovering, but he now has a bad diaper rash. What is the most likely cause of this rash?
    1. Poor hygiene.
    2. Cellulitis.
    3. Seborrheic diaper dermatitis.
    4. *Candida albicans.*

92. A school-age child presents with erythematous, papular lesions, and scaly plaques in the antecubital and popliteal fossae and on the neck, wrists, and ankles. The mother states that the child has been scratching the areas, especially at night. History reveals that the child also has been treated for asthma. What diagnosis would the family nurse practitioner make?
    1. Scabies.
    2. Atopic dermatitis.
    3. Tinea corporis.
    4. Contact dermatitis.

93. A toddler is brought to the clinic with a history of an insect bite last evening. What presenting symptom would be associated with the bite of a brown recluse spider?
    1. Paresthesias in all extremities.
    2. Edematous, erythematous area with coalescing macules.
    3. Tissue sloughing in the bite area within 8–10 hours.
    4. Development of a central black eschar of "sinking infarct" within 12–24 hours.

94. The family nurse practitioner understands that cat bites become infected more often than dog bites because:
    1. Dogs have a "cleaner mouth" than cats.
    2. Cat bites are often deep puncture wounds.
    3. Dog bites are usually on the face, which makes them less susceptible to infection.
    4. Cat bites are usually associated with clawing and spreading of microorganisms.

95. An adolescent was bitten by a neighbor's dog 3 days ago. He has developed an infection in a large wound on his lower leg. What would be an appropriate management for the patient?
    1. Prescribe amoxicillin-clavulanate (Augmentin).
    2. Approximate the edges of the wound together with suture.
    3. Prescribe cephalexin (Keflex).
    4. Have the adolescent return to the clinic for follow-up in 2 weeks.

96. A young adolescent has been bitten by a black widow spider while doing yard work. He is having a severe reaction. What does the family nurse practitioner expect?
    1. Hypotension and shock.
    2. Localized pain, erythema, and edema in the area.
    3. Black eschar of sloughing tissue within 4 hours of the bite.
    4. Abdominal cramping, nausea, and headache.

Childhood Diseases

97. Phone consultation with a mother reveals that her child has been taking trimethoprim-sulfamethoxazole (Septra) for 3 days for a urinary tract infection. She has been treated with the drug previously with no problems. Currently, the child is experiencing blister-like sores in the skinfold areas (axilla and groin), oral ulceration, and a few genital sores. Her temperature is 104°F (40°C), and she is very weak. Differential diagnosis includes:
    1. Kawasaki disease.
    2. Erythema multiforme (major).
    3. Viral exanthem.
    4. Early scalded-skin syndrome.

98. A day care center director calls to confirm when a child can return to the center after having fifth disease (erythema infectiosum). The family nurse practitioner's response is based on the knowledge that the period of communicability lasts until:
    1. The rash is gone.
    2. The rash appears.
    3. Upper respiratory symptoms are gone.
    4. The transient joint pain disappears.

99. Exam of a nontoxic but ill-appearing 6 year old reveals vesicular and ulcerative oral lesions and a maculopapular rash on the hands and feet; temperature is 100.4°F (38°C), and the child has feelings of malaise. What does the differential diagnosis include?
    1. Hand-foot-and-mouth disease.
    2. Roseola.
    3. Drug rash.
    4. Varicella.

100. The family nurse practitioner understands that the rash of roseola differs from that of rubella. Which statement is correct?
    1. Rash of roseola starts on the trunk.
    2. Rash of rubella is pruritic.
    3. Rash of roseola fades in 3–5 days.
    4. Rash of rubella clears on the extremities, when facial rash erupts.

101. What is an appropriate treatment for a child with roseola?
    1. Antiviral medications, fluids, and rest.
    2. Antipyretics, rest, and hydration.
    3. Antibiotics, hydration, and rest.
    4. Hospitalization, antipyretics, and IV fluid replacement.

102. In treatment of severe inflammatory acne for a female adolescent, the family nurse practitioner understands that:
    1. Isotretinoin (Accutane) provides an effective first-line therapy.

2. The benefits of treatment will be noted in 5–7 days.
    3. Counseling on stringent dietary changes is important.
    4. Systemic antibiotics are effective treatment.

103. A young mother brings her infant to the family nurse practitioner with a complaint of diaper rash present for about 1 week. The diaper area appears beefy red with sharply marginated dermatitis. Satellite lesions are also noted. What does the family nurse practitioner recommend?
    1. Changing from disposable diapers to cloth diapers with plastic pants.
    2. Nystatin cream (Mycostatin) after each diaper change.
    3. Wet soaks three times daily.
    4. Liberally applying oil after bathing.

104. The family nurse practitioner is examining lesions around a child's nose and mouth. His mother states that the lesions appeared several days ago and now seem worse. Some of the vesicular, edematous, red, and tender lesions have yellow crusts and an erythematous base. What is the recommended treatment for this child?
    1. Mupirocin ointment (Bactroban) qid × 10 days.
    2. Gently soaking the lesions with antibacterial soap and removing the crusts.
    3. Amoxicillin-clavulanate (Augmentin).
    4. Diphenhydramine (Benadryl) to decrease itching and spreading.

105. A mother brings her 1-year-old child to the clinic for problems with a "rash." She states the child has not been feeling well since the rash started 2 days ago. The family nurse practitioner observes numerous macules and vesicles in clusters over the child's trunk and mucous membranes; some are clear, some are crusting. The child is irritable but does not have a fever. What would be the diagnosis and treatment for the child?
    1. Varicella; immunize with varicella-zoster vaccine to decrease symptoms and begin acyclovir (Zovirax) therapy to prevent/decrease complications.
    2. Impetigo; treat with amoxicillin-clavulanate (Augmentin) for 10 days and return to clinic in 2 weeks.
    3. Contact dermatitis; apply diphenhydramine (Benadryl) spray over rash, cut child's fingernails to decrease scratching, and thoroughly review any changes in care with the mother.
    4. Varicella; treat first with diphenhydramine (Benadryl) in age-appropriate dose, apply hydroxyzine (Atarax) for itching, and give daily baths with colloidal oatmeal (Aveeno).

106. A 6-month-old infant is brought to the clinic for a rash on the face and diaper area that consists of linear erythematous burrows. An older sibling has a similar rash on his wrists and between his fingers. What would be an appropriate intervention?
    1. Bacitracin ointment.
    2. Mycitracin ointment.
    3. Acitretin (Soriatane).
    4. Permethrin 5% cream (Elimite).

107. An adolescent female presents to the office with a long history of facial acne. She has been seen by several dermatologists and has been treated over the last 3 years with multiple therapies, including topical antibiotics, drying agents, intralesional injections of corticosteroids, and multiple systemic antibiotics, without success. After consulting with the collaborating physician, the family nurse practitioner prescribes isotretinoin (Accutane). What would teaching/counseling related to the use of this medication include?
    1. No dietary/alcohol restrictions are necessary.
    2. Exposure to sunlight without burning can be helpful in hastening the healing process.
    3. Eliminate all fat from the patient's diet.
    4. Emphasize the importance of effective contraception if the patient is sexually active.

108. A father brings in his 4-year-old son to the emergency department immediately after the boy ingested a small bottle of aspirin. What is the family nurse practitioner's priority?
    1. Insert a nasogastric tube and attach to low suction.
    2. Give 16 oz of orange juice.
    3. Give 8 oz of milk.
    4. Give activated charcoal.

109. The family nurse practitioner is aware that the toxic symptoms of salicylate poisoning are:
    1. Tinnitus and nausea.
    2. Itching and blurred vision.
    3. Fruity odor to the breath.
    4. Fever and chills.

Musculoskeletal

110. The family nurse practitioner is assessing a preadolescent girl for scoliosis. How is this test conducted?
    1. Have the girl bend at the waist and look for asymmetry in the back and hip area.
    2. Examine the child fully clothed, paying particular attention to the hips and back.
    3. Have the child walk heel-to-toe and observe the gait and pelvis.

    4. Place the child on her back and flex the knees and observe for misalignment.

111. In doing a physical assessment on a newborn, the family nurse practitioner notes a "hip click." What other findings are associated with this condition?
    1. Shortened quadriceps.
    2. Lateral deviation of patella.
    3. Limited abduction.
    4. Lax hamstrings.

112. An adolescent complains of right knee pain immediately after running in track practice. On exam, the knee is warm to touch, and a tender, swollen tibial tuberosity is noted. What does the family nurse practitioner suspect?
    1. Osgood-Schlatter's disease.
    2. Rheumatoid arthritis.
    3. Acute tendinitis.
    4. Posttraumatic knee effusion.

113. Nighttime extremity pain in school-age children that is deep but not present in the joints and that may be caused by inflammation of the muscle bodies in tight fascial sheaths and by periods of high activity is:
    1. Osgood-Schlatter's disease.
    2. Patellofemoral stress syndrome.
    3. Growing pains.
    4. Shin splints.

114. The family nurse practitioner is teaching crutch walking to an adolescent with a lower leg cast for a fractured tibia. What would instructions for assisting the adolescent to walk up the stairs include?
    1. Place both crutches on the upper step and step up with unaffected leg while balancing on crutches.
    2. Position the affected leg on the upper step and use the crutches to move up.
    3. Place the unaffected leg on the upper step and move affected leg and crutches up together.
    4. Position the affected leg and the crutch on the upper step and bring the unaffected leg up with the crutch.

115. An adolescent patient is being evaluated by the family nurse practitioner for knee pain. The patient is active in sports in his school but can recall no specific injury to the knee. On exam, the family nurse practitioner finds unilateral swelling of the anterior aspect of the tibial tubercle, which is tender. What is the most likely diagnosis?
    1. Stress fracture.
    2. Patellar dislocation.
    3. Osgood-Schlatter's disease.
    4. Neuman's syndrome.

116. Which of the following is the most accurate statement about juvenile rheumatoid arthritis (JRA)?
    1. Symptoms present in much greater severity than in adult RA.
    2. Complete remission occurs in three-fourths of patients.
    3. More than 90% of cases progress to severe joint destruction.
    4. Cytotoxic drugs should be initiated as early as possible in the treatment regimen.

117. What must children with juvenile rheumatoid arthritis (JRA) be screened regularly for?
    1. Ulcerative colitis.
    2. Iridocyclitis.
    3. Diabetes mellitus.
    4. Adrenal insufficiency.

118. An adolescent who twisted his knee while skateboarding comes to the clinic complaining of knee pain. He also states that in the past few weeks his knee has "locked up a couple of times." On exam, a positive McMurray's test is elicited. What diagnosis is this consistent with?
    1. Anterior cruciate ligament tear.
    2. Dislocated patella.
    3. Medial meniscus tear.
    4. Chondromalacia patella.

119. In young children, a complaint of hip pain without a history of trauma suggests several differential diagnoses. Which diagnosis is considered a true orthopedic emergency?
    1. Toxic synovitis of the hip.
    2. Legg-Calvé-Perthes disease.
    3. Increased femoral anteversion.
    4. Avascular necrosis of the femoral head.

120. Differentiation between structural and functional scoliosis can be done by placing the child in Adam's position. Which of the following occurs in this position?
    1. Structural scoliosis disappears, and functional scoliosis is enhanced.
    2. Persistent functional scoliosis is indicated.
    3. Functional scoliosis disappears, and structural scoliosis is enhanced.
    4. Curves greater than 10 degrees are indicated.

Neurology

121. In infants, especially preterm infants, seizures can present as:
    1. Coughing spells.
    2. Poor feeding.
    3. Awake apnea.
    4. Regurgitation.

122. The family nurse practitioner is caring for a 10-year-old child with meningitis. How would the family practitioner assess for the presence of nuchal rigidity?
    1. Have the child bend forward at the waist and observe the line of the spine.
    2. Place hand on child's forehead and ask child to press nurse's hand with his head.
    3. With the child relaxed, attempt to move his head side to side.
    4. Place hand on back of child's head and assist him to put his chin on his chest.

123. An adolescent girl is accompanied to the clinic by her mother, who states the school reports that she "stares off into space a lot" and does not seem to pay attention during these brief periods, which typically last 1–3 minutes. The neurologic exam is within normal limits. What should the family nurse practitioner suspect in the patient?
    1. Grand mal seizure.
    2. Complex partial seizure.
    3. Absence seizure.
    4. Simple partial seizure.

124. A child is admitted to the rural clinic after a car accident in which she sustained a closed head injury and fractured femur. The child is lethargic and follows commands slowly, and her pupils are equal and reactive. The child is to be transferred to a hospital by air ambulance. In assessing the child, what would the family nurse practitioner consider as a significant change in her condition?
    1. Urine output is less than 500 mL in 24 hours.
    2. She complains of a headache in the frontal area.
    3. She is able to move her lower extremities to command.
    4. Vital signs are blood pressure of 130/50 mm Hg and pulse of 70 beats/min.

125. Which three statements made by a 5-month-old infant's caregiver would make the family nurse practitioner consider shaken baby syndrome?
    1. "He's not breathing like usual."
    2. "He hit his head last night when sitting on our floor."
    3. "He won't wake up for me no matter what I do."
    4. "He feels hot to me, but I don't have a thermometer."
    5. "I left him with the babysitter like usual when I worked today."

126. Febrile seizures in young children are expected to disappear by approximately what age?
    1. 12 months of age.
    2. Two years of age.
    3. Three years of age.
    4. Five years of age.

127. A parent whose son was recently diagnosed with Tourette's syndrome asks the family nurse practitioner about the condition. The family nurse practitioner understands that:
    1. Tourette's syndrome is usually treated with antianxiety agents, such as diazepam (Valium).
    2. The tics may occur often throughout the day and may change over time.
    3. Children rarely have attention deficit/hyperactivity disorder (ADHD) in conjunction with Tourette's syndrome.
    4. Tics are typically neuromuscular (e.g., facial grimacing, tongue protruding, neck twitching) and rarely vocal.

128. A 3-week-old infant has been diagnosed with bacterial meningitis. The family nurse practitioner is aware that the most common causative organism is:
    1. *Streptococcus pneumoniae.*
    2. *Escherichia coli.*
    3. *Neisseria meningitidis.*
    4. Group B *streptococcus.*

129. The family nurse practitioner is seeing a 3-year-old child with a history of hospitalization at 18 months for bacterial meningitis and treatment with ampicillin and gentamicin. Which test should the family nurse practitioner make sure to include in the exam?
    1. Vision testing.
    2. Hearing testing.
    3. Lumbar puncture.
    4. Electrocardiogram (ECG).

130. Which is considered a likely cause of seizures in adolescents and young adults?
    1. Congenital abnormalities and metabolic disturbances.
    2. Metabolic disorders, central nervous system (CNS) infection, and fever.
    3. Idiopathic disease, trauma, and substance abuse.
    4. Trauma, malignant tumor, and cerebrovascular accident.

131. A child presents with a history of a purpuric rash with a centrifugal distribution and a fever. After the family nurse practitioner examines this child, what would be the most important condition to rule out at this time?
    1. Rubella.
    2. Lyme disease.
    3. Meningococcemia.
    4. Roseola.

132. A mother brings her 5-year-old son to the clinic with complaints that he is "acting funny." She states there are brief periods when he does not respond to her, and then he suddenly responds and acts as if nothing has happened. The nurse would initially evaluate the child further for the presence of:
    1. Petit mal or absence seizures.
    2. Attention deficit disorder.

    3. Horner's syndrome.
    4. Avoidance disorder of childhood.

133. Which finding would lead the family nurse practitioner to consider shaken baby syndrome in an infant?
    1. Visible head trauma.
    2. Subconjunctival hemorrhages.
    3. Anisocoria.
    4. Retinal hemorrhages.

134. Which statement about autism is correct?
    1. Autism has no gender preference.
    2. There is no genetic predisposition.
    3. Delay in motor development is an expected comorbidity.
    4. Language skills are delayed or underdeveloped.

135. Which of the following statements is true regarding cerebral palsy (CP)?
    1. CP can be reversed.
    2. It is more common in females than in males.
    3. Delayed motor milestones is the hallmark of the disorder.
    4. Cognitive impairment is an expected finding.

136. During physical exam of a child diagnosed with chronic recurrent seizures who is currently receiving antiepileptic medication, the family nurse practitioner notes hyperplasia of the gums. The nurse understand that hyperplasia of the gums is:
    1. An unusual side effect of phenobarbital.
    2. A common side effect of phenytoin.
    3. Common with chronic recurrent seizures.
    4. Caused by poor oral hygiene.

Gastrointestinal

137. The viral gastroenteritis seen in older children and adults has a short incubation (18–72 hours) and short duration (24–48 hours), is characterized by abrupt onset of nausea and abdominal cramps, followed by vomiting and diarrhea, and is often accompanied by headache and myalgia. What causes this disorder?
    1. Enteric adenovirus.
    2. Enteric calicivirus (Norwalk).
    3. *Rotavirus.*
    4. *Cytomegalovirus.*

138. The family nurse practitioner is interpreting the notation of "string sign" on an upper gastrointestinal (GI) series performed on an infant. What diagnosis is this associated with?
    1. Intussusception.
    2. Hirschsprung's disease.
    3. Pyloric stenosis.
    4. Gastroesophageal reflux.

139. The family nurse practitioner identifies the following condition as most conducive to the development of metabolic alkalosis in a child:
    1. Severe anxiety resulting in hyperventilation.
    2. Excessive vomiting related to gastroenteritis.
    3. Depressed respirations from excessive narcotics ingestion.
    4. Decreased renal function with glomerular damage.

140. The family nurse practitioner in the emergency department examines a child with severe diarrhea and vomiting, which results in dehydration. One of the orders is to start an IV line of 500 mL normal saline with 10 mEq potassium to run at 23 mL/hr. The child takes nothing by mouth. What would be a priority action before initiating the IV fluid with potassium?
    1. Weigh the child.
    2. Obtain serum electrolyte values.
    3. Make sure the child is voiding adequately.
    4. Determine amount of previous fluid loss.

141. An 18-month-old child is brought to the clinic by her mother and is complaining of abrupt onset of vomiting, followed by more than 10 liquid stools with mucus for the last 48 hours. The temperature is 100°F (37.8°C) orally. The stool smear obtained by the family nurse practitioner is negative for white blood cells (WBCs). What is the most likely etiologic pathogen for this young child's gastroenteritis?
    1. *Rotavirus.*
    2. *Shigella dysenteriae.*
    3. *Campylobacter jejuni.*
    4. *Salmonella.*

142. What are the symptoms of abdominal discomfort after meals, diarrhea or constipation, anorexia, weight loss, and failure to grow most often associated with?
    1. Ulcerative colitis.
    2. Irritable bowel syndrome.
    3. Carcinoma of the colon.
    4. Crohn's disease.

143. What are the most consistent clinical findings in children with acute appendicitis?
    1. An elevated white blood cell (WBC) count and pyuria.
    2. High fever and tenderness around the umbilicus.
    3. Low-grade fever and periumbilical abdominal pain.
    4. Nausea, vomiting, and diarrhea.

144. What question by the family nurse practitioner would be appropriate to ask the parents of an infant suspected of intussusception?
    1. "Does the infant have clay-colored stools?"
    2. "Does the infant have projectile vomiting?"
    3. "Does the infant have constant abdominal pain?"
    4. "Does the infant have red currant jelly stools?"

145. What is the major symptom of reflux in infants?
    1. Vomiting or regurgitation, especially after feeding.
    2. Poor weight gain in infants.
    3. Hyperirritability and refusal of feeding.
    4. Fever and diarrhea.

146. What does the optimal medical therapy for young infants with vomiting or regurgitation of gastroesophageal reflux disease (GERD) consist of?
    1. Frequent small feedings and burping after each feeding.
    2. Placing the infant prone after frequent feedings.
    3. Placing the infant supine after feedings.
    4. Thickening the feedings and using proton-pump inhibitors.

147. What is true regarding the management of an infant born to an hepatitis B surface antigen (HBsAg)-positive mother?
    1. No prophylaxis against hepatitis B is required because the infant is not at risk for the development of hepatitis B based on exposure to mother.
    2. One dose of hepatitis B immunoglobulin should be administered by 36 hours after birth.
    3. The family nurse practitioner should administer one dose of hepatitis B vaccine.
    4. One dose of hepatitis B immunoglobulin should be administered within 12 hours of birth and a complete three-dose immunization of hepatitis B vaccine administered at the usual recommended intervals.

148. What physical findings would lead the family nurse practitioner to suspect Hirschsprung's disease in a 6-month-old infant?
    1. Rectal bleeding, diarrhea, and prolonged jaundice at birth.
    2. History of constipation and current abdominal distention.
    3. Irritability, vomiting, and dehydration.
    4. History of colic, bloody diarrhea, and nausea.

149. What is a common cause of acute abdominal pain in children under 5 years old?
    1. Appendicitis.
    2. Intussusception.
    3. Incarcerated hernias.
    4. Gastroenteritis.

150. The family nurse practitioner understands that common causes of recurrent abdominal pain in children are:
    1. Intussusception, gastroenteritis, and right lower lobe pneumonia.
    2. Psychogenic pain, trauma, and urinary tract infection.
    3. Parasitic infestation, lactose intolerance, and chronic stool retention.
    4. Incarcerated hernia, appendicitis, and inflammatory bowel disease.

151. An older adolescent is being seen for evaluation after a dirt-bike accident. The patient states that the bike flipped over and struck him on the abdomen. He has a hematoma just below the left anterior rib area. The family nurse practitioner must be particularly aware of which possibility?
    1. Ruptured bowel caused by blunt trauma.
    2. Bladder trauma caused by blunt trauma.
    3. Hypovolemia caused by ruptured spleen.
    4. Arrhythmias.

152. A 2-year-old Asian American comes to the clinic with her parents and infant brother. The chief complaint is abdominal pain with flatulence and diarrhea after eating. Until 3 months ago, the patient had continued to be breast-fed twice a day. What would the family nurse practitioner suspect?
    1. Irritable bowel syndrome (IBS).
    2. Hirschsprung's disease.
    3. Lactose intolerance.
    4. Food allergy.

153. A 10-year-old girl comes to the clinic with complaints of nausea, vomiting, and right upper quadrant pain during vigorous play. She is also more tired than usual. Serologic tests for immunoglobulin (Ig)M antibodies are ordered to rule out:
    1. Cholecystitis.
    2. Hepatitis A.
    3. Infectious mononucleosis.
    4. Hepatitis B.

154. A 2-year-old child is seen for a foreign body in the gastrointestinal tract. The family nurse practitioner pays particular attention to the size of the object, knowing that passing the ligament of Treitz is difficult with objects larger than:
    1. 5 cm.
    2. 8 cm.
    3. 10 cm.
    4. 12 cm.

155. A 2-month-old infant presents with coughing, which results in emesis that occurs when laid supine after eating. The infant has lost 1.3 lb since birth with a birth weight of 7.5 lb. The family nurse practitioner focuses the assessment toward the possibility of:
    1. Suck-swallow incoordination.
    2. Gastroesophageal reflux.
    3. Tracheoesophageal fistula.
    4. Infantile colic.

156. Shigellosis is diagnosed in a young child with bloody diarrhea. The family nurse practitioner knows *Shigella* is a bacteria that is transmitted by the fecal-oral route or swimming in contaminated water and is treated by:
    1. Amoxicillin in weight-based dosing for 10 days.
    2. Symptomatic treatment and antidiarrheal agent loperamide (Imodium) as needed.
    3. Symptomatic treatment, including fluid replacement, such as Pedialyte, and avoid any antidiarrheals.
    4. Trimethoprim-sulfamethoxazole (TMP-SMX; Bactrim) dosed age appropriately for 7 days.

157. A 3-year-old child is seen in the clinic for chronic, relapsing diarrhea. A stool for ova and parasites is obtained and is positive for *Giardia*. What is the most appropriate pharmacologic intervention?
    1. Ampicillin (Omnipen).
    2. Erythromycin (E-Mycin).
    3. Metronidazole (Flagyl).
    4. Tetracycline (Achromycin).

Urinary

158. A 5-year-old male patient is brought to the outpatient clinic with the child's mother complaining he has not urinated in the last 24 hours. The child had nausea, diarrhea, abdominal pain, and a low-grade fever for 3 days, which he states started improving yesterday. Physical exam reveals no abnormalities. Laboratory analysis reveals hemoglobin 10.1 g/dL, hematocrit 26%, and platelets 90,000 mm^3. Urinalysis is unable to be obtained initially. Which of the following should the family nurse practitioner suspect?
    1. Urinary retention.
    2. Viral syndrome.
    3. Nephrotic syndrome.
    4. Hemolytic uremic syndrome (HUS).

159. Which clinical finding is *not* associated with acute glomerulonephritis in a child?
    1. Urine culture *Escherichia coli* greater than or equal to 50,000 colony-forming units/mL.
    2. Hypertension.
    3. Proteinuria.
    4. Tea-colored urine.

160. Congenital genitourinary anomalies may place a child at risk for:
    1. Lifelong urinary incontinence, dysmotility, and pain.
    2. Infection, impaired fertility, and impaired renal function.
    3. Constipation, tethered spinal cord, and delayed ambulation.
    4. Chronic diarrhea, kidney stones, and poor nutrition.

161. The family nurse practitioner suspects acute pyelonephritis in an older child. What clinical finding is *not* found?
    1. Flank pain.
    2. Hematuria.
    3. Fever.
    4. Frequency and urgency.

162. A child has a history of several episodes of acute pyelo-nephritis and has known renal scarring. What should be performed on follow-up visits? (Select 2 responses.)
    1. Blood pressure measurement.
    2. Urine culture and sensitivity.
    3. Urine dipstick for leukocyte esterase.
    4. Urine test for proteinuria.
    5. Streptozyme test.

163. Which of the following patients would the family nurse practitioner refer to a urologist? (Select 3 responses.)
    1. Infant aged 2 months with possible urinary tract in-fection (UTI).
    2. Boys after third UTI.
    3. Girls after second UTI.
    4. All children with gross hematuria.

Male Reproductive

164. Circumcision can prevent which of the following?
    1. Paraphimosis.
    2. Epididymitis.
    3. Sexually transmitted disease.
    4. Prostatitis.

165. A 15-year-old male presents with complaints of severe scrotal pain for the last 2 hours. The scrotum is swollen and extremely tender; palpation of the epididymis is not possible. What does the family nurse practitioner rec-ognize as the immediate treatment?
    1. Narcotic analgesics and bed rest.
    2. Warm packs and scrotal support.
    3. Antibiotics, ice packs, and analgesics.
    4. Referral to a surgeon for exploration.

166. Cryptorchidism is most commonly found in the:
    1. Infant with history of 25 week prematurity.
    2. Infant with history of 43 week postmaturity.
    3. Term infant.
    4. Toddler who is potty training.

Female Reproductive

167. While assessing a 16-year-old girl, the family nurse practitioner was asked about douching. What informa-tion would be used in the family nurse practitioner's teaching plan?
    1. Douching during menstruation is safe.
    2. Daily douching is important because the patient has copious vaginal discharge.
    3. Hypoallergenic douches include flavored or per-fumed types.
    4. Douching removes natural mucus and upsets nor-mal vaginal flora.

168. A high school athlete presents to the clinic with con-cerns regarding her menstrual periods. She states she has not had a period in the last 2 months. She has been in training and running about 3 miles a day for the last 3 months. She has lost approximately 15 lb. Her height is about 63 inches, and she currently weights 100 lb. What is the best response by the family nurse practitioner?
    1. Determine the patient's percentage of body fat and body mass.
    2. Obtain follicle-stimulating hormone serum levels.
    3. Determine serum levels of human chorionic gonad-otropin (hCG).
    4. Order thyroid function tests.

169. During a gynecologic exam at the family planning clinic, an underweight 17-year-old presents with bruis-ing around her upper torso and genitalia. She is mini-mally interactive and avoids eye contact as much as possible. Priority intervention should focus on:
    1. Laboratory work to rule out bleeding disorder.
    2. Nutritional assessment to determine possible anemia.
    3. Determination of possible physical abuse.
    4. Finding out if she has a support system.

Newborn

170. The family nurse practitioner is measuring a newborn's frontal-occipital circumference. What does the correct technique involve?
    1. Placing the paper tape measure at the maximal occipital prominence and just above the eyebrows.
    2. Placing the cloth tape measure at a level 2 inches above the ears.
    3. Using a cloth tape to prevent inaccuracy caused by stretchable materials.
    4. Having another person hold the tape in the center of the forehead and repeating the measurement.

171. Which newborn screening tests are mandatory state requirements?
    1. Complete blood count and urinalysis.
    2. Thyroid function test and phenylketonuria (PKU).
    3. PKU and alpha-fetoprotein.
    4. Glucose and thyroid function tests.

172. The family nurse practitioner notes an undescended testicle on a newborn. She understands that testicular function and the ability to produce healthy sperm as an adult may be impaired if the repair is not made by age:
    1. 6 years.
    2. 2 years.
    3. 1 year.
    4. 6 months.

173. The family nurse practitioner is examining a full-term infant who developed physiologic jaundice and is being treated with phototherapy. What is the mechanism of action of phototherapy in the treatment of this infant?
    1. The light is absorbed by bilirubin and promotes the conversion of a toxic bilirubin to an unconjugated product that can be excreted in the bile.
    2. It increases hemolysis of the excessive red blood cells that are received by the full-term infant during labor and delivery.
    3. The ultraviolet light decreases sensitivity to the destruction of red blood cells secondary to the Rh incompatibility.
    4. It increases enzymatic activity in breaking down the unconjugated bilirubin to a nontoxic form to be eliminated by the kidney.

174. A 4-day-old infant who is being breast-fed begins to develop jaundice. What is a common theory regarding the precipitating cause of this jaundice?
    1. Decreased intake in the first few days and the subsequent weight loss.
    2. Decreased tolerance and digestion of the breast milk.
    3. Increased destruction of red blood cells with release of bilirubin.
    4. Antigen-antibody reaction that increases destruction of fetal red blood cells.

175. Which infant is at an increased risk for development of "bronze baby syndrome"?
    1. Premature infant with ABO incompatibility.
    2. Asian infant who is bottle-fed.
    3. Caucasian infant who is breast-fed.
    4. Presence of obstructive liver disease.

176. A mother brings her 6-week-old infant to the office with concern over the child's "constant crying." She states she did not have this problem with her other two children. She is bottle-feeding the infant, and there is no problem with feeding. The infant has a bowel movement every day, and the stools are soft. The infant is afebrile with no evidence of ear, throat, lung, or abdominal problems. What is the best diagnosis for this infant?
    1. Infantile colic.
    2. Spastic colon.
    3. Infant stress syndrome.
    4. Lactose intolerance.

177. The family nurse practitioner suspects infantile colic in a 2-month-old infant. A complete physical exam reveals no abnormalities. What further study might the family nurse practitioner order?
    1. Chest radiograph.
    2. Complete blood count and differential.
    3. Blood culture.
    4. None of the above.

178. The family nurse practitioner is discussing with the parents the care of their 1-month-old infant, who has been diagnosed with infantile colic. What is important to explain to the parents?
    1. The problem may be decreased by not feeding the infant more often than every 3 hours.
    2. No specific medication is indicated to treat the problem.
    3. The problem is often related to increased stress in the home; family therapy may be indicated.
    4. The formula should be changed from a milk-based to a soy-based formula.

179. The family nurse practitioner is assessing an infant who was delivered by cesarean section. What is a complication frequently associated with cesarean delivery?
    1. Increased levels of serum bilirubin.
    2. Respiratory distress.
    3. Meconium aspiration.
    4. Hypoglycemia.

180. The family nurse practitioner is assessing an infant's respiratory status immediately after birth. Breath sounds are normal, no retractions present, acrocyanosis present, respirations of 70 breaths/min and irregular with 5-second periods of apnea, pulse regular at 160 beats/min, and first and second heart sounds normal with no murmurs. What is the initial interpretation of these findings?
    1. Normal newborn findings for immediately after birth.
    2. Symptoms suggestive of respiratory distress syndrome.
    3. Increased probability of neonatal asphyxia.
    4. Presence of choanal atresia.

181. The family nurse practitioner is performing a newborn assessment on a full-term infant approximately 6 hours after birth. When evaluating the infant's head, the family nurse practitioner identifies an edematous area that crosses the cranial suture lines, is soft, and varies with size. The cranial suture lines have minimal space between them. What is the family nurse practitioner's interpretation of these findings?
    1. A cephalhematoma is present.
    2. The cranial suture lines indicate premature closing.
    4. Molding of the infant's head is present.
    5. A caput succedaneum is present.

182. The nurse is evaluating an infant 8 hours after delivery. The infant was full term, weighed 10 lb at birth, and is being breast-fed. The mother has a history of gestational diabetes during the pregnancy. What findings indicate the need for further evaluation?
    1. Blood glucose of 50 mg/dL with glucose screening strips.
    2. Respirations of 70 breaths/min, tremors, and jitteriness.
    3. Bilirubin level 3 mg/dL.
    4. No passage of meconium stool.

Mental Health

183. While taking a history, the family nurse practitioner is aware that the following drug is most commonly the first one that an adolescent uses:
    1. Nicotine.
    2. Alcohol.
    3. Marijuana.
    4. Crystal methamphetamine.

184. A mother brings her young child to the clinic, stating she fell off the porch swing. What assessment finding would cause the family nurse practitioner to consider the possibility of child abuse?
    1. Mother is very upset and stroking her daughter's hair.
    2. Child is crying and says her head and arm hurt.
    3. Child has red-, blue-, and green-colored bruised areas on her trunk.
    4. Child has a bruised, edematous area on forehead and shoulder.

185. In evaluating a 16-year-old female patient, which symptom would indicate anorexia nervosa?
    1. Refuses to discuss questions pertaining to food.
    2. Reflects a positive body image.
    3. States she is eating very well but has episodes of vomiting.
    4. The family states she refuses to stop her severe dieting.

186. A mother is concerned about her child having nightmares. The family nurse practitioner understands the difference between nightmares and night terrors is:
    1. Nightmares are vivid, frightening dreams recalled by the child.
    2. Nightmares rarely occur in children before age 4.
    3. Nightmares are accompanied by gross motor movements, labored breathing, and enuresis.
    4. Nightmares and night terrors are essentially the same and are unrelated to stressful events.

187. A 16-year-old adolescent boy is 54 inches in height. The family nurse practitioner identifies the following as a positive, effective coping behavior:
    1. Acts as the class clown.
    2. Has a rehearsed reply to teasing comments.
    3. Spends most of his free time watching television.
    4. Has predominantly friends that have short stature.

188. The family nurse practitioner is examining an older adolescent who has been a long-term intravenous cocaine user. What other findings would alert the family nurse practitioner to a frequent complication?
    1. Epistaxis and chronic rhinorrhea.
    2. Cardiac arrhythmias and hypertension.
    3. Chest congestion and wheezing.
    4. Hepatitis and cellulitis.

189. The family nurse practitioner is comparing the typical signs of depression in the adolescent with the adult patient. The depressed adolescent would present with:
    1. Lonely feelings.
    2. Sad, flat affect.
    3. Anger and acting-out behavior.
    4. Feelings of powerlessness and anxiety.

190. The effects of prenatal cocaine exposure on newborns includes:
    1. Increased incidence of prematurity.
    2. Large for gestational age.
    3. Caput succedaneum.
    4. Hypotonia and lethargy.

191. While interviewing a teenager to determine her level of health, the family nurse practitioner recognizes symptoms of anorexia nervosa. Which characteristics of anorexia nervosa would be noted in the admission assessment interview?
    1. Below-to-average intelligence.
    2. Increased libido.
    3. Vigorous daily exercise.
    4. Tachycardia.

192. What does the family nurse practitioner expect a preschool child with attention deficit/hyperactivity disorder (ADHD) to have?
    1. Delayed growth and development, especially language skills.
    2. Negativism, overactivity, and active curiosity.
    3. Diminished fine motor skills and frequent mood swings.
    4. Easy distractibility, impulsiveness, and fidgeting.

193. The family nurse practitioner is completing a history and physical exam on a child whom she suspects may be autistic. Which of the following findings is associated with autism?
    1. Delay in language development.
    2. Delay in physical growth.
    3. Overprotective parents who provide minimal social interaction for the child.
    4. Warm, cuddling child with excessive need for interaction.

194. The mother of a preschooler is concerned because her child has begun to stutter. What should the family nurse practitioner do?
    1. Refer the child to a speech pathologist.
    2. Encourage the mother to correct the child when she stutters.
    3. Give the child verbal exercises to perform at home.
    4. Reassure the mother that stuttering is normal in a preschooler.

195. A teenage female patient is brought to the family nurse practitioner for evaluation by her grandmother with whom she lives. The teenager has been vomiting and her grandmother believes that she is becoming confused. The grandmother relates that the patient has been upset lately over a breakup with her boyfriend. What will the family nurse practitioner investigate as a possible cause for the teenager's symptoms?
    1. Appendicitis.
    2. Ectopic pregnancy.
    3. Drug overdose.
    4. Sexually transmitted disease.

196. A teenager comes to the office of the family nurse practitioner and states that she was raped several hours ago by her boyfriend. What immediate action should be taken by the family nurse practitioner?
    1. Perform a pelvic exam to determine injuries to the patient.
    2. Accompany her to the emergency department for an exam.
    3. Send her immediately for counseling to help her deal with this situation.
    4. Call the patient's parents so they can be with her.

197. The parents of a 7-year-old boy ask advice regarding sugar intake, stating the teacher has said not to allow the child to have any sugar products, such as cookies at lunch, because of behavior problems. Advice would include:
    1. The child needs further assessment for attention deficit/hyperactivity disorder (ADHD).
    2. Moderate sugar consumption rarely produces inappropriate behavior.
    3. Increase the protein and fat in his diet to decrease nerve overstimulation.

    4. Research has shown increased sugar intake directly affects cognitive performance.

198. What condition of a child would the family nurse practitioner identify as most likely to be the result of abuse?
    1. Concussion in a 4 year old.
    2. Fractured wrist in a 6 year old.
    3. Femur fracture in a 6 month old.
    4. Scald burn on the arm of a 1 year old.

199. While interviewing an adolescent female presenting with her mother for birth control counseling and exam, you detect signs of family tension. During the physical exam, while the mother is out of the room, the daughter admits to frequent marijuana use and occasional drinking. What assessment information would most confirm the presence of active or potential violence in the home?
    1. Signs of general neglect.
    2. Injuries at different stages of healing.
    3. Patient's response to a direct question.
    4. Admitted fear of mother's boyfriend.

200. The family nurse practitioner's physical exam on an adolescent is as follows: disheveled appearance, 5-lb weight loss since the last visit 2 months ago, pulse strong and regular at 128, +4 deep tendon reflexes, and nasal mucosa erythematous and ulcerated. His mother relates that he has been getting in trouble at school, avoids the family, has no appetite, and is not sleeping much at night. The family nurse practitioner suspects drug use of:
    1. Heroin.
    2. Marijuana.
    3. Lysergic acid diethylamide (LSD).
    4. Crack cocaine.

18 Pediatrics Answers & Rationales

Endocrine

1. Answer: 3

Rationale: Thyroid replacement is lifelong maintenance therapy and should be given as one dose in the morning and absorbs best 1 hour before or 2 hours after a meal. Weight loss, diarrhea, and tachycardia are signs of overmedication.

2. Answer: 1

Rationale: This is the best choice for the initial exam because the history may reveal normal variation in pattern of growth related to race, heredity, size of other family members, and psychosocial status. Skeletal maturation ("bone age") can be assessed through radiography if child is in the 5th growth percentile or lower. Other choices are inappropriate without history and physical exam, and growth hormone would not be administered without laboratory evaluation.

3. Answer: 3

Rationale: Pubertal (physiologic) gynecomastia is a visible or palpable glandular enlargement of the male breast that can occur in healthy adolescents. Typically, the breasts are unequal in size and may be tender, nipples are often irritated from rubbing against clothing, and Tanner stages II–IV of pubertal development are noted. The symptoms of lymphadenopathy, goiter, asymmetric testes, and repaired hypospadias are associated with pathologic gynecomastia.

4. Answer: 2

Rationale: Hyperthyroidism in children most often affects girls and is an autoimmune disorder (Graves' disease) in which the body produces antibodies that stimulate thyroid-stimulating hormone receptors, causing overproduction of thyroid hormones and goiter. Hypothyroidism is associated with iodine deficiency.

5. Answer: 4

Rationale: The following findings are consistent with Turner's syndrome: short stature, gonadal dysgenesis, lymphedema (usually appearing in infancy), left-sided heart or aortic abnormalities, primary amenorrhea, and delayed onset of puberty. Fragile X syndrome is an inherited condition usually affecting males and characterized by a long, narrow face and prominent ears, mild to profound mental retardation, hyperactivity and poor attention span, and autistic-type behavior. Marfan's syndrome is a connective tissue disorder of tall and thin adolescents that is characterized by long limbs; narrow

hands; long, slender fingers; and nearsightedness. Klinefelter's syndrome is characterized by small testes, sterility, gynecomastia, and long legs.

6. Answer: 4

Rationale: Hypogonadism, associated with delayed sexual development, sexual infantilism, and small testes, is most often the contributing factor to growth retardation after age 10 years for girls and 12 years for boys. Other causes of decelerated growth or short stature include hypothyroidism, diabetes, and hypopituitarism. Chromosomal abnormalities would be noted at an earlier age.

7. Answer: 3

Rationale: The American Diabetes Association recommends most children have a pre-meal target range for blood glucose between 90–130 mg/dL if they can recognize the symptoms of hypoglycemia. A blood glucose of 60–75 mg/dL is too low and may predispose the child to hypoglycemia. The other options are too high.

8. Answer: 1

Rationale: Type 1 diabetes usually (but not always) appears before age 30 and is heralded by the three "P's": polydipsia, polyuria, and polyphagia.

9. Answer: 4

Rationale: Tight glycemic control is contraindicated in infants less than 2 years of age and should be instituted with extreme caution in children less than 7 years of age to avoid severe hyperglycemia injuring the developing brain.

10. Answer: 1

Rationale: Infants with hypothyroidism often have an abnormally pitched cry because of lethargy and delayed mental responsiveness. Hypertelorism does not produce an abnormal cry unless accompanied by microcephaly.

11. Answer: 3

Rationale: A low temperature and pulse, constipation, and fatigue are all signs of hypothyroidism; therefore the dose of levothyroxine needs to be increased. Levothyroxine toxicity would manifest with signs of hyperthyroidism. Constipation is a symptom of hypothyroidism and is not related to the child's fluid intake. Congenital hypothyroidism requires lifelong drug therapy.

Hematology

12. Answer: 4

Rationale: This clinical presentation would make the family nurse practitioner consider the diagnosis of leukemia, necessitating a workup. CBC with differential, along with platelet count (indicators of bone marrow function), is the diagnostic approach for leukemia. Further testing may be necessary, but the workup should always include a CBC.

13. Answer: 1

Rationale: The findings associated with iron-deficiency anemia include low MCV, decreased hemoglobin/hematocrit, and low reticulocyte count. Elevated MCV is associated with macrocytic anemias (e.g., pernicious anemia).

14. Answer: 4

Rationale: Dolls and puppets are effective teaching tools for the preschool child. Using the doll reflects the child's understanding of the procedure. Children will often withdraw and appear calm when they have feelings of anxiety.

15. Answer: 3

Rationale: Early presenting symptoms of ALL include pallor, bleeding, pain, and fever associated with infiltration of the bone marrow of proliferative lymphocytic cells, which ultimately leads to bone marrow failure. The symptoms splenomegaly, facial rash, cough, expiratory wheezing, bleeding, and hepatomegaly are often found in juvenile chronic myelogenous leukemia (CML). Bone pain, fever, and night sweats are often noted in CML.

16. Answer: 3

Rationale: With iron-deficiency anemia, the amount of oxygen-carrying hemoglobin is reduced. Long-term oxygen deprivation can lead to impaired cognitive and motor development. Pernicious anemia is associated with lack of intrinsic factor. Crohn's disease has a familial incidence and leads to diarrhea-related problems. The liver and spleen are both involved in red blood cell production.

17. Answer: 4

Rationale: Sickle cell disease is an autosomal recessive inherited disease transmitted by both parents, who are carriers of the sickle cell trait or have disease. Each pregnancy carries a 25% chance of sickle cell disease, a 25% chance of an unaffected child, and a 50% chance of the child carrying the trait. Depending on the country and state in which the parent was born and the parents' age, a hemoglobin electrophoresis would diagnose sickle cell disease and/or trait on a newborn screen.

18. Answer: 3

Rationale: Iron-deficiency anemia is often found in this age group, especially in infants who do not eat a balanced diet that includes foods rich in iron (e.g., iron-fortified cereals). This is a microcytic, hypochromic anemia with a decrease in serum iron (ferritin). MCV would be decreased.

19. Answer: 4

Rationale: The normal, full-term infant is born with sufficient iron stores to prevent iron deficiency for the first 6 months of life.

Urinary/Renal

20. Answer: 2

Rationale: Acute hypertension in children and adolescents is usually caused by an identifiable secondary cause, such as glomerulonephritis, because of a streptococcal infection.

21. Answer: 2

Rationale: The facial edema and increased BP are common. Generally, the child does not have a high fever, and the urine is not concentrated, but it may be decreased in amount.

22. Answer: 2

Rationale: Gross hematuria may occur for 1–2 weeks after the diuresis and microscopic hematuria for up to 2 years. It is essential that parents be educated about poststreptococcal glomerulonephritis to ensure they know what to expect and to ensure that they know what is considered abnormal. Appropriate education will ensure that the parent will know when to notify a health care professional.

23. Answer: 1

Rationale: The family nurse practitioner should contact the pediatrician immediately; this is frequently the first sign of a Wilms' tumor, which can be malignant. Because a Wilms' tumor is very fragile, the abdomen should not be examined. The family nurse practitioner should not wait for a referral because the child may not be seen immediately. The family nurse practitioner should contact the hospital pediatrician, radiologist, or surgeon by telephone to discuss the clinical findings and to arrange for radiologic testing. A UA and blood testing can be done, but often these tests are negative.

24. Answer: 1

Rationale: The clinical presentation indicates a urinary tract infection (UTI). The dipstick is positive for bacteria. The child may have had a reaction to sulfisoxazole, so it would be best to avoid sulfa drugs at this time. The other appropriate medication for UTI in children is amoxicillin. Ciprofloxacin is not recommended for children under 18 years old, and clarithromycin is not a first-line drug for UTI.

Cardiac

25. Answer: 2

Rationale: Weak or absent pulses are associated with coarctation of the aorta and are not indicative of the other cardiovascular diseases. Patent ductus arteriosus may present with a widened pulse pressure and a consistent murmur; pulmonary stenosis with fatigue, tachycardia, cyanosis or syncope.

26. Answer: 2

Rationale: A continuous murmur is consistent with PDA. The turbulent flow of blood from the aorta through the PDA to the pulmonary artery results in this characteristic murmur. Coarctation presents with upper extremity hypertension, systolic murmur, and weak or absent femoral pulses. Ventricular septal defect is characterized by a loud, harsh, pansystolic murmur heard best at the lower left sternal border. Aortic stenosis has a systolic murmur.

27. Answer: 4

Rationale: Most cases of HF in children result from congenital heart disease, and most occur during the first year of life. Although the clinical presentation of a child with CHD will vary with the specific defect, the clinical manifestations usually relate to the degree of HF or cyanosis.

28. Answer: 3

Rationale: Most cases of HF in infants result from congenital heart disease during the first 12 months of life. Symptoms result from the decreased cardiac output and the infant's compensatory mechanisms. Symptoms include tachypnea, dyspnea, tachycardia, pallor, and easy fatigability. Additional symptoms include periorbital edema, hepatomegaly, difficult feeding, and persistent cough. Diaphoresis, central cyanosis, and peripheral edema are not necessarily associated with HF but may be manifestations of the underlying congenital heart defect.

29. Answer: 1

Rationale: Congenital heart disease is usually classified as increased pulmonary blood flow, decreased pulmonary blood flow, or mixed or obstructive lesions. Tetralogy of Fallot is a decreased pulmonary blood flow lesion caused by pulmonary stenosis and shunting right to left (causing cyanosis). Children with cyanotic heart disease develop polycythemia to increase the oxygen-carrying capacity of the blood. Additionally, the child with a cyanotic heart defect should have a Hgb of at least 16 g/dL.

30. Answer: 1

Rationale: Although all these conditions can lead to hypertension, the most common in infants and young children is secondary hypertension because of renal disease (e.g., glomerulonephritis; polycystic kidneys; nephrosis). Endocrine-induced hypertension is the second most common cause.

31. Answer: 1

Rationale: The two major conditions known to play a causative role in the development of cardiovascular disease in children are untreated streptococcal infections involving group A β-hemolytic streptococci (leads to cardiac valve dysfunction) and Kawasaki disease (leads to coronary artery aneurysm).

32. Answer: 3

Rationale: Procedures for which endocarditis prophylaxis is recommended include dental procedures known to induce gingival bleeding. It also is recommended for surgical procedures that involve the respiratory mucosa such as tonsillectomy/adenoidectomy. Endocarditis prophylaxis is not recommended for insertion of tympanostomy tubes, cardiac catheterization, simple dental procedures, or endotracheal intubation. Cardiac catheterizations are done under sterile conditions, and prophylactic treatment is not recommended because of a very low incidence of infection. Endocarditis prophylaxis is for patients with prosthetic valves, prosthetic rings or chords used in cardiac repair, previous infective endocarditis, unrepaired critical congenital heart disease or repaired congenital heart disease with shunts, valvular regurgitation or prosthetic device, and cardiac transplant with valve regurgitation.

33. Answer: 4

Rationale: Metal detectors and electric fences have an electromagnetic field that could alter the pacemaker's function temporarily. In addition, the alarm will be set off as a result of the metal in the pacemaker. For the child with a pacemaker, an electric shock may irreparably damage the pacemaker, and immediate surgical replacement would be necessary. There is no risk of electromagnetic interference between the permanent pacemaker and household items such as electrical appliances, radios, electronic equipment, cellular phones, or microwave ovens. Most electrical appliances have filtering systems that prevent interference with the pacemaker's function, and pacemakers utilize shielding, filters, and bipolar leads to mitigate electromagnetic interference.

34. Answer: 1

Rationale: According to the Jones Criteria, in addition to two major manifestations (carditis, polyarthritis, Sydenham's chorea, erythema marginatum, and subcutaneous nodules) or one major and two minor manifestations (arthralgia, fever, elevated ESR, C-reactive protein, and prolonged PR interval), a diagnosis of rheumatic fever is highly likely if there is evidence of a previous group A β-hemolytic streptococcal infection.

35. Answer: 2

Rationale: Nausea, vomiting, and anorexia are common side effects of many medications. The first-degree AV block confirms the ingestion of digoxin in this situation. Tricyclic antidepressant toxicity is characterized by agitation and anticholinergic symptoms; furosemide toxicity is characterized by hypokalemia, weakness, and cardiac dysrhythmias; and aspirin toxicity is characterized by tinnitus, confusion, gastrointestinal symptoms, and rapid, deep respirations

Respiratory

36. Answer: 2

Rationale: Sweat chloride test is positive for cystic fibrosis (CF) because of the abnormal amount of sodium chloride in the sweat. Hemoccult is a test for blood in the stool. Sputum culture and sensitivity help determine which medication is effective against an organism. Glucose tolerance test is performed to diagnose diabetes. Genetic testing can be used. There are more than 1700 mutations of the CFTR gene, with likely more gene mutations that have not yet been discovered; thus a sweat test remains the "gold standard."

37. Answer: 1

Rationale: The child has the symptoms and history that are consistent with a partial airway obstruction from aspiration of a foreign body. Direct laryngoscopy or bronchoscopy is necessary to remove the foreign body. Chest physiotherapy may dislodge the object and force it farther into the airway. Antibiotics and epinephrine will not be effective. There is no need to intubate the infant if the foreign body can be removed.

38. Answer: 4

Rationale: Croup, epiglottitis, and tracheitis are all middle respiratory tract infections with a rapid onset. Bronchiolitis is a lower respiratory tract infection that has a more gradual onset and no "barking" sound to the cough. Diagnosis can be made on clinical picture or with a viral panel. Treatment is supportive therapy such as nasal suctioning, fluids, and antipyretics.

If oxygen saturations are low or infant cannot feed, the child may require hospitalization.

39. Answer: 4

Rationale: In CF, the stools are large, bulky, and foul smelling (steatorrhea) with insufficient pancreatic enzymes. Yellow stools are indicative of liver or gallbladder problems. Green stools often indicate a rapid transit time and may be associated with an infection.

40. Answer: 2

Rationale: In children too young to use a peak flowmeter properly, the inability to cry or complete a sentence may indicate an acute asthma attack. Obtaining an ABG is usually not performed in office settings, and a chest x-ray will most likely agitate the child and take too long to process.

41. Answer: 4

Rationale: Maintaining a high-caloric intake is important in the care of infants with BPD to promote growth and nourishment of developing lung tissue. Infants may have gastroesophageal reflux after feedings. Initially, positioning should be tried, and then feedings may be thickened or given in smaller amounts more frequently. If the problem persists or weight gain is inadequate, referral to a pediatrician is indicated.

42. Answer: 3

Rationale: If the child is up to date on immunizations, he should have had his vaccine for *Haemophilus influenzae* type b (Hib), the most common cause of epiglottitis. A dramatic decline in the incidence of epiglottis and *H. influenzae* type b infections is associated closely with the history of Hib vaccines. Considering the age of this child and the suddenness of the onset, the most likely diagnosis is foreign body aspiration.

43. Answer: 4

Rationale: A β-agonist (albuterol) by MDI is the first line of treatment to decrease airflow obstruction. Aminophylline by mouth would take too long to be effective. Epinephrine is used predominantly for anaphylactic reaction. Beclovent is a steroid inhaler that is most effective when used prophylactically rather than in acute episodes.

44. Answer: 3

Rationale: These are the common drugs used for combination therapy for the treatment of TB in children. Rimantadine is an antiviral, and pyrimethamine is an antimalarial. Montelukast therapy is not indicated because of the virulence of the tubercle bacillus.

45. Answer: 4

Rationale: Close contacts of patients with an active case of TB should be placed on isoniazid single-drug therapy, even if the tuberculin skin test is negative. This early treatment will destroy the tubercle bacilli before hypersensitivity develops. The isoniazid should be continued for 4 months for those whose skin test remains negative and who show no evidence of disease. If there is a positive skin test conversion, isoniazid (10–20 mg/kg) should be continued for 1 year. If the child develops TB symptoms, he should be given isoniazid and rifampin (10 mg/kg) for 1 year.

46. Answer: 3

Rationale: Rhinitis and a productive cough are common and are not cause for concern unless the mucus begins to change color and is accompanied by a high fever. The wheezes are also common, if the mucus is loose. A high fever and crackles after initially improving indicate further deterioration and possible bacterial infection (secondary pneumonia).

47. Answer: 2

Rationale: Pyridoxine (vitamin B_6) is added to prevent peripheral neuropathy. Foods containing tyramine and histamine (e.g., tuna, aged cheese, yeast, vitamin supplements) cause interaction with monoamine oxidase inhibitors. Anorexia, jaundice, malaise, and fatigue would be signs of hepatic involvement.

48. Answer: 1

Rationale: Bronchodilators are strongly discouraged in current evidence-based bronchiolitis guidelines. Antibiotics and antihistamines are not effective and should not be used. The condition is usually treated symptomatically. If oxygen saturations are low or infant cannot feed, the child may require hospitalization.

49. Answer: 1

Rationale: Medications should be taken only when the child is planning to exercise and anticipates respiratory difficulty. Cromolyn and beclomethasone are steroids and do not provide immediate relief. Theophylline should be avoided unless symptoms progressively worsen and cannot be controlled with inhalation therapy.

50. Answer: 2

Rationale: In all states CF newborn screening starts with evaluating infants for an elevated serum IRT, which is a biomarker for trypsinogen. When there is blockage in the pancreatic exocrine ducts, which occurs in CF, this prevents the release of trypsinogen in the small intestine. The increased circulating trypsinogen is because of blockage caused by decreased cystic fibrosis transmembrane conductance regulator activity, which is a protein that acts on the chloride channel. If the infant's serum IRT is elevated, a second step is required, which is DNA analysis looking for common mutations. If one or more mutations are found, the infant is referred to a Cystic Fibrosis Foundation–accredited care center for sweat chloride confirmative testing. The sweat chloride test has been the primary way to confirm a diagnosis of CF. A sweat chloride test measures the amount of chloride in the infant's sweat. A chloride value of 60 mmol/L or greater has been considered positive for a diagnosis of CF.

Immune and Allergy

51. Answer: 3

Rationale: A positive PPD for an immunocompetent child is 15 mm. A child who is HIV positive, immunocompromised, or exposed to an active case of TB is considered positive at 5 mm. The child (less than 4 years of age) who has chronic disease or has been exposed to HIV-positive individuals or persons born in a foreign country is considered positive at 10 mm.

52. Answer: 2

Rationale: The typical allergic facies consists of allergic shiners (black eyes), Dennie-Morgan lines (extra crease below the lower eyelids), and mouth breathing. Nasal polyps are uncommon in childhood allergic rhinitis. The nasal discharge with allergies is usually clear.

53. Answer: 3

Rationale: In adolescent and through adult atopic dermatitis, common sites are the popliteal and antecubital fossae, face, neck, upper arms and back, dorsa of the hand, feet, fingers, and toes.

54. Answer: 2

Rationale: Epinephrine would be the first-line drug to be injected for the treatment of the respiratory distress associated with an anaphylactic reaction. The dose for epinephrine (1:1000, SC) is 0.01 mL/kg for a child and 0.3–0.5 mL/kg for an adult. The onset of action of Benadryl elixir is not fast enough. Antiinflammatory drugs would not be given initially but may be given later, if needed, for generalized discomfort or pain at the sting site.

55. Answer: 4

Rationale: Although diphenhydramine, brompheniramine, and chlorpheniramine are antihistamines and could be prescribed, loratadine would have less central nervous system–sedating effects.

56. Answer: 3

Rationale: Although diphenhydramine could be administered for itching after the child's distress is relieved, the immediate concern is to prevent respiratory arrest from swelling of the throat's mucosa. The usual epinephrine dose for children is 0.01 mL/kg of the 1:1000 solution.

57. Answer: 3

Rationale: The most common food allergy worldwide is cow's milk, with egg and peanut as the second- and third-most common, respectively. Wheat allergy is in the top eight of food allergens, but milk must be ruled out first through an elimination diet. Dust mite and internal mold allergy as an inhalant trigger is unlikely in this age group and may be present by 4 or 5 years of age.

58. Answer: 4

Rationale: Type IV hypersensitivity reactions are delayed hypersensitivity disorders with symptoms that start after 1 day of exposure, such as with poison ivy contact; symptoms are not immediate. Flowering plants are nonallergenic because their pollen is heavy and spread by insects, not the wind as in grass and tree and weed pollen. Tree and grass pollen result in a type I hypersensitivity reaction that is immediate on exposure, resulting in atopic dermatitis, allergic rhinitis, asthma, or urticaria.

HEENT

59. Answer: 3

Rationale: Dental fluorosis causes surface pitting and staining, especially to the central and lateral permanent incisors. Tetracycline would have caused staining of all the teeth. Dental caries would be more indicative of poor dental hygiene. "Baby teeth," not the permanent teeth, would be affected by going to bed with a bottle.

60. Answer: 4

Rationale: Strabismus (malaligned eyes) can be a precursor for amblyopia (decreased visual acuity). It is important to detect strabismus as early as possible in preschool children. Checking pupils and assessing for double vision (diplopia) are components of a neurologic assessment. Tonometry exams are performed to assess for glaucoma.

61. Answer: 3

Rationale: Pure-tone audiometry is appropriate after age 3 years; 0–25 dB = normal, 26–40 dB = mild hearing loss, and 41–55 dB = moderate hearing loss.

62. Answer: 3

Rationale: Low-set or obliquely set ears occur more frequently in children who also have genitourinary defects. None of the other defects is associated with low-set ears.

63. Answer: 3

Rationale: Enlarged tonsils are common in young children. As the child grows older, the tonsils recede in size. Only about 25%–30% of tonsillitis is caused by the β-hemolytic streptococcus. Having large tonsils does not make a child more prone to tonsillitis.

64. Answer: 2

Rationale: The patient in this situation had risk factors (age) and symptoms of mononucleosis, so the monospot or heterophile antibody test should be conducted. The classic triad of mononucleosis symptoms includes sore throat, fever, and posterior cervical lymphadenopathy with or without mild tenderness. Rapid screening for streptococcal infection can be done from throat swab with antigen agglutination kits and would be obtained first, but it would probably be negative. WBC count would be ordered for bacterial pharyngitis; an increased WBC is found with bacterial infection and a decreased WBC with viral agents.

65. Answer: 2

Rationale: A fluoridated dentifrice should be used in a small amount (pea-size), and children under 6 should be supervised so that they do not swallow too much toothpaste, which would put them at risk for fluorosis. The dose of fluoride rinse is too high, and it is inappropriate to prescribe to a preschooler. Bottled water does not contain fluoride. Topical application, although appropriate, is not the best answer.

66. Answer: 3

Rationale: Generalized, diffuse swelling and erythema of the eyelid is associated with an insect bite. Blepharitis is a chronic inflammatory condition characterized by erythema and scaling of the lid margins. Hordeolum, or stye, is an acute, purulent inflammation of the sebaceous glands (usually the glands of Zeis or the meibomian glands) of the eyelids and usually does not involve the entire eyelid. It may be painful, especially over the gland. Dacryocystitis is an inflammation of the lacrimal sac that is characterized by erythema and swelling over the lacrimal duct.

67. Answer: 1

Rationale: Nasolacrimal obstruction occurs in up to 6% of infants. Signs and symptoms include a wet eye with mucoid discharge. Irritated skin and conjunctivitis also may be associated with this condition. There is no redness, which would suggest conjunctivitis. Congenital dacryocystocele presents at birth as a bluish subcutaneous mass. There would be more signs of irritation and pain with a corneal abrasion.

68. Answer: 1

Rationale: Strabismus is not an uncommon or abnormal occurrence in infants up until 3 months of age.

69. Answer: 4

Rationale: Classic signs of bacterial conjunctivitis include those symptoms listed along with complaints of eyelids being "glued shut" on awakening. Severe itching, moderate tearing, and minimal discharge symptoms are indicative of allergic conjunctivitis. Minimal itching, moderate tearing, and mucoid exudate symptoms are indicative of viral conjunctivitis.

70. Answer: 4

Rationale: Steroid (dexamethasone) medications are not used to treat nasolacrimal obstruction in infancy. Because of the yellow discharge in the eye, it would be appropriate to prescribe an antibiotic to prevent or treat conjunctivitis. Cleansing the eye with warm water and massaging the lacrimal duct are both appropriate interventions.

71. Answer: 1

Rationale: The diagnosis of AOM is clinical, made by otoscopy based on the appearance of the TM. The bony landmarks are absent or decreased. The TM may be full, bulging, or retracted, with pus, and the light reflex is distorted. A pneumatic otoscopy reveals decreased or absent TM mobility. Erythema is an inconclusive finding, especially in children, because the redness may be caused by crying rather than infection.

72. Answer: 4

Rationale: The patient has the clinical findings of otitis externa, an inflammation and infection of the external ear canal predisposed by excessive wetness, such as swimming. Common organisms responsible for otitis externa include *Pseudomonas aeruginosa, Proteus mirabilis,* and *Enterobacter aerogenes* or fungal organisms of the *Aspergillus* or *Candida* species. Sinusitis clinical findings focus on sinus tenderness and a purulent nasal discharge. Clinical findings of otitis media include ear pain, full or bulging tympanic membrane, decreased or negative mobility, and possible erythema. Findings associated with serous otitis media include opaque or translucent tympanic membrane with air bubbles; landmarks may be absent, and the light reflex may be diffuse or absent.

73. Answer: 1

Rationale: AOM occurs more during the fall, winter, and spring than summer. American Indians and Eskimos have more repetitive and severe otitis media than members of other races. Children who attend day care centers have more frequent infections than those who do not. Members of lower socioeconomic levels are more at risk than those at higher levels. Other risk factors are children who live with many siblings or in homes with smokers, children who have developmental abnormalities, and male gender.

74. Answer: 3

Rationale: The patient with otitis externa, "swimmer's ear," or inflammation of the external auditory canal presents with ear pain. The most common clinical findings include redness and swelling of the external ear canal, pain with manipulation of movement of auricle, no swelling or pain over mastoid, and usually no involvement of the TM. The TM is involved in AOM. No evidence indicated that the child placed a foreign body in the ear. The most significant distinction between OME and AOM is that clinical findings of acute infection (e.g., fever, otalgia) are lacking in OME. Clinical findings of OME, the most common cause of hearing loss in children, include relatively asymptomatic, decreased mobility, and bulging, opaque TM with no visible landmarks.

75. Answer: 3

Rationale: Transmission of cold viruses is indirect (e.g., self-inoculation from virus on surfaces of inanimate objects to mucous membranes of nose and mouth). Virus is less likely to be spread by the aerosol route; thus the patient should avoid touching the nose and mouth unless the hands have been thoroughly washed. It is impractical to avoid contact because cold viruses are found everywhere. Although many individuals believe vitamin C prevents colds, research to support this claim is minimal.

76. Answer: 4

Rationale: Amoxicillin with clavulanic acid is effective against β-lactamase production. Cephalexin, cefuroxime, or cefixime can be used as alternatives. Erythromycin-sulfisoxazole has recently been reported as less effective. Cephalosporins are effective against β-lactamase production by *H. influenzae* and *M. catarrhalis.* Amoxicillin is ineffective against β-lactamase production, as is penicillin V.

77. Answer: 3

Rationale: The recommended treatment for otitis media in a child is amoxicillin 75–90 mg/kg/day, or for this child (18 kg), 250 mg/5 mL, 2.75 tsp bid × 10 days. The other drugs and doses listed are not appropriate treatment for acute otitis media.

78. Answer: 4

Rationale: The patient is experiencing symptoms of moderately severe acute sinusitis based on the symptoms of facial pressure, headache, and postnasal discharge. The first-line antibiotic to prescribe is amoxicillin/clavulanate for its safety and efficacy. Oral antihistamines, such as diphenhydramine, should not be used unless the patient has allergies. Oral decongestants (pseudoephedrine) are not as effective in patients with sinusitis as are topical agents. Erythromycin is not a first-line antibiotic for sinusitis.

Integumentary

79. Answer: 4

Rationale: This best describes mongolian spots, which are characteristic in newborns of African, Asian, or Latin descent. When closely evaluated, these spots do not resemble the ecchymoses that occur with trauma. Telangiectatic nevi are commonly known as "stork bites" and are deep-pink lesions most often found on the back of the neck. Cutis marmorata is the transient mottling that occurs when an infant is cold.

80. Answer: 1

Rationale: The location and appearance of the lesions are typical of scabies: short, irregular runs that are approximately 2–3 mm long and the width of a hair. A rash causes little bumps that often form a line that is approximately 2 to 3 mm long and the width of a hair. The inflammatory lesions are erythematous and pruritic papules most commonly located in the finger webs, flexor surfaces of the wrists, elbows, axillae, buttocks, genitalia, feet, and ankles. The older adult may itch more severely with fewer cutaneous lesions and is at risk for extensive infestations, probably related to a decline in cell-mediated immunity. In addition, there may be back involvement in those who are bedridden.

81. Answer: 1

Rationale: Food allergies and other causative triggers should be identified and avoided. Excessive bathing dries the skin, which irritates the atopic dermatitis. Bubble baths can irritate skin, as can sweating.

82. Answer: 2

Rationale: This is the correct procedure for the permethrin cream rinse. After rinsing, remove nits with a nit comb. Repeat shampoo treatment after 7 days if living lice are still observed. Clothing and bedding should be washed or dry-cleaned.

83. Answer: 2

Rationale: Nonintentional scalding is usually splash-related and occurs on the front of the body. The family nurse practitioner should be suspicious of any burns on the back of the body or any well-defined, uniform burn areas on the buttocks or extremities, which may indicate physical abuse. Immersion burns on the buttocks may be seen as punishment for toileting or wetting "accidents."

84. Answer: 3

Rationale: The cornstarch or Aveeno baths will temporally help relieve the itching, followed by application of a heavy cream emollient (the thicker and greasier the emollient, the more effective). The shorts and short-sleeved shirt would expose too much skin, which would be scratched by the infant. Wool irritates the skin. Salt would also be an irritant.

85. Answer: 3

Rationale: The most common treatment is observation because most hemangiomas resolve over time, usually beginning about 18 months of age. The other treatments may be performed, especially for hemangiomas proliferating rapidly. Treatment with propranolol, topical, or laser therapy may be used. Propranolol is generally initiated inpatient, with nursing supervision of blood pressure and heart rate and blood glucose.

86. Answer: 2

Rationale: Infantile atopic dermatitis, as contrasted to atopic dermatitis in older children and adolescents, is a moist, oozing, crusting pruritic rash found mainly on the extensor surfaces of the body and the face. It usually begins about 2 months of age, often with a family history of atopy.

87. Answer: 1

Rationale: In prepubertal children, café-au-lait spots larger than 1 cm and present in more than five areas are a concern and may be associated with neurofibromatosis. The child should be referred to a pediatric neurologist for further evaluation.

88. Answer: 1

Rationale: Seborrheic dermatitis is usually salmon in color and has a yellowish, greasy appearance. It occurs in infants under 6 months of age. It does not itch. The distribution is mainly to the face, postauricular scalp, axillae, and groin. Rashes in atopic dermatitis and eczema are pink, or red if inflamed, and have a whiter, nongreasy appearance. Rash may begin at 2–12 months and continues through childhood and is associated with a family history of allergy. Itching may be severe. The distribution is to the cheeks, trunk, and extensors of extremities. Erythema toxicum consists of yellow or white papules on the face. It occurs in 30%–50% of term infants and disappears in 2 weeks.

89. Answer: 3

Rationale: Given the distribution of the rash, the most likely cause is a contact dermatitis, such as that caused by the use of baby wipes. Allergy to disposable diapers would involve the entire diaper area. Seborrheic dermatitis presents as large, confluent, sharply marginated bright plaque on the anterior surface of the groin. *Candida* rashes are bright red with satellite lesions that involve the deep folds and may spread to the entire diaper area.

90. Answer: 2

Rationale: Impetigo presents with honey-colored crusted lesions with an erythematous base. Staphylococci and group A streptococci are important pathogens in this disease. Scabies presents with linear burrows about the wrists, ankles, finger webs, anterior axillary folds, genitalis, or face (in infants). Pityriasis rosea presents as erythematous papules that coalesce to form oval plaques preceded by a large oval plaque with central clearing and a scaly border (the herald patch). Varicella (chickenpox) presents as crops of red macules that rapidly become tiny vesicles with surrounding erythema that form pustules. The pustules become crusted, and then scabs form. The rash appears predominantly on the trunk and face.

91. Answer: 4

Rationale: After a course of antibiotics, the normal flora is destroyed, making the child a prime target for *Candida albicans*. The classic signs of a yeast infection include a beefy red, sharply marginated, maculopapular rash with satellite lesions. Poor hygiene and a contact dermatitis would present as erythema and thickening of the skin in the perianal area. Seborrheic dermatitis consists of an erythematous, scaly dermatitis, accompanied by overproduction of sebum in areas rich in sebaceous glands (face, scalp, and perineum).

92. Answer: 2

Rationale: Atopic dermatitis typically presents in the flexural areas of children. The lesions are characteristically erythematous and papular, with scales and pruritus often noted. A personal or family history of atopy is noted in about 70% of patients with atopic dermatitis. Scabies lesions appear as gray or skin-colored ridges, vesicles, and papules. Tinea corporis lesions are generally distributed over the body and face, with an area of clearing in the center of the lesion. Contact dermatitis usually produces vesicular lesions in the shape of the object causing the reaction.

93. Answer: 4

Rationale: Brown recluse spiders produce sharp pain at the instant of the bite, with subsequent minor swelling and erythema. Tissue necrosis may occur within the next 24–96 hours. A blue-gray to black macular halo may surround the bite, with eventual widening and sinking of the center of the lesion, leading to a sinking infarct" This leaves a deep ulcer that requires weeks or months to heal.

94. Answer: 2

Rationale: Deep puncture wounds are more likely to become infected with anaerobic organisms. The narrow, sharp feline incisors deeply puncture tissue and may easily penetrate a bone or joint. Bites on the hand have the highest infection rate, whereas bites on the face have the lowest rate.

95. Answer: 1

Rationale: Amoxicillin-clavulanate is an excellent choice for the empiric treatment of animal bites. Cephalexin is not indicated because of resistant strains of *Pasteurella multocida*, an organism present in 25% of dog bites and 50% of cat bites. Avoid first-generation cephalosporins (e.g., cephalexin), penicillinase-resistant penicillins (e.g., dicloxacillin), macrolides (e.g., erythromycin), and clindamycin when it is not administered with another medication, as these medications are not effective against *P. multocida*. An infected bite should be followed up daily until the infection clears. Open wound management is indicated, not suturing.

96. Answer: 4

Rationale: In addition to these symptoms, bronchospasm, hypertension, seizures, and altered mental status may occur. Black eschar is associated with a brown recluse spider bite. Rash with bump or boil is typical of a bug bite.

Childhood Diseases

97. Answer: 2

Rationale: Erythema multiforme is a major side effect of sulfa drug use that presents with a sudden onset of high fever, weakness, blisters, bulla, and ulcerations of the mucous membranes. Kawasaki disease presents with a more diffuse erythematous rash. Viral exanthems are centrally located and do not resemble blisters. Scalded-skin syndrome is staphylococcal in origin and causes the skin to peel off and turn bright red.

98. Answer: 2

Rationale: The incubation period for erythema infectiosum is 4–14 days, with communicability until the rash appears.

99. Answer: 1

Rationale: The symptoms are indicative of coxsackievirus 5 or 16 group A (usually A16), called hand-foot-and-mouth disease. The lesions may appear in one or all three areas. Children are usually uncomfortable, but not seriously ill, and may refuse fluids with severe oral lesions. Varicella lesions begin on the trunk with classic "teardrop" vesicles.

100. Answer: 1

Rationale: In roseola, an erythematous, maculopapular rash appears on the trunk after abrupt onset of fever and spreads to the extremities, neck, and face. It fades within 24 hours. The pink maculopapular rash of rubella begins on the face and spreads down the trunk. Often the facial rash will disappear as the rash erupts on the extremities, clearing in 3–5 days.

101. Answer: 2

Rationale: The primary treatment for roseola is supportive, including control of fever, adequate rest, and hydration. No preventive measure or immunization is available.

102. Answer: 4

Rationale: Systemic antibiotics (e.g., tetracycline) offer the most effective treatment in inflammatory acne. Isotretinoin is also very effective but, because of serious teratogenic side effects, it is not first-line treatment. Improvement in acne will not be noted for 4–8 weeks, and dietary changes have not been demonstrated to have any beneficial effect.

103. Answer: 2

Rationale: The appearance is indicative of *Candida albicans,* which is best treated with nystatin. The other choices would aggravate the diaper rash by promoting overhydration.

104. Answer: 3

Rationale: The child's lesions are characteristic of impetigo and should be treated with an antibiotic if present on the face; amoxicillin-clavulanate (Augmentin) is considered the first-line medication. The ointment, soaking, and Benadryl will not stop the spread of the infection, which could lead to post-streptococcal glomerulonephritis.

105. Answer: 4

Rationale: Varicella (chickenpox) should be treated symptomatically unless the child is at high risk secondary to other medical problems. Acyclovir is not recommended for routine treatment of uncomplicated varicella. The current bathing therapy is with colloidal oatmeal products, taking preference over the traditional baking soda baths. Impetigo usually occurs on the face and neck with no diffuse lesions over the trunk. Contact dermatitis is characterized by erythema and scaling, possibly with weeping vesicles. The area of distribution of rash offers clues to diagnosis.

106. Answer: 4

Rationale: Permethrin 5% cream is used in infants but is not recommended in those under 2 months of age. Bacitracin could be used to treat secondary infections but would not help eradicate the scabies. Mycitracin is also not effective for the treatment of scabies. Acitretin is used for the treatment of psoriasis.

107. Answer: 4

Rationale: Because isotretinoin is extremely teratogenic, sexual assessment and pregnancy testing (as appropriate) and contraceptive counseling should be done for all patients. The combination of alcohol and isotretinoin can cause a disulfiram-like reaction, so alcohol should be avoided. Isotretinoin can cause photosensitivity, so the family nurse practitioner should counsel the patient to avoid sunlight, wear protective clothing and sunglasses, and apply sunscreen to all sun-exposed areas that are without acne. No conclusive relationship between diet and acne has been established.

108. Answer: 4

Rationale: An age-appropriate dose of activated charcoal (1g/kg of body weight) would be indicated. Gastric lavage may be of little benefit if used later than 1 hour after ingestion.

109. Answer: 1

Rationale: Tinnitus and nausea are toxic symptoms of salicylate poisoning. Fruity odor to the breath is usually associated with diabetic ketoacidosis.

Musculoskeletal

110. Answer: 1

Rationale: The child should remove her shirt (leave on bra or swimsuit top) and bend at the waist. The family nurse practitioner should examine for uneven hips and shoulders.

111. Answer: 3

Rationale: Typical findings include Ortolani's (hip click) sign, limited abduction, shortening of the extremity on the affected side, and asymmetric gluteal folds. The lax hamstrings allow for full extension of the hip when the knee is fully flexed. This child may need further evaluation (with a hip ultrasound) for congenital hip dysplasia. Babies at highest risk are females, breech delivery, firstborn, family history of congenital hip dysplasia, or oligohydramnios.

112. Answer: 1

Rationale: Osgood-Schlatter's disease (tibial tubercle apophysitis) is characterized by a painful, self-limiting tibial tubercle swelling that leads to knee pain, especially during periods of rapid growth. Extension of the knee against resistance or application of pressure over the tibial tubercle aggravates the pain. Pain worsens with activity and subsides with rest.

113. Answer: 3

Rationale: Growing pains usually occur at night and resolve by morning. The pain is deep and does not involve the joints. Osgood-Schlatter's disease results from degeneration of the tibial tubercle because of overuse and a rapid growth spurt. Pain and swelling occur over the tibial tubercle. Symptoms are exacerbated by activities that involve the quadriceps muscle. Another form of overuse syndrome is patellofemoral stress syndrome. Pain of a dull, aching quality is present in the knee, sometimes with clicking. Long periods of sitting or activities that involve knee flexion and compression of the patella in the groove cause increased pain. In shin splints, inflammation of muscles along the medial shaft of the tibia results from overuse and causes aching pain. Rest improves the pain. Improper warm-up exercises or extended exercise by an unconditioned person, especially in unsuitable shoes, can lead to this pain.

114. Answer: 3

Rationale: The unaffected leg goes up the step first, and then the crutches, followed by the affected leg. This allows for stability and weight bearing on the unaffected leg, with the crutches supporting the affected leg.

115. Answer: 3

Rationale: Osgood-Schlatter's disease is common in late childhood and adolescence. The risk for disease increases in patients who are involved in strenuous activity, especially involving the quadriceps muscle. The usual treatment is nonsteroidal antiinflammatory drugs and rest.

116. Answer: 2

Rationale: Most do not have disease persistent into adulthood. JRA symptoms present very similar to adult arthritis. Most disease activity diminishes with age; although some do have some residual joint damage, the percentage is not this high. Nonsteroidal antiinflammatory drugs (previously aspirin) are the treatment of choice, and cytotoxic drugs are reserved for patients in whom other therapies have failed.

117. Answer: 2

Rationale: Development of iridocyclitis may be insidious and asymptomatic and, if untreated, may cause blindness. Although children may develop any of the other listed diseases, there is no correlation with JRA.

118. Answer: 3

Rationale: A positive McMurray's test (palpable click and pain when rotating the foot laterally and extending the leg) along with the symptoms is indicative of a medial meniscus tear. The drawer test evaluates for anterior cruciate ligament tears (knee flexed with foot on table, sit on foot and grasp both sides of tibia at knee, pull tibia forward, abnormal if movement of tibia away from the joint).

119. Answer: 4

Rationale: Avascular necrosis results in death of the femoral head with revascularization. Toxic synovitis and increased femoral anteversion, while causing pain, are not bone threatening. Legg-Calvé-Perthes disease results in necrosis of the proximal femoral epiphysis; however, there is later revascularization.

120. Answer: 3

Rationale: In Adam's position (forward bending, arms loose at side, and thumbs hooked together), true scoliosis (structural) is demonstrated (by an elevated rib hump), whereas the functional type related to other conditions is not apparent. Persistent functional scoliosis can eventually become structural.

Neurology

121. Answer: 3

Rationale: Although it is important to investigate all episodes of apnea in infants, premature infants may not exhibit the typical tonic-clonic type seizures but may have awake apnea.

122. Answer: 4

Rationale: Nuchal rigidity is a stiff neck; the child cannot move his head forward and cannot bring his chin in contact with his chest. Movement of the head from side to side does not elicit nuchal rigidity.

123. Answer: 3

Rationale: This accurately fits the description of a petit mal or absence seizure, which is a type of generalized seizure that begins in childhood and usually ends in early adulthood (30s). There is usually impairment of consciousness, automatic symptoms, and mild tonic-clonic symptoms. Classically, staring off into space is the reporting symptom.

124. Answer: 4

Rationale: An increase in the pulse pressure and decrease in pulse rate are indications of increasing cerebral edema and intracranial pressure, which would necessitate immediate intervention. A child's urine output should be 20–30 mL/hr.

125. Answer: 1, 3, 4

Rationale: Shaken baby syndrome is associated with lethargic behavior and changes in breathing patterns. Fever is also an associated finding with brain injury. The infant should not have had a significant injury if the head was injured when falling over from a seated position on the floor. Any caregiver can be responsible, including parents.

126. Answer: 4

Rationale: Febrile seizures are most common between the ages of 6 months to 5 years. The peak incidence occurs between 12 and 18 months of age. Tonic-clonic seizure activity is the most common.

127. Answer: 2

Rationale: Tourette's syndrome is a hereditary, chronic neuromuscular disorder consisting of various motor and vocal tics. Tics are sudden, involuntary, brief, repetitive motor movements that often begin in childhood and change over time. ADHD frequently occurs concomitantly with Tourette's syndrome.

128. Answer: 4

Rationale: The most common cause of bacterial meningitis in the first month of life is group B streptococci. *S. pneumoniae* and *N. meningitides* are usually associated with meningitis after age 1 month in areas in which the conjugate *Haemophilus influenzae* type b (Hib) vaccines are used.

129. Answer: 2

Rationale: A formal hearing acuity test is most important in a child with a history of bacterial meningitis because of the ototoxic medications used to treat the disease. A vision test should be done on all children but is not specific for a child with a history of meningitis. A lumbar puncture or ECG would not be appropriate.

130. Answer: 3

Rationale: The most likely causes of seizures in adolescents and young adults are idiopathic disease, trauma, and substance abuse. Congenital abnormalities are the likely cause of seizures in newborns. In children under 6 years old, metabolic causes, CNS infection, and fever can cause seizures. Trauma, malignant tumor, and stroke are likely causes of seizures in elderly patients.

131. Answer: 3

Rationale: The most common finding in children with meningococcemia (71%) is fever and a purpuric rash. The rash of rubella, Lyme disease, and roseola is finer, and none of these problems is life-threatening, unlike with meningococcemia, which makes it a "do not miss" diagnosis.

132. Answer: 1

Rationale: The description is that of a petit mal or absence seizure. Although the etiology of the majority of seizures is unclear, the patient should be referred for neurologic evaluation to determine whether an underlying abnormality is present.

133. Answer: 4

Rationale: Retinal hemorrhages may be evident on fundoscopic assessment. This finding should lead the family nurse practitioner to suspect shaken baby syndrome or hypertension. Visible head trauma would typically be absent in shaken baby syndrome. Subconjunctival hemorrhages are not an associated finding. Anisocoria is a common finding in up to 20% of the population and not associated with increased intracranial pressure.

134. Answer: 4

Rationale: Delayed language development is an early sign of autism, along with impaired social interactions. Males are diagnosed more commonly than females, and there is a genetic influence with the genome responsible for early brain development. Motor skills are not affected in autism.

135. Answer: 3

Rationale: Delayed motor milestones and posture irregularities are the hallmark of the condition. CP affects males more often than females. It is not a reversible condition. Cognitive impairment is not always present in CP.

136. Answer: 2

Rationale: Hyperplasia of the gums is a common side effect of phenytoin (Dilantin). The child should have regular dental prophylactic hygiene to deal with the problem.

Gastrointestinal

137. Answer: 2

Rationale: Gastroenteritis is a common cause of abdominal pain in children. Symptoms vary depending on the type of viral infection. *Rotavirus* mainly affects infants 3–15 months of age in the winter months, causing voluminous watery diarrhea without leukocytes. Enteric adenoviruses are the second most common viral infection in infants, with symptoms similar to *rotavirus* except the duration of the illness may be longer. Enteric calicivirus (Norwalk) mainly causes vomiting but also diarrhea in older children and adults. Duration of symptoms is short, usually 24–48 hours. *Cytomegalovirus* rarely causes diarrhea and is common after bone marrow transplants and in late stages of HIV infection.

138. Answer: 3

Rationale: The string sign is indicative of a narrow pyloric channel and is associated with pyloric stenosis. Intussusception would be evaluated by a barium enema. Hirschsprung's disease (congenital aganglionic megacolon) can be diagnosed with a Wagensteen-Rice series (air rises in the inflated colon). Gastroesophageal reflux is usually diagnosed by clinical findings in infants. Barium swallow will reveal free regurgitation of barium from stomach to esophagus. An upper GI series would be performed to rule out causes of vomiting.

139. Answer: 2

Rationale: Excessive vomiting with loss of acid and gastric juice is the most common cause of metabolic alkalosis. Respiratory problems do not precipitate primary metabolic acid-base imbalance, and renal disease most often causes metabolic acidosis. Severe anxiety resulting in hyperventilation results in respiratory alkalosis. Hyperventilation results in an increase in pH.

140. Answer: 3

Rationale: It is critical that a child void before starting an IV solution with potassium. The problem with renal compromise is always a possibility, and adequate output should be established before initiating fluid therapy with potassium. The other three options are important but not the priority in this situation. Clinical evaluation of the child patient with dehydration should be prioritized as the volume of fluid intake, urine output, fever, and underlying medical conditions. Weight is also important in estimating dehydration but needs to be compared with prior weights. Important laboratory values include urine specific gravity, blood urea nitrogen, creatinine, hematocrit, and serum albumin.

141. Answer: 1

Rationale: *Rotavirus* is the most frequent cause of gastroenteritis in children 6 months to 2 years of age. The Norwalk virus is more predominant in school-age children. Up to 58% of diarrhea in children results from viral infections, causing vomiting and then diarrhea. The stool smear is negative for WBCs in viral causes and positive in bacterial causes. In viral diarrhea, the fever is mild, and diarrhea is watery and nonbloody.

142. Answer: 4

Rationale: Clinical features of Crohn's disease include severe weight loss, abdominal pain, growth failure, and weight loss. In irritable bowel syndrome, abdominal pain predominates. Altered bowel habits with either diarrhea or constipation are also seen. Clinical findings associated with carcinoma of the colon include mild occult blood loss with intermittent episodes of acute bleeding. Ulcerative colitis clinical features include diarrhea, rectal bleeding, and moderate weight loss.

143. Answer: 3

Rationale: Appendicitis usually begins as periumbilical abdominal pain accompanied by anorexia and nausea but not necessarily vomiting or diarrhea. Within hours the patient may develop a low-grade fever. Most laboratory tests are normal. A WBC count greater than 15,000/mm³ is often noted but neither confirms nor excludes the diagnosis of appendicitis. Pyuria is not indicative of appendicitis and suggests renal disease.

144. Answer: 4

Rationale: Red currant jelly stools are seen in intussusception and are caused by a mixture of stool, mucus, and blood. Clay-colored stools are seen with hepatitis. Projectile vomiting is associated with pyloric stenosis. Infants with intussusception usually have periods of severe pain, followed by intervals in which they appear comfortable. Constant or recurrent abdominal pain is experienced by about 10% of healthy children 5–15 years of age. School phobia may be associated with the etiology of the pain. An organic etiology is found in less than 10% of patients.

145. Answer: 1

Rationale: The major symptom of reflux is vomiting or regurgitation. It may occur during sleep, and frequently after feeding. Poor weight gain, hyperirritability, and refusal of feeding may be signs in some infants but are not the major symptoms. Fever or diarrhea may be present in patients with acute otitis media, gastroenteritis, or urinary tract infections.

146. Answer: 1

Rationale: The optimal therapy for GERD should include small, frequent feedings, burping after each feeding, and placing the baby on an inclined surface at 30 degrees. The prone position is not advocated because it allows gravity to promote reflux and sudden infant death syndrome. The supine position leads to more reflux compared with the prone position. The effectiveness of thickened feedings has not been demonstrated because it is believed to delay gastric emptying and thus promotes reflux. Proton-pump inhibitors are useful in controlling esophagitis, but long-term effects in infants are not defined. Pharmacologic therapy in young infants has received scant justification in research literature.

147. Answer: 4

Rationale: The recommendations for an infant born to an HBsAg-positive mother are that the baby should have one dose of hepatitis B immunoglobulin (by 12 hours after birth) and a complete three-dose immunization of hepatitis B vaccine. The vaccine will stimulate the newborn's active immunity.

148. Answer: 2

Rationale: Classic signs and symptoms of Hirschsprung's disease in later infancy include alternating diarrhea and constipation and abdominal distention. The stools are offensive and ribbon-like, the abdomen is enlarged, and the veins are prominent. The other listed physical findings are not usually found in Hirschsprung's disease but are prevalent in other gastrointestinal disorders.

149. Answer: 4

Rationale: Gastroenteritis is the most common cause of abdominal pain in all age groups. The incidence of appendicitis increases after age 5 and peaks between ages 15 and 30. Intussusception and incarcerated hernia are uncommon and certainly occur less often than gastroenteritis in children.

150. Answer: 3

Rationale: Parasitic infestations cause recurrent episodes of abdominal pain, often with diarrhea, nausea, and vomiting, depending on the type of infestation. Lactose intolerance can cause recurrent abdominal pain in the lower abdomen with cramping and distention. Chronic stool retention occurs in a child with a history of ineffective toilet training. There is often a family history of constipation. All other conditions present with acute symptoms, except for psychogenic pain, which is recurrent and is a diagnosis of exclusion.

151. Answer: 3

Rationale: The location of the injury suggests a ruptured spleen. Hypovolemia can quickly occur because there can be a large amount of internal bleeding and is a medical emergency. The rupture occurs when there is a severe direct blow to the abdomen. Common causes of the trauma are motor vehicle accidents, contact sports, bicycle accidents, and domestic violence. Diseases such as lymphoma, infectious mononucleosis, and hemolytic anemia increase the risk of rupture. Although bowel and bladder injuries are possible with blunt trauma to the abdomen, the upper abdominal location, noted by the hematoma location, makes a spleen injury more likely. Older adolescents may complain of dizziness, fatigue, chest pain, and palpitations because of arrhythmias, but hematomas are not usually present.

152. Answer: 3

Rationale: Lactose intolerance is common among Asian patients. The primary symptoms are bloating, flatulence, abdominal cramps, and diarrhea 2 hours after eating food containing lactose. Symptoms of IBS include abdominal pain and diarrhea, alternating with constipation. IBS is more common during late adolescence. Hirschsprung's disease is four times more common in boys than girls; 10%–15% of patients have Down syndrome. Food allergies are common in children under age 3 years. Clinical findings occur minutes to 2 hours after ingestion of the food. Clinical findings include hives, facial angioedema, flushing, and throat itching.

153. Answer: 2

Rationale: Right upper quadrant pain during exercise, malaise, nausea, and vomiting are early signs of hepatitis A. Elevated IgM antibodies indicate a recent or current infection. Clinical findings of cholecystitis include colicky pain in the right upper quadrant with radiation to the flanks after a large meal. Mononucleosis, common in college-age adults and young children, has the classic triad of fever, exudative pharyngitis, and adenopathy (particularly posterior cervical). Hepatitis B causes symptoms ranging from asymptomatic seroconversion to acute illness with malaise, anorexia, and nausea to fatal hepatitis.

154. Answer: 1

Rationale: Objects 5 cm or larger have difficulty passing the ligament of Treitz and other points of narrowing, such as the gastroesophageal junction. Ingested foreign bodies tend to lodge in areas of natural constriction.

155. Answer: 2

Rationale: When the infant is in a supine position, increased abdominal pressure after eating can result in passage of gastric contents into the esophagus, which often would be aspirated during sleep, and result in the forceful coughing, resultant emesis, and esophageal reflux. Suck-swallow incoordination can cause the same problems regardless of position, as can tracheoesophageal fistula. Colic is characterized by severe crying in healthy, well-fed infants for more than 3 hours a day.

156. Answer: 3

Rationale: Shigellosis usually is self-limited, lasting 5–7 days. Prevention of hydration is key, and fluid replacement should be diligent. For children, the most common age is 2–4 years for *Shigella* infection; a mild case can be managed with fluids, such as Pedialyte, and good handwashing. Antidiarrheals should not be used because the course could worsen. Treatment with TMP-SMX (Bactrim) shortens the course and prevents further spread of the organism but is not required in mild cases. Prevention of dehydration also includes a clear liquid diet for 24–48 hours, no dairy products, electrolyte-rich sports drinks, and advance to a bland diet as tolerated.

157. Answer: 3

Rationale: The drug of choice for treating *Giardia* is metronidazole 5 mg/kg (up to 250 mg) tid × 5 days (80%–95% effective). This drug is well tolerated in children. Metronidazole has a disulfiram-like effect and should not be used in children or adolescents receiving ethanol-containing medications. All other drugs are ineffective for *Giardia*. Tetracycline should not be prescribed to children under age 8 for any reason.

Urinary

158. Answer: 4

Rationale: HUS is most often caused by Shiga toxin-producing *Escherichia coli* (STEC) or *Shigella* and less commonly by *Streptococcus pneumoniae.* Urinary symptoms and thrombocytopenia in HUS typically do not manifest until several days after the presentation of nausea, vomiting, and diarrhea (which is often bloody). Immediate supportive therapy is indicated, including transfusions and dialysis based on the severity of symptoms.

159. Answer: 1

Rationale: There is usually evidence of a prior β-hemolytic *Streptococcus* infection. An infection with *E. coli* is associated with acute pyelonephritis. Macroscopic hematuria (tea-colored urine), hypertension, proteinuria, decreased urine output, edema, dyspnea, fatigue, lethargy, and headache are common clinical findings.

160. Answer: 2

Rationale: Congenital genitourinary anomalies can place a patient at risk for urinary tract infection, which include obstruction, impaired renal function, impaired fertility, and psychosocial difficulties.

161. Answer: 2

Rationale: Hematuria is not a usual clinical finding. Fever may be the only presenting complaint in the child. Older children are more likely to present with flank pain, dysuria, frequency, urgency, and incontinence.

162. Answer: 1, 4

Rationale: If a child has suffered several episodes of acute pyelonephritis or has known renal scarring, measure blood pressure at follow-up visits and consider a urine specimen for proteinuria. Leukocyte esterase is a screening test used to detect white blood cells in the urine, which may indicate a urinary tract infection. A urine culture and sensitivity would be done if a urinary tract infection is suspected. A streptozyme test is a test for β-hemolytic *Streptococcus*, which is associated with glomerulonephritis, not pyelonephritis.

163. Answer: 1, 3, 4

Rationale: It is important to refer to a urologist the following patients: a boy after first UTI and girl after second UTI and all children with gross hematuria; all infants aged less than 3 months with possible UTI should be transferred to the emergency department.

Male Reproductive

164. Answer: 1

Rationale: Paraphimosis is a retraction disorder related to a constricted prepuce that can be relieved through circumcision.

165. Answer: 4

Rationale: This involves the differential diagnosis between epididymitis and testicular torsion. Irreversible damage will be done to the testicles if torsion is not released in 3–4 hours. Time should not be wasted with other treatments if torsion is strongly suspected.

166. Answer: 1

Rationale: Cryptorchidism is the result of undescended testes, either bilateral or, more often, affecting the right testis. Normally, descent is in the seventh to eighth month of gestation; therefore it more often affects premature infants.

Female Reproductive

167. Answer: 4

Rationale: Douching is never necessary. It changes the normal pH and upsets the normal vaginal flora. Douching during menstruation could cause "retrograde menstruation," a potential precursor to endometriosis. Copious vaginal discharge can be a symptom of infection and warrants workup.

168. Answer: 3

Rationale: Pregnancy is the most common cause of amenorrhea in young women. It is important to rule out pregnancy by obtaining a serum hCG level in patient with a problem of amenorrhea, even if she is very athletic. Interviewing the patient regarding her sexual practices is unreliable. The presence or absence of pregnancy should be determined before other diagnostic studies.

169. Answer: 3

Rationale: The presence of bruising, particularly on genitalia, should raise suspicion of abuse. Combined with her nonverbal behavior, the bruising should prompt the family nurse practitioner to explore the possibility of abuse.

Newborn

170. Answer: 1

Rationale: Using a paper or a plastic tape, rather than cloth, prevents error because of the stretching of the fabric. Measurements should be repeated to confirm accuracy. The tape should not lie over the ears.

171. Answer: 2

Rationale: Neonatal screening for PKU and congenital hypothyroidism is done in all states. Other tests are generally mandated by the state or obtained by the provider because of family history. Alpha-fetoprotein is usually a maternal blood test done during the prenatal period to screen for genetic defects, primarily neural tube anomalies.

172. Answer: 3

Rationale: Normal morphology and testes tissue development will be impaired if the testes are not descended by age 1 year. These children are at higher risk for development of testicular cancer in the young adult male (20–30 years old).

173. Answer: 1

Rationale: Phototherapy is effective secondary to the absorption of the light by bilirubin across the infant's skin. The light energy is absorbed by bilirubin and promotes the conversion of bilirubin to a nontoxic form that can be excreted in the bile and eliminated in the urine and stool. The increase in hemolysis will increase the bilirubin level; this is physiologic jaundice that is not associated with an Rh-incompatibility problem.

174. Answer: 1

Rationale: Neonatal jaundice is more common in breast-fed infants and is thought to result from the decreased intake in the first few days. It usually begins between 4 and 7 days after birth, and the bilirubin levels range from 10–30 mg/dL. Increasing the infant's intake of water does not improve the condition. Breast-feeding may be temporarily interrupted, but phototherapy is usually unnecessary.

175. Answer: 4

Rationale: Bronze baby syndrome describes a grayish-brown pigmentation that occurs in neonates. It may occur in infants undergoing phototherapy but is usually associated with infants who have obstructive liver problems. The pigmentation is not permanent but may last for several months.

176. Answer: 1

Rationale: Infantile colic is unexplained crying and restlessness that lasts longer than 3 hours per day, 3 days a week. Most often it stops spontaneously at about 3 months. Other causes, particularly infections, should be ruled out. Spastic colon and lactose intolerance are unlikely and would include problems with diarrhea and constipation. Infant stress syndrome is not a valid problem.

177. Answer: 4

Rationale: With a normal physical exam, in the absence of fever or sepsis, the listed laboratory tests are not necessary to diagnose colic. If there were positive findings or fever, the complete laboratory workup should be obtained, with the addition of urinalysis and lumbar puncture.

178. Answer: 2

Rationale: After the infant has been carefully evaluated and there is no evidence of other problems, it is important to explain to the parents that no medication is available to treat the condition. The condition is not resolved by changing the feeding schedule of the infant nor is it related to stress within the home, and a change to soy formula will not solve the problem. The parents must be informed that the colic most often resolves with no residual problems by age 3 months.

179. Answer: 2

Rationale: The physiology of normal vaginal delivery causes pressure against the infant's thorax and helps remove amniotic fluid. If the cesarean section was done as an emergency before term, the infant may have inadequate surfactant for good pulmonary function. Increased levels of bilirubin, meconium aspiration, and hypoglycemia are not associated with an increase in cesarean delivery.

180. Answer: 1

Rationale: These are normal newborn findings. The respiratory rate is increased but is usually increased immediately after birth (transient tachypnea) and during the second period of reactivity. Continued tachypnea is abnormal. The respiratory rate should be counted for a full minute because of the irregularity of the infant's breathing. Periodic pauses may occur for up to 10 seconds, but apnea lasting longer than 20 seconds is abnormal. Acrocyanosis is normal immediately after birth. Choanal atresia occurs when one or both of the nasal passages are blocked by an abnormality of the septum. In respiratory distress syndrome, the infant exhibits other symptoms that are consistent with hypoxia.

181. Answer: 4

Rationale: Caput succedaneum results from pressure against the mother's cervix during labor. The edematous area crosses the suture lines and will resolve within hours to days after birth. There is normally a space between the cranial suture lines; if there is no space or an overriding suture line, it may be caused by molding. Widening of the suture line may indicate increased intracranial pressure. Cephalhematoma is characterized by bleeding between the bone and the periosteum, and it does not cross the suture line.

182. Answer: 2

Rationale: Early signs of hypoglycemia are jitteriness, poor muscle tone, tremors, and symptoms of respiratory difficulty. The blood sugar of 50 mg/dL is within normal limits at this time (40–60 mg/dL the first 24 hours). If blood sugar levels are less than 45 mg/dL on the screening strip, a follow-up serum glucose should be done. The meconium stool should be passed within the first 24 hours, and the bilirubin level is normal.

Mental Health

183. Answer: 1

Rationale: Nicotine is known as the "gateway drug" and is commonly the first drug used by adolescents.

184. Answer: 3

Rationale: The family nurse practitioner must determine whether the bruised areas match the type of trauma the parent describes. Bruises in various stages of healing turn different colors and are indicative that the injuries did not occur at the same time, which could be indicative of child abuse.

185. Answer: 4

Rationale: Adolescents with anorexia nervosa will severely reduce their nutritional intake by dieting constantly on high fiber and low calories. They usually have an inappropriate body image and may admit to occasional episodes of vomiting.

186. Answer: 1

Rationale: Nightmares peak in incidence around ages 3–4 years and are often associated with abandonment issues and posttraumatic stress disorder (following gun shootings, fires, and abuse). Night terrors are typically accompanied by gross motor movements (sleepwalking and enuresis), tachypnea, labored breathing, and tachycardia.

187. Answer: 2

Rationale: Role playing and planning a rehearsed reply to teasing comments about short stature are helpful tools to deal with this issue. Although humor can be effective, constantly clowning around for attention is not positive coping behavior. Withdrawal (i.e., watching television or reading) is not effective coping and may indicate depression. Spending time and associating only with younger adolescents who are his height is not a positive coping behavior and may hinder normal maturation.

188. Answer: 4

Rationale: More than 50% of intravenous cocaine users develop hepatitis, phlebitis, endocarditis, and AIDS. Epistaxis, rhinorrhea, and nasal congestion are seen most often in intranasal users of cocaine. Chest congestion, wheezing, and eventual emphysema occur with chronic freebase (crack) smokers. Although cardiac arrhythmias, hypertension, and respiratory arrest can occur, they are not the common complications.

189. Answer: 3

Rationale: Adolescents often act out to protect themselves from feelings of vulnerability and dependency. It is important to evaluate signs of anger and frustration in the adolescent because the significance of the behavior may indicate symptoms of depression. Adults who are depressed typically display findings noted in the other three options.

190. Answer: 1

Rationale: The newborn exposed to cocaine is often premature, small for gestational age, has low birth weight, and has a low Apgar score. Intrauterine growth retardation occurs along with symptoms of hypertonia, irritability, tremulousness, irregular sleeping patterns, and frequent gaze aversion.

191. Answer: 3

Rationale: People with anorexia nervosa will exercise up to 4 hours a day. They are above average intelligence in most cases, suffer from bradycardia, and have decreased libido.

192. Answer: 4

Rationale: In a preschool child, it may be difficult to distinguish ADHD because problems of overactivity, inattention, and negativism are common. Problems with language-skill development, along with fine motor skills, are more likely found with learning disabilities. Active curiosity and negativism are normal behaviors for preschoolers.

193. Answer: 1

Rationale: Autism is a developmental disorder that starts early in a child's life and is characterized by avoidance of eye contact, indifference to caregivers, language and communication delays, failure to develop a social smile, repetitive movements, and an excessive need for routine.

194. Answer: 4

Rationale: Repetition of whole words and phrases is normal for preschoolers; therefore it would be inappropriate to refer to a speech pathologist at this time. Parents should not correct or criticize the child because it could contribute to low self-esteem. Verbal exercises are unnecessary and could be very stressful to the child and contribute to low self-esteem.

195. Answer: 3

Rationale: The grandmother's concern is warranted. In teenage girls, the most common form of suicide attempt is by drug overdose. The combination of vomiting and confusion suggests a drug overdose, and the family nurse practitioner should run a toxicology screen.

196. Answer: 2

Rationale: This patient should be examined by emergency department personnel, many of whom are specially trained to collect the evidence needed to testify in court about rape. The exam should not be done in the office unless the family nurse practitioner has been trained in evidence collection and has a rape evidence collection kit. The exam must be done quickly, before evidence is destroyed. The patient decides who should be called for support. Although she is encouraged to call her parents, she is also offered the support of rape crisis and other resources.

197. Answer: 2

Rationale: Woraich's 1994 study failed to demonstrate a link between sugar and behavior or cognitive performance. Further assessment is indicated before labeling as ADHD.

198. Answer: 3

Rationale: Based on developmental levels, a 6 month old is not walking or pulling up. A 4 year old is beginning to run and jump, a 6 year old is playing outside and riding a bicycle, and a 1 year old is beginning to pull up and cruise around cabinets and tables.

199. Answer: 4

Rationale: Although all answers may contribute to a family nurse practitioner's suspicion of family violence, the admission of genuine fear of a household member is considered an excellent indicator of actual or potential violence and the level of danger in a home. The family nurse practitioner should involve Social Services to assist the adolescent female in this situation.

200. Answer: 4

Rationale: Often, the first indication of drug use in adolescents is a sudden change in behavior or school performance. Symptoms of heroin use are constricted pupils, respiratory depression, needle tracks, and poor nutrition. Symptoms of marijuana use are slow reflexes, tachycardia, conjunctival injection, nasal congestion, and increased appetite. Symptoms of LSD use are dilated pupils, reddened eyes, hypertension, increased appetite, and hallucinations. The use of central nervous system stimulants, such as crack cocaine, leads to hypertension, weight loss, anorexia, insomnia, hyperreflexia, and a perforated or ulcerated nasal septum.

19

Mental Health

Psychosocial Exam & Diagnostic Tests

1. What does the mental status exam enable the family nurse practitioner to identify?
   1. Intelligence quotient (IQ) and reasoning.
   2. Abstract thinking and memory functioning.
   3. Reasoning and coordination.
   4. Memory functioning and IQ.

2. **QSEN** The family nurse practitioner understands the following concerning direct questioning about intimate partner violence in the home:
   1. Direct questioning should be avoided for fear of offending the patient.
   2. It should be a routine component of history taking with all patients presenting as an initial visit to primary care clinicians.
   3. Direct questioning should be used only when there are obvious findings noted on physical exam.
   4. It should be used only once a year when the patient is seen for a routine physical exam.

3. A patient with a history of psychiatric problems arrives at the clinic shouting that he is a messenger of God and knows the meaning of the prophecies in Revelations. This behavior is assessed as:
   1. A delusion.
   2. A hallucination.
   3. Magical thinking.
   4. An illusion.

4. Which of the following is a tool used to screen adolescents for alcoholism?
   1. CRAFFT.
   2. CAGE questionnaire.
   3. PACES tool.
   4. HITS screening tool.

5. What would an assessment of a patient experiencing auditory hallucinations most likely reveal?
   1. Patient mumbling to self, tilted head, eyes darting back and forth.

2. Performance of obsessive-compulsive rituals of turning off and on a radio, talking to self.
   3. Hyperactivity, expansive mood, easy distractibility.
   4. Cool, aloof, unapproachable, avoiding enclosed areas.

6. CAGE (Cut down, Annoyed, Guilty, Eye Opener) is a screening instrument for which disease process?
   1. Glaucoma.
   2. Depression.
   3. Alcoholism.
   4. Diabetes.

7. When receiving records from another agency, the family nurse practitioner notes on the summary sheet that the patient has a dual diagnosis. This means the patient has:
   1. Both manic and depressive symptoms of bipolar affective disorder.
   2. Two closely related psychiatric disorders (e.g., panic disorder and bulimia nervosa).
   3. Coexistence of both a psychiatric disorder (e.g., depression) and a substance abuse disorder (e.g., alcohol dependence).
   4. Coexistence of a personality disorder (e.g., borderline personality) and a psychiatric disorder (e.g., panic disorder).

8. When the family nurse practitioner asks the patient to explain the meaning of a proverb or metaphor, the family nurse practitioner is assessing which of the following?
   1. Impaired judgment.
   2. Memory.
   3. Abstract reasoning.
   4. Level of consciousness.

9. While completing the history on an older adult, the family nurse practitioner understands that when a patient "makes up stories or answers" to questions, it is known as:
   1. Perseveration.
   2. Confabulation.
   3. Echolalia.
   4. Alcoholic encephalopathy.

10. **QSEN** In taking a history from a patient with depression, which is the most important question for the family nurse practitioner to ask?
    1. Have you ever experienced hallucinations, delusions, or illusions?
    2. Have you ever been hospitalized in a psychiatric facility?
    3. Do you regularly take antidepressants or other medications?
    4. Have you thought about or attempted suicide?

11. The family nurse practitioner asks the patient to follow a series of short commands to assess:
    1. Judgment.
    2. Abstract reasoning.
    3. Attention span.
    4. Cooperation.

12. What is a common laboratory finding associated with bulimia nervosa?
    1. Hyperkalemia.
    2. Hypochloremia.
    3. Elevated liver enzymes.
    4. Platelet abnormalities.

13. The family nurse practitioner is testing recent memory on an older adult client. Select the response that can be used to test for recent memory.
    1. Ask the patient to recall three items after a delay of 3–5 minutes.
    2. Ask the patient to solve a simple math problem.
    3. Ask the patient to name the past four presidents.
    4. Ask the patient his or her mother's maiden name.

14. An 85-year-old woman comes in with her daughter with the primary complaint of worsening confusion over 6 months. The family nurse practitioner has already ordered a urine analysis, which was negative. The basal metabolic panel was unremarkable. Complete blood count showed a mild anemia. What other tests might the family nurse practitioner consider ordering for this patient?
    1. A1c, folic acid, thyroid-stimulating hormone (TSH).
    2. TSH, lipid panel, vitamin B_{12}, vitamin D.
    3. Folic acid, vitamin B_{12}, TSH.
    4. Lipid panel, A1c, vitamin D.

15. The family nurse practitioner knows drug tolerance is suggested when a patient gives a history of:
    1. Reduced effects with the same dose of the drug.
    2. Less of the medication produces the desired effects.
    3. No withdrawal symptoms when the drug is stopped.
    4. Increasing side effects with an increase in the dose of the drug.

16. When doing a mental status exam, which questions would be helpful to assess the patient for the ability to think abstractly?
    1. Can you repeat the following numbers: 1, 3, 5, 7, 9?
    2. What is today's date?
    3. How are a carpet and a hardwood floor alike?
    4. Can you tell me the names of three past U.S. presidents?

Psychiatric Disorders

17. An older adult patient is experiencing a recent onset of confusion. The family nurse practitioner is trying to determine whether the confusion is related to depression or dementia. In evaluating the patient, what specific assessment finding would be helpful in making this distinction?
    1. Determining whether confusion worsens in the evening.
    2. Assessing early morning agitation, hyperactivity, and insomnia.
    3. Noting signs of anger, hostility, and loss of control.
    4. Assessing reality distortions and preoccupation with family matters.

18. **QSEN** A patient calls the clinic and asks to speak to the family nurse practitioner. When the family nurse practitioner answers the telephone, the patient states that he is going to commit suicide. The priority goal is to:
    1. Refer the patient to an appropriate treatment facility.
    2. Encourage ventilation of angry and depressed feelings.
    3. Assess the lethality of the suicide plan.
    4. Establish rapport with the patient.

19. During an intake interview with a 26-year-old man diagnosed with generalized anxiety disorder, the family nurse practitioner might observe what type of behavior?
    1. An inflated sense of self.
    2. Constant relation to future events.
    3. Inability to concentrate and irritability when questioned.
    4. Nervousness and fear of the family nurse practitioner during the interview.

20. An older adult woman answers the family nurse practitioner's questions by mumbling in low tones with answers that seem inappropriate. What would be initial findings associated with a diagnosis of dementia?
    1. Sees people floating across the ceiling of her room.
    2. Has problems with cognition and confusion.
    3. Hears voices at night telling her to change her clothes.
    4. Shows fear when the nurse makes any movements toward her.

21. An older patient comes to the office with the complaint of confusion. The daughter is concerned that her mother is developing Alzheimer disease. Which of these assessments would indicate the patient is experiencing delirium versus dementia?
    1. The confusion has been slowly developing.
    2. The confusion started after the patient started taking over-the-counter cimetidine (Tagamet).
    3. The patient's attention span has been affected.
    4. The patient's memory has been impaired.

22. When the family nurse practitioner talks with a patient about his chemical dependency, the patient states, "I wish I would have never used cocaine. It has ruined my life!" What would be the most appropriate response by the family nurse practitioner?
    1. "You should think before you do something."
    2. "Things will work out, don't worry."
    3. "It sounds like you've thought a lot about your cocaine use."
    4. "You shouldn't be so hard on yourself. You can change."

23. The family nurse practitioner would expect which symptoms in a patient with a diagnosis of schizophrenia?
    1. High energy with varying sleep patterns and nonstop conversation.
    2. Extreme and frequent mood swings with hyperactivity and difficulty concentrating.
    3. Paranoia, delusions, hallucinations, and diminished self-care.
    4. Antisocial behavior, manipulative behavior, charisma, and ability to lie convincingly.

24. How can dementia be distinguished from delirium?
    1. Dementia lasts days to weeks compared with delirium, which lasts months to years.
    2. Dementia is often associated with medications or systemic illness.
    3. Dementia exhibits a disturbance in attention that is not present in delirium.
    4. Dementia is a chronic medical condition and delirium is an acute illness.

25. An older adult patient is brought to the family nurse practitioner by his family for evaluation of increasing confusion over the past few days. The patient has a history of dementia; however, the family states that there is a definite change. What course of action would the family nurse practitioner consider?
    1. Help the family look for a nursing home.
    2. Order a magnetic resonance imaging scan.
    3. Order a noncontrast head computerized tomography.
    4. Order a urinalysis (UA).

26. **QSEN** A middle-aged, upper-middle-class, married woman presents to your clinic for the third time in 2 months with a complaint of headache, gastrointestinal upset with abdominal pain, and difficulty sleeping. Past exams have been essentially negative. You suspect the patient suffers from depression, but she has been reluctant to complete even the briefest of screenings for this. Today, the patient requests "something for sleep," again stating that she "doesn't have time to take a bunch of tests." Which tentative diagnosis seems most likely?
    1. Hypochondriasis.
    2. Domestic violence.

3. Addiction.
4. Irritable bowel syndrome.

27. An older adult patient was taken to the clinic in a confused state that began suddenly 24 hours ago. She fails to be oriented to person, time, or place. She was incontinent of urine because of her confusion. She looks apathetic and is drowsy. What would the family nurse practitioner suspect?
    1. Delirium.
    2. Dementia.
    3. Depression.
    4. A psychotic disorder.

28. **QSEN** Which of the following groups of patients fall under mandatory reporting laws for abuse and neglect in most states in the United States?
    1. Children, adult women, dependent older adults.
    2. Children, disabled individuals, adult women.
    3. Disabled individuals, adult women, dependent older adults.
    4. Children, disabled individuals, dependent older adults.

29. Which patient statement would be the most reassuring when considering early diagnosis of dementia?
    1. "I have forgotten where I put my keys about three times in the past year."
    2. "I have been in three little car accidents in the past few years."
    3. "My family tells me I am forgetful and don't cook like I should."
    4. "I remember my prom dress, but I can't remember what I had for lunch."

30. Which are physical findings of cocaine abuse?
    1. Bradycardia, miosis, hypertension.
    2. Hypertension, tachycardia, tremor.
    3. Hypotension, bradycardia, abdominal cramps.
    4. Decreased level of consciousness, tachycardia, excessive salivation.

31. An older adult patient's wife is concerned about her husband's increasing confusion and agitation. Not only has he exhibited symptoms of increased confusion, but he also is unable to care for his physical needs. He has been incontinent of urine and feces and sometimes is totally unaware of other people. What would be an assessment priority for the patient?
    1. Evaluate changes in social habits.
    2. Assess for hallucinations and impaired reality testing.
    3. Evaluate his orientation to person, place, and time.
    4. Determine whether he is experiencing a problem with impaired judgment.

32. **QSEN** A 42-year-old male presents to the office with his friend. The friend states that he found the patient confused with some shaking and seeing things that are not there. The patient typically drinks two six packs of beer every day. The patient decided to stop drinking 2 days ago. Vital signs show elevated blood pressure, fever, and tachycardia. The family nurse practitioner transfers the patient to the hospital as he:
    1. Is overdosing on heroin.
    2. Has thyroid storm.
    3. Is septic from pneumonia.
    4. Has delirium tremens.

33. It is important for the family nurse practitioner to use evidence-based contemporary terminology when talking with patients to ameliorate stigma and health disparities faced by vulnerable populations. Which statement is reflective of nonjudgmental, empowering language?
    1. A diabetic patient having an episode of hyperglycemia.
    2. An illegal who needs housing.
    3. A transsexual who has a urinary infection.
    4. A patient who declined to sign an informed consent.

34. When assessing a patient who has a diagnosis of major depressive disorder, which would be considered cognitive symptoms of depression? (Select 2 responses.)
    1. Decreased energy.
    2. Hopelessness.
    3. Memory impairment.
    4. Inability to make decisions.
    5. Loss of pleasure in previously enjoyable things.
    6. Guilt or hopelessness.

35. A young adult male patient is seen by the family nurse practitioner for complaints of abdominal pain and early morning nausea. The patient reports on some days he has severe bouts of vomiting and over the past month has lost 5 pounds. After a thorough history and physical, the family nurse practitioner notices that the patient relates a 4-year history of chronic daily cannabis use. The family nurse practitioner suspects cannabinoid hyperemesis syndrome. What other finding is associated with this diagnosis?
    1. Binging and purging.
    2. Hyperpigmentation of the skin.
    3. Compulsive bathing in hot water.
    4. Unilateral headache.

36. What is a helpful acronym to use when assessing sleep patterns?
    1. Beers.
    2. CAGE.
    3. BEARS.
    4. BATTED.

Pharmacology

37. **QSEN** A patient has been receiving fluphenazine (Prolixin) for the last 3 weeks. The family nurse practitioner's assessment notes the following: temperature elevated 105.8°F (41°C), marked muscle rigidity, agitation, and confusion. The family nurse practitioner understands these findings are often associated with which diagnosis?
    1. Acute dystonia.
    2. Tardive dyskinesia.
    3. Neuroleptic malignant syndrome.
    4. Extrapyramidal disorder.

38. What is the preferred antidepressant for an older adult patient?
    1. Amitriptyline (Elavil).
    2. Citalopram (Celexa).
    3. Trazodone (Desyrel).
    4. Haloperidol (Haldol).

39. A patient has been referred to the family nurse practitioner. The patient's medical history reveals long-term use of benzodiazepines, which the patient considers harmless. The family nurse practitioner understands that benzodiazepines can:
    1. Cause drug dependency.
    2. Produce nephrotoxicity.
    3. Lead to functional damage of the cardiopulmonary system.
    4. Cause profound dissociative personality problems.

40. Which medication group is considered first-line treatment for anxiety disorders in older adult patients?
    1. Benzodiazepines.
    2. Selective serotonin reuptake inhibitors (SSRIs).
    3. Tricyclic antidepressants (TCAs).
    4. Atypical antipsychotics.

41. The family nurse practitioner is prescribing an antidepressant medication for an older adult. What is an important consideration about starting doses?
    1. Reduce starting doses by 50%.
    2. Reduce starting doses by 10%.
    3. Increase starting doses by 25%.
    4. Order the normal therapeutic dose.

42. What is the best initial treatment plan for a sleep disorder in the older adult patient?
    1. Medicate with amitriptyline (Elavil).
    2. Medicate with trazodone (Desyrel).
    3. Discuss the importance of daily naps.
    4. Decrease noise and light in the environment.

43. An older adult patient presents with a new symptom of acute confusion over the past 24 hours. Which assessment would be a priority for the family nurse practitioner to evaluate during the exam?
    1. Medication review.
    2. Electrocardiogram.
    3. Mini-Mental status exam.
    4. Thyroid profile.

44. The family nurse practitioner is aware that the following class of drugs is most likely to precipitate a hypertensive crisis in the older adult:
    1. Narcotic analgesics.
    2. Monoamine oxidase (MAO) inhibitors.
    3. Barbiturates.
    4. Phenothiazines.

45. The family nurse practitioner knows that the following class of drugs would have the greatest effect on memory in the older adult patient:
    1. Phenothiazines.
    2. Tricyclic antidepressants.
    3. Benzodiazepines.
    4. Monoamine oxidase inhibitors.

46. The family nurse practitioner understands that adolescents who use lysergic acid diethylamide (LSD):
    1. Experience withdrawal symptoms within 24 hours.
    2. Will quickly become addicted.
    3. Experience flashbacks and depression.
    4. Experience disorientation and delusional feelings.

47. Of the following antidepressants, which one has the most sedating side effects, making it a good sleeping agent?
    1. Fluoxetine (Prozac).
    2. Doxepin (Sinequan).
    3. Trazodone (Desyrel).
    4. Paroxetine (Paxil).

48. Which three laboratory results would be important to assess before placing a patient on lithium?
    1. Thyroid-stimulating hormone, T_4, T_3.
    2. Fasting lipids.
    3. Blood urea nitrogen, creatinine.
    4. Electrolytes.
    5. Erythrocyte sedimentation rate (ESR).
    6. Alanine transaminase, aspartate transaminase, lactate dehydrogenase.

49. **QSEN** A patient comes to the rural clinic having taken an undetermined amount of heroin. Before transferring the patient to a psychiatric treatment facility, the family nurse practitioner anticipates the drug of choice for an opioid overdose is:
    1. Clonidine (Catapres).
    2. Methadone (Dolophine).

3. Naloxone (Narcan).
4. Naltrexone HCl (Revia).

50. Benzodiazepines are useful in the treatment in which three of the following disorders:
    1. Alcohol withdrawal.
    2. Schizophrenia.
    3. Anxiety.
    4. Obsessive-compulsive disorder.
    5. Seizures.
    6. Bipolar affective disorder.

51. When starting a psychotropic medication in the older adult, what is a good rule of thumb?
    1. Start low, go slow.
    2. Higher doses are almost always needed.
    3. Side effects of psychotropic medications will usually not affect other medications.
    4. The same adult dosages can be used initially without any problems.

52. A patient is a 20-year, two-pack-a-day smoker with a history of chronic bronchitis. In addition to counseling, what is the prescription to give the patient who wishes to stop smoking?
    1. Nicotine polacrilex (Nicorette) gum 2-mg piece, chew for 30 minutes, q1–2h × 6 weeks, then q2–4h × 3 weeks, then q4–8h × 3 weeks, and then discontinue.
    2. Nicotine patch (Nicoderm) 21 mg/24 hr qd × 6 weeks, then 14 mg/24 hr qd × 2 weeks, then 7 mg/24 hr qd × 2 weeks, and then discontinue.
    3. Bupropion HCl (Zyban) 150 mg qd × 3 days, then 150 mg bid for 7–12 weeks, and then stop smoking when medication is started.
    4. Nicotine patch (Nicoderm) 14 mg/24 hr qd × 6 weeks, then 7 mg/24 hr qd × 6 weeks, and then discontinue.

53. A young woman tells the family nurse practitioner that she no longer wants to be on sertraline (Zoloft). She had a traumatic event a few years ago but has been doing much better and has a strong support structure from family and friends. What does the family nurse practitioner advise her to do?
    1. Stop taking the medication.
    2. Taper the dose slowly.
    3. Keep taking the medication.
    4. Switch to citalopram (Celexa).

54. A patient with bipolar disorder is on divalproex sodium (Depakote) for mania. What test(s) would the family nurse practitioner monitor?
    1. Liver function test and complete blood count.
    2. Pulmonary function test.
    3. Electrocardiogram.
    4. Urinalysis with culture and sensitivity.

55. A 75-year-old female comes to see the family nurse practitioner to follow-up on an upper respiratory infection that she has had for 1 week. She has been taking diphenhydramine (Benadryl). The family nurse practitioner knows this is a poor medication for older adult patients because it can cause:
    1. Confusion.
    2. Prolonged QT.
    3. Bradycardia.
    4. Hypertension.

56. **QSEN** What is the maximum dose of citalopram (Celexa) for a patient over 60 years old?
    1. 40 mg once daily by mouth.
    2. 20 mg twice daily by mouth.
    3. 20 mg once daily by mouth.
    4. 10 mg once daily by mouth.

57. The family nurse practitioner understands the following about the use of benzodiazepines in the older adult:
    1. Withdrawal symptoms may occur within 24 hours of abruptly stopping the medication.
    2. Adverse effects are minimal and rarely lead to falls or other injury.
    3. Long-acting medications (e.g., chlordiazepoxide [Librium]) are preferred over the shorter acting medications (e.g., lorazepam [Ativan]).
    4. Larger doses are needed to maintain therapeutic levels for the anxious or agitated patient.

19 Mental Health Answers & Rationales

Psychosocial Exam & Diagnostic Tests

1. Answer: 2

Rationale: The mental status exam provides a basic assessment of the patient's intellectual functioning (reasoning, abstract thinking, and memory). The IQ is determined by neuropsychologic evaluation. Coordination is part of a neurologic exam and can be tested by rapid alternating movements and heel-to-shin or finger-to-nose tests.

2. Answer: 2

Rationale: The personal nature of intimate partner violence (IPV) often influences a victim's decision to report the crime; thus victimizations by intimate partners are highly underreported for both men and women. Given the lack of harm and potential benefits of screening, routine screening is recommended on initial visits to primary care clinicians, to obstetrician-gynecologists, to the emergency department, and on hospital admission. All pregnant women and patients presenting with concerning symptoms or signs including women with injuries, women with chronic unexplained abdominal pain, women with sexually transmitted diseases, older adults with evidence of neglect, and older adults with injuries should be asked about IPV. For those patients who screen positive, the family nurse practitioner should offer resources, reassure confidentiality, and provide close follow-up.

3. Answer: 1

Rationale: Delusions are false, fixed beliefs that can be of a persecutory or grandiose nature. In this instance the patient is experiencing a delusion of grandeur. Often older adults with a diagnosis of dementia will have delusions, which worsen with acute illnesses. A person may have delusions as a symptom of a disorder, such as schizophrenia. They may also occur as part of a delusional disorder, such as grandiose, jealousy, persecutory, somatic, or mixed. A hallucination is a false sensory experience. An illusion is a misinterpretation of reality. Magical thinking is when the patient feels that his or her thoughts or wishes can control other people.

4. Answer: 1

Rationale: The CRAFFT is a behavioral health screening tool that consists of a series of six questions developed to screen adolescents for high-risk alcohol and other drug use disorders simultaneously. The CAGE questionnaire is a screening tool that asks four questions and is widely used for screening adults about problem drinking and potential alcohol problems. PACES is a reliable tool for assessing enjoyment of physical activity and has been used with all age groups. HITS is a screening tool and scale that stands for Hurt, Insult, Threaten, and Scream that consists of four questions to assess risk for IPV.

5. Answer: 1

Rationale: The patient experiencing auditory hallucinations will often look out into space and act as if he or she is listening to someone talking. This is associated with behaviors such as tilting the head, mumbling, and eye movement.

6. Answer: 3

Rationale: CAGE (Cut down, Annoyed, Guilty, Eye opener) is a screening instrument used to alert providers to the possibility of alcoholism.

7. Answer: 3

Rationale: Dual diagnosis involves both a psychiatric diagnosis and a substance abuse diagnosis.

8. Answer: 3

Rationale: Abstract thinking is the ability to think about concepts, objects, principles, and ideas that are not physically present. Using a metaphor or an analogy is an example of assessing abstract thinking, for example, "America is a melting pot." Judgment refers to the person's capacity to make good decisions and act on them. Memory is the ability to recall something. Level of consciousness is a measurement of arousability and responsiveness.

9. Answer: 2

Rationale: Patients who experience confabulation are fabricating, distorting, or misinterpreting memories about oneself or the world without the conscious intention to deceive. Confabulation is usually the result of memory disorders, brain injuries, and certain psychiatric disorders. Echolalia is the parroting or automatic, meaningless repeating of another's words. Perseveration is the involuntary persistent repetition of an idea or response (e.g., patient keeps repeating the same phrase over and over).

10. Answer: 4

Rationale: Although it is important to know whether the patient has ever experienced hallucinations, delusions, or illusions and has ever been hospitalized in a psychiatric facility, the single most important factor to ascertain is whether or not the patient has contemplated suicide. In addition, determination of a specific plan and the means to do it also are involved in the questioning about suicidal ideation. Asking a patient whether or not he or she is suicidal does not increase the risk of the patient committing suicide. It is also important for the family nurse practitioner to determine whether the patient regularly takes antidepressants or other medications. Patients may have stopped taking their antidepressant, causing an acute exacerbation of their depression, or starting another medication that may be causing an increase in their depression.

11. Answer: 3

Rationale: A patient's attention span is the length of time the patient can keep their thoughts and interest fixed on something. Although patient cooperation is a necessity for following a series of short commands, it is not measuring attention span. Abstract thinking is the ability to think about concepts, objects, principles, and ideas that are not physically present. Judgment refers to the person's capacity to make good decisions and act on them.

12. Answer: 2

Rationale: The other abnormalities are not usually associated with bulimia. The hypochloremia is associated with the purging (self-induced vomiting). Other fluid and electrolyte imbalances that may be seen include hyponatremia, hypokalemia, and metabolic alkalosis and acidosis.

13. Answer: 1

Rationale: Recent memory is tested by asking the patient to recall something after a brief delay. Testing for remote memory is usually related to historical events (past presidents or maiden name). Thinking and cognition can be assessed by asking the patient to solve a simple math problem.

14. Answer: 3

Rationale: It is appropriate to check for other conditions that cause confusion, such as hypothyroidism, folic acid deficiency, and vitamin B_{12} deficiency. The other tests listed are important for patient health but will not help determine the cause of confusion.

15. Answer: 1

Rationale: Drug tolerance exists when the same dose of the drug produces reduced effects and is usually seen with the development of physical dependence on any medication. Addiction occurs when there is a deep-seated psychologic need for the drug/medication.

16. Answer: 3

Rationale: Abstract thinking requires the patient to compare and tell how two things are alike or different, involving the thought process that is oriented toward the development of an idea without application to a particular object; it is independent of space and time. Today's date assists to determine orientation, listing the names of past presidents demonstrates long-term memory, and repetition of numbers demonstrates short-term memory.

Psychiatric Disorders

17. Answer: 1

Rationale: Confusion can occur in both dementia and depression. However, with dementia, symptoms worsen at night and are commonly referred to as sundowning. Additionally, the family nurse practitioner must also ensure that the increased confusion is not a result of an acute illness. Often the only sign or symptom the demented older adult may present with is confusion. Usually the culprit is a urinary tract infection. The family nurse practitioner should order a urinalysis to ensure that the confusion is not the result of an acute illness and is reversible.

18. Answer: 4

Rationale: The family nurse practitioner must first establish trust and rapport with the caller before an assessment can be made. If rapport is not established, the patient will hang up the phone. The family nurse practitioner understands that, by keeping the patient talking, he is prevented from acting out the suicidal threat. On the side while talking with the patient, the family nurse practitioner can signal for assistance to send additional emergency assistance to the home of the caller.

19. Answer: 3

Rationale: Impaired concentration and irritability are major characteristics of generalized anxiety disorder. Other symptoms of generalized anxiety disorder include excessive anxiety and worry; inability to control the worry and restlessness; easily fatigued; difficulty concentrating; muscle tension; and sleep disturbance. Patients often pace the exam room because of their irritability; they are more focused on the here and now and have low self-esteem.

20. Answer: 2

Rationale: Confusion and cognitive function problems (e.g., short-term memory loss) are initial signs of dementia. Other signs of early-stage Alzheimer dementia include time and spatial disorientation, poor judgment, personality changes, depression or withdrawal, and perceptual disturbances. The severity of the symptoms depends on what stage of cognitive degeneration the patient is manifesting. The other options are characteristic of hallucinatory experiences and may occur later. This patient also may be exhibiting signs and symptoms of an acute illness. The culprit is commonly a urinary tract infection and the family nurse practitioner should order a urinalysis to ensure that the cause of the confusion is not related to a reversible cause.

21. Answer: 2

Rationale: Cimetidine (Tagamet) is not tolerated well in the older adult patient and should be avoided, as reversible central nervous system effects can occur, such as disorientation, mental confusion, agitation, psychosis, depression, anxiety, and hallucinations. It is important to obtain a thorough history of all over-the-counter medications, and those prescribed. Any time a new medication is added to an older adult patient's medication regimen, an abrupt onset of confusion must be reviewed closely because it may be attributed to the new medication or a drug–drug interaction with an existing medication. Another possibility is the onset of an acute illness, which often manifests as acute confusion in the older adult patient. Most often the culprit is a urinary tract infection (UTI); therefore in addition to a careful medication review, obtaining a urinalysis also could rule out a UTI. When a patient has true dementia, the onset of confusion develops slowly, over a longer time period and not acutely, which would indicate that there is another underlying problem causing the acute confusion. Attention span and memory may be affected in each diagnosis.

22. Answer: 3

Rationale: The family nurse practitioner's statement acknowledges the patient's feelings and is open ended, which promotes open discussion and helps the patient clarify feelings and thoughts. Telling the patient to think before doing something is condescending and punitive. Telling the patient to not worry and things will work out offers false reassurance. When the family nurse practitioner tells the patient to not be so hard on himself or herself, it tends to discount the patient's feelings.

23. Answer: 3

Rationale: The characteristics of schizophrenia are paranoia, delusions, tangential thought, suspiciousness, disorganized behavior, and hallucinations.

24. Answer: 4

Rationale: Dementia lasts for months to years, and the patient never recovers. Delirium is an acute process that is often associated with medications or a systemic illness and is reversible once the acute problem is addressed and resolved.

25. Answer: 4

Rationale: One of the most common reasons for an acute change in mental status in the demented older adult patient is an acute infection. This is usually a urinary tract infection (UTI). Usually the demented older adult patient is incontinent, and, because of the changes of aging, does not recognize the normal signs or symptoms of a UTI (burning, urgency, frequency, and suprapubic tenderness). Older adults also do not typically run elevated temperatures. The family nurse practitioner should order a UA to ensure that an acute infectious process is not the cause of the acute confusion. The family nurse practitioner should also conduct a medication review to ensure that no new medications have been added or that no new over-the-counter or herbal medications have been added because this is the second major reason for acute confusion in the older adult patient.

26. Answer: 2

Rationale: The indicators to domestic violence in this case are the multiple vague physical complaints without supporting objective data, the suspected depression, and the reluctance to wait around in the clinic for extended periods of time. This patient is on the verge of disclosing if a provider would only ask her about domestic violence.

27. Answer: 1

Rationale: Based on the state of acute confusion and the incontinence, she is experiencing delirium. This is most likely secondary to sepsis, with a urinary tract infection as the source of infection. The fact that she has mental status changes (disoriented to person, place, or time, in addition to the acute confusion, delirium, and incontinence) gives you the clues to sepsis. Dementia is more insidious versus acute. Depression and psychosis are not consistent with the assessments. The major symptoms in depression would include loss of interest, sleep disorder, decreased appetite, loss of concentration, inactivity, guilt, lack of energy, and potential suicidal thoughts. Psychotic disorders include thoughts and behavior indicating the patient is not in touch with reality.

28. Answer: 4

Rationale: The laws in most states require the reporting of suspected or actual abuse and neglect of any person considered to be dependent or with a reduced ability to make life choices. Children, disabled individuals, and dependent older adults fall into these categories. Very few states require reporting for adult women unless a weapon is involved; this is a different situation, requiring a report.

29. Answer: 1

Rationale: Patients admitting to forgetfulness are not as much of a concern for the diagnosis of cognitive impairment as those who have been in motor vehicle accidents or deny any level of memory loss. Dementia is associated with loss of short-term/recent memory more than long-term/remote memory loss.

30. Answer: 2

Rationale: Bradycardia and excessive salivation are not found with cocaine abuse. There are no drug antagonists that can be used for cocaine overdose, although benzodiazepines are used to treat effects of cocaine toxicity such as seizures, tachycardia, and hypertension. Naloxone is given to reduce the concurrent toxic effects of other narcotic drugs that may be in the patient's body system but is not effective against cocaine toxicity.

31. Answer: 4

Rationale: Although all the items listed are appropriate to assess in the patient, it is most important to determine judgment. If he cannot make safe judgments, he is at high risk for unsafe behaviors, such as driving, walking along the sidewalk, running the bath water, and so forth.

32. Answer: 4

Rationale: The history supports a diagnosis of delirium tremens. Delirium tremens is severe alcohol withdrawal that typically develops 24–72 hours after the last drink. The patient may be confused, disoriented, and have hallucinations, tremors, elevated blood pressure, tachycardia, a rise in body temperature, and tonic-clonic seizures. A patient with heroin overdose may also be confused, but he or she would have hypotension, slowed respirations, and a decreased pulse. A patient septic from pneumonia may present with cough, chills, low oxygen saturation, fever, hypotension, and tachycardia. Thyroid storm is severe hyperthyroidism that presents with elevated temperature, weakness, sweating, confusion, tachycardia, and gastrointestinal symptoms.

33. Answer: 4

Rationale: Using the words "declined, chose not to, or is not in agreement with" are preferable to saying that the patient is noncompliant, resistant, or refusing treatment. Terminology often heard in the media may be inappropriate in the clinical setting. For example, in the case of immigrants who are residing without legal status, "undocumented" is preferable to "illegal" or "foreigner." It is preferable to use "person-first language," such as a person with diabetes rather than "diagnosis-first" language—a diabetic patient. Transgender is preferred rather than transsexual.

34. Answer: 3, 4

Rationale: Cognitive deficits associated with depression include deficits in executive function (problem solving, decision making, impaired judgment), memory loss, and lack of concentration and attention to daily activities. The symptoms of major depressive disorder include feelings of sadness, tearfulness, emptiness, helplessness or hopelessness, inappropriate guilt, loss of interest in previously enjoyable activities, sleep disturbances, decreased energy, tiredness, appetite and weight changes, psychomotor retardation or agitation, and preoccupation with death or thoughts of suicide.

35. Answer: 3

Rationale: Compulsive bathing in hot water is reported by most patients with cannabinoid hyperemesis syndrome. Patients experience rapid, transient relief of nausea, vomiting, and abdominal pain and may spend up to half their waking hours bathing or showering in hot water. The other three symptoms are part of the differential diagnosis—binging and purging (bulimia nervosa), hyperpigmentation of the skin (Addison's disease), and unilateral headache (migraine headache).

36. Answer: 3

A simple and useful guide to organize sleep assessment is the BEARS screening tool (Bedtime problems, Excessive sleepiness, Awakenings, Regularity of sleep, and Sleep-disordered breathing). Testing tip—think "sleep like a bear." The Beers Criteria is a compendium of medications potentially to avoid or consider with caution because they often present an unfavorable balance of benefits and harms for older people. CAGE is a four-question survey to identify potential alcohol dependence (felt the need to Cut back on drinking, Annoyed by someone criticizing your drinking, Guilt about drinking, and Eye-opening morning drinking). The acronym BATTED is for assessing activities of daily living (Bathing, Ambulation, Transfers, Toileting, Eating, Dressing).

Pharmacology

37. Answer: 3

Rationale: The patient is experiencing a rare problem called neuroleptic malignant syndrome. The patient would require immediate referral and hospitalization. This can also occur with the medication prochlorperazine. Acute dystonia, parkinsonism, and akathisia are associated with extrapyramidal disorder or acute movement disorder. Tardive dyskinesia occurs late in therapy and is often irreversible. Slow, worm-like movements of the tongue are the earliest symptom, followed by grimacing, lip smacking, and involuntary limb movements.

38. Answer: 2

Rationale: The favorable side effect profile of citalopram (Celexa), which is a selective serotonin reuptake inhibitor, makes it a useful antidepressant in the older adult because it has a short half-life. Amitriptyline (Elavil) has the most anticholinergic and sedating side effects of the antidepressants. There may be pronounced effects on the cardiovascular system (hypotension). Geropsychiatrists agree it is best to avoid amitriptyline (Elavil) in the older adult; however, low dose (10 mg, PO every evening) is low cost and can be effective at controlling neuropathic pain. Trazodone (Desyrel) is very sedating for the older adult patient but can be used for insomnia and for behavioral issues with dementia patients. Haloperidol (Haldol) is an antipsychotic medication and is not to be used at all in long-term care facilities.

39. Answer: 1

Rationale: Physical dependence can occur, even with low doses of benzodiazepines. This is a particular problem in the older adult, who is sensitive to low-dose ranges. If possible, it is better to slowly taper the patient from benzodiazepines; often they can be tapered to a much lower dose.

40. Answer: 2

Rationale: Antidepressants, such as SSRIs and serotonin-norepinephrine reuptake inhibitors (SNRIs), are considered first-line treatment for anxiety disorders. Benzodiazepines are not helpful in the older adult patient because of problems associated with this class of medications, including increased risk of falls, confusion, and memory problems. TCAs and older monoamine oxidase inhibitors have indications for management of some of the anxiety disorders but are not considered first line because of tolerability and carry a high risk of cardiac dysrhythmias. Atypical antipsychotics are not first-line therapy and include significant side effects (metabolic syndrome, extrapyramidal effects, sedation), which can be problematic for the older adult.

41. Answer: 1

Rationale: It is important to reduce starting doses of antidepressants by 50% in older adults, people with impaired renal function, or those especially sensitive to side effects.

42. Answer: 4

Rationale: Correction of environmental factors and treatment of underlying iatrogenic and medical problems should be addressed initially. Amitriptyline (Elavil) can cause excessive somnolence. Trazodone (Desyrel) may be of particular use when sleep disturbance is prominent; however, it does not address the best initial plan. The goal is to begin with good sleep hygiene before pharmacologic therapy. Eliminating naps during the day may be useful in facilitating sleep.

43. Answer: 1

Rationale: Drug–drug interactions are a common cause of acute confusion in the older adult patient. This medication review assessment can minimize the need to do further costly interventions if the patient needs only medication adjustment. The other options should be included in the plan after the medication review history is completed and has been ruled out as a potential problem. The family nurse practitioner must always consider that an acute illness, such as a urinary tract infection, may be the cause of acute confusion. A urinalysis should also be obtained because the patient can quickly progress to sepsis.

44. Answer: 2

Rationale: In combination with tyramine-rich foods that have undergone an aging process, such as cheese, wine, beer, salami, and yogurt, catecholamines are released from the nerve endings, causing a hypertensive crisis. The other drugs listed cause hypotension.

45. Answer: 3

Rationale: The benzodiazepines cause sedation and decreased attention, which, in turn, affect the memory. Although phenothiazines and antidepressants may also cause sedation, they do not affect memory.

46. Answer: 3

Rationale: Flashbacks, depression, and psychotic behavior can occur with LSD use. There are no withdrawal symptoms or physical dependence associated with use; however, tolerance develops quickly. Commonly, the adolescent remains oriented but experiences hallucinations and altered bodily sensations.

47. Answer: 3

Rationale: Trazodone (Desyrel) has sedation as a side effect, which has made it less popular as an antidepressant; however, it is commonly prescribed for insomnia.

48. Answer: 1, 3, 4

Rationale: Lithium has adverse side effects on renal, cardiac, and thyroid function. Baseline electrolytes are also important to obtain. It is not important to evaluate liver function, fasting lipids, and ESR before initiating treatment with lithium.

49. Answer: 3

Rationale: Naloxone (Narcan) is a narcotic antagonist and is used for the reversal of narcotic depression, including respiratory depression. Clonidine (Catapres) is a central-acting α_2 agonist and is indicated for treatment of hypertension. Methadone is used in the treatment of opioid addiction. The Food and Drug Administration has placed methadone in a special drug category that allows medically supervised administration of the drug to addicts with chronic, intractable addiction to heroin. In addition, methadone can be used for pain management. The therapeutic classification of naltrexone (Revia) is as a narcotic detoxification adjunct.

50. Answer: 1, 3, 5

Rationale: Seizures, alcohol withdrawal, and anxiety are commonly treated with benzodiazepines. They are not the first drug of choice for obsessive-compulsive disorder; selective serotonin reuptake inhibitors are usually used. Schizophrenia and bipolar affective disorder are treated with antipsychotics.

51. Answer: 1

Rationale: The rule of thumb for starting medications in the older adult patient is to start low and go slow; therefore doses should be reduced by 30%–50% to start therapy and gradually increased as necessary. Adverse effects are likely to occur because of slowed drug metabolism, which occurs with aging. These include hypotension, arrhythmias, and sedative and anticholinergic effects.

52. Answer: 2

Rationale: A highly nicotine-dependent patient benefits from intense counseling and prescription of alternative nicotine delivery during the smoking cessation process. The nicotine patch is usually the preferred form of replacement because the gum is noncontinuous and withdrawal symptoms may occur during nonchewing times. The nicotine patch delivers a fixed dose of nicotine on a continual basis, is applied once daily, and eliminates the gastrointestinal upset that often occurs with the gum. If this patient insisted on using the gum, the dose should be 4 mg, not 2 mg. A nicotine patch with 14 mg is too low a dose to start on this patient and is not the correct dosing schedule. Underdosing can cause patients to start smoking again. Zyban (bupropion HCl) would be used in conjunction with the nicotine patch, and patients are to quit smoking 1–2 weeks after starting the Zyban, not immediately.

53. Answer: 2

Rationale: When stopping a selective serotonin reuptake inhibitor, such as sertraline (Zoloft), it is important to taper the dose over at least 2 weeks. Stopping the medication abruptly can lead to flulike symptoms. There is no need to continue the medication or switch to a different antidepressant because the patient was assessed for safety and it is reasonable to stop the medication. The family nurse practitioner should make a follow-up appointment to assess how the patient is doing off the medication.

54. Answer: 1

Rationale: Divalproex sodium (Depakote) is an antiepileptic used to treat seizures, treat mania in bipolar disorder, and prevent migraine headaches and is used for agitation in dementia patients. It can cause hepatotoxicity, especially in the first 6 months of starting the medication. It can also cause thrombocytopenia and pancreatitis in some incidences.

55. Answer: 1

Rationale: Diphenhydramine (Benadryl) is an antihistamine with anticholinergic properties. Anticholinergic drugs may cause confusion, urinary retention, orthostatic hypotension, tachycardia, dry mouth, constipation, sedation, and blurred vision. Anticholinergic drugs are particularly dangerous in the older adult because they can lead to falls and confusion.

56. Answer: 3

Rationale: The maximum dose of citalopram (Celexa) for a patient older than age 60 is 20 mg. Celexa has a risk of prolonged QT interval, which can lead to torsades de pointes. Torsades de pointes is a ventricular dysrhythmia that can lead to sudden death.

57. Answer: 1

Rationale: Benzodiazepines should be tapered in all patients but especially in the older adult. Withdrawal symptoms may include sweating, vomiting, muscle cramps, tremors, and/or seizures. Rebound or withdrawal symptoms occur within 24 hours in patients taking the shorter-acting medications and may not occur for several days in patients taking long-acting medications. The adverse effects of oversedation—dizziness, confusion, and orthostatic hypotension—contribute to falls and other injuries in the older adult. Short-acting medications are preferred. Typically, larger doses are not needed but rather small initial doses with gradual increases.

20

Research & Theory

Research

1. A family nurse practitioner has read a nursing research article in which there were no statistically significant findings. In interpreting these findings, what would be the family nurse practitioner's most appropriate response?
   1. "Because there were no statistically significant findings, there are no relationships between the study groups."
   2. "Because there were no statistically significant findings, there is no reason to conduct similar studies."
   3. "Because there were no statistically significant findings, further study is warranted to compare results."
   4. "Because there were no statistically significant findings, the sample size was too large."

2. What is the primary purpose of using evidence-based practice (EBP) in clinical research and practice management?
   1. To ensure credible resources are used in clinical decision-making.
   2. To further advance the peer review process.
   3. To provide quality care to patients by closing the gap among theory, experience, and best practice guidelines.
   4. To arrive at a consensus of opinion.

3. In a recent study, the researcher reports that "the statistical analysis used was Pearson's product-moment correlation." When is it appropriate to use Pearson's product-moment correlation as the statistical analysis for analyzing data in research? (Select 2 responses.)
   1. Pearson's product-moment correlation can be used for comparing interval or ratio levels of measurement among two or more variables.
   2. Pearson's product-moment correlation actually determines whether a causal relationship exists between one or more variables.
   3. Pearson's product-moment correlation can be used only when there is a single variable.
   4. Pearson's product-moment correlation is used to identify the relationship between two or more variables.

4. When might a qualitative research design be used over a quantitative or mixed methods research design?
   1. Qualitative research is the appropriate methodology for exploring and understanding a particular phenomenon of interest.
   2. Qualitative research does not require rights of research subjects to be protected.
   3. Qualitative research will provide precise measures for statistical analysis.
   4. Qualitative research ensures tight control during data collection and data analysis.

5. A family nurse practitioner is reviewing a research article that refers to a study of elderly patients who received different treatment protocols regarding fall risk assessments. Based on this information, what type of research design is being represented?
   1. Historical.
   2. Experimental.
   3. Correlational.
   4. Descriptive.

6. Variance is a key statistical concept. How would current research methods change if there was no variance?
   1. Nurse researchers would need to increase the sample size in all research studies to 100 research subjects or greater.
   2. Because current research methods do not depend on the presence of variance, researchers would not need to change current methods.
   3. Nurse researchers would need to decrease the sample size of all research studies to 15 research subjects.
   4. Because current research methods are based on the presence of variance, researchers would not be able to use current methods.

7. A family nurse practitioner is reviewing a behavioral pain assessment tool to determine whether the tool should be used in the clinical practice setting. Which statistical measure would indicate that the tool can be used?
   1. Two-tailed t-test.
   2. Descriptive statistics.
   3. Cronbach's alpha.
   4. Factor analysis.

8. A family nurse practitioner understands that an incidence rate is: (Select 2 responses.)
   1. Often a percentage and describes the characteristics of a population.
   2. A sensitive indicator of the changing health of a community.
   3. The number of new cases of a disease in those exposed to a disease.
   4. The number of cases of a specific disease or condition in a population at a specified point in time relative to the population at the same point in time.
   5. The occurrence of new cases of a disease or condition in a population over a period of time relative to the size of the population at risk for the disease of condition in the same time period.

9. A state public health region reported 21 cases of influenza in adults 65 years of age and older to date this year, with two adults who died. The total population for this geographic region is 11,533, of whom 4420 are adults 65 years of age and older. What is the prevalence rate of influenza in the region thus far in the current year?
   1. 1.8/1000.
   2. 2/1000.
   3. 21/1000.
   4. 4.7/1000.

10. What are the major sequential steps in evidence-based practice (EBP)?
    1. Establish a patient relationship, perform a health assessment, make a diagnosis, devise a plan of care, perform prescribed treatments, and evaluate efficacy of the treatments.
    2. Identify the problem and generate a clinical question, conduct a literature review of scholarly research articles, critically appraise published research, implement useful findings in practice and clinical decision making, and disseminate findings.
    3. Review the popular literature, review the institution's policy and procedures, summarize the findings from the literature review and policies and procedures, and evaluate applicability of the study findings to practice setting.
    4. Review the patient's laboratory reports, complete a thorough health assessment, diagnose, collaborate with the health care provider in developing a treatment plan, implement the treatment, and evaluate the efficacy of the treatment.

11. A family nurse practitioner is planning to conduct a study to examine the efficacy of a high-protein, high-fiber diet in weight reduction of obese patients. The family nurse practitioner develops the following research question to guide the study: What is the effect on the weight of obese patients who follow a high-protein, high-fiber diet compared with the weight of obese patients who do not follow a high-protein, high-fiber diet over a 12-week period? What are the independent variable and the dependent variable in the research question?
    1. The independent variable is the 12-week time frame and the dependent variable is the high-protein, high-fiber diet.
    2. The independent variable is the high-protein, high-fiber diet and the dependent variable is the patients' weight.
    3. The independent variable is the patients' weight and the dependent variable is the high-protein, high-fiber diet.
    4. The independent variable is the high-protein, high-fiber diet and the dependent variable is the 12-week time frame.

12. The family nurse practitioner is evaluating research reports on the efficacy of cognitive-behavioral therapy (CBT) on anxiety in patients with Alzheimer's disease. When reviewing the literature, which type of research study does the family nurse practitioner recognize as the highest level of evidence?
    1. A quantitative research study using a case-control design.
    2. A quantitative research study using a correlational research design.
    3. A quantitative research study using a randomized-controlled trial design.
    4. A qualitative research study using a phenomenologic approach.

13. When the family nurse practitioner questions whether being exposed to secondhand smoke leads to lung cancer in a group of residential home patients with another group of residential patients who have not been exposed to secondhand smoke, what is the family nurse practitioner determining?
    1. Prevalence rate.
    2. Incidence rate.
    3. Confidence interval.
    4. Relative risk.

14. The state public health department reported a total of 423 cases of tuberculosis between 2016 and 2018. During that same time, 17 deaths were attributed to tuberculosis. Based on this information, what is the death-to-case ratio?
    1. 4.05.
    2. 2.08.
    3. 2.48.
    4. 4.01.

15. The family nurse practitioner is conducting a meta-analysis on the effectiveness of patient teaching on how to use a metered-dose-inhaler in the treatment of asthma patients. Which three statements are accurate concerning a meta-analysis?
    1. Assesses clinical effectiveness of health care interventions.
    2. Provides a precise estimate of the treatment effect.
    3. Focuses on a few targeted studies with homogeneity.
    4. Adds potential bias to the review of specific research studies.
    5. Provides a qualitative review of pertinent research literature.
    6. Provides highest level of evidence because of statistical analysis and integration of many studies.

16. The family nurse practitioner is working with a team of colleagues on a research study that will involve patients as study participants. The research team understands which of the following must be included in the written consent to participate?
    1. Role of the primary research investigator.
    2. Anticipated date for publication of the completed research report.
    3. Assurance of patient privacy and confidentiality.
    4. Number of previously published research studies about this topic.

17. A family nurse practitioner is trying to determine whether a group of elderly patients are at increased risk for falls and wants to design a research study to examine the concerns of both patient and family member relative to the effect that falls in the elderly population have on physical and emotional lifestyle changes. What type of research design should be used?
    1. Quantitative research design looking at number of falls and hospital admissions as a result of complications.
    2. Mixed methods design looking at physical variables related to falls, hospital admissions, and focus group discussions to gather information about lifestyle changes experienced by patients and families after a fall.
    3. Qualitative research using focus groups to obtain information for analysis.
    4. Quasi-experimental design to examine relationships among participants.

18. The family nurse practitioner understands that when determining whether to incorporate a new procedure into a clinical practice based on the findings of a recent quantitative research study, which of the following should be considered? (Select 2 responses.)
    1. Statistical significance of the findings.
    2. Statistical relevance of the findings.
    3. Statistical software program used.
    4. Statistical background of the researcher.
    5. Methodological limitations of the study.

19. Which of the following statements made by the family nurse practitioner indicates an understanding of descriptive and inferential statistics? (Select 2 responses.)
    1. Inferential statistics are used for assigning participant code numbers.
    2. Descriptive statistics are used for assigning participant code numbers.
    3. Descriptive statistics are used to provide information about the study sample.
    4. Inferential statistics are used for hypothesis testing.
    5. Descriptive statistics are used for hypothesis testing.

20. The family nurse practitioner is preparing to participate in a research study and is considering the key differences between qualitative and quantitative research designs. What are the key differences between these two research designs?
    1. Qualitative research is a process in which the researcher attempts to stay far removed from the process to control for potential bias.
    2. Quantitative research design aims to search for themes collected during the research process.
    3. Qualitative research methods use research questions and/or hypotheses to test for relationships or cause and effect.
    4. Quantitative researchers use controls during the research process to minimize the effect of the results of the study.

21. The scientific method for conducting research uses the null hypothesis, which is statistically based. What is the correct format for stating the null hypothesis?
    1. There is no relationship between the independent and dependent variables.
    2. There is a significant relationship between the independent and dependent variables.
    3. There is a moderate relationship between the independent and dependent variables.
    4. There is an opposite relationship between the independent and dependent variables.

22. When evaluating claims made in advertisements, such as "Drug X has been used for 5 years with over 1 million doses administered in the United States, Canada, and Great Britain. Drug X stops heartburn, aids in digestion, and prevents esophageal reflux, and is the 'treatment of choice' to relieve GERD," the family nurse practitioner realizes that the claim is:
    1. Invalid; there is no control or comparison group, and no statistics are stated.
    2. Valid; there are sufficient numbers of users who have had success.
    3. Invalid; the level of significance is not mentioned to be at the 0.05 level or higher.
    4. Valid; the Hawthorne effect clearly demonstrates the relationship between the drug and the outcome.

23. The family nurse practitioner is critiquing several research articles to evaluate causality of an intervention to improve patient health. The nurse practitioner will consider what three questions to evaluate causality?
    1. Did the independent variable(s) have an effect on the dependent variable(s)?
    2. Did the influence of the intervention occur before the outcome?
    3. Did the researcher provide their credentials in the study report?
    4. Did the researcher control for extraneous variable(s) that may have affected the effect?

24. What is the difference between univariate and multivariate studies?
    1. Number of subjects in the sample.
    2. Number of statistical hypotheses.
    3. Number of sites for collecting data.
    4. Number of variables being studied.

25. The family nurse practitioner is compiling monthly statistics for the practice. One piece of data that is collected is the ethnicity of patients. What level of measurement data can be used to analyze the variable of ethnicity?
    1. Nominal level.
    2. Ordinal level.
    3. Interval level.
    4. Ratio level.

26. Quantitative research articles provide a section containing descriptive findings because descriptive data analysis:
    1. Provides the basis for making inferences about the findings.
    2. May yield statistically significant findings that were unexpected.
    3. Provides a clearer understanding of study participants and variables.
    4. Is conducted for predicting patient outcomes in nursing settings.

27. A family nurse practitioner is compiling statistics at the end of the month for an older adult patient population with coronary artery disease. The family nurse practitioner and physician in the general practice want to know the average total cholesterol level of their patients. Which would be the most appropriate statistical measure of the average cholesterol level for the patient population?
    1. The mean.
    2. The median.
    3. The mode.
    4. The range.

28. A family nurse practitioner is evaluating research articles for a research utilization project. The majority of the articles report that randomization was used. The practitioner understands that the purpose of randomization in many quantitative research studies is to:
    1. Be sure that subjects can choose whether they receive the intervention or not.
    2. Select research subjects who fit certain demographic criteria.
    3. Attempt to control for threats to internal validity by allowing research subjects to choose either the control or treatment group.
    4. Attempt to control for threats to internal validity by randomly assigning research subjects to either a control or a treatment group.

29. The ability to predict outcomes of care is desirable both in research and in practice. If a family nurse practitioner wanted to determine the effect of the independent variables of exercise and diet on the dependent variable of blood pressure, which statistical analysis method would be most appropriate to analyze the clinical data?
    1. Descriptive statistics.
    2. Paired t-test.
    3. Multiple regression.
    4. Chi-squared (χ^2) test.

30. The family nurse practitioner is reviewing information about incidence and prevalence rates among different populations in the United States. Which statement is accurate?
    1. Prostate cancer is more prevalent in Asian American men than African American men.
    2. African Americans have higher rates of hypertension than do white or Hispanic adults.
    3. Hispanic men have the lowest incidence of diabetes.
    4. American-Indians and Alaska Natives have a lower incidence of asthma than white persons.

31. When reviewing a research study, which three statements are correct regarding the use of symbols?
    1. χ^2 represents the correlation coefficient.
    2. p = .05 is used to identify the confidence interval.
    3. Confidence interval (CI) represents the chi-square test.
    4. n is the sample size.
    5. r is the correlation coefficient of a sample.
    6. H_o is the symbol for the null hypothesis.

32. When developing a research question, which statement has the correct format for correlational research?
    1. Is there a difference in Y (dependent variable) between people who have X characteristic (independent variable) and those who do not have X characteristic?
    2. Is there a difference in Y (dependent variable) between Group A, who received X (independent variable), and Group B, who did not receive X?
    3. Is there a relationship between X (independent variable) and Y (dependent variable) in the specified population?
    4. What is it like living with X (independent variable)?

33. What is the role of the Institutional Review Board (IRB)?
    1. Secures permission for obtaining grants.
    2. Maintains control over the researcher and the institution's access to funding.
    3. Evaluates the research study in accordance with clinical practice guidelines.
    4. Assesses that ethical standards are met in relation to the protection of the rights of human subjects.

Theory

34. Which statement provides best practice approach toward the development of nursing theory?
    1. Nursing theory should be integrated with other disciplines to arrive at a consensus of opinion.
    2. Nursing theory must be based solely on relevant clinical practice.
    3. Continued research must be encouraged to support the body of nursing research as a professional discipline.
    4. Nursing theory should be realigned to focus solely on middle range theory.

35. Martha Rogers' theory of principles of homeodynamics focuses on several principles that explain how individuals interact with the environment. Which of the following three principles are included in Rogers' theory of principles of homeodynamics?
    1. Carative factors.
    2. Resonancy.
    3. Primary prevention.
    4. Integrality.
    5. Helicy.

36. Using the Transtheoretical Model (TTM) as a framework for a behavioral change process, the family nurse practitioner knows that the patient who has expressed a desire to quit smoking, has begun to examine their tobacco use, and is weighing the pros and cons of quitting is in which stage of change?
    1. Precontemplation.
    2. Contemplation.
    3. Determination or preparation.
    4. Action.

37. What does King's Theory of Goal Attainment specifically focus on?
    1. Effective communication among patient, family, and health care provider.
    2. Reducing stressors that may contribute to illness and disease.
    3. Interaction, transactions, and mutually shared outcomes between the nurse and patient.
    4. The nurse assisting the patient with improving and meeting self-care needs.

38. What is the theoretical basis for nursing practice?
    1. A recent development in nursing practice.
    2. Developed from the medical model.
    3. Traced back to Florence Nightingale.
    4. Unrelated to the practice of nursing.

39. What is the verification of the more abstract nursing theories (e.g., of Martha Rogers) often hampered by?
    1. Lack of adequate instrumentation for the theoretical concepts.
    2. Prior studies that did not support the theory.
    3. Lack of adequate settings for conducting experiments.
    4. Prior studies that were conducted in other countries.

40. The family nurse practitioner is aware that basing nursing practice on nursing theory contributes to the professionalization of nursing practice by: (Select 2 responses.)
    1. Exploring relationships among person, health, environment, and nursing.
    2. Limiting the choice of treatments for patients, families, and communities.
    3. Determining what type of patients will be seen by the family nurse practitioner.
    4. Providing a consistent perspective for providing nursing care to patients.

41. Which nursing theory focuses on the transaction interaction between nurse and patient?
    1. Watson's Theory of Caring.
    2. Neuman's Systems Model.
    3. Martha Roger's Science of Unitary Beings.
    4. King's Theory of Goal Attainment.

42. A family nurse practitioner has decided to incorporate a theoretical nursing model into the ambulatory care practice, which emphasizes patients doing as much as possible independently to maintain their own health. Which nursing model is most applicable to this setting?
    1. Orem's Self-Care Deficit Theory of Nursing.
    2. Roy's Adaptation Model.
    3. Roger's Science of Unitary Human Beings.
    4. King's Theory of Goal Attainment.

43. Which of the following nursing theorists is considered to have general systems theory as the philosophic orientation to her model?
    1. Callista Roy.
    2. Martha Rogers.
    3. Rosemarie Parse.
    4. Betty Neuman.

44. Which nursing conceptual model addresses interventions in terms of primary, secondary, and tertiary prevention?
    1. Roy's Adaptation Model.
    2. Neuman's Systems Model.
    3. Levine's Conservation Model.
    4. Johnson's Behavioral System Model.

45. The family nurse practitioner is planning to conduct an educational program to facilitate smoking cessation in a group of adult smokers. The family nurse practitioner will use interventions that facilitate the participant's recognition of the health risk associated with continued smoking to facilitate the participant's desire to use the proposed interventions to improve overall health. Based on the goals and desired outcomes of the educational program, the family nurse practitioner knows that the most appropriate theoretical model to guide the development of the program would be:
    1. Roy's Adaptation Model.
    2. The Health Belief Model.
    3. The Conservation Model.
    4. The Intersystem Model.

46. Many biologic theories have been developed to explain aging. Which theory supports the idea of the "biologic clock"?
    1. Programmed Aging Theory.
    2. Autoimmune Theory.
    3. Wear-and-Tear Theory.
    4. Oxidative Stress Theory.

47. The family nurse practitioner is conducting a follow-up home visit for a patient who underwent a transpelvic amputation of the left leg for femoral osteomyelitis. The patient's past medical history includes type 2 diabetes, chronic kidney disease, diabetic neuropathy, and heart failure. The patient states, "I'll never be the same again without my leg. What is the point in trying to learn how to walk again? My life is over." Using the middle-range theory of chronic sorrow to this patient case scenario, the family nurse practitioner knows that the theory of chronic sorrow is composed of which major concepts? (Select 3 responses.)
    1. Trigger events.
    2. Person.
    3. Environment.
    4. Nursing.
    5. Management strategies.
    6. Disparity.

48. Using the framework of Benner's Theory of Novice to Expert, which statement describes a family nurse practitioner who is just starting his or her professional practice but has over 10 years' experience as a registered nurse?
    1. Advanced beginner.
    2. Expert.
    3. Novice.
    4. Proficient.

49. The family nurse practitioner is discussing methods to facilitate independence with a patient who has recently had a stroke and who is experiencing residual hemiplegia. The family nurse practitioner is using which concept of Orem's Self-Care Deficit Theory during this interaction?
    1. Universal self-care requisites.
    2. Developmental self-care requisites.
    3. Health deviation self-care deficits.
    4. Nursing system.

50. The family nurse practitioner is working in a culturally diverse medical clinic and would like to develop an educational program to facilitate improvement in health in the patient population. Based on the patient population and the purpose of the program, which of the following nursing theorists would be most appropriate to consider when developing the educational program?
    1. Calista Roy.
    2. Dorothea Orem.
    3. Margaret Newman.
    4. Madeleine Leininger.

51. A family nurse practitioner has been practicing for 2 years in the current role. Professional role evaluations have indicated that the practitioner is assuming an interactive role in the interdisciplinary team, demonstrating leadership skills and management skills with minimal direction. Based on the framework of Benner's Theory of Novice to Expert, the practitioner is functioning at which practice level?
    1. Competent.
    2. Expert.
    3. Proficient.
    4. Advanced beginner.

52. The family nurse practitioner understands the following about the Donabedian Model:
    1. Measures only nurse practitioner effectiveness.
    2. Is a model used for developing informatic systems.
    3. Provides a structure for nurse practitioners to plan patient care.
    4. Is a framework for assessing the quality of care that draws information about structure, process, and outcomes.

53. Which of the following principles applies to the Theory of Self-Transcendence?
    1. End-of-life transition.
    2. Rehabilitation.
    3. Parenting.
    4. Addiction.
    5. Neglect.

20 Research & Theory Answers & Rationales

Research

1. Answer: 3

Rationale: The lack of significant findings is an important piece of information in the study findings. Particularly when findings are not statistically significant, additional studies need to be conducted about this topic to determine whether the data are inconclusive. Threats to validity may cause a relationship to exist between study groups with no statistically significant findings. Ideally, changes in practice are based on the findings of more than one study, and a small sample size makes it more difficult to find statistically significant findings, not a large sample size.

2. Answer: 3

Rationale: The primary purpose of using EBP in clinical research and practice management is focused on the ability to provide quality care to patients by closing the gap among theory, experience, and best practice guidelines. Although credible resources are important, this relates more to the systematic process and ranking of research. The peer review process is also used in conjunction with EBP, but again this relates to the evaluation process rather than the primary purpose. Last, arriving at a consensus of opinion relates to the overall evaluation of the presented research. It is not an expectation of purpose.

3. Answer: 1, 4

Rationale: Pearson's product-moment correlation is the preferred statistical analysis to use for variables that consist of ratio or interval levels of measurement, whereas Spearman's correlation would be an appropriate statistical test to use when the research variables are ranked. Pearson's product-moment correlation also identifies the relationships between variables, not causal relationships between variables. Two or more variables are used for Pearson's product-moment correlation.

4. Answer: 1

Rationale: The purpose of qualitative research designs is to learn more about a particular phenomenon of interest by exploring the beliefs, values, and experiences of individuals. Qualitative designs do not yield precise measures, are usually not analyzed statistically, and carry the same concerns about the rights of subjects as all other research designs. Quantitative research designs ensure tight control over data collection and analysis.

5. Answer: 2

Rationale: Based on the provided information, the research design is based on quantitative methods using an experimental approach because there are different treatment protocols provided. Historical design is an example of qualitative research looking at prior information in terms of predicting possible future outcomes. Correlational design is an example of quantitative research looking at relationships between specific factors within a sample group. Descriptive design is an example of quantitative research providing information about specific factors in a data set providing summary information.

6. Answer: 4

Rationale: All current research and statistical analysis methods rely on the presence of variance or variation. Variance is a statistical measure used to identify how spread out scores are from the mean. If variance is no longer present, current methods could no longer be used. If there is no variance, a sample of one would be adequate.

7. Answer: 3

Rationale: Cronbach's alpha is a statistical tool that helps to determine reliability by examining internal consistency. A two-tailed t-test is a statistical measurement based on observation of two independent groups. Descriptive statistics provides information related to data sets. Factor analysis is used to assess relative effects of variables as to which is most important.

8. Answer: 2, 5

Rationale: The incidence rate is the occurrence of new cases of a disease or condition in a population over a period of time relative to the size of the population at risk for the disease or condition in the same time period. Incidence rates are helpful for monitoring short-term changes in a disease (influenza, chickenpox, measles, etc.) and are a sensitive indicator of the changing health of a community because the rate captures the fluctuations of a disease. A prevalence rate is the number of cases of a specific disease or condition in a population at a specified point in time relative to the population at the same point in time. An attack rate is the number of new cases of a disease in those exposed to the disease.

9. Answer: 4

Rationale: A prevalence rate is the total number of cases of a disease existing in a population divided by the total population. The number of existing cases is 21 and the total geriatric population is 4420. The formula to calculate is:

$$\frac{number\ of\ existing\ cases}{total\ population} \times 1000$$

10. Answer: 2

Rationale: Identify the problem and generate a clinical question, conduct a literature review of scholarly research articles, critically appraise published research, implement useful findings in practice and clinical decision making, and disseminate findings containing the published steps of EBP. All other options are nursing actions taken on behalf of the patient (in no particular order).

11. Answer: 2

Rationale: The independent variable is the measure that can be manipulated in a study: the high-protein, high-fiber diet. The dependent variable is the response from the independent variable and is measurable, for example, the obese patients' weight. The population of interest is the obese patient and the length of the study is 12 weeks.

12. Answer: 3

Rationale: A randomized-controlled trial is one of the highest levels of evidence in determining whether a cause-and-effect relationship exists between an experimental intervention (treatment) and dependent variable (outcome). By randomizing participants into either a control or a treatment group, rigor is increased. A quantitative case-control study is a type of observational study in which the researcher compares risk factors or exposure in study participants who have a disease or medical condition with study participants who do not have the disease to determine whether an association exists. In this type of research, no intervention or treatment is given. A quantitative correlational research design examines the relationship between one or more variables; correlational research does not predict causality. Qualitative research designs are lower on the hierarchal level of evidence pyramid because they do not attempt to predict causality or determine the effectiveness of an intervention.

13. Answer: 4

Rationale: The relative risk or risk ratio is a measure of the risk of a certain event (getting lung cancer) happening in one group exposed to a factor (secondhand smoke) compared with the risk of the same event happening in another group not exposed to a factor. A prevalence rate is the total number of cases of a disease existing in a population divided by the total population. The incidence rate is a measure of the frequency with which a disease occurs in a population over a period of time. The confidence interval describes the amount of uncertainty associated with a sample estimate of a population parameter, usually at 95% level, and assists in representing how good an estimate is.

14. Answer: 4

Rationale: The death-to-case ratio is the number of deaths caused by a certain disease during a specific period of time divided by the number of new cases of that disease identified during the same time period and is calculated as follows:

$$\frac{\text{Number of deaths caused by a disease during specific time period}}{\text{Number of new cases of the same disease identified during the same time period}} \times 100$$

15. Answer: 1, 2, 6

Rationale: A meta-analysis is a summary of a number of independent studies focused on one question or topic, and it uses a specific statistical methodology to synthesize the findings to draw conclusions about the area of focus that ultimately seeks new knowledge, as well as confirming knowledge, from existing research data. It is used to assess clinical effectiveness of health care interventions and is helpful in providing a precise estimate of a treatment or intervention outcome. Meta-analysis provides level I evidence, which is considered the highest level of evidence, because it statistically analyzes and integrates the results of many independent studies. An effective, robust meta-analysis aims for complete coverage of all relevant studies, examines for the presence of heterogeneity in the studies, and explores the studies' main findings using sensitivity analysis. Meta-analysis, when performed as a rigorous systematic review, can overcome inherent bias by offering an unbiased synthesis of the empirical data. Meta-analyses offer a systematic and quantitative (not qualitative) approach to synthesizing research evidence to analyze clinical interventions.

16. Answer: 3

Rationale: By federal law, the rights of human research subjects must be protected. Patients must be assured of their privacy and confidentiality through informed consent. The researchers may include the other information; however, it is not required by federal law.

17. Answer: 2

Rationale: The situation described relates to looking at both physical and emotional components of the subject groups. Because of this, a mixed methods design should be used that looks at both physical and emotional variables across the population. Descriptive statistics (quantitative) would be needed to look at number of falls and hospital admissions as a result of complications, but this is just one aspect of the research design. Similarly, using only focus groups (qualitative) would not address the other relevant factors expressed by the family nurse practitioner. A quasi-experimental design would not be applicable in this situation because it would not address the patient's and family's experience as provided and there is no attempt to control for variables.

18. Answer: 1, 5

Rationale: In published research reports, of the options listed, statistical significance of the findings and methodological limitations of the study are consistently reported by researchers. The statistical significance of a study's findings provides consumers of research with information about the likelihood that the results may have occurred by chance. It is also equally important to have knowledge of a study's limitations, such as sample size, to determine whether the findings could be applicable in a different population or setting. The clinical relevance is considered, not the statistical relevance. The specific statistical software program used does not make a difference because all are based on the same statistical formulas. Researchers frequently work with statistical consultants, so a researcher's background is not a limitation to a published study.

19. Answer: 3, 4

Rationale: Neither type of statistics is used to assign participant code numbers. Descriptive statistics use statistical methods to describe the study sample and variables. Inferential statistics are used for hypothesis testing to analyze data from a sample to determine whether the study findings could be generalized to an entire population.

20. Answer: 4

Rationale: Quantitative researchers remain as removed from the research process as possible and use controls to mitigate influencing test results or introducing potential bias. Quantitative research tests for relationships and cause an effect through a statistical analysis and reporting to test hypotheses or research questions. Qualitative researchers are integrated into the research process and, through analysis of dialog and observations, search for themes.

21. Answer: 1

Rationale: The correct format for the null hypothesis is "There is no relationship between the independent and dependent variables." If a relationship does exist, the null hypothesis would be rejected. The alternate or research hypothesis may take the other forms.

22. Answer: 1

Rationale: Even though the claims detail extensive use of "Drug X," there must be statistical evidence reported. Additionally, randomization, as demonstrated through the use of control or comparison groups, should be implemented that will render a level of significance. The Hawthorne effect is a limitation and threat to a study's validity because the study participants' behaviors and responses are changed because they are in the study, not necessarily from the intervention or treatment performed.

23. Answer: 1, 2, 4

Rationale: When evaluating for causality, the consumer of research should consider the following: did the intervention precede the effect, did the intervention affect the outcome, and what, if any, impact did extraneous variable(s) have on the effect. Although the experience and credentials of the researcher are important when evaluating the strength of the study, they have little influence on the interventions(s) and outcomes of the study.

24. Answer: 4

Rationale: Variate refers to the number of variables in the study. A univariate study has one variable and a multivariate study has two or more variables. Variate does not relate to the number of participants, hypotheses, or a description of the study setting.

25. Answer: 1

Rationale: The variable of ethnicity is categorical data or nominal-level data. Ordinal-level measurements are also categorized, but the categories can be ranked. Interval-level measurements of data are categorized, ranked, and have equal interval scales in which the distance between intervals is always the same. Ratio-level measurement has all of the criteria as interval-level data and has an absolute zero point.

26. Answer: 3

Rationale: Descriptive data analysis organizes the data, and it facilitates understanding of the participants who participated in the study and variables of the study. Descriptive statistics cannot be used for significance testing or for making inferences; instead, inferential statistics are used. Predictions or causality are made from studies that use inferential statistics.

27. Answer: 1

Rationale: In light of the fact that the practitioner is looking for the average, the mean would provide for the average of all values. The median is the middle score, the mode is the most frequent score, and the range provides the difference between the highest and lowest scores in a set.

28. Answer: 4

Rationale: Randomization is a research technique used to increase the amount of control and reduce potential threats of internal validity in any research design. The other three options do not decrease potential threats to internal validity.

29. Answer: 3

Rationale: Of the options, only multiple regression examines the relationship between two or more independent variables on a dependent variable. Descriptive statistics provide information about the study variables and sample. A paired t-test is used to determine differences between two groups (e.g., control and experimental group) on an outcome. The chi-squared (χ^2) test compares whether the frequency in each category is different from what would be expected by chance.

30. Answer: 2

Rationale: African American adults have higher rates of hypertension than do white or Hispanic adults through age 75. African Americans have a higher incidence of cardiovascular, stroke, and renal complications and have a higher mortality rate related to hypertension than do people of other ethnic backgrounds. This is in part caused by enhanced renal sodium reabsorption that occurs in 57% of African Americans compared with 27% in other groups. This salt sensitivity contributes to the problem of high blood pressure among African Americans. The majority of prostate cancer cases are diagnosed in men older than 65 years, with incidence rates higher in African American men than in Asian American and non-Hispanic white men. The prevalence of diabetes increases with age and is higher in Hispanics than in non-Hispanic whites. African Americans and American Indian or Alaska Native races have a higher asthma prevalence compared with white Americans.

31. Answer: 4, 5, 6

Rationale: Sample size is denoted by a lower case "n." A capital N represents the total population in the study. The small case "r" represents the correlation coefficient of a sample. H_o is the symbol for the null hypothesis. χ^2 is the symbol for chi-squared test. The symbol, p = .05, stands for significance, not CI. The smaller the p value; the more significant the results. Most studies use a cutoff of p = .05 for significance.

32. Answer: 3

Rationale: A research question should clearly identify the variables under consideration. When exploring relationships between variables, a correlation or degree of association is examined. An independent variable, usually symbolized by X, is the variable that has the presumed effect on the dependent variable (symbol Y). In experimental research studies, the researcher manipulates the independent variable (Option #2). Option #4 is an example of a qualitative research study question. Option #1 is an example of a comparative research study question.

33. Answer: 4

Rationale: IRBs are boards that review studies to assess that ethical standards are met in relation to the protection of the rights of human subjects and typically consist of at least five members of various backgrounds to provide a complete and adequate review of a proposed research study. The primary role of an IRB, often called a human subjects' committee, is to review research projects and protect the rights of the human subjects.

Theory

34. Answer: 3

Rationale: The best practice approach toward the development of nursing theory is to build on research that directly relates to the professional discipline of nursing. Although it is important to work with other disciplines, integration of nursing theory should not be subject to restriction and limitation. Nursing theory should be based on hypothesis-generating and experience-generating issues. No one theoretical model should be used for any professional discipline because it will limit/restrict original thought.

35. Answer: 2, 4, 5

Rationale: Resonancy, integrality, and helicy are principles of homeodynamics that Rogers developed and defined to explain how individuals interact with their environment. Carative factors refer to Jean Watson's 10 carative factors under the Theory of Human Caring, and primary prevention relates to Neuman's Systems Model.

36. Answer: 2

Rationale: The TTM developed by Prochaska and DiClemente is used to conceptualize the process of intentional behavior change, such as quitting smoking, losing weight, or exercising regularly. There are five steps: precontemplation (not ready), contemplation (getting ready), determination or preparation (ready), action (change is made), maintenance (sustains change). The patient who expresses a desire to quit smoking, has begun to examine tobacco use, and is weighing the pros and cons of quitting is in the contemplation stage.

37. Answer: 3

Rationale: King's Theory of Goal Attainments focuses on human interaction between the nurse and patient. During this interaction, information sharing and mutual patient goal setting occurs between the nurse and patient. Although King's Theory focuses on communication, additional factors make up King's Theory. Minimizing stressors in the patient's environment refers to Neuman's Systems Model. Orem's Self-Care Theory focuses on assisting the patient with meeting self-care needs.

38. Answer: 3

Rationale: The theoretical basis for nursing practice began with Florence Nightingale and has been used in practice and research for more than a century. Nursing theories are specifically developed for nursing.

39. Answer: 1

Rationale: The lack of adequate tools and instruments for theoretical concepts is a major roadblock in many areas of research, and particularly so with the more abstract theories. Prior studies always provide information about the theory, even when conducted in other countries. The setting of the study plays no role in testing the theory.

40. Answer: 1, 4

Rationale: Theory-based practice contributes the consistent perspective that permits the comparison of care across settings. This practice does not necessarily limit treatments or determine patient types. Theory-based practice specifically eliminates reliance on the medical model and provides nursing with a method to explain and explore the relationships between phenomena specific to nursing; specifically, the following four concepts: person, health, environment, and nursing.

41. Answer: 4

Rationale: King's Theory of Goal Attainment focuses on the transactional interactions between the nurse and the patient. The other theories do not examine transactional relationships between the nurse and patient as the primary measurement parameter. Watson's Theory of Caring focuses on health promotion and restoration applied to the delivery of nursing care. Neuman's Systems Model examines the individual in the context of environmental systems. Martha Roger's Science of Unitary Beings focuses on nursing phenomenon characteristics.

42. Answer: 1

Rationale: Orem's theory focuses on the patient participating in their own health care. Roy's model focuses on adaptation. Roger's theory focuses on the synchronicity between the patient and the environment. King's theory is focused on the patient and nurse working together to achieve health-related goals.

43. Answer: 4

Rationale: Neuman's Systems Model is based on general systems theory. Roy's Adaptation Model is based on stress and adaptation as the framework. The theories of Martha Rogers and Rosemarie Parse are based on a humanistic developmental framework.

44. Answer: 2

Rationale: Betty Neuman identified the need to implement nursing interventions through the use of one or more of three modalities: primary, secondary, and tertiary prevention. Roy,

Levine, and Johnson do not use these concepts in their nursing models.

45. Answer: 2

Rationale: The Health Belief Model recognizes that an individual's desire to use health-promoting interventions is directly related to his or her perceived risk of developing a negative outcome if the intervention is not used. The Intersystem Model, the Conservation Model, and Roy's Adaptation Model do not use the risk and benefit concepts to facilitate participation in improving health or participating in health promotion activities.

46. Answer: 1

Rationale: The Programmed Aging Theory postulates that each cell has a preprogrammed life span, that is, the biologic clock, and that the number of cell reproductions was limited. The Wear-and-Tear Theory proposes that cellular errors were the result of "wearing out" over time because of continued use, in which the damage was caused by pollutants and metabolic by-products, that is, free radicals. Oxidative Stress Theory postulates that stress appears to be random and unpredictable, varying from one cell to another, from one person to another. Oxidative stress theories and their associated mitochondrial theories of aging are among the most studied and most widely accepted. The Autoimmune Theory postulates that aging is a result of an accumulation of damage caused by changes in the activities and function of the immune system (immunosenescence), which leads to the decreased ability of lymphocytes to withstand oxidative stress and appears to be a key factor in the aging process.

47. Answer: 1, 5, 6

Rationale: The theory of chronic sorrow is composed of three major concepts: chronic sorrow (disparity), trigger events, and management strategies. Person, environment, and nursing are concepts within the nursing metaparadigm.

48. Answer: 3

Rationale: Even though the individual has clinical work experience as a registered nurse, the fact that the individual is beginning/assuming an advanced practice role would indicate, according to Benner's Theory of Novice to Expert, that they would be classified as a novice. An advanced beginner would have some experience within the advanced practice role. An expert level would represent the highest level of knowledge, skill integration, and application in practice. A proficient level would indicate flexibility and fluid use of nursing judgment.

49. Answer: 3

Rationale: Health deviation self-care deficits relate to facilitating self-care when a health care deficit exists. Universal self-care requisites relate to general human needs. Developmental self-care deficits refer to necessary developmental processes that occur throughout life. Nursing systems, according to Orem's Self-Care Deficit Theory, refers to the relationship between the nurse and the patient.

50. Answer: 4

Rationale: Madeleine Leininger's Theory of Transcultural Nursing explores cultural diversity and aims to recognize similarities and differences with various cultures and the role of nursing in working with these cultures in the health care setting. Calista Roy's Adaptation Model, Dorothea Orem's Self-Care Deficit Theory, and Margaret Newman's Health as Expanding Consciousness Theory all explore the interrelationship of nursing and the patient, but only Leininger's Theory of Transcultural Nursing explores the aspect of cultural diversity in addition to these concepts.

51. Answer: 1

Rationale: The noted findings of assuming an interactive role within the interdisciplinary team and demonstrating leadership and management skills with minimal direction point to the level of competency. An expert would represent the highest level of knowledge, skill integration, and application in practice. A proficient level would indicate flexibility and use of nursing judgment. An advanced beginner would have some experience within the advanced practice role but would still rely on other guidelines.

52. Answer: 4

Rationale: The Donabedian Model is about health care quality. According to the model, information about quality of care can be drawn from three health care quality measures or categories: structure, process, and outcomes. Donabedian believed that structure measures have an effect on process measures, which in turn affect outcome measures. Essentially, structure measures are physical and organization characteristics in which health care occurs, process measures focus on the care delivered to patients (services, treatments, diagnostic texts), and outcome measures are the effect of health care on the status of patients and populations. Role description studies focus on defining and describing role components and job attributes of nurse practitioners.

53. Answer: 1

Rationale: The Theory of Self-Transcendence focuses on the person's experience at the end of life. The other focus areas are not unique to the Theory of Self-Transcendence.

21

Professional Issues

Legal and Ethical

1. Which authority regulates the scope of practice of family nurse practitioners?
   1. Federal law.
   2. Academic institutions.
   3. Individual state law.
   4. Individual practice settings.

2. A family nurse practitioner is obtaining informed consent for a 78-year-old female patient with a clinical diagnosis of dementia for a minor incision and drainage procedure. Which option would provide best practice for obtaining informed consent?
   1. Have the patient sign the form.
   2. Inquire as to whether there is an individual who is a power of attorney (POA) for the patient.
   3. Have the patient sign the form in the presence of a witness who can substantiate informed consent and that information has been provided.
   4. Reschedule the procedure until next week until the patient's daughter can be contacted.

3. What priority action should the family nurse practitioner take when assessment findings on an older adult patient indicate potential physical abuse during a scheduled office visit?
   1. Admit patient to the hospital for observation.
   2. Review patient's chart to see if there were any other documented findings that would indicate abuse.
   3. Report case to appropriate agency based on state law.
   4. Arrange for home health to assess and monitor patient.

4. Why is an occurrence-form professional liability insurance policy preferred?
   1. The amount of insurance money available to pay a claim increases with each renewal of the policy.
   2. The policy proceeds are available to pay claims regardless of when the claim is reported to the carrier.
   3. The carrier will be notified of a potential claim during the policy period.

4. The coverage is broader than that provided by a claims-made policy form.

5. Why is the early reporting of a potential professional liability claim advantageous?
   1. Insurance carriers have a 10-day reporting window, after which the coverage is canceled.
   2. Documents and witnesses needed to defend the claim are more likely to be available at the time of the event.
   3. Insurance premiums will be reduced with a good-faith showing of cooperation with the carrier.
   4. Risk management personnel require such reporting to comply with Joint Commission on the Accreditation of Healthcare Organizations mandates.

6. Why might a family nurse practitioner's nursing license be in jeopardy?
   1. The family nurse practitioner appropriately delegates medication administration to a trusted registered nurse (RN) employee, who administers a fatal dose.
   2. The family nurse practitioner delegates patient assessment tasks to a licensed practical nurse (LPN), who has been "floated" to the outpatient clinic for the day.
   3. The family nurse practitioner provides nursing care services consistent with established standards of practice in the jurisdiction.
   4. The medical assistant in the supervising physician's office exceeds the scope of her authority, but the family nurse practitioner takes prompt action to correct the problem.

7. A 46-year-old mentally challenged man has been diagnosed with colon cancer. Consent for his corrective surgery should be obtained from:
   1. The patient himself.
   2. The patient's 84-year-old mother, who is his closest relative.
   3. The patient's court-appointed guardian.
   4. The administrator of the group home where the patient lives.

8. A family member calls the office to speak to the family nurse practitioner who is taking care of her father, who is 65 years old and has since left the office. The family member asks for specific information related to the patient's medical history and clinical diagnosis. What action should be taken at this time by the family nurse practitioner?
   1. Answer all of the questions that the family member has with regard to the patient.
   2. Acknowledge the family member's concerns, but do not answer any questions unless the patient has given documented consent to release information.
   3. Call the patient at home and ask if the patient gives consent to answer the family member's questions.
   4. Contact the patient and have him come back to the office to fill out a medical release of information form.

9. A family nurse practitioner has a 75-year-old female patient with metastatic cancer. Her affairs are in order; she has arranged all her finances and her own funeral rites. She has systematically secured enough barbiturates to successfully end her life. The patient asks the family nurse practitioner to mix the drugs for her in some pudding to make them palatable for ingestion. What would be the family nurse practitioner's best course of action?
   1. Mix the medications as requested and stay with her while she consumes the preparation.
   2. Consult with the attending physician to warn them about the patient's proposed course of action.
   3. Seek an immediate order for an antidepressant.
   4. Sit down with the patient and conduct a physical and psychologic assessment.

10. The Patient Self-Determination Act passed by the U.S. Congress in 1990 resulted in which of the following policy changes?
    1. Hospitals are mandated to assist every patient to create a "living will."
    2. Federally funded managed care organizations (MCOs) are required to inform subscribers about their rights under state law to create "advance directives."
    3. Home health agencies are required to have "do not resuscitate" orders on file for all terminally ill patients.
    4. Hospitalized patients are obligated to select a surrogate decision maker to make health care decisions for them if they become incapacitated.

11. If served with a summons and complaint (lawsuit documents), the family nurse practitioner should take which of the following actions as the first step?
    1. Call the patient to determine the basis for the action and nature of the alleged wrongdoing.
    2. Call the patient's lawyer (listed on first page of lawsuit) to obtain more information.
    3. Call their insurance company/malpractice carrier for instructions on how to proceed.
    4. Confer with colleagues and review the chart to determine whether notes need to be clarified.

12. A family nurse practitioner in an impoverished rural area frequently encounters a female patient in a situation of domestic violence with few community options for referral. To address the situation, the family nurse practitioner participates in community education forums and fundraising for a safe house. The family nurse practitioner's participation is an example of applying what ethical principle?
    1. Autonomy.
    2. Nonmaleficence.
    3. Justice.
    4. Veracity.

13. The confidentiality of medical records is always a valid concern, especially with widespread computerization and fax machines. Release of medical information to third parties is:
    1. A "creature of state law," meaning that state statutes control the processing of such requests.
    2. Prohibited without the informed consent of the patient.
    3. Automatic when the requesting party is a third-party payer or insurer.
    4. Disallowed if the records contain proof of a diagnosis of AIDS.

14. Which population is not included in the definition of disability under the Americans with Disabilities Act (ADA)?
    1. Profoundly deaf employees.
    2. Persons who are wheelchair bound.
    3. Current users of illegal drugs.
    4. Persons with mental retardation.

15. If a patient is having a problem with a managed care plan, the family nurse practitioner can offer to assist in which of the following ways?
    1. Suggest that the patient contact the customer service department (or "member services") for the care plan to resolve the issue; a formal grievance filing may be necessary.
    2. Remind the patient, who is a member of the "senior" plan for Medicare recipients, that he or she may complain to the federal Office of Personnel Management.
    3. Remind the patient that the state's insurance department also investigates complaints against health plans.
    4. All the above.

16. If a piece of equipment malfunctions while being used on a hospitalized patient, the risk manager would probably recommend which of the following courses of action?
    1. Return the item to the manufacturer with a description of the problem and a request for analysis.
    2. Tag and sequester the item at the facility and defer analysis pending risk management review of the litigation potential.
    3. Send the item to the biomedical engineering department with a request for immediate equipment breakdown and troubleshooting.
    4. Repair the item, either in-house or by an outside contracted firm, and return it to service as soon as possible.

17. Nurse expert witnesses are essential in the adjudication of most professional negligence claims against nurses. Which of the following criteria do attorneys use in selecting family nurse practitioner experts?
    1. Appropriate professional education, preferably at the technical level.
    2. Relevant and recent professional work experience.
    3. Ability to understand and articulate the legal issues involved in the claim.
    4. Published authors of medical texts in the clinical subject areas.

18. Which federal law mandates the tracking of implantable medical devices?
    1. Administrative Procedures Act (APA).
    2. Patient Self-Determination Act (PSDA).
    3. Safe Medical Devices Act (SMDA).
    4. Omnibus Budget Reconciliation Act (OBRA) of 1987.

19. What type of insurance coverage is purchased (or self-insured) by an organization to address employee job-related injuries?
    1. Professional liability insurance.
    2. Business interruption insurance.
    3. Directors and officer's insurance.
    4. Workers' compensation insurance.

20. While driving your personal vehicle on a job-related errand, you are struck by a semitrailer on the interstate. The car is deemed "totaled," and you are severely injured. Which insurance policies will respond to these losses?
    1. Your personal auto policy and your employer's workers' compensation policy.
    2. The employer's business auto policy and workers' compensation policy.
    3. Your homeowner's policy.
    4. The semitrailer driver's personal auto policy.

21. Family nurse practitioners with hospital privileges may be affected by the part of the Health Care Quality Improvement Act known as the National Practitioner Data Bank (NPDB). Which of the following statements about the Data Bank is **not** true?
    1. Professional liability insurance claims payments made on behalf of family nurse practitioners are reported to the NPDB.
    2. The facility granting medical staff privileges must query the NPDB before approving a practitioner's privileges.
    3. The purpose of the NPDB is as a nationwide flagging system that provides information about malpractice claims, licensure actions, and restrictions on privileges so that practitioners may not easily move from one jurisdiction to another to escape quality review.
    4. Insurance companies report all malpractice payments made on behalf of affected family nurse practitioners within 30 days of the date the payment was made, if the amount of the claim is in excess of $11,000 and no matter how it was settled.

22. In 1985, the U.S. Congress took action against a phenomenon known as "patient dumping" by enacting what was known at the time as the Consolidated Omnibus Budget Reconciliation Act law, now referred to the Emergency Medical Treatment and Labor Act (EMTALA). Which three statements about EMTALA are true?
    1. The original purpose of the statute was to prohibit the transfer of uninsured and untreated patients from the emergency department of one hospital to another (usually the county hospital).
    2. Subsequent rules and case law have expanded the statute so that almost any unauthorized transfer of a patient from one facility to another is potentially problematic.
    3. To effect a proper transfer, the forwarding facility need not notify or secure the acquiescence of the receiving facility.
    4. The transferring facility must use appropriate transport methods and send copies of patients' medical records.
    5. The patient can be transferred by family members to another facility awaiting the patient's arrival.

23. A family nurse practitioner who wants to effect change in the state's laws regarding the dispensing of prescription medications by family nurse practitioners would take this case to the:
    1. State legislature.
    2. State board of nursing.
    3. State board of pharmacy.
    4. Nursing specialty organization.

24. Under the Safe Medical Devices Act of 1990, which of the following health care providers or organizations are required to report the death of a patient to the U.S. Food and Drug Administration if the death is related to the use of a medical device?
    1. Physician office staff.
    2. Hospitals, home health agencies, and ambulance companies.
    3. Nurse family members treating patients without compensation.
    4. Physicians making home visits.

25. A patient receives a medication that was intended for another person. Which is an appropriate way for the family nurse practitioner to document this event in the medical record?
    1. "Patient was given X mg of Y drug in error."
    2. "X mg of Y drug administered to patient. No adverse effects noted. Physician notified."
    3. "Patient received wrong medication. Incident report filed. Practitioner disciplined."
    4. "Practitioner inadvertently administered Y drug to wrong patient. Supervisor notified. Family threatening litigation."

26. What is the primary reason that patients are the reasons for suing family nurse practitioners for medical negligence?
    1. The care they received was substandard.
    2. The provider made an honest mistake.
    3. The patient was not "heard" when attempting to communicate with the provider.
    4. The patient participated fully in all aspects of medical decision making, but the results were disappointing.

27. Which ethical principal is informed consent based on?
    1. Beneficence.
    2. Respect for persons.
    3. Nonmaleficence.
    4. Autonomy.

28. What are the four elements of a professional negligence claim?
    1. Duty, fulfillment of duty, professional relationship, and wrongful act.
    2. Professional responsibility, fault, harm to patient, and wrongful act.
    3. Duty, breach of duty, causal connection between act and harm, and harm to patient.
    4. Professional relationship, intentional wrongful act, proximate cause, and damage to patient.

29. Why is an expert witness usually required in a nursing negligence case?
    1. Knowledge of medical or nursing facts is not considered intuitive to a lay jury.
    2. Jurors are allowed to use their "sixth sense" regarding the facts presented to them.
    3. Fact witnesses are not able to present an unbiased account of the circumstances in dispute.
    4. Appropriately credentialed experts have more credibility in the eyes of lay jurors.

30. The standard of care for a family nurse practitioner will be established by an expert witness(es) in a trial. The expert opinion will be based on which three items?
    1. National norms for the specialty.
    2. Facility policies and procedures.
    3. Professional literature.
    4. Opinions of other nurse practitioners.
    5. Current events.

31. Alternative dispute resolution (ADR) is a process in which the parties to a dispute resolve their differences outside of a court trial. What are three advantages to this system of problem solving?
    1. The parties usually prefer the process because they have their opportunity to be heard in a less formal and less intimidating environment.
    2. The process is often less time consuming and less costly than traditional litigation.

    3. Damage awards are less likely to include nonfinancial compensation.
    4. Insurers are amenable to working with mediators with a track record of fairness and successful case resolution.
    5. The losing party may appeal the ADR decision to the court system.

32. What is the statute of limitations?
    1. The state law that prescribes the time frames within which a nursing negligence action may be filed.
    2. The law that states that minors have no legal authority to sue nurses for malpractice.
    3. The law that limits the right of patients to sue family nurse practitioners for negligent acts.
    4. The federal law that limits a family nurse practitioner's right to countersue a patient for malicious prosecution.

33. A family nurse practitioner is driving to a nursing seminar on an interstate highway. The nurse practitioner observes a head-on collision and decides to stop to render aid. Which three statements are accurate with respect to the family nurse practitioner's potential liability for malpractice?
    1. There is no legal obligation to stop to render assistance; if the family nurse practitioner had driven by the accident, there would be no liability on the nurse's part.
    2. If appropriate nursing care is provided, gratuitously, the family nurse practitioner will be protected from liability under that state's Good Samaritan Law.
    3. Even if the family nurse practitioner acts in a grossly negligent manner, the Good Samaritan Law will shield the nurse from liability.
    4. The protections afforded by the Good Samaritan Law may differ from state to state; the family nurse practitioner should research the state's law on the subject.
    5. The family nurse practitioner must stop and render aid.

34. If a family nurse practitioner is subpoenaed to appear for a deposition in a nursing negligence case, appropriate preparation is prudent. Which advice from the attorney is appropriate? (Select 3 responses.)
    1. "Discreetly chew gum to calm your nerves, and dress for dinner because depositions usually take all day and you won't have time to change."
    2. "Review the patient's medical record and other pertinent material before appearing for questioning."
    3. "Take as much time as needed to think about your responses before answering; don't let the other lawyer put words in your mouth."
    4. "Be straightforward and truthful; remember that 'I don't know' and 'I don't remember' are acceptable responses."
    5. "Try to confuse the other attorney by displaying sophisticated medical knowledge and information."

35. Which four of the following suggestions for documentation are recommended?
    1. "Carefully document your criticism of a fellow provider's clinical decision in the patient's medical record. This will protect you if your treatment decisions need to be defended later."
    2. "Use standard abbreviations in the medical record so that subsequent readers will have no doubt as to your meaning and intent."
    3. "Document telephone conversations with the patient and family nurse practitioner in the medical record. Be particularly vigilant about recording changes in the patient's medications."
    4. "Document noncompliant patient behaviors in the medical record; be thorough, yet factual."
    5. "Always make notation of errors in the medical record according to agency policy."

36. If a patient is under the "age of majority" for the state, what three factors would be considered to determine whether the patient is "emancipated" and able to consent to medical treatment?
    1. The patient is married.
    2. The patient is in the military.
    3. The patient is living outside the "care, custody, and control" of a parent or guardian.
    4. The patient has a child.

37. A family nurse practitioner is employed in a private medical office. There is constant activity at the front desk, with patients checking in for appointments, staff scheduling tests, and telephone advice triage in progress. To preserve patient confidentiality, what changes should be implemented? (Select 3 responses.)
    1. Orient the computer monitor and printer, so that persons other than staff cannot read incoming reports and other data.
    2. Do all telephone scheduling from a more secure location, such as a conference room in the back office.
    3. Create a more private space to confer with patients who need follow-up information or explanations of tests or treatments.
    4. Confirm only the patient's name, date of birth, and social security number in the front desk.

38. Which activity could be considered grounds for a sexual harassment claim?
    1. A male employee tells an off-color joke to another man. The joke is overheard by a female coworker who seems to appreciate the humor in it. The joke telling is an isolated incident.
    2. A nurse supervisor conducts an employee performance review. The supervisor does not mention a prior social relationship with the employee. The ratings are appropriate for the level of performance, and the employee receives a salary increase.

3. A coed locker room is decorated with multiple centerfold photos from a popular men's magazine. The female employees find this offensive and have filed several complaints.
4. A nurse is complimented on her appearance and asked on a date by her boss. She informs the boss that she is married and not seeking another relationship. The incident is forgotten.

39. A comatose female patient requires a feeding tube inserted for long-term nutritional needs. Her husband presents the family nurse practitioner with a document that he says is his wife's living will. It is signed by him, and he says that it sets out the wishes of his wife with respect to the feeding tube. He does not have a document verifying her health care representative. Why is this living will not a legally binding document?
    1. The wife did not sign the document.
    2. The husband is not authorized to execute a living will on behalf of his wife.
    3. This type of advance directive must be signed by the individual (wife/patient) while this person is legally competent to execute the documents.
    4. All the above.

40. A family nurse practitioner is volunteering at a clinic for homeless women. A diabetic patient in her third trimester of pregnancy has been reasonably compliant with respect to insulin therapy. Now, however, she has announced her intent to abandon her insulin regimen because she has heard from her friends that some drugs "hurt your baby." Which option is **not** legally appropriate for the family nurse practitioner, as this patient's health care provider, to consider?
    1. Seek the support of the clinic's attorney to file a petition for court-ordered treatment for the patient.
    2. Attempt to engage the patient in dialog to provide her with accurate medical information.
    3. Detain the patient in the homeless shelter and administer the insulin, with or without her consent.
    4. Confer with social services to find an appropriate interim placement for the patient until her medical and legal issues can be addressed.

41. What is the purpose of the Americans with Disabilities Act (ADA)?
    1. "Level the playing field" with respect to employment and other opportunities for disabled persons.
    2. Create a federal entitlement program for AIDS patients.
    3. Guarantee wheelchair access to every residential and commercial building.
    4. Authorize interpreters for deaf employees at all private businesses.

42. As a result of the U.S. Supreme Court's ruling on assisted suicide, which of the following is the current state of the law on this topic?
    1. Assisted suicide is still a criminal offense in most jurisdictions.
    2. A physician may prescribe a fatal dose of medication with the concurrence of the ethics committee.
    3. A family nurse practitioner may prescribe a fatal dose of medication with the concurrence of the supervising physician.
    4. A pharmacist may instruct a patient on how to mix and ingest a fatal dose of prescription medication.

43. A professional negligence or medical malpractice case is a civil action. What is the difference between a civil lawsuit and a criminal lawsuit?
    1. The damages sought in a civil suit are monetary; one private party sues another for money.
    2. If convicted in a criminal case, you are still covered by your professional liability insurer.
    3. In a criminal case, your state sues you for money; other penalties do not apply.
    4. In a civil suit, if you do not prevail, you could be incarcerated.

44. Which of the following are three forms of alternative dispute resolution (ADR)?
    1. Court or bench trial (judge's decision).
    2. Binding and nonbinding arbitration.
    3. Settlement conference.
    4. Jury trial.
    5. Mediation.

45. Why is it especially important for family nurse practitioners caring for children to have adequate professional liability insurance coverage?
    1. Damages are always higher when a child is the injured party.
    2. Juries tend to award fewer dollars to injured children because the children are eligible for a variety of social programs that cover their medical expenses.
    3. The statute of limitations is often tolled (put on hold) until the minor reaches majority, so the time frame within which the child can file a lawsuit is extended.
    4. Insurers are sensitive to the increased risk posed by minor claimants, so the coverage is difficult to obtain.

46. A health care provider has a duty to disclose certain information to the patient as part of the informed consent process. Exceptions to this duty would include all the following *except:*
    1. The patient has waived the right to receive the data.
    2. It is a bona fide emergency situation.

3. The provider believes that the information would be harmful to the patient and invokes the therapeutic privilege.
4. The patient is 80 years old, and older adult persons are unable to comprehend complex medical facts.

47. What is the primary purpose of a preemployment physical exam?
    1. Identify existing health problems that might adversely affect the company's insurance rates.
    2. Determine the mental status of the applicant.
    3. Determine whether the applicant is physically capable of doing the job.
    4. Document any existing disabilities and recommend accommodations.

48. A family nurse practitioner involved in work-related surveillance knows all employers must report, according to Occupational Safety and Health Administration (OSHA), the following: (Select 2 responses.)
    1. Keep all OSHA records for 5 years.
    2. Report all work-related fatalities within 8 hours.
    3. Report all work-related inpatient hospitalizations, amputations, and losses of an eye within 24 hours.
    4. Report hospital-employee fatalities occurring 90 days following a work-related incident.

49. When treating a work-related injury, what is the family nurse practitioner required to do?
    1. Document thoroughly because of the high probability of legal action.
    2. Communicate directly with the patient's employer.
    3. File a report with the industrial commission documenting the injury and treatment.
    4. Notify the Occupational Safety and Health Administration (OSHA).

50. Which of the following situations would be considered a reportable employee injury under the Occupational Safety and Health Administration (OSHA)?
    1. A 3-cm abrasion of forearm.
    2. Warehouse worker with back strain reassigned to office work for a week.
    3. Twisted ankle that responded to ice and ACE wrap.
    4. Minor closed-head injury with no loss of consciousness.

51. The purpose of an Occupational Health and Safety Administration 300 log is to record:
    1. Occupational injuries and illnesses.
    2. Only work-related deaths.
    3. Dangerous workplace situations.
    4. Lost work days.

52. The family nurse practitioner understands which of the following about the Health Insurance Portability and Accountability Act (HIPAA) of 1996?
    1. HIPAA allows health insurance providers to deny insurance to patients because of preexisting medical conditions.
    2. HIPAA provides easier access to all providers to obtain secure and private health information.
    3. A National Provider Identifier and Employer Identifier facilitates enrollment, eligibility, and claims processing and provides a mechanism to identify a specific provider, insurer, or patient.
    4. Health care organizations, insurers, and payers using electronic storage of patient data and performing claims submission must comply with the Final Rule for National Standards for Electronic Transactions.

53. Bioethical practice dilemmas are best described as situations in which proposed treatment alternatives are:
    1. Ranked from most acceptable to least acceptable.
    2. Not appealing to involved parties.
    3. Lacking acceptance by anyone.
    4. Less-than-perfect approaches to the situation.

54. What is the difference between the electronic medical record (EMR) and the electronic health record (EHR)? (Select 2 responses.)
    1. There is no difference.
    2. The EHR is more efficient and effective.
    3. The EMR is more comprehensive.
    4. The EMR communicates information within a facility.
    5. The EHR communicates information among multiple facilities.
    6. The EHR is a relatively new system that started after the year 2000.

55. What should the family nurse practitioner do to reduce liability while using either an electronic health record (EHR) or electronic medical record (EMR) system?
    1. Clone or copy and paste notes and details from a previous exam or patient history into a current visit record.
    2. Refuse to enter information into the EHR or EMR with which you do not agree.
    3. Share your log-in ID with colleagues who are also entering information into the EHR or EMR.
    4. Avoid making late entries and changes in the EHR or EMR.

56. Which of the following are components of the Licensure, Accreditation, Certification and Education (LACE) network that support implementation of the consensus model for advanced practice registered nurse (APRN) regulation? (Select 4 responses.)
    1. Accreditation.
    2. Licensure.
    3. Compliance.
    4. Certification.

    5. Education.
    6. Excellence.

57. What do family nurse practitioners need to do to validate their knowledge, skills, and abilities to practice as advanced practice nurses? (Select 3 responses.)
    1. Become licensed.
    2. Obtain certification.
    3. Participate in credentialing.
    4. Follow regulations.
    5. Understand accreditation.

58. Which of the following is true regarding obtaining prescriptive authority? (Select 3 responses.)
    1. Varies among individual states and regulatory agencies.
    2. Requires an additional pharmacology course for continuing education after graduation.
    3. Requires a Drug Enforcement Administration number (DEA) for prescribing controlled substances.
    4. Continues to be a regulatory hurdle for advanced practice registered nurses (APRNs).
    5. Requires an application for a national provider identifier (NPI) number.

59. The family nurse practitioner understands the following about Drug Enforcement Administration (DEA) numbers: (Select 2 responses.)
    1. DEA numbers are site specific.
    2. DEA authority is federal.
    3. DEA number is automatically provided on receiving prescriptive authority.
    4. DEA numbers are required for all prescriptions.
    5. DEA numbers remain with nurse practitioners for their lifetime, like the advanced practice license number.

60. The family nurse practitioner understands that the following illustrates a breach in patient confidentiality:
    1. Using the electronic health record to document clinical findings.
    2. Having health care records subpoenaed by a local court.
    3. Releasing the patient's health record to an insurance company.
    4. Discussing a patient's laboratory findings with the patient's family.

Issue and Trends

61. An older adult patient has decided to start hospice care. What are the eligibility criteria for hospice care as required by Medicare?
    1. Continue with curative care and chemotherapy.
    2. Have a terminal illness and a prognosis of 6 months or less to live.
    3. Choose to continue to use Medicare benefits.
    4. Pay a small daily fee to receive 24-hour on-call hospice care.

62. Considering the four advanced practice roles of the clinical nurse specialist (CNS), nurse practitioner, certified nurse-midwife, and nurse anesthetist, which role became accepted by and included into the practice arena without significant controversy?
    1. CNS.
    2. Nurse practitioner.
    3. Certified nurse-midwife.
    4. Nurse anesthetist.

63. To facilitate exchange of information in the clinical practice setting, the family nurse practitioner should provide educational materials that:
    1. Contain evidenced-based practice recommendations.
    2. Provide auditory and written instruction.
    3. Determine patient readiness to learn.
    4. Meet health literacy standards.

64. What would be considered to be an expectation of the professional role of a family nurse practitioner based on practitioner competencies established by the American Association of Colleges of Nursing (AACN) 2010 standards?
    1. Teaching classes related to health promotion and disease prevention.
    2. Observing and maintaining professional boundaries.
    3. Providing mentorship to other practitioners.
    4. Prescribing medications within legally defined practice regulations.

65. Historically, who was one of the most outspoken opponents of the family nurse practitioner role?
    1. Loretta Ford.
    2. Hildegard Peplau.
    3. Martha Rogers.
    4. Dorothea Orem.

66. Who started the first family nurse practitioner program?
    1. Hildegard Peplau.
    2. Mary Breckenridge.
    3. Agnes McGee.
    4. Loretta Ford.

67. Which is the most important action in developing health policy skills in the family nurse practitioner?
    1. Develop political allies in the U.S. Congress.
    2. Work on a campaign.
    3. Support causes (e.g., teen pregnancy; AIDS).
    4. Write letters and editorials.

68. Which is the least important barrier to collaborative advanced nursing practice?
    1. Prescriptive authority.
    2. Reimbursement privileges.
    3. Legal scope of practice.
    4. Political activism.

69. According to the advanced practice registered nurse (APRN) Consensus Model, what is the family nurse practitioner categorized as?
    1. An APRN role.
    2. Representing a specialty.
    3. Specifies a practice population focus.
    4. Nurse practitioner.

70. To obtain reimbursement, the family nurse practitioner must understand which of the following?
    1. Minimum Nursing Data Set (MNDS).
    2. International Classification of Diseases (ICD-10), Current Procedural Terminology (CPT), and Health Care Financing Administration Common Procedure Coding (HCPC).
    3. HCPC and North American Nursing Diagnosis Association (NANDA) diagnoses.
    4. Medicare and Medicaid numbers.

71. Which four items are included in the advanced practice registered nurse (APRN) Consensus Model and should be included in the curriculum for a family nurse practitioner program?
    1. Completion of graduate studies.
    2. Meeting accreditation standards.
    3. Maintaining compliance with core competencies.
    4. Maintaining licensure.
    5. Nurse Residency Program.

72. According to Kurt Lewin, steps in the change process are as follows:
    1. Unsolving, mobilizing, recruiting, and finalizing.
    2. Building relationships, acquiring resources, choosing solution, and stabilizing.
    3. Unfreezing, moving, and refreezing.
    4. Forming, storming, and norming.

73. What was the major impetus for family nurse practitioner development?
    1. Need for an expert nurse clinician.
    2. Shortage of primary care physicians.
    3. Trend for specialized nurses to diagnose and manage unstable acute and chronic patients.
    4. Movement of graduate nursing education to diagnosis and treatment of major illness.

74. The family nurse practitioner understands that Medicare B provides:
    1. Hospitalization costs for insured patients.
    2. Health insurance benefits for low-income families.
    3. Benefits that cover physicians, family nurse practitioners, medical equipment, and outpatient services.
    4. Outpatient laboratory services, radiography services, and skilled nursing care in appropriate facilities.

75. What was the effect of the Balanced Budget Act of 1997 on family nurse practitioner practice?
    1. Authorized all states to provide family nurse practitioners prescriptive authority.
    2. Provided for only well visits and primary care services.
    3. Prevented a physician from billing 100% for an family nurse practitioner's services.
    4. Allowed direct Medicare payments to family nurse practitioners in both rural and urban settings.

76. In the clinic, the family nurse practitioner must resolve a conflict between two medical assistants. The nurse has observed that one assistant is usually pleasant and helpful and the other is often abrasive and angry. What is the most important guideline that the family nurse practitioner must observe in resolving such a conflict?
    1. Require the medical assistants to reach a compromise.
    2. Weigh the consequences of each possible solution.
    3. Encourage ventilation of anger and use humor to minimize the conflict.
    4. Deal with issues, not personalities.

77. Which of the following is the name of an initiative that is part of the Affordable Care Act of 2009, which affects all health providers who practice in or admit patients to a hospital setting?
    1. Advanced Practice Registered Nurse (APRN) Compact Licensure Act.
    2. Interprofessional Education Collaborative (IPEC).
    3. Accountable Care Organization.
    4. Value-Based Purchasing (VBP).

78. A family nurse practitioner approaches his friend, another family nurse practitioner, and tells him that a female physician at the clinic often follows him into the supply room and tells him how "good looking" he is. Yesterday she patted his hand and said, "I wish we would get to know each other better. I would make it worth your while; better benefits at the clinic, more money." The staff nurse asks his friend, "What do I do? I don't want to date her, but I don't want to lose my job. I just want her to leave me alone." What would be the friend's best reply?
    1. "Tell her that her behavior makes you feel uncomfortable and that you want her to stop."
    2. "Go for it; date her and see if you get what she promises."
    3. "Go to the human relations office at the agency right away and relate to them the entire situation."
    4. "Contact your lawyer and get advice as soon as possible, in case she decides to turn the tables and accuse you of advances."

79. The family nurse practitioner understands that "incident to" services are reimbursed at which percentage?
    1. 75%.
    2. 80%.
    3. 85%.
    4. 100%.

80. What is the purpose of the Agency for Healthcare Research and Quality (AHRQ)?
    1. Develop cost-cutting strategies for health care.
    2. Provide assessment and treatment protocols and algorithms.
    3. Promote health care policy by lobbying efforts.
    4. Produce evidence to make a safer health care that is equitable and affordable.

81. In 1999, the Institute of Medicine (IOM) reported that at least 44,000 people die in hospitals each year as a result of which of the following?
    1. Hospital-acquired infections.
    2. Falls.
    3. Lack of access to affordable primary care treatment.
    4. Medical errors.

82. What three courses are required in an advanced practice education program to comply with the advanced practice registered nurse (APRN) Consensus Model?
    1. Informatics.
    2. Advanced physiology/pathophysiology.
    3. Social policy and political action.
    4. Advanced health assessment.
    5. Legal and ethical issues.
    6. Advanced pharmacology.

83. What is the purpose of the Technology Informatics Guiding Education Reform (TIGER) Competencies as applicable for a family nurse practitioner?
    1. Identify tools and procedures to address specific quality outcomes and metrics in health care agencies.
    2. Improve nursing practice, education, and delivery of patient care through the use of health information technology (HIT).
    3. Set the stage to increase awareness of family nurse practitioners needing a national provider identifier number.
    4. Identify population health literacy in specific metropolitan areas regarding use of technology and the electronic health record.

84. Which of the following is a common competency for all doctorally prepared advanced practice nurses?
    1. Provide care to children through young adult.
    2. Perform a comprehensive evidence-based assessment.
    3. Advocate only for the patient.
    4. Focus on adult group of health issues.

85. What are three specific aspects of the Consensus Model for Advanced Practice Registered Nurse (APRN) Regulation?
    1. Full practice authority.
    2. State-to-state mobility.
    3. Restricts practice authority to nurse practitioners only.
    4. Removes practice barriers.
    5. Increases cost burden to nurse practitioners.

86. Since the development of the nurse practitioner role, there have been studies comparing nurse practitioner care to physician care. What have been the findings of these studies?
    1. Nurse practitioner care is equivalent to physician care.
    2. Nurse practitioner care is inferior to physician care.
    3. Nurse practitioner and physician care is equivalent across all measurement indicators.
    4. Nurse practitioner and physician care is mostly equivalent with the indicator of patient satisfaction higher for nurse practitioners.

87. Which two statements are accurate about the creation of the doctorate of nursing practice (DNP) degree?
    1. Was developed by the National Council State Boards of Nursing (NCSBN).
    2. Was created to provide for better reimbursement of services for advanced practice registered nurses (APRNs).
    3. Was effective in 2015 throughout the country and encompasses all graduate programs in standardization of advanced practice entry requirements.
    4. Had as its primary purpose to ensure a strong educational preparation for APRNs.
    5. Had a focus to compete with the clinical nurse specialist and midwifery advanced practice roles.

88. Which of the following is covered under Medicare Plan A? (Select 2 responses.)
    1. Ambulance services.
    2. Diagnostic testing.
    3. Skilled nursing facility care.
    4. Obtaining a second opinion before surgery.
    5. Medical supplies and medications during hospitalization.

89. According to the American Association of Colleges of Nursing (AACN), what are the clinical hour requirements for completion of the doctorate of nursing practice (DNP) program?
    1. 500 supervised clinical hours.
    2. 900 supervised clinical hours.
    3. 1000 supervised clinical hours.
    4. 1500 supervised clinical hours.

90. What is the purpose for reporting patient outcomes? (Select 3 responses.)
    1. Increase revenue stream and expenditures.
    2. Improve patient care outcomes.
    3. Required by state and federal regulatory agencies.
    4. Relaxes requirements imposed by certification agencies.
    5. Promote effective patient care delivery.

91. The family nurse practitioner understands the following about quality improvement (QI): (Select 2 responses.)
    1. QI needs to be realistic and achievable.
    2. QI involves large-scale projects for best outcomes.
    3. QI is action research.
    4. QI generates new ideas and knowledge.
    5. QI avoids replicating strategies used by others.
    6. QI uses existing tools and evidence to change and improve nursing practice.

92. Which of the following legislation changed Medicare payments beginning January 1, 2019, away from the existing fee-for-service system to one that is based on the quality and effectiveness of the care the health care provider delivers?
    1. Medicare Access and CHIP Reauthorization Act (MACRA).
    2. Consumer Assessment of Health Care Providers.
    3. Sustainable Growth Rate (SGR) Formula Values-Based Modifier.
    4. Meaningful use.

93. The family nurse practitioner participates in a hospital-based quality improvement project. When the family nurse practitioner records an assessment of the patient's skin status using the Braden Scale for Predicting Pressure Score Risk, this process is:
    1. Peer review.
    2. Risk analysis.
    3. Force field analysis.
    4. Benchmarking.

21　Professional Issues Answers & Rationales

Legal and Ethical

1. Answer: 3

Rationale: Family nurse practitioners' scope of practice is regulated by individual state law. Federal law does not address scope of practice. Academic institutions provide the necessary training for individuals to obtain an academic degree and assist in preparation for required certification in the specialty area. Scope of practice is not regulated by individual practice settings.

2. Answer: 2

Rationale: A clinical diagnosis of dementia for a patient indicates that to provide and obtain informed consent, an individual who has been designated as a health care surrogate and/or is acting as a POA should be contacted to provide informed consent. The family nurse practitioner should not allow the individual patient to sign the form because the informed consent process cannot be verified. Having a witness present when signing the form does not convey informed consent has taken place. Delaying medical treatment would not represent prudent practice.

3. Answer: 3

Rationale: If the family nurse practitioner suspects that physical abuse has occurred, then he or she is legally obligated to report the case to the appropriate agency based on state law. Admitting the patient to the hospital is not indicated unless confirmation of injury or trauma is justified. Reviewing the patient's chart for past history of abuse may be warranted, but it is not the priority action. Arranging for home health to assess and monitor the patient does not preclude the legal responsibility of taking action to report the incident.

4. Answer: 2

Rationale: The most important advantage of an occurrence policy is that the coverage is available regardless of how long it takes to become aware of a claim (the long "tail" of a medical malpractice claim). The limits do not automatically increase. The carrier need not be notified during the policy period as is required with claims-made coverage. The coverage under each policy may be as broad as the carrier allows.

5. Answer: 2

Rationale: Fact witnesses and necessary paperwork are always easier to discover the sooner they are sought after a medical misadventure. Memories are fresh, and documents are less likely to be misplaced or destroyed. No rigid reporting window is required by insurance carriers, although they do want to be notified in a timely manner. Insurance premiums may be reduced if the insured's track record is clean (i.e., no claims), but not by mere compliance with policy requirements. Risk management employees prefer early notification so that damage-control efforts may be implemented promptly, not for regulatory reasons.

6. Answer: 2

Rationale: Assessment skills are presumed to be within the purview of the professional nurse, not those with fewer years of nursing education. Also, in this option, the LPN is an unknown entity to the delegator. Delegating to the LPN should be done cautiously after determining that person's skill level. The family nurse practitioner's license is not in jeopardy as they delegated appropriately to the RN, but an error was made and is attributed to the delegatee (RN). Activities such as providing nursing services and intervening when medical assistant personnel exceed their authority are appropriate for the role.

7. Answer: 3

Rationale: The patient's capacity to consent is questionable, so alternatives must be sought. If the patient has a court-appointed guardian, that person is the decision maker. The court has already made a determination of the patient's legal incapacity and appointed the person to whom the nurse will look for consent. If there were no guardian, the family nurse practitioner would analyze whether the patient himself may be able to consent or whether to look to his mother as the most appropriate surrogate decision maker. The group home employee has no automatic legal authority to consent to treatment for any resident.

8. Answer: 2

Rationale: Release of medical information by a patient to others requires documentation of intent and approval within the patient's chart. Because the patient has left the office and there is no documentation related to medical release of information, the family nurse practitioner is bound by patient confidentiality and privacy laws (Health Care Insurance Portability and Accountability Act [HIPAA]) to not answer any questions. Calling the patient to obtain verbal approval for release of medical information and/or having the patient come in to fill out a medical release form for release of information is not an expectation at this time.

9. Answer: 4

Rationale: Assisted suicide is still a criminal activity in most states (and in legal limbo in others). Circumventing the patient may seem to be an appealing option, but it substitutes paternalism for the autonomy we all claim as our due. A diagnosis of depression cannot be made with inadequate data; the necessary information can be determined only by conferring with the patient herself.

10. Answer: 2

Rationale: MCOs are one group of health care organizations affected by this law. All subscribers must be provided with the stated information at the time of enrollment. Advance directive documents, although extremely helpful in the health care setting, are never mandatory.

11. Answer: 3

Rationale: Insurance carriers are thoroughly familiar with the processes of handling a claim. They will assist with every step, first by meeting their obligation to put the family nurse practitioner in contact with a lawyer. Conferring with the patient or the patient's lawyer is never a wise move. Colleagues can only offer moral support at this stage and can be called to testify if they have knowledge about the case; the lawyer is the professional of choice at this time. The family nurse practitioner must never consider altering a record; it can turn a defensible case into a nondefensible one.

12. Answer: 3

Rationale: Lobbying for underserved patients is an example of justice, which is the duty to treat all patients fairly, without regard to age, socioeconomic status, or other variables. Autonomy is the patient's right to self-determination without outside control. Nonmaleficence is the duty to prevent or avoid doing harm, whether intentional or unintentional. Veracity is the duty to tell the truth.

13. Answer: 1

Rationale: State law must be examined to define the circumstances under which confidential medical information may be disclosed. There may be additional requirements imposed by federal regulations (e.g., the handling of certain psychiatric records), but the bulk of the rule making on this issue is accomplished at the state level. Exceptions to the requirement of patient consent include communicable disease reporting to public health authorities and court-ordered record production. Third-party payers, although powerful with their fiscal controls, must produce some proof of patient consent to acquire records. An AIDS diagnosis does not shield a record

from production, although many states have enacted extra levels of protection for this information. Again, knowledge of state laws is crucial.

14. Answer: 3

Rationale: The ADA does not protect this population. In fact, employers may test for illegal drug use; this is not considered a medical exam, which ordinarily is subject to specific requirements under the law.

15. Answer: 4

Rationale: These are all ways to achieve satisfaction from a health plan. The family nurse practitioner could also offer to help explain clinical issues to personnel who may not be clinically oriented.

16. Answer: 2

Rationale: The best immediate solution is to identify the item and remove it from service to avoid further patient injury. Then the risk manager, in consultation with the facility's attorneys and insurers, will determine how to proceed with equipment analysis. Returning the item to the manufacturer removes it from the nurse's control and diminishes the opportunity to defend against a charge of user error. Immediate repair may fail to uncover the real cause of the patient injury and impair a successful defense of a claim. If the litigation potential is high, the parties may want to pool their efforts (and costs) to conduct a third-party review of the equipment. If litigation is likely, it is also likely that the manufacturer and others in the distribution chain will be codefendants with the facility and staff.

17. Answer: 2

Rationale: The level of education preferred is that of a master's or doctoral of nursing practice degree with family nurse practitioner specialization, not an associate's degree conferred on the technical nurse. The legal issues are the province of the attorneys and the judge; the nurse is expected to be the expert in the clinical issues. Published authorship on nursing issues does add an aura of credibility; specific work experience coupled with the educational credentials are more desirable.

18. Answer: 3

Rationale: The SMDA of 1990 mandates the regulation and tracking of medical devices. The APA describes the workings of federal agencies. The PSDA deals with advance directives, and the OBRA of 1987 changed the rule dealing with long-term care.

19. Answer: 4

Rationale: Liability insurance is acquired to protect the organization from suits by patients arising from negligent acts of employees. Business interruption coverage is usually purchased in tandem with fire insurance. It reimburses an organization for losses sustained while the business is partially or completely shut down after a catastrophic event. The organization's management team (chief executive officer and senior staff) is insured against losses based on business judgment errors through directors and officers coverage. Workers' compensation is the line of coverage that protects employees after on-the-job injuries. It is a no-fault system (negligence is not a factor) that covers employee medical bills and pays a percentage of wages while an employee is unable to work.

20. Answer: 1

Rationale: You were driving your personal vehicle, so your own auto insurer is "primary" (i.e., responds first to a loss). Because you were on company business, your injuries were sustained "within the course and scope of your employment," so there is coverage under the employer's workers' compensation policy for your medical bills and wage replacement. Depending on the circumstances and policy definitions, there could be some "excess" or additional coverage available under the employer's auto policy, but in no event would that carrier be primarily responsible for your losses. This is not the type of incident that homeowner's insurance is intended to cover. The semitrailer, presumably in use as a business vehicle, would not be insured under a driver's personal auto policy.

21. Answer: 4

Rationale: The intent of the NPDB is to improve the quality of health care by encouraging state licensing boards, hospitals, and other health care entities and professional societies to identify and discipline those who engage in unprofessional behavior and to restrict the ability of incompetent physicians, dentists, and other health care practitioners to move from state to state without disclosure or discovery of previous medical malpractice payment and adverse action history. Adverse actions can involve licensure, clinical privileges, professional society membership, and exclusions from Medicare and Medicaid.

22. Answer: 1, 2, 4

Rationale: The forwarding facility needs to know whether the receiving facility has space for the new arrival and, more importantly, the ability to treat the particular illness for which the patient needs therapy. The receiving agency needs to be contacted and agree on the transfer. The transferring agency must send the patient's medical records. The transfer must be with qualified personnel and transportation equipment. A familiar example of a patient transfer is that of the burn victim, for whom specialty care is mandatory, and the locations of that specialty care are usually limited.

23. Answer: 1

Rationale: Health care policy within the states is codified or enacted into law by the respective state legislature. The state boards of nursing and pharmacy should have significant input in the process, providing the research data and expert "testimony" that the legislature needs to make informed decisions. Nursing organizations should also be willing to provide background information and nurse experts to educate the lawmakers.

24. Answer: 2

Rationale: These are three of the agencies required to report. Events occurring in the other settings are exempt from reporting requirements under this federal law.

25. Answer: 2

Rationale: This is the most factual note; the writer does not apportion blame or assume liability. The other notes would be "red flags" for a chart reviewer. The mention of an incident report makes it virtually impossible to protect these documents from disclosure, especially in those jurisdictions still affording protection to these internal early warning documents that seek to alert risk management personnel to a potential claim.

26. Answer: 3

Rationale: Patients are often unable to evaluate the quality of the care they receive, but they do react to the way in which the care is delivered. Patient perceptions of rudeness or "uncaring" actions by the provider often spur patients to pursue legal action. Patients tend to be more forgiving of less-than-optimal outcomes if they have been involved in the process and are treated with respect.

27. Answer: 4

Rationale: Making one's own decisions is the basis for informed consent and the ethical underpinning of the Patient Self-Determination Act. "Doing good" (beneficence) and its corollary, "avoiding harm" (nonmaleficence), are ethical principles that are usually cited as the basis for other health care activities, such as maintaining professional competency. Respect for persons is a more global ethical principle supporting much of a nurse's personal philosophy of caring.

28. Answer: 3

Rationale: Usually phrased as duty, breach, proximate cause, and damages, these are the four elements of proof required to prevail in a medical negligence action. Intentional acts are not synonymous with negligent acts. Duty presumes a professional relationship and obligation to provide services. The breach is the error or mistake ascribed to the provider that results in the harm to the patient.

29. Answer: 1

Rationale: Lay jurors are not expected to know the clinical facts and circumstances involved in a professional negligence claim. The expert witness is necessary to educate the jurors about the medical facts and to testify to the standard of care to be applied. Witnesses with direct involvement in the case are no less credible because of their involvement; their testimony and personal bias, if any, will be evaluated by the jurors in the context of their roles.

30. Answer: 1, 2, 3

Rationale: With respect to nursing specialties, the standard of care is usually a national one. Facility policies, books, and journals are important to review, and physician input may be sought. In some cases, physicians may even be allowed to testify about the standard of care. Opinions of other nurse practitioners and current events are not considered a component of expert opinion.

31. Answer: 1, 2, 4

Rationale: One advantage of alternative dispute resolution (ADR) is the flexibility of the system. In mediation, for example, the mediator can assist with crafting a solution package that meets all the needs of a party, including an apology from the health care provider. Money is not always the only answer. Insurers' goals, however, usually do focus on cash, avoiding huge damage awards to plaintiffs. If a mediator is successful in facilitating case settlements, the costs are usually significantly lower than the costs of a court trial. Insurers focusing on the bottom line are not averse to these advantages. Damage awards in the ADR process are generally financial awards. The parties may invest substantial time and money in the ADR process. The arbiter's decision can then be appealed to the district court, which is a disadvantage.

32. Answer: 1

Rationale: Statutes of limitations set out each state's rules for the timing of the filing of lawsuits, including malpractice actions. These statutes are procedural laws in that they describe the "how-to" parameters within which legal rights may be exercised. Minority is considered a legal disability; other state laws usually define it and describe its effects. Rights to sue are not governed by statutes of limitations.

33. Answer: 1, 2, 4

Rationale: Statutes may indeed differ from state to state with respect to the breadth of the protection, but most statutes will protect a family nurse practitioner who renders aid, without expectation of compensation and in a competent manner.

Gross negligence will usually void the statutory protections. The family nurse practitioner is not required to stop and render aid.

34. Answer: 2, 3, 4

Rationale: A professional appearance boosts credibility as a witness. Inappropriate attire and gum chewing detract from the nurse's professional demeanor. Preparation is critical before the practitioner's words are recorded and transcribed as part of the official litigation transcript. The nurse should review documents but should refrain from bringing any materials to the deposition without the attorney's approval. The nurse should always ask for clarification of ambiguous questions. Speculation and trying to use sophisticated language and knowledge to confuse the other attorney are not appropriate. Questions about professional work history are always asked, so a copy of the family nurse practitioner's curriculum vitae is a useful tool to bring to a deposition.

35. Answer: 2, 3, 4, 5

Rationale: Jousting in the patient's medical record is never a good approach; it provides fodder for plaintiffs' lawyers and does not contribute to quality nursing care. The family nurse practitioner who has a conflict with another provider should deal with the provider directly, preferably in person. Another arena for resolving such disputes is the quality review process. The remaining options are good practice for documentation.

36. Answer: 1, 2, 3

Rationale: All these factors enter into an analysis of whether it is appropriate to accept a minor's consent to treatment. Another factor to consider is the type of treatment sought. Some states have statutes allowing minors to consent to specific therapies, such as treatment for venereal disease. A statement from a third party without supporting documentation to show that the patient is emancipated is not a factor. Parenthood does not constitute emancipation for a minor.

37. Answer: 1, 2, 3

Rationale: Family nurse practitioners can become careless with information management and the way they interact with patients and their personal data. The often wide-open and frantic front desk atmosphere of an office does little to calm patient fears that their information will be too easily accessible to those without a need to know. Verbally disclosing an individual's patient information in a public setting places the patient at risk for identity theft.

38. Answer: 3

Rationale: The coed locker room with centerfold photos seems to fit the criteria for a hostile environment, a form of sexual harassment. The harassment seems to be pervasive and longstanding; the women have complained, and apparently no action has been taken. The isolated incident and single date request do not rise to the level of harassment. The participants did not find the actions objectionable, and job performance was not affected. Although the potential was there for the nurse to use the prior relationship either to downgrade the employee or to deny a benefit during the employee performance review, this result did not occur.

39. Answer: 4

Rationale: Advance directives are documents crafted by individuals who personally decide how they wish their future health care decisions to be handled. The documents must be prepared while the signer is fully capable of understanding their content and importance. Because the wife in this scenario is already comatose, she has missed her opportunity to prepare advance directives. This does not mean that the spouse is unable to decide on her medical treatment, only that a different consent process needs to be used.

40. Answer: 3

Rationale: The option of detaining the patient would create liability potential for the family nurse practitioner under at least two legal theories, battery and false imprisonment. Talking with the patient would be the first prong of a planned approach to convince this patient that she needs the prescribed medical therapy. Conferring with social services would be the next choice. Court-ordered treatment is a consideration with a viable fetus.

41. Answer: 1

Rationale: This is the overall goal of the ADA. It is not another entitlement program, and it cannot impose wheelchair ramp requirements on every building owner in America. Access ramps and interpreters may be required as a "reasonable accommodation" to qualified people in certain defined circumstances. No across-the-board mandate exists for these types of aid to the handicapped population.

42. Answer: 1

Rationale: The U.S. Supreme Court essentially deferred to the states to legislate on this topic. In most states, the activity is not permitted. In one of the states involved in the high court's case, a statute permitting assisted suicide is being challenged. Family nurse practitioners need to look at their state laws on this topic for guidance. The providers referenced in the other options would act at their peril if their state laws followed the current majority view.

43. Answer: 1

Rationale: The purpose of a medical malpractice action is to make the claimant whole by the awarding of money damages. The award compensates the claimant or plaintiff for the wrong (or tort) he or she has suffered at the hands of the defendant. On the criminal side, the state sues on behalf of society for violations of society's criminal laws. The punishments are fines, imprisonment, or both. Professional liability insurance usually excludes criminal and intentional acts, so coverage for these types of activities is unlikely.

44. Answer: 2, 3, 5

Rationale: The full-blown jury trial and a bench or court trial are what ADR seeks to avoid. Mediation and arbitration are the most well-known forms of ADR. Some jurisdictions use the settlement conference as a technique to attempt settlement after a lawsuit has been filed but before a trial begins. ADR hybrids include "med-arb," in which a proceeding starts out as a mediation, but if the case does not settle, it is referred to an arbitrator for resolution.

45. Answer: 3

Rationale: This is the so-called "long tail" of professional liability; there is always a time lag from the date of injury to the date a claimant files a malpractice action. In the case of an infant, the time lag may be many years because of the statute of limitations. This extends the period of potential risk to the nurse who cares for children. Although a sympathy factor may be involved when jurors decide damages awards, the judgment is usually proportional to the injury and not the age of the claimant. Insurance coverage for pediatric providers is no less available than for other specialties; insurers adjust premiums to account for the level of risk.

46. Answer: 4

Rationale: All patients are entitled to medical information to make an informed decision about treatment. Age, in and of itself, is not an exclusionary criterion. Providers may treat in the other circumstances.

47. Answer: 3

Rationale: The purpose is to determine the appropriateness of the applicant for the job. Identifying health problems to prevent hiring an individual is discriminatory. The mental status and disabilities may also be a part of the preemployment physical but are not the primary purpose.

48. Answer: 2, 3

Rationale: As of January 1, 2015, OSHA requires that all employers must report all work-related fatalities within 8 hours and all work-related inpatient hospitalizations, all amputations, and all losses of an eye within 24 hours. Fatalities occurring within 30 days of a work-related incident must be reported to OSHA.

49. Answer: 3

Rationale: It is required by law that a report of any work-related injury be filed with the industrial commission of the state in which the injury occurred. OSHA requires the report of any injury or illness that requires more than first-aid treatment and/or involves loss of work time, limited work status, loss of consciousness, or death.

50. Answer: 2

Rationale: OSHA requires the report of any injury or illness that requires more than first-aid treatment and/or involves loss of work time, limited work status, loss of consciousness, or death.

51. Answer: 1

Rationale: The purpose is to record occupational injuries and illnesses, including mortality reports and lost workdays, which could also reveal dangerous working conditions.

52. Answer: 4

Rationale: The four major goals of HIPAA of 1996 are to ensure health insurance portability by eliminating "job-lock" because of preexisting medical conditions, reduce health care fraud and abuse, enforce standards for health information, and guarantee security and privacy of health information. Because of protests from civil libertarians and others concerned about privacy issues, the National Individual Identifier has been put on hold until some compromise can ensure that no abuses of such an identifier system will occur. The first compliance HIPPA rule relates to national standards for electronic transactions.

53. Answer: 4

Rationale: The crux of a bioethical dilemma is that the proposed solutions are not perfect and, therefore, create some aspect of moral conflict.

54. Answer: 4, 5

Rationale: The EMR communicates information within a facility and the EHR communicates information among multiple facilities. They are both efficient and effective. The EHR systems originated back in the 1960s and 1970s when medical centers developed electronic data systems with the idea of compiling patient health information so that it could be centrally managed and shared. Development work also was underway by industry and the federal government, which instituted an EHR in the U.S. Department of Veterans Affairs in the 1970s, a pioneering initial effort of electronic documentation.

55. Answer: 4

Rationale: It is important to maintain the integrity of the EMR or EHR because it is a legal and medical record and must meet federal and state regulations. Avoiding late entries or changes to the record, such as postvisit addendums, corrections, retractions, deletions, or others, can reduce the family nurse practitioner's legal liability exposure. Cloning records or copying and pasting information from previous visits can lead to inaccurate documentation and should be avoided. The log-in ID should never be shared with other colleagues. The EHR or EMR is a legal document and must reflect the accurate entry of information related to the patient and their care, whether or not the family nurse practitioner agrees with it.

56. Answer: 1, 2, 4, 5

Rationale: The LACE Network is a communication network that includes organizations that represent licensure, accreditation, certification, and education components of APRN regulation. They work together to move forward the process of implementation of the APRN Consensus Model. LACE is the implementation mechanism for the APRN Consensus Model. LACE is intended to be a transparent process for communicating about APRN regulatory issues, facilitating implementation of the APRN Consensus Model, and involving all above stakeholders in advancing APRN regulation.

57. Answer: 1, 2, 3

Rationale: Licensure is completed by state agencies to provide authorization to practice as a family nurse practitioner. Certification is often a prerequisite to licensure, depending on the state nurse practice act. Certification involves a formal process, usually an examination, to review a candidate's knowledge, skills, and abilities to perform as a family nurse practitioner. Accreditation involves educational institutions and is performed by outside agencies that review the processes and strategies of the institution, creating a metric of the quality of education. Credentialing is a general term that refers to regulatory mechanisms and process of establishing qualifications of licensed professionals. The two credentialing bodies for family nurse practitioners are American Nurses Credentialing Center and the American Academy of Nurse Practitioners, which provide a certification exam.

58. Answer: 1, 3, 5

Rationale: Requirements for obtaining prescriptive authority vary among states, along with specific requirements to maintain licensure. Most states and all certification programs require a core advanced pharmacotherapeutics course during the advanced practice program, which is a requirement of the APRN Consensus Model. The DEA number, as required by federal and state policies, is issued to nurse practitioners to prescribe or dispense controlled substances. In addition to prescriber and DEA registration, APRNs will need to apply for an NPI number, which is issued by the National Plan & Provider Enumeration System that collects identifying information on health care providers.

59. Answer: 1, 2

Rationale: A DEA number authorizes prescription of controlled substances and is applied for by the family nurse practitioner. DEA numbers are site specific. Family nurse practitioners practicing at more than one site will need to obtain an additional DEA number for each site, if they are dispensing controlled substances. The DEA's authority is federal; states have specific regulations pertaining to controlled substance authority. A family nurse practitioner who does not prescribe controlled substances is not required to obtain a DEA number.

60. Answer: 4

Rationale: The Health Insurance Portability and Accountability Act of 1996 mandates confidentiality about and protection of patients' personal health information. The legislation defines the rights and privileges of patients for protection of privacy. The release of a patient's medical information to an unauthorized person such as a member of the press, the patient's employer, or the patient's family, or online is a breach in patient confidentiality. The information that is in a patient's medical record is confidential and may be shared with health care providers for the purpose of medical treatment only. A patient must authorize the release of information and designate to whom the health care information may be released.

Issue and Trends

61. Answer: 2

Rationale: If a patient has Medicare Part A and meets all of the following conditions, the patient can receive hospice care: (1) health care provider must certify the patient is terminally ill (with a life expectancy of 6 months or less), (2) patient accepts palliative care instead of curative care, and (3) patient must sign a statement choosing hospice care instead of other Medicare-covered benefits to treat the terminal illness and related conditions. Patients do not pay for hospice care. There may be a small copayment (less than $5) for prescription medications.

62. Answer: 1

Rationale: According to the National Commission on Nursing (1983) and the Task Force on Nursing Practice in Hospitals (1983), the CNS role was accepted quite rapidly. The psychiatric CNS role is considered the oldest and most highly developed of the CNS specialties and helped initiate the growth of other CNS specialties.

63. Answer: 4

Rationale: Educational materials given to patients should be based on meeting established health literacy standards to facilitate exchange of information. Although evidenced-based practice recommendations provide credible information, the reading level at which information is provided enables understanding. Providing auditory and written instruction addresses learning styles but does not specifically indicate that the information provided as written or discussed meets health literacy standards. Determination of a patient's readiness to learn helps to identify increased likelihood of interest but it does not address how the content of the information is provided in terms of meeting health literacy standards.

64. Answer: 3

Rationale: The family nurse practitioner should act as a mentor while acting within the professional role competency as identified by the AACN 2010 standards. Teaching classes is part of the teaching competency. Observing and maintaining professional boundaries is part of the nurse practitioner–patient relationship. Prescribing medications is part of the management of patient health/illness status.

65. Answer: 3

Rationale: Martha Rogers argued that the development of the family nurse practitioner role was a ploy to lure nurses out of nursing and into medicine, thus weakening and undermining nursing's unique role in health care. This led to a major division within nursing, hindering the establishment of family nurse practitioner educational programs within the mainstream of graduate nursing education.

66. Answer: 4

Rationale: Loretta Ford, RN, PhD, and Henry Silver, MD, established the first pediatric nurse practitioner program at the University of Colorado. Hildegard Peplau started the first psychiatric Clinical Nurse Specialist program at Rutgers University. Mary Breckenridge established the Frontier Nursing Service in the depressed, rural mountain area of Kentucky, which led to training nurse-midwives. Agnes McGee is credited with offering the first postgraduate program for the nurse anesthetist role at St. Vincent's Hospital in Portland, Oregon.

67. Answer: 1

Rationale: Although all these answers are important for the family nurse practitioner in developing policy skills, the most important is developing political allies. Having political allies in decision-making places (legislature) will enable the family nurse practitioner to be active and informed regarding issues of regulation, limitations on admitting privileges and prescriptive authority, and managed care.

68. Answer: 4

Rationale: Three major issues are central to the expansion of the family nurse practitioner role: prescriptive authority, reimbursement privileges, and legal scope of practice. Although political activism is important, it is not specific to collaborative practice.

69. Answer: 3

Rationale: According to the APRN Consensus Model, there are four APRN roles: nurse anesthetist, nurse midwife, clinical nurse specialist, and a nurse practitioner. Specialty areas include but are not limited to clinical areas of practice/health care needs rather than patient populations. The family nurse practitioner represents one of the six practice population foci that addresses specific populations across the life span.

70. Answer: 2

Rationale: The ICD-10 diagnostic codes identify the condition, illness, or injury to be treated and are used for billing insurance carriers. Physicians' CPT codes specify the procedure or medical service given. Medicare and state Medicaid carriers are required by law to use CPT codes. The HCPC is used for reporting supplies and medical equipment. MNDS is a classification system of a set of items of essential nursing data with specific definitions and categories related to nursing and nursing care. Having a Medicare and Medicaid number is important, but additional information is required for reimbursement.

71. Answer: 1, 2, 3, 4

Rationale: Requirements for building an APRN curriculum reflecting a Consensus Model include completing graduate studies, meeting accreditation standards, maintaining compliance with core competencies, and maintaining licensure. Nurse Residency Programs are used in reference to new graduates who have just obtained licensure.

72. Answer: 3

Rationale: Lewin described three processes of change. Unfreezing involves "breaking the habit" or "disturbing the equilibrium." Moving involves development of new responses based on new information, with a change in attitudes, feelings, behaviors, or values. Refreezing involves reaching a new status quo by stabilizing and integrating new behaviors, with appropriate support to maintain the change. Forming, storming, and norming refer to the stages of group process development. Building relationships, acquiring resources, choosing a solution, and stabilizing are steps in Havelock's change theory.

73. Answer: 2

Rationale: According to most sources, the family nurse practitioner role developed as a result of a shortage of primary care physicians in the 1960s and 1970s, when medical specialization was the trend.

74. Answer: 3

Rationale: Medicare is regulated by the federal government and Plan B includes the services described (services or supplies that are needed to diagnose and treat a medical condition and preventive services), plus outpatient laboratory, radiography, durable medical equipment, ambulance services, mental health care (both inpatient and outpatient services, along with partial hospitalization), and obtaining a second opinion before surgery. Hospitalization costs, skilled nursing facility care, hospice care, and home health care are covered under Medicare Plan A.

75. Answer: 4

Rationale: The Balanced Budget Act is a crucial piece of legislation that allows direct payments to family nurse practitioners at "80% of the lesser of either the actual charge or 85% of the fee schedule amount of the same service if provided by a physician." This does not change the "incident to" rule, which allows a physician to bill for 100% of a family nurse practitioner's services, provided the physician is in the suite at the time of the service and readily available to provide assistance.

76. Answer: 4

Rationale: Conflict must be addressed directly by the family nurse practitioner. The personal characteristics of the medical assistants must not enter into the conflict resolution process. The family nurse practitioner should determine the issue of conflict, and then work on possible solutions to resolve the issue. Compromise, in which both parties must be willing to give up something, is only one method of conflict resolution.

77. Answer: 4

Rationale: VBP is an initiative that affects all providers who practice in or admit patients to a hospital setting. VBP is part of the Affordable Care Act of 2009 with the goal to improve quality of patient care by linking payment from the Centers for Medicare and Medicaid Services for inpatient services to successful outcome measures. Essentially, the VBP program adjusts payments to hospitals based on the quality of care they deliver using hospital-quality metrics. Accountable care organizations are groups of health care providers who come together voluntarily to give coordinated high-quality care to their Medicare patients based on performance measures. The APRN Compact from the National Council of State Boards of Nursing allows APRNs within the compact states who meet the compact requirements to obtain a multistate license, expanding advanced nursing practice and mobility for APRNs. The purpose of IPEC is to connect various health professions to advance interprofessional learning.

78. Answer: 1

Rationale: There are two ways to deal with sexual harassment at work: informally and formally through a grievance procedure. The harassed person should always start with the direct approach and ask the person to stop. The male family nurse practitioner should tell the female physician in clear terms that her behavior makes him uncomfortable and that he wants it to stop immediately.

79. Answer: 4

Rationale: The family nurse practitioner is reimbursed at 100% of "incident to" services. Medicare services provided entirely by the family nurse practitioner are reimbursed at 80% of the lesser of the actual charge or 85% of the fee schedule amount of physicians.

80. Answer: 4

Rationale: The AHRQ purpose or mission statement is to produce evidence-based practice and research to make health care that is of higher quality, more accessible, equitable, and affordable safer for all individuals. The AHRQ works within the U.S. Department of Health and Human Services and with other agencies to make sure that the evidence-based research is understood and used.

81. Answer: 4

Rationale: The 1999 IOM report "To Err Is Human: Building a Safer Health System" revealed that at least 44,000 and as many as 98,000 people die in hospitals each year because of preventable medical errors. Medical errors were defined as failure of a planned action to be completed as intended or the use of a wrong plan to achieve an aim.

82. Answer: 2, 4, 6

Rationale: The APRN Consensus Model stipulates that an APRN education program must include at a minimum three separate comprehensive graduate-level courses known as the APRN core, which are advanced physiology/pathophysiology, advanced health assessment, and advanced pharmacology. Social policy and political action and ethical/legal issues would be included in other courses and are not part of the APRN core.

83. Answer: 2

Rationale: The TIGER initiative was formed in 2004 to bring together nursing groups to collaborate to improve nursing practice, education, and delivery of patient care using HIT. This included recommendations for basic computer competencies, information literacy, and information management (including use of an electronic health record). In 2011 the group published a landmark report titled "Informatics Competencies for Every Practicing Nurse: Recommendations from the TIGER Collaborative."

84. Answer: 2

Rationale: The doctorally prepared advanced practice nurse performs a comprehensive evidence-based assessment and demonstrates competent and efficient assessment of patients with multiple comorbidities. Advanced practice nurses advocate not only for the patient, but for other populations and advancing nursing practice in general. They also advocate for improved access; quality and cost-effective health care; and ethical policies that promote access, equity, quality, and cost. Providing care to children through young adults focuses only on the pediatric nurse practitioner. The family nurse practitioner provides care to individuals and families across the life span. The adult-geriatric primary care nurse practitioner provides patient care across the adult-older lifespan, inclusive of adults (young adults, adults, and older adults).

85. Answer: 1, 2, 4

Rationale: The Consensus Model for APRN Regulation strives to standardize APRN regulations, which include education, accreditation, certification, and licensure. There are 23 states with full practice authority, 16 states with reduced practice authority, and 12 states with restricted practice authority. Each aspect of the model will standardize the regulatory process for APRNs, increasing state-to-state mobility for practicing, and will provide an increased access to APRN care nationwide. In addition, the Consensus Model was designed to create unity in the standards of practice for APRNs across the United States and will increase access to health care. It is not meant to restrict practice authority or increase cost burden for advanced practice nurses.

86. Answer: 4

Multiple studies over the last 10 years have shown that nurse practitioner care compared with physician care is equivalent and in some outcome indicators, such as patient satisfaction, nurse practitioner care is higher.

87. Answer: 2, 4

Rationale: The DNP degree was created and introduced to nurse educators by the American Association of Colleges of Nursing in 2004, not the NCSBN, which is nursing's regulatory body. The purpose was to ensure a strong educational preparation for APRNs. The DNP program was to address the reality of increasing curricular requirements in master's degree programs throughout the country. It was planned that the DNP would standardize practice entry requirements for all APRNs by the year 2015. Although 2015 has passed, the issue of requiring the practice doctorate remains unsettled among advanced practice faculty across the country. The projected year of implementation is now 2025.

88. Answer: 3, 5

Rationale: Hospitalization costs, skilled nursing facility care, hospice care, and home health care are covered under Medicare Plan A. Medicare Plan B includes the services described (services or supplies that are needed to diagnose and treat a medical condition and preventive services), plus outpatient laboratory, radiography, durable medical equipment, ambulance services, mental health care (both inpatient and outpatient services, along with partial hospitalization), and obtaining a second opinion before surgery.

89. Answer: 3

Rationale: To achieve the DNP competencies, advanced practice programs should provide a minimum of 1000 hours of supervised clinical practice as part of the academic program. The credentialing body, the American Academy of Nurse Practitioners, requires a minimum of 500 faculty-supervised direct patient care clinical hours for eligibility to take the certification exam. The credentialing body, the ANCC, requires completion of school-stated faculty-supervised clinical practice hours for degree completion. In addition, the ANCC states, "All practice requirements must have been met while holding an active professional license (RN licensure for nursing certifications or applicable license, certification, registration or organizational documentation for interprofessional specialties) in a U.S. state or territory or the professional, legally recognized equivalent in another country."

90. Answer: 2, 3, 5

Measuring outcomes is a required component of health care by federal and state regulatory agencies, practice guidelines, employers, and consumer groups. Health care organizations monitor outcomes of patient care as a means of evaluation and meeting requirements for accreditation and certification. Measuring outcomes does not correlate with additional revenue but with the maximum revenue available and should reduce expenditures.

91. Answer: 1, 6

Rationale: QI needs to be realistic and achievable. Large QI studies are not necessary and can be intimidating or overwhelming to those engaging in a QI project; small projects with available resources and tools are best. QI is not research; the intent is not to generate new ideas and knowledge for publication and dissemination but to use existing tools and evidence to change and improve nursing practice and patient care.

92. Answer: 1

Rationale: The MACRA took effect on January 1, 2017, with final implementation on January 1, 2019. MACRA repeals the SGR Formula that has determined Medicare Part B reimbursement rates for physicians and replaces it with new ways of paying for care. MACRA combines three existing programs: Physician Quality Reporting System, Value-Based Payment Modifier, and meaningful use into one system that provides both financial incentives and penalties based on quality of care, outcomes, and efficiencies. The initial 2 years are focused on collecting and analyzing data and for hospital systems and providers to see the future impact to their reimbursement.

93. Answer: 4

Rationale: Benchmarking is an important component of a quality improvement project because it helps identify when performance is below an agreed-on standard, and it signals the need for improvement. If the score falls below a set standard, indicating high risk for pressure ulcer development, interventions can be initiated. In addition, after an intervention is implemented, changes can be tracked in the Braden Scale score to determine whether the interventions were effective in reducing risk for pressure ulcer development. Using standardized measurement tools can inform the family nurse practitioner when changes in care are needed and whether implemented interventions have resulted in actual improvement of patient outcomes. Peer review is an evaluation of work by another person with similar competencies. Risk analysis is the process of identifying and analyzing potential issues that could negatively affect key initiatives or critical projects to help organizations avoid or mitigate those risks. Force field analysis is a strategic method used to understand what is needed for change to take place in both a business and a personal environment by listing and evaluating forces for and against a situation.

Academy of Nurse Practitioners Certification Program (AANPCP). (2018). *Candidate handbook and renewal of certification handbook.* Austin, TX: AANPCP.

Adams, M., Holland, N., & Urban, C. (2014). *Pharmacology for nurses: A pathophysiologic approach* (4th ed.). Boston, MA: Pearson.

Advisory Committee on Immunization Practices. (2019.). Retrieved from http://www.immunize.org/acip/.

Aletaha, M., Salour, H., Bagheri, A., Raffati, N., & Amouhashemi, N. (2012). Oral propranalol for treatment of pediatric capillary hemangiomas. *Journal of Opthalmic and Vision Research, 7*(2), 130–133.

Allen, P. J., Vessey, J., & Schapiro, N. (2010). *Primary care of the child with a chronic condition* (5th ed.). St. Louis, MO: Mosby.

Alligood, M. R. (2014). *Nursing theory: Utilization and application* (5th ed.). St. Louis, MO: Elsevier.

American Academy of Endodonics. (2017). Antibiotic prophylaxis 2017 update. Retrieved from https://www.aae.org/specialty/wp-content/uploads/sites/2/2017/06/aae_antibiotic-prophylaxis-2017update.pdf.

American Academy of Orthopedic Surgeons. (2015). How to use crutches, canes, and walkers. Retrieved from http://orthoinfo.aaos.org/topic.cfm?topic=a00181.

American Academy of Pediatrics. (2015). Car seats: Information for families for 2015. Retrieved from https://www.healthy-children.org/English/safety-prevention/on-the-go/Pages/Car-Safety-Seats-Information-for-Families.aspx?nfstatus=401&nftoken=00000000-0000-0000-0000-000000000000&nfstatusdescription=ERROR:+No+local+token

American Academy of Pediatrics. (2014). Clinical practice guideline: The diagnosis, management and prevention of bronchiolitis. *Pediatrics, 134*(5), e1474–e1502.

American Academy of Pediatrics (Bright Futures). (2018). Recommendations for preventive pediatric health care. Retrieved from https://www.aap.org/en-us/Documents/periodicity_schedule.pdf.

American Academy of Pediatrics, Report of the Committee on Infectious Diseases. (2015). *Red book* (30th ed.). Elk Grove, IL: American Academy of Pediatrics.

American Cancer Society. (2018). American Cancer Society guidelines for the early detection of cancer. Retrieved from https://www.cancer.org/healthy/find-cancer-early/cancer-screening-guidelines/american-cancer-society-guidelines-for-the-early-detection-of-cancer.html.

American Cancer Society. (2017). Limitations of mammograms. Retrieved from https://www.cancer.org/cancer/breast-cancer/screening-tests-and-early-detection/mammograms/limitations-of-mammograms.html.

American Cancer Society. Ovarian cancer statistics: How common is ovarian cancer. (n.d.). Retrieved from https://www.cancer.org/cancer/ovarian-cancer/about/key-statistics.html.

American Cancer Society. (2015). What are the risk factors for oral cavity and oropharyngeal cancers? Retrieved from http://www.cancer.org/cancer/oralcavityandoropharyngealcancer/detailed-guide/oral-cavity-and-oropharyngeal-cancer-risk-factors.

American College of Obstetricians and Gynecologists. (2017). Routine tests during pregnancy. Retrieved from https://www.acog.org/Patients/FAQs/Routine-Tests-During-Pregnancy?IsMobileSet=false.

American College of Radiology Appropriateness Criteria. (2019). ACR appropriateness criteria: Cranial neuropathies. Retrieved from https://acsearch.acr.org/docs/69509/Narrative/.

American Diabetes Association. (2019). 14. Management of diabetes in pregnancy: Standards of medical care in diabetes—2019. *Diabetes Care, 42*(suppl 1), S165–S172.

American Geriatrics Society. (2012). AGS Beers criteria for potentially inappropriate medication use in older adult. Retrieved from http://www.americangeriatrics.org/files/documents/beers/2012AGSBeersCriteriaCitations.pdf.

American Nurses Credentialing Center (ANCC). (2019). *Certification: General testing and renewal handbook.* Silver Spring, MD: American Nurses Association.

American Psychiatric Association. (2013). *Diagnostic and statistical manual of mental disorders* (5th ed.). Arlington, VA: American Psychiatric Association.

American Society for Colposcopy and Cervical Pathology (ASCCP). (2013). Management guidelines. Retrieved from http://www.asccp.org/Guidelines-2/Management-Guidelines-2.

American Society of Clinical Oncology. (2015). Head and neck cancer: Risk factors and prevention. Retrieved from http://www.cancer.net/cancer-types/head-and-neck-cancer/risk-factors-and-prevention.

Anderson, B. (2014). General evaluation of the adult with knee pain. In T. W. Post (Ed.), *UpToDate.* Waltham, MA.

Arabi, Z., Aziz, N. A., Abdul Aziz, A. F., Razali, R., & Wan Puteh, S. E. (2013). Early dementia questionnaire (EDQ): A new screening instrument for early dementia in primary care practice. *BMC Family Practice, 14*(49).

Arnett, K., Blumenthal, R. S., Albert, M. A., et al. (2019). 2019 ACC/AHA guideline on the primary prevention of cardiovascular disease: A report of the American College of Cardiology/American Heart Association task force on clinical practice guidelines. *Journal of the American College of Cardiology* (accepted manuscript). Retrieved from http://www.onlinejacc.org/content/accj/early/2019/03/07/j.jacc.2019.03.010.full.pdf?_ga=2.251653702.1342542142.1564246931-2145731604.1560714896.

Askgaard, G., Grønbæk, M., Mette, S., et. al. (2015). Alcohol drinking pattern and risk of alcoholic liver cirrhosis: A prospective cohort study. *Journal of Hepatology, 62*(5), 991–1220.

Asthma in Schools: Asthma facts. (2017). Retrieved from https://www.cdc.gov/healthyschools/asthma/index.htm.

Augenbraun, M. H., & McCormack, W. M. (2015). Urethritis. In J. E. Bennett, R. Dolin, & M. J. Blaser (Eds.). *Mandell, Douglas, and Bennett's principles and practice of infectious disease* (8th ed.) (pp. 1349-1357). Philadelphia, PA: Elsevier.

Ball, J., Dains, J., Flynn, J., Solomon, B., & Stewart, R. (2015). *Seidel's guide to physical examination*. (8th ed.) St. Louis: Elsevier.

Bartlett, J. (2014). Diagnostic approach to community-acquired pneumonia in adults. *UpToDate*. Waltham, MA.

Beitz, J. (1997). Unleashing the power of memory: the mighty mnemonic. *Nurse Educator 2*(22), 25–28.

Bickley, L. S., & Szilagyi, P. G. (2007). *Bates' guide to physical examination* (9th ed.). New York, NY: Lippincott Williams & Wilkins.

Bloomingfield, R. (1982). *Mnemonics, rhetorics, and poetics for medics*. Salem, NC: Harbinger Medical Press.

Boisoneau, D. S. (2015). The lump in the neck: Evaluation and management. CT Academy of Family Physicians. Retrieved from https://ctafp.org/wp-content/uploads/2015/08/Session-1 The-Lump-in-the-Neck.pdf.

Brown, W. J., & McCarthy, M. S. (2015). Sarcopenia: What every NP needs to know. *Journal for Nurse Practitioners, 11*(8), 753–760.

Burns, C. (2013). *Pediatric primary care* (5th ed.). Elsevier: Saunders.

Buttaro, T., Trybulski, J., Bailey, P., & Sandberg-Cook J. (2016). *Primary care: A collaborative practice* (5th ed.). St. Louis: Mosby.

Cash, J. C., & Glass, C. A. (2017). *Family practice guidelines* (4th ed.). New York, NY: Springer Publishing.

Centers for Disease Control and Prevention. (2015). *Hepatitis B FAQ's for health professionals*. Retrieved from www.cdc.gov/hepatitis/hbv/hbvfaq.htm.

Centers for Disease Control and Prevention. (2015). *Immunization schedules*. Retrieved from http://www.cdc.gov/vaccines/schedules/index.html.

Centers for Disease Control and Prevention. (n.d.). *Improving the nation's vision health: A coordinated public health approach*. Retrieved from http://www.cdc.gov/visionhealth/pdf/improving_nations_vision_health.pdf.

Centers for Disease Control and Prevention. (2014). *Latent tuberculosis infection: A guide for primary health care providers*. Retrieved from http://www.cdc.gov/tb/publications/ltbi/diagnosis.htm#3.

Center for Disease Control and Prevention. (2015). *Meningococcal vaccination*. Retrieved from http://www.cdc.gov/vaccines/vpd-vac/mening/default.htm.

Centers for Disease Control and Prevention. (2015). *Pneumococcal vaccination*. Retrieved from http://www.cdc.gov/vaccines/vpd-vac/pneumo/default.htm.

Centers from Disease Control and Prevention. (2019). *Preventing intimate partner violence*. Retrieved from https://www.cdc.gov/violenceprevention/intimatepartnerviolence/fastfact.html.

Center for Disease Control and Prevention. (2015). *Shingles (Herpes zoster)*. Retrieved from http://www.cdc.gov/shingles/about/transmission.html.

Centers for Disease Control and Prevention. (n.d.). *Preventing lead poisoning in young children: Chapter 6*. Retrieved from http://www.cdc.gov/nceh/lead/publications/books/plpyc/chapter6.htm.

Centers for Disease Control and Prevention. (2018). *Treating for two: Medicine and pregnancy*. Retrieved from https://www.cdc.gov/pregnancy/meds/treatingfortwo/index.html.

Centers for Disease Control and Prevention. (2012). *Tuberculosis fact sheet*. Retrieved from http://www.cdc.gov/tb/publications/factsheets/testing/skintesting.htm.

Centers for Disease Control and Prevention. (2013.) *Varicella vaccination: Information for health care providers*. Retrieved from http://www.cdc.gov/vaccines/vpd-vac/varicella/default-hcp.htm.

Chalasani, N., Younossi, Z., Lavine, J. F., et al. (2018). The diagnosis and management of nonalcoholic fatty liver disease: Practice guidance from the American Association for the Study of Liver Diseases. *Hepatology, 67*(1), 328–357.

Chan, E., & Talmadge, K. (2018). Amiodarone pulmonary toxicity. Retrieved from https://www.uptodate.com/contents/amiodarone-pulmonary-toxicity

Chernecky, C., & Berger, B. (2013). *Laboratory tests and diagnostic procedures* (6th ed.). St. Louis: Saunders.

Chey, W. D., Leontiadis, G. I., Howden, C. W., & Moss, S. F. (2017). ACG clinical guideline: Treatment of *Helicobacter pylori* infection. *American Journal of Gastroenterology, 112*(2), 212–239.

Chinn, P. L., & Kramer M. K. (2011). *Integrated theory and knowledge development in nursing* (8th ed.). St. Louis: Mosby.

Choose My Plate. (2018). Nutritional needs during pregnancy. Retrieved from https://www.choosemyplate.gov/nutritional-needs-during-pregnancy.

Chow, A. W., & Doron, S. (2015). Evaluation of acute pharyngitis in adults. Aronson, M.D. (Ed.). *UpToDate*. Waltham, MA.

Constantine, G. D., Kessler, G., Graham, S., & Goldstein, S. R. (2019). Increased incidence of endometrial cancer following the women's health initiative: An assessment of risk factors. *Journal of Women's Health, 28*(2), 237–243.

Cotler, K., Yingling, C., & Broholm, C. (2018). Preventing new human immunodeficiency virus infections with pre-exposure prophylaxis. *Journal for Nurse Practitioners, 14*(5), 376–382.

Creanga, A. A., Shapiro-Mendoza, C. K., Bish, C. L., Zane, S., Berg, C. J., & Callaghan, W. M. (2011). Trends in ectopic pregnancy mortality in the United States: 1980-2007. *Obstetrics & Gynecology, 117*(4), 837-843.

Cystic Fibrosis Foundation. (n.d.). Role of genetics in CF. Retrieved from https://www.cff.org/What-is-CF/Role-of-Genetics-in-CF/.

Diekema, D. S. (2005; AAP: 2013). Responding to parental refusals of immunization of children. *Pediatrics, 115*(5), 1428–1431. American Academy of Pediatrics. (2013). Rereaffirmed: Responding to parental refusals of immunization of children. *Pediatrics, 131*:5, e1696; originally published online April 29, 2013, doi:10.1542/peds.2013-0430.

Dos Santos, J., Lopes, R., & Koyle, M. (2017). Bladder and dowel dysfunction in children: An update on the diagnosis and treatment of a common, but underdiagnosed pediatric problem. *Canadian Urologic Association Journal, 11*(1-2 [suppl 11]), S64–S72.

Dunphy, L. M., Winland-Brown, J. E., Porter, B. O., & Thomas, D. J. (2011). *Primary care: The art and science of advanced practice nursing* (3rd ed.). Philadelphia: F.A. Davis.

Edmunds, M., & Mayhew, M. (2014). *Pharmacology for the primary care provider* (4th ed). Retrieved from http://online.vitalsource.com/#/books/9780323087902/pages/232443p963.

El-Ghar, M., Refaie H., Sharaf, D., & El-Diasty, T. (2014). Diagnosing urinary tract abnormalities: Intravenous urography or CT urography? *Reports in Medical Imaging, 7*, 55-63.

Eltorai, A. E., Ghanian, S., Adams, C. A., Born, C. T., & Daniels, A. H. (2014). Readability of patient education materials on the American Association for Surgery of Trauma website. *Archive of Trauma Research, 3*(2), e18681. Retrieved from https://www.ncbi.nlm.nih.gov/pmc/articles/PMC4139691/.

Estes, M. (2010). *Health assessment & physical examination* (4th ed.). Independence, KY: Delmar Cencage Learning.

Faes, M. C., Spigt, M. G., & Rikkert O. (2007). Dehydration in geriatrics. *Geriatrics and Aging, 10*(9), 590–596.

Fenstermacher, K., & Hudson, B. T. (2019). *Practice guidelines for family nurse practitioners* (5th ed.). St. Louis: Elsevier.

Ferri, F. (2013). *Ferri's Clinical Advisor*. St. Louis: Mosby.

Fihn, S. D., Gardin J. M., Abrams J., et al. (2012). 2012 ACCF/AHA/ACP/AATS/PCNA/SCAI/STS guideline for the diagnosis and management of patients with stable ischemic heart disease: A report of the American College of Cardiology Foundation/American Heart Association task force on practice guidelines and the American College of Physicians, American Association for Thoracic Surgery, Preventive Cardiovascular Nurses Association, Society for Cardiovascular Angiography an Interventions and the Society of Thoracic Surgeons. *Journal of the American College of Cardiology, 60*(24), e44–e164.

File, T. (2019). Treatment of community-acquired pneumonia in adults in the outpatient setting. Retrieved from https://www.uptodate.com/contents/treatment-of-community-acquired-pneumonia-in-adults-in-the-outpatient-setting.

Final recommendation statement: Breast cancer screening. (2016). Retrieved from https://www.uspreventiveservicestaskforce.org/Page/Document/RecommendationStatementFinal/breast-cancer-screening1.

Fischer, B. L., Gleason, C. E., Gangnon, R. E., Janczewski, J., Shea, T., & Mahoney, J. E. (2014). Declining cognition and falls: role of risky performance of everyday mobility activities. *Physical Therapy, 94*(3), 355–362.

5 Minute Consult. (2015). Philadelphia, PA: Wolters Kluwer.

Fragoso, C. (2018). Diagnosis and management of asthma in older adults. Retrieved from https://www.uptodate.com/contents/diagnosis-and-management-of-asthma-in-older-adults.

Freda, M. C. (2004). Issues in patient education. *Journal of Midwifery & Women's Health, 49*, 203–209.

Fuller, K. (2014). Diagnosis of testicular cancer. *Journal for Nurse Practitioners, 10*(6), 438.

Garcia-Tsao, G., Sanyal, A. J, Grace, N. D., et al. (2007). Prevention and management of gastroesophageal varices and variceal hemorrhage in cirrhosis. *Hepatology, 46*(3), 922–938.

Garneau, A. M. (2015). Nursing theory. In J. Zerwekh, & A. M. Garneau. (Eds.). *Nursing today: Transition and trends* (pp. 170-187). St. Louis: Elsevier.

Geoffrey, R. S., Cynthia, B., Graham 3rd, A. B., Brown, O. W., Hardin, A., Lessin, H. R., & Rodgers, C. T. (2014). 2014 Recommendations for pediatric preventive health care. *Pediatrics, 133*(3), 568.

Gilbert, D. N., Chambers, H. F., Eilopoulos, G. M., & Saag, M. S. (2015). *The Sanford guide to antimicrobial therapy 2015* (45th ed.). Sperryville, VA: Antimicrobial Therapy.

Global Initiative for Asthma. (2015l). *Pocket Guide for Asthma Management and Prevention*. Retrieved from Ginasthma.org http://www.ginasthma.org/.

Global Initiative for Chronic Obstructive Lung Disease. (2019). *Global strategy for the diagnosis, management, and prevention of chronic obstructive pulmonary disease*. Retrieved from Global Initiative for Chronic Obstructive Lung Disease www.goldcopd.org.

Gomella, L. G. (2010). *The 5 minute urology consult* (2nd ed.). Philadelphia: Lippincott Williams & Wilkins.

Grove, S. K., Burns, N., & Gray, J. R. (2013). *The practice of nursing research: Appraisal, synthesis, and generation of evidence* (7th ed.). St. Louis, MO: Saunders.

Grove, S. K., Gray, J. R., & Burns, N. (2015). *Understanding nursing research: Building an evidence-based practice* (6th ed.). St. Louis: Elsevier.

Grundy, S., et al. (2018). AHA/ACC/AACVPR/AAPA/ABC/ACPM/ADA/AGS/ASPC/NLA/PCNA guideline on the management of blood cholesterol: A report of the American College of Cardiology/American Heart Association task force on the clinical practice guidelines. *Journal of the American College of Cardiology, 73*(24), e285–e350.

Hall, M. A. (2013). Sinusitis. In T. M. Buttaro, J. Trybulski, P. P Bailey, & J. Sandberg-Cook (Eds.). *Primary care: A collaborative practice* (pp. 376–379). St. Louis: Elsevier.

Halter, J. G., Ouslander, J. G., Tinetti, M. E., Studenski, S., High, K. P., & Asthana, S. (2009). *Hazzard's geriatric medicine and gerontology* (6th ed.). New York: McGraw-Hill.

Hamric, A. B., Hanson, C. M., Tracy, M. F., O'Grady, E. T. (2014). *Advanced practice nursing: An integrative approach* (5th ed.). St. Louis: Elsevier.

Hartig, M. T. (2013). Otitis media. In T. M. Buttaro, J. Trybulski, P. P Bailey, & J. Sandberg-Cook (Eds.). *Primary care: A collaborative practice* (pp. 359-363). St. Louis: Elsevier.

Heller, J. (2013). Heroin overdose. *US National Library of Medicine: Medline Plus*. Retrieved from http://www.nlm.nih.gov/medlineplus/ency/article/002861.htm.

Hill, D. L. (2015). Infant constipation. Retrieved from https://healthychildren.org/English/ages-stages/baby/diapers-clothing/Pages/Infant-Constipation.aspx.

Hollier, A. (Ed.) (2016). *Clinical guidelines in primary care* (2nd ed.). Scott, LA: Advanced Practice Education Associates.

Hsu, S., Le, E., & Khoshevis, M. (2001). Differential diagnosis of annular lesions. *American Family Physicians, 64*(2), 289–297.

Hwang, P. H., & Patel, Z. M. (2015). Acute sinusitis and rhinosinusitis in adults: Treatment. In D. G. Deschler & S. B. Calderwood. (Eds.). *UpToDate*. Waltham, MA.

Institute of Medicine. (2009). Weight gain during pregnancy: Reexamining the guidelines. Retrieved from http://iom.nationalacademies.org/~/media/Files/Report%20Files/2009/Weight-Gain-During-Pregnancy-Reexamining-the-Guidelines/Report%20Brief%20-%20Weight%20Gain%20During%20Pregnancy.pdf.

Isaac, A. (2015). Treatment of neck pain. In T. W. Post (Ed.). *UpToDate*. Waltham, MA.

Issa, I. A., & Noureddine, M. (2017). Colorectal cancer screening: An updated review of the available options. *World J Gastroenterol, 23*(28), 5086–5096.

Jacobs, D. S. (2015). Cataract in adults. In J. Trobe (Ed.). *UpToDate*. Waltham, MA.

Jacobs, D. S. (2015). Open-angle glaucoma. In J. Trobe (Ed.). *UpToDate*. Waltham, MA.

Jacobs, D. S. (2015). Photokeratitis. In J. Trobe (Ed.). *UpToDate*. Waltham, MA.

James, P. A., Oparil, S., Carter, B. L., et al. (2014). Evidence-based guideline for the management of high blood pressure in adults: Report from the panel members appointed to the Eighth Joint National Committee (JNC 8). *JAMA, 311*(5), 507–520.

January, C. T., Wann, L. S., Calkins, H., et al. (2019). 2019 AHA/ACC/HRS focused update of the 2014 AHA/ACC/HRS guideline for the management of patients with atrial fibrillation: A report of the American college of Cardiology/American Heart Association task force on clinical practice guidelines and Heat Rhythm Society. *Journal of the American College of Cardiology* (accepted manuscript). Retrieved from http://www.onlinejacc.org/content/early/2019/01/21/j.jacc.2019.01.011?_ga=2.42871653.1342542142.1564246931-2145731604.1560714896.

Jarvis, C. (2016). *Physical examination & health assessment* (7th ed.). St. Louis: Elsevier.

Kaji, A., & Hockberger, R. (2015). Evaluation of thoracic and lumbar spinal column injury. In T. W. Post (Ed.). *UpToDate*. Waltham, MA.

Katz, P. O., Gerson, L. B. & Vela, M. F. (2013). Guidelines for the diagnosis and management of gastroesophageal reflux disease. *American Journal of Gastroenterology, 108*(3), 308–328.

Keltner, N., & Steele, D (Eds.). (2014). *Psychiatric nursing* (7th ed.) (pp. 401–417).

Kern, B., & Rosh, A. J. (2014). Hyperventilation syndrome treatment & management. Retrieved from http://emedicine.medscape.com/article/807277-treatment#d10.

Klompas, M. (2019). Risk factors and prevention of hospital-acquired and ventilator-associated pneumonia in adults. Retrieved from https://www.uptodate.com/contents/risk-factors-and-prevention-of-hospital-acquired-and-ventilator-associated-pneumonia-in-adults.

Kossler, A. L., & Banta, J. T. (2013). Blepharitis, hordeolum, and chalazion. In T. M. Buttaro, J. Trybulski, P. P Bailey, & J. Sandberg-Cook (Eds.). *Primary care: A collaborative practice* (pp. 324-326). St. Louis: Elsevier.

Kozy, M., & Halter, M. (2014). Depressive disorders. In M. Halter (Ed.). *Varcarolis' foundations of psychiatric mental health nursing: a clinical approach* (7th ed.) (pp. 249–276).

Lemaine V Cayci C Simmons P Petty P 2013 Gynecomastia in adolescent males.Lemaine, V., Cayci, C., Simmons, P., & Petty, P. (2013). Gynecomastia in adolescent males. *Seminars in Plastic Surgery, 27*(1), 56–61.

Lewinsohn, D. M., Leonard M. K., LoBue P. A., et al. (2017). Official American Thoracic Society/Infectious Diseases Society of America/Centers for Disease Control and Prevention clinical practice guidelines: diagnosis of tuberculosis in adults and children. Retrieved from https://www.thoracic.org/statements/resources/tb-opi/diagnosis-of-tuberculosis-in-adults-and-children.PDF.

Lin, K. W. (2019). Diagnostic tests: What physicians need to know: m*SEPT9* blood test (Epi proColon) for colorectal cancer screening. *American Family Physician, 100*(1), 10–11.

Lindenmeyer, C. C., & McCullough, A. J. (2018). The natural history of nonalcoholic fatty liver disease—An evolving view. *Clinics in Liver Disease, 22*, 11–21.

LoBiondo-Wood, G. & Haber, J. (2014). *Nursing research: Methods and critical appraisal for evidence-based practice* (8th ed.). St. Louis: Mosby

Logical Images. (2013). *Psoriasis*. Retrieved from http://www.skinsight.com/adult/psoriasis.htm.

Lowdermilk, D. L., Perry, S. E., Cashion, K., & Alden, K. R. (2016). *Maternity & women's health care* (11th ed.). St. Louis: Elsevier.

Mack, R. (2018). Increasing access to health care by implementing a consensus model for advanced practice registered nurse practice. *Journal for Nurse Practitioners, 14*(5), 419–424.

Mandell, L. A., Wunderink, R. G., Anzueto, A., et al. (2007). Infectious Diseases Society of America/American Thoracic Society consensus guidelines on the management of community-acquired pneumonia in adults. *Clinical Infectious Diseases, 44*(suppl 2), S27–S72.

Marcdante, K. J., & Kliegman, R. M. (2015). *Nelson essentials of pediatrics* (7th ed.). St. Louis: Saunders.

Margulis, V., & Sagalowsky, A. I. (2011). Assessment of hematuria. *Medical Clinics of North America, 95*, 153–159.

Mast, E. E., Margolis, H. S., Fiore, A. E., et al. (2005). A comprehensive immunization strategy to eliminate transmission of Hepatitis B virus infection in the United States. Recommendations of the Advisory Committee on Immunization Practices. National Center of Infectious Diseases, Division of Viral Hepatitis. *Morbidity and Mortality Weekly Report, 54*(RR-16), 1–37.

Matsumoto E., Carlson J. R., & Xu A. (2017). Management of recurrent *Clostridium difficile* infection: A case-based approach. *Consultant, 57*(10), 583–587.

Maughan, K. (2015). Ankle sprain. In T. W. Post (Ed.). *UpToDate*. Waltham, MA.

McCaffrey, R., & Youngkin, E. Q. (2014). *NP notes* (2nd ed.). Philadelphia, PA: F.A. Davis.

McCance, K. & Huether, S. (2015). *Pathophysiology: The biological basis for disease in adults and children* (7th ed.). St. Louis: Mosby.

McDonagh, A. F. (2011). Bilirubin, copper-porphyrins and bronze baby syndrome. *Journal of Pediatrics, 158*(1), 160–164.

Medicare.gov (2019). Hospice care. Retrieved from https://www.medicare.gov/coverage/hospice-care.

Merriam-Webster Medical Dictionary. (2015). *Erythroplasia*. Retrieved from http://www.merriam-webster.com/medical/erythroplasia.

Michaelson, M. D., & Oh, W. K. (2015). Epidemiology of and risk factors for testicular germ cell tumors. In P. W. Kantoff & M. E. Ross (Eds.). *UpToDate*. Waltham, MA.

Midthun, D. (2019). Overview of the risk factors, pathology, and clinical manifestations of lung cancer. Retrieved from https://www.uptodate.com/contents/overview-of-the-risk-factors-pathology-and-clinical-manifestations-of-lung-cancer.

Millichap, J. J. (2019). Clinical features and evaluation of febrile seizures. Retrieved from https://www.uptodate.com/contents/clinical-features-and-evaluation-of-febrile-seizures.

Mitchell, L. (2012). Long QT syndrome and torsades de pointes ventricular tachycardia. *Merck Manuals*. Retrieved from http://www.merckmanuals.com/professional/cardiovascular-disorders/arrhythmias-and-conduction-disorders/long-qt-syndrome-and-torsades-de-pointes-ventricular-tachycardia.

Moayyedi, P. M., Lacy, B. E., Andrews, C. N., Enns, R. A., Howden, C. W., & Vakil, N. (2017). ACG and CAG clinical guideline: Management of dyspepsia. *American Journal of Gastroenterology, 112*(7), 988–1013.

Mohan, R., & Schellhammer, P. F. (2011). Treatment options for localized prostate cancer. *American Family Physician, 84*(4), 414–420.

Munsell, D. S. (2013). Pharyngitis and tonsillitis. In T. M. Buttaro, J. Trybulski, P.P Bailey, & J. Sandberg-Cook (Eds.). *Primary care: A collaborative practice* (pp. 399-403). St. Louis: Elsevier.

Murphree, D. D., & Thelen, S. M. (2010). Chronic kidney disease in primary care. *Journal of the American Board of Family Medicine, 22*(4), 542–550.

National Cancer Institute (2013). Head and neck cancers. Retrieved from http://www.cancer.gov/types/head-and-neck/head-neck-fact-sheet#q1.

National Cancer Institute. (2018). Secondhand smoke and cancer. Retrieved from https://www.cancer.gov/about-cancer/causes-prevention/risk/tobacco/second-hand-smoke-fact-sheet#doesnbspsecondhand-smoke-cause-cancer.

National Institute on Drug Abuse. (2014) Drug Facts: Hallucinogens–LSD, peyote, psilocybin, and PCP. Retrieved from http://www.drugabuse.gov/publications/drugfacts/hallucinogens-lsd-peyote-psilocybin-pcp.

National Institute of Neurological Disorders and Stroke. (n.d.) *Febrile seizures fact sheet.* Retrieved from http://www.ninds.nih.gov/disorders/febrile_seizures/detail_febrile_seizures.htm.

National Institutes of Health, National Cholesterol Education Program Expert Panel. (2001). *Detection, evaluation and treatment of high blood cholesterol in adults (Adult Treatment Panel III).* Retrieved from http://www.nhlbi.nih.gov/files/docs/guidelines/atp3xsum.pdf.

National Occupational Research Agenda: Disease and injury: NIOSH Publication & Products. (2014). Retrieved from https://www.cdc.gov/niosh/docs/96-115/diseas.html.

National Osteoporosis Foundation. (2019). Bone density exam/testing. Retrieved from https://www.nof.org/patients/diagnosis-information/bone-density-examtesting/.

Niederhuber, J. E. (2014). *Abeloff's clinical oncology* (5th ed.). Philadelphia, PA: Elsevier.

Nopper, A., Markus, R., & Esterly N. (1998). When it's not ringworm: Annular lesions of childhood. *Pediatrics Annuals, 27*(3), 136–148.

O'Connor, P. (2008). Cocaine. *Merck manual.* Retrieved from http://www.merckmanuals.com/professional/special-subjects/drug-use-and-dependence/cocaine.

O'Doherty, L., Hegarty, K., Ramsay, J., Davidson, L. L., Feder, G., & Taft, A. (2015). Screening women for intimate partner violence in healthcare settings. *Cochrane Database of Systemic Reviews. 22*(7), CD007007.

Oeffinger, K. C., Fontham, E., & Etzioni, R. (2015). 2015 Breast cancer screening recommendations for women at average risk. Retrieved from https://jamanetwork.com/journals/jama/fullarticle/2463262.

O'Neil, J. (2018). Zoonotic infections from common household pets. *Journal for Nurse Practitioners, 14*(5), 363–370.

Parkinson's Foundation. (2014). *Parkinson's toolkit.* Retrieved from http://toolkit.parkinson.org/content/physical-examination.

Peterson, N. E. (2019). Exercises for older adults with knee and hip pain. *Journal for Nurse Practitioners,15*(4), 263–267.

Pezaro, C., Woo, H. H., & Davis, I. D. (2014). Prostate cancer: Measuring PSA. *Internal Medicine Journal, 44*(5), 433–440.

Pozniak, A. (2019). Clinical manifestations and complications of pulmonary tuberculosis. Retrieved from https://www.uptodate.com/contents/clinical-manifestations-and-complications-of-pulmonary-tuberculosis.

Prescriber's letter. (2018). Managing NSAID risks. *Pharmacist letter/prescriber's letter.* Retrieved from Prescribersletter.com.

Radhakrishnan, N., & Sacher, R. A. (2017). Bone marrow aspiration and biopsy. *Medscape.* Retrieved from https://emedicine.medscape.com/article/207575-overview#a1.

Ramirez, J. (2019). Overview of community-acquired pneumonia in adults. Retrieved from https://www.uptodate.com/contents/overview-of-community-acquired-pneumonia-in-adults.

Rayner, A. O'Brien, J. Schoenbachler, B. (2006). Behavior disorders of dementia: Recognition and treatment. *American Family Physician, 73*(4), 647–652.

Remedy Health Media. (2015). Allergy testing overview, types of allergy tests. Retrieved from http://www.healthcommunities.com/allergy-testing/overview-types-of-allergy-tests.shtml.

Reuben, D. B., Herr, K. A., Pacala, J. T., Pollock, B. G., Potter, J. F., & Semla, T.P. (2019). *Geriatrics at your fingertips.* (21st ed.). New York, NY: American Geriatrics Society.

Rex, D., Boland, R., Dominitz, J.A., et al. (2017). Colorectal cancer screening: Recommendations for physicians and patients from the U.S. multi-society task force on colorectal cancer. *American Journal of Gastroenterology, 112*(7), 1016–1030.

Rich, P., & Jefferson, J. (2015). Overview of nail disorder. In T. W. Post (Ed.). *UpToDate.* Waltham, MA.

Richardson, B. (2016). *Pediatric primary care: Practice guidelines for nurses* (3rd ed.). Burlington, MA: Jones & Bartlett.

Riddle, M. S., Connor, B. A., Beeching, N. J., et al. (2017). Guidelines for the prevention and treatment of travelers' diarrhea: A graded expert panel report. *Journal of Travel Medicine, 24*(suppl 1), S63–S80.

Ross, D. S. (2015). Overview of the clinical manifestations of hyperthyroidism in adults. In D. S. Cooper (Ed.). *UpToDate.* Waltham, MA.

Schrier, S., Camaschella, C. (2015). Anemia of chronic disease. In T. W. Post (Ed.). *UpToDate.* Waltham, MA.

Seidel, H. M., Ball, J. W., Dains, J. E., Flynn, J. A., Solomon, B. S., & Stewart, R. W. (2019). *Mosby's guide to physical exam* (9th ed). St. Louis: Elsevier.

Shekelle, P. G. (2018). Clinical practice guidelines: What's next? *JAMA, 320*(8), 757–758.

Sherry, D. (2019). Juvenile idiopathic arthritis treatment and management. Retrieved from https://emedicine.medscape.com/article/1007276-treatment.

Silberberg, C. (2013). Nephrotic syndrome. *MedlinePlus encyclopedia.* Retrieved from http://www.nlm.nih.gov/medlineplus/ency/article/000490.htm.

Simpson, K. R., & Creehan, P. A. (2014). *Perinatal nursing* (4th ed.). Philadelphia, PA: Wolters Kluwer/Lippincott Williams & Wilkins.

Smikle, C., & Khetarpal, S. (2019). Asherman syndrome. Retrieved from https://www.ncbi.nlm.nih.gov/books/NBK448088/.

Smith, R. J. H., & Gooi, A. (2015). Hearing impairment in children: Evaluation. In G. C. Isaacson (Ed.). *UpToDate.* Waltham, MA.

Soma-Pillay, P., Nelson-Piercy, C., Tolppanen, H., & Mebazaa, A. (2016). Physiological changes in pregnancy. *Cardiovascular Journal of Africa, 27*(2), 89–94.

Stanford School of Medicine (2015). *Fundoscopic exam.* Retrieved from http://stanfordmedicine25.stanford.edu/th25/fundoscopic.html.

Stausmire, J. M., & Ulrich, C. (2015). Making it meaningful: Finding quality improvement projects worthy of your time, effort and expertise. *Critical Care Nurse, 35*(6), 57-61.

Storker, S., & Skaggs, D. (2006). Developmental dysplasia of the hip. *American Family Physician, 74*(8), 1310–1316.

Strohl, K. (2018, April 13). Overview of obstructive sleep apnea in adults. Retrieved from https://www-uptodate-com.contentproxy.phoenix.edu/contents/overview-of-obstructive-sleep-apnea-in-adults?source=history_widget.

Swantz, M. H. (2014). *Textbook of physical diagnosis* (7th ed.). Philadelphia, PA: Elsevier.

Taketomo, C. K., Hodding, J. H., & Kraus, D. M. (2014). *Pediatric & neonatal dosage handbook.* Hudson, OH: Lexi-Comp.

Thompson, B. T., Kabrhel, C., Pena, C. (2019). Clinical presentation, evaluation, and diagnosis of the nonpregnancy adult with suspected acute pulmonary embolism. Retrieved from https://www.uptodate.com/contents/clinical-presentation-evaluation-and-diagnosis-of-the-nonpregnant-adult-with-suspected-acute-pulmonary-embolism.

Thornhill, M. H., Dayer, M., Lockhart, P. B, & Prendergast, B. (2017). Antibiotic prophylaxis of infective endocarditis. *Current Infectious Disease Reports, 19*(9), 1–9.

U.S. Department of Health & Human Services. (2015). Office for Human Research Protections (OHRP). Retrieved from http://www.hhs.gov/ohrp/policy/consentckls.html.

U.S. Department of Health & Human Services, National Institutes of Health, National Kidney and Urologic Diseases Information Clearinghouse (2007). Urinary incontinence in men (NIH publication no. 07-5280). Retrieved from http://www.niddk.nih.gov/health-information/health-topics/urologic-disease/urinary-incontinence-in-men/Documents/uimen_508.pdf.

U.S. Preventive Services Task Force. (2016). Final recommendation statement latent tuberculosis infection: Screening. Retrieved from https://www.uspreventiveservicestaskforce.org/Page/Document/RecommendationStatementFinal/latent-tuberculosis-infection-screening.

U.S. Preventive Services Task Force. (2013). Final recommendation statement lung cancer screening. Retrieved from http://www.uspreventiveservicestaskforce.org/Page/Document/RecommendationStatementFinal/lung-cancer-screening.

U.S. Preventive Services Task Force. (2012). Final recommendation statement prostate cancer: Screening. Retrieved from http://www.uspreventiveservicestaskforce.org/Page/Document/RecommendationStatementFinal/prostate-cancer-screening.

U.S. Preventive Services Task Force. (2011). Final recommendation statement testicular cancer: Screening. Retrieved from http://www.uspreventiveservicestaskforce.org/Page/Document/RecommendationStatementFinal/testicular-cancer-screening.

Varcarolis, E. (2014). Communication and the clinical interview. In M. Halter (Ed.). *Varcarolis' foundations of psychiatric mental health nursing: A clinical approach* (7th ed.) (pp. 147–165).

Vasavada, S. P. (2014). Urinary incontinence: Practice essentials, background, anatomy. *Medscape reference: drugs, diseases & procedures*. Retrieved from http://emedicine.medscape.com/article/452289-overview.

Wallace, M., & Fulmer, T. (2008). Fulmer SPICES: An overall assessment tool for older adults. *Annals of Long Term Care, 15*(3).

Wang, L., Mannalithara, A., Singh, G., & Ladabaum, U. (2018). Low rates of gastrointestinal and non-gastrointestinal complications for screening or surveillance colonoscopies in a population-based study. *Gastroenterology, 154*(3), 540–555.

Weber, P. C. (2000). Noise-induced hearing loss. *American Family Physician, 61*(9), 2749–2756.

Wein, A. J., Kavoussi, L. R., Novick, A. C., Partin, A. W., & Peters, C. A. (2012). *Campbell-Walsh urology* (10th ed.). Philadelphia, PA: Elsevier.

Weiss, B. D., Mays, M. Z., Martz, W., et al. (2005, November). Quick assessment of literacy in primary care: The newest vital sign. *Annals of Family Medicine, 3*(6), 514–522.

Weizer, J. S. (2015). Angle-clsoure glaucoma. In J. Trobe (Ed.). *UpToDate*. Waltham, MA.

Whelton, P. K., Carey R. M., Aronow W. S., et al. (2018). 2017 ACC/AHA/AAPA/ABC/ACPM/AGS/APhA/ASH/ASPC/NMA/PCNA guideline for the prevention, detection, evaluation and management of high blood pressure in adults: A report of the American College of Cardiology/American Heart Association task force on clinical practice guidelines. *Journal of the American College of Cardiology, 71*(10), e127–e268.

Whitcomb, B. W, Purdue-Smithe A. C., Szegda K. L., et al. (2018, April 10). Cigarette smoking and risk of early natural menopause. *American Journal of Epidemiology, 187*(4), 696–704.

Williams, M. E. (2007). Examining the ears, nose and oral cavity in the older patient. Retrieved from http://www.medscape.org/viewarticle/556144_2.

Wolf, J. S. (2014). Nephrolithiasis treatment & management. *Medscape: drugs and diseases*. Retrieved from http://emedicine.medscape.com/article/437096-overview.

Woo, T., & Robinson, M. (2016). *Pharmacotherapeutics for advanced practice nurse prescribers* (4th ed.). Philadelphia, PA: F.A. Davis.

World Health Organization. (2014). *Children: Reducing mortality*. Retrieved from http://www.who.int/mediacentre/factsheets/fs178/en/.

World Health Organization. *Measles*. (2019). Retrieved from https://www.who.int/news-room/fact-sheets/detail/measles.

Yancy, C., Jessup M., Bozkurt B., et al. (2017). 2017 ACC/AHA/HFSA focused update of the 2013 ACCF/AHA guideline for the management of heart failure: A report of the American College of Cardiology/American Heart Association task force on clinical practice guidelines and the Heart Failure Society of America. *Journal of the American Heart Association, 70*(6), 776–803.

Youngkin, E. Q., Davis, M. S., Schadewald, D. M., & Juve, C. (Eds.). (2013). *Women's health: A primary care clinical guide* (4th ed.). Upper Saddle River, NJ: Pearson/Prentice Hall.

Zakrison, T. L., Rattan, R., & Miljan Valdes D., et al. (2018). Universal screening for intimate partner and sexual violence in trauma patients—What about the men? An Eastern Association for the Surgery of Trauma multicenter trial. *Journal of Trauma and Acute Care Surgery, 85*(1), 85–90.

Zerwekh, J. (2019). Test-taking strategies. In *Illustrated study guide for the NCLEX-RN® Exam* (10th ed.). St. Louis: Elsevier.

Zerwekh, J., Garneau, A., & Miller C. J. (2017). *Digital collection of the memory notebook of nursing* (4th ed). Chandler, AZ: Nursing Education Consultants Publishing.